Birkhäuser Advances in Infectious Diseases

BAID

Series Editors

Axel Schmidt
University Witten/Herdecke
Faculty of Medicine
Alfred-Herrhausen-Str. 50
58448 Witten
Germany

Manfred H. Wolff
University Witten/Herdecke
Faculty of Biosciences
Stockumer Str. 10
58448 Witten
Germany

Stefan H.E. Kaufmann
Max-Planck-Institut für Infektionsbiologie
Department of Immunology
Schumannstrasse 21/22
10117 Berlin
Germany

The Grand Challenge for the Future

Vaccines for Poverty-Related Diseases from Bench to Field

Edited by S. H. E. Kaufmann and P.-H. Lambert

Birkhäuser Verlag
Basel · Boston · Berlin

Editors
Stefan H.E. Kaufmann
Max Planck Institute for Infection Biology
Schumannstrasse 21-22
D-10117 Berlin
Germany

Paul-Henri Lambert
CMU – Centre of Vaccinology
1 rue Michel Servet
CH-1211 Geneva 4
Switzerland

A CIP catalogue record for this book is available from the Library of Congress, Washington, D.C., USA

Bibliographic information published by Die Deutsche Bibliothek
Die Deutsche Bibliothek lists this publication in the Deutsche Nationalbibliografie; detailed bibliographic data is available in the internet at http://dnb.ddb.de

ISBN 3-7643-7175-7 Birkhäuser Verlag, Basel - Boston - Berlin

Part of Springer Science+Business Media
Printed on acid-free paper produced from chlorine-free pulp. TFC ∞
Cover design: Micha Lotrovsky, CH-4106 Therwil, Switzerland
Cover illustration: With the friendly permission of Alice Greenwood and Philippe Beutels (see pages 9 and 256).
Printed in Germany
ISBN-10: 3-7643-7175-7
ISBN-13: 978-3-7643-7175-3
9 8 7 6 5 4 3 2 1

www. birkhauser.ch

Contents

Regulatory issues

Clinical trials

Vaccination programmes

List of contributors

Carl R. Alving, Department of Vaccine Production and Delivery, Division of Retrovirology, Walter Reed Army Institute of Research, U.S. Military HIV Research Program, 1600 East Gude Drive, Rockville, MD 20850, USA; e-mail: calving@hivresearch.org

Ann M. Arvin, Departments of Pediatrics and Microbiology and Immunology, Stanford University School of Medicine, Stanford, CA 94305-5164, USA; e-mail: Aarvin@stanford.edu

Adwoa D. Bentsi-Enchill, Vaccine Assessment and Monitoring, Department of Immunization, Vaccines and Biologicals, World Health Organization, 20 Avenue Appia, 1211 Geneva 27, Switzerland; e-mail: bentsienchilla@who.int

Philippe Beutels, Department of Epidemiology and Community Medicine, University of Antwerp, Universiteitsplein 1, 2610 Antwerpen, Belgium, and National Centre for Immunisation Research

Royal Alexandra Hospital for Children & University of Sydney, Australia, e-mail: philippe.beutels@ua.ac.be

Bjarne Bjorvatn, Centre for International Health, University of Bergen, Armauer Hansen Building, Haukeland University Hospital, 5021 Bergen, Norway; e-mail: bjarne.bjorvatn@cih.uib.no

John D. Clemens, International Vaccine Institute, SNU Research Park, San 4-8 Bongcheon-7-dong, Kwanak-gu, Seoul, Korea 151-818; e-mail: jclemens@ivi.int

Philippe Duclos, Vaccine Assessment and Monitoring, Department of Immunization, Vaccines and Biologicals, World Health Organization, 20 Avenue Appia, 1211 Geneva 27, Switzerland; e-mail: duclosp@who.int

Brian Greenwood, Department of Infectious and Tropical Diseases, London School of Hygiene and Tropical Medicine, Keppel St., London WC1E 7HT, UK; e-mail: brian.greenwood@lshtm.ac.uk

Arnd Hoeveler, European Commission, Unit for Poverty-related Diseases, DG Research, 1049 Brussels, Belgium; e-mail: arnd.hoeveler@cec.eu.int

Luis Jodar, International Vaccine Institute, SNU Research Park, San 4-8 Bongcheon-7-dong, Kwanak-gu, Seoul, Korea 151-818; e-mail: ljodar@ivi.int

Maria Lattanzi, Chiron Vaccines, Via Fiorentina 1, 53100 Siena, Italy; e-mail: maria-lattanzi@chiron.com

David B. Lewis, Department of Pediatrics and Program in Immunology, Stanford University School of Medicine, Stanford, CA 94305-5164, USA; e-mail: dblewis@stanford.edu

Gary R. Matyas, Department of Vaccine Production and Delivery, Division of Retrovirology, Walter Reed Army Institute of Research, U.S. Military

HIV Research Program, 1600 East Gude Drive, Rockville, MD 20850, USA; e-mail: GMatyas@hivresearch.org

Hanna M. Nohynek, National Public Health Institute, Department of Vaccines, Clinical Unit, Mannerheimitie 166, 00300 Helsinki, Finland; e-mail: hanna.nohynek@ktl.fi

R. Leon Ochiai, International Vaccine Institute, SNU Research Park, San 4-8 Bongcheon-7-dong, Kwanak-gu, Seoul, Korea 151-818; e-mail: rlochiai@ivi.int

Ole F. Olesen, European Commission, Unit for Poverty-related Diseases, DG Research, 1049 Brussels, Belgium; e-mail: ole.olesen@cec.eu.int

Dina Pfeifer, Vaccine Assessment and Monitoring, Department of Immunization, Vaccines and Biologicals, World Health Organization, 20 Avenue Appia, 1211 Geneva 27, Switzerland; e-mail: pfeiferd@who.int

Stanley A. Plotkin, University of Pennsylvania, and Sanofi Pasteur, 4650 Wismer Road, Doylestown, PA 18901, USA; e-mail: Stanley.Plotkin@Sanofipasteur.com

Rino Rappuoli, Chiron Vaccines, Via Fiorentina 1, 53100 Siena, Italy; e-mail: rino_rappuoli@chiron.com

James M. Robinson, Industrial Operations, Sanofi Pasteur, Inc, Discovery Drive, Swiftwater, PA 18370, USA

Veronica L. Tallo, Research Institute for Tropical Medicine, Department of Health, Filinvest Corporate City, Alabang, Muntinlupa 1781, The Philippines; e-mail: vltallo@pacific.net.ph

François Verdier, Sanofi Pasteur, Campus Mérieux, 1541 avenue Marcel Mérieux, 69280 Marcy l'Etoile, France; e-mail: francois.verdier@sanofipasteur.com

Introductory remarks: Towards relevant vaccinology

It is a dream for all scientists engaged in vaccine research to quickly identify a gene product or genetically engineer a microorganism and to find out that this product represents a potential vaccine against a major infectious disease. It is often a nightmare for the same scientist to experience the hurdles that have to be overcome to move this marvellous product towards clinical trials. Most distressful may even be the rising awareness that a fully successful candidate may end up on the list of vaccines waiting for the unlikely introduction into vaccination programs.

The main goal of this book is to review various aspects related to vaccinology and to appreciate how they apply to major infectious diseases associated with poverty. This approach will take us from vaccine research and development efforts for malaria, AIDS and tuberculosis vaccines to issues critical to introduction of these candidates into national vaccination programs.

These reviews show how, within a few decades, vaccinology has emerged as a unique discipline through the increasing confrontation of the scientists who deal with vaccine research with the intricate network of multiple obstacles to be overcome. Issues range from immunology to epidemiology, from genetics to ecology, from economics to industrial engineering, from social sciences to primary health care. Until a few years ago, a vaccine would largely be developed on the basis of its technical feasibility within a decent time frame. Surprisingly little consideration was given at onset to the relative need for the vaccine at public health level or to specific practical issues that could direct its future use. This often led to wrong market analyses. For example, initial marketing studies for a hepatitis B vaccine concluded that use in high-risk groups and medical personnel would be the primary indications. The mere fact that this vaccine was becoming available, however, led public health experts to realize its potential benefit for developing countries where the disease is highly endemic, and to recommend universal vaccination programs.

This development has had remarkable consequences. It is now inconceivable to engage at any level of vaccine R&D for poverty-associated infectious diseases without some knowledge of the broad range of related issues which have to be considered.

Novel vaccination strategies for poverty-related diseases must deal at a global and comprehensive level with the specific issues related to both the target microorganism and the target population.

Antigenic diversity, naturally occurring mutations and microbial selection under immunological pressure do influence the global epidemiology of microbial pathogens targeted by novel vaccination strategies. This is well appreciated for influenza and a major impediment to the design of optimal vaccination strategies for diseases intrinsically associated with antigenic variation, including HIV and malaria. The multiplicity of antigenic variants may open the way to "replacement" strains. For example, new pneumococcal vaccines, which only prevent a limited number of dominant serotypes, can effectively decrease the infant carrier rate for the serotypes covered by the vaccine. However, this may lead to colonization by pneumococci of different serotypes not included in the vaccine formulation. Such replacement phenomena necessitate the continuing monitoring of pneumococcal strains and, if needed, regular changes in the vaccine formulation.

Equally important, the nature of the target population influences the selection of vaccination strategies in conjunction with the definition of epidemiological patterns. For a number of childhood diseases, the period of greatest vulnerability to infection and disease is within the first few years after birth. Vaccine-induced long-term memory is not always critical, since after a basic level of vaccination, re-exposure to the antigens or re-infection can 'boost' the immune response. However, when dealing with poverty-related diseases, one has to face the fact that infants and adults, throughout much of their lifetime, can be at risk for infection. How long can a vaccine given in early life confer protection? Can we expect that infant immunization protects against HIV/AIDS for 20–30 years? How can immunological memory be generated and sustained? Can it be achieved with subunit vaccines, or will immunization with live, attenuated vectors be necessary, with potentially greater risks of adverse effects? Or should we favour combinatory strategies comprising heterologous prime-boost regimes? These are just a few of the questions that do await answers in the near future.

We have learned a great deal about how to deliver vaccines to toddlers and infants to protect them against childhood infectious diseases. Extraordinary logistical challenges had to be solved and ways of integrating immunization programs into public health and primary care programs had to be developed. As one of the results of these efforts, the level of vaccine coverage in developing countries is now far better for vaccines given soon after birth (e.g., BCG, hepatitis B, polio) than for those given later in life. Thus, in addition to protecting against early-occurring infections, any new poverty-related disease vaccine that is found to be efficacious in the first weeks of life will have a remarkable competitive advantage. As discussed in this book, the immunological challenge of engendering potent protective immune responses in newborns is far from negligible.

Vaccination of immunodeficient individuals also poses unique problems. The risk of adverse events needs to be carefully evaluated, particularly if live attenuated vaccines cannot be controlled and cause disease in immunocompromised vaccinees. Because of the long latency of HIV infection before symptoms of AIDS develop, the possibility exists to induce significant protection prior to major immunodeficiency. However, should the level of vaccine-induced immunity fall short of that achieved in the general population, potential implications for transmission and persistence of infection need to be assessed.

Additional challenges reside in the pressing need for rapid assessment of clinical efficacy. Vaccine trials represent a long, complex and expensive endeavour. Surrogates of protection do exist for a number of vaccines currently in use, because they are thought to provide protection by means of neutralizing antibodies which can be easily assessed. However, protection against major poverty-related disease is likely to require multiple and complex mechanisms, including antibodies and cell-mediated immunity. The definition of relevant correlates of protection in these infections remains an area of considerable concern which needs to be addressed in the near future.

In several industrialized countries, public resistance to the addition of new vaccines to the existing paediatric schedule is on the rise. This is often reflected by parental rejection of what is resented as medical "aggression" for their healthy child. It is also directly related to the number of injections required for completing infant vaccination plans. In several European countries, this feeling is reinforced by particular medical groups, who are proponents of new "natural" preventive or therapeutic approaches. These negative reactions partly mirror a decreased perception of the risk of infectious disease in countries where efficient disease control or elimination strategies have been successful.

Although it is likely that such considerations have a lower penetration in developing countries, misperceptions of vaccine safety increasingly contribute to vaccine failures as illustrated by the recent re-emergence of polio in Kano (Nigeria/Niger) following suspension of polio vaccination. Better information is the key to success in this area and this is the topic of an important chapter of this volume.

Finally, numerous challenges are economic in nature. At the industrial level, vaccines increasingly appear as low-profit products, with an increasing litigation risk, as compared to some of the new high-return blockbusting drugs, often produced by another section of the same giant pharmaceutical company. In many developing countries, economic obstacles still limit the use of existing vaccines and no rapid solution can be expected without international aid and significant financing plans. It is hoped that the true value of preventive vaccination will be taken into proper consideration at political and general public levels in both developing and industrialized countries. Greater recognition of the social value of prophylactic vaccination will be essential in order to let humankind benefit from the considerable scientific and economic efforts that underpin the development of new vaccines against poverty-related diseases.

We are now at a time when relevant vaccinology should prevail. The scientific community is developing an understanding of how to engage the immune response in molecular and cellular terms to provide protection against the target disease. However, the specific needs for the vaccine, the various epidemiological patterns to be faced, the target population foreseen for vaccination and related economic aspects should be equally considered at the time of vaccine design. How will the new and effective vaccine be used? How will target populations be reached? What could be the public acceptance? Will high priority be given to this vaccine in public health policies? These are the realms of knowledge that we see as the "grand challenge" for vaccines and vaccination.

We would like to sincerely thank the staff of Birkhäuser Publishers, and notably Dr. Beatrice Menz, for editing this volume of the "Advances in Infectious Diseases" series, as well as our secretaries Yvonne Bennett, Souraya Sibaei and Gaby Roetzer for their extraordinary help. Most of all we would like to thank all our colleagues who generously shared their knowledge in the broad interdisciplinary field of relevant vaccinology with us. It is only through their in-depth knowledge and their willingness to share their experience with us that we were able to compile this volume on the grand challenge for the future, namely vaccine development for poverty-related diseases from the bench to the field.

Berlin/Geneva, January 2005

Stefan H. E. Kaufmann
Paul-Henry Lambert

Background

The Grand Challenge for the Future
ed. by Stefan H.E. Kaufmann and Paul-Henri Lambert

Economic aspects of vaccines and vaccination: a global perspective

Philippe P.A. Beutels

Centre for the Evaluation of Vaccination, Department of Epidemiology and Community Medicine, University of Antwerp, Universiteitsplein 1, 2610 Antwerpen, Belgium, and National Centre for Immunisation Research Royal Alexandra Hospital for Children & University of Sydney, Australia

Introduction

A basic principle of economic decision-making is that in an environment of scarce resources choices have to be made in the allocation of these resources. This principle also applies to the provision of health care. The share of health-care expenditures in the Gross Domestic Product (GDP) of most industrialised countries has increased from 3%-5% in the early sixties to 7%–11% in 2001 (from 5% to 14% in the USA) [1] This rise has been attributed to medical advances (increasing the number and technological complexity of medical interventions), population aging, sociological changes (more, but smaller families and less familial support for the elderly) and insufficient productivity increases in the services sector. In less wealthy economies, medical decision-makers are faced with a smaller margin, and such a rise in health-care spending has not been observed yet. Basically, the richer a country, the more it can afford (in nominal and in relative terms) to spend on health care.

The two-way interaction between health and economic development is generally explained as follows. The healthier the population, the more adults can contribute to society by productive activity (i.e., work creating a surplus value in terms of capital gains and human resources), as well as by raising children in a stable environment, thus ensuring continued economic development. The process of economic development itself creates conditions (education, employment, infrastructure (including safe water and sanitation)), which provide a basis for continued improvement in longevity and health-related quality of life [2]. Individual good health can be seen as the product of some unknown complex function to which health care is only one of the inputs. Other important inputs are: life-style variables (eating habits, smoking, etc.), environmental factors (urbanisation, climatic conditions, etc.), income, education and genetic predestination. Furthermore, expenditures on health are not necessarily put to use in the most efficient way. In this respect a distinction can be made between technical efficiency (providing maximal health care for a given cost, or delivering a certain service at minimal cost) and allocative efficiency (the distribution of resources across alternative services so as to maximise health gains, in accordance with preferences). Finally, though much may be spent on health care, not all people may have equal access to health care of the same quality. Indeed inequities in the consumption of health care may also interfere with the overall allocative efficiency of the system, and create inequities in health *per se*. Therefore greater expenditures on health care are no guarantee for more global health. It should be noted that these observations do not plead for a reduction or containment of health-care budgets, but rather for a way of spending that ensures that societal goals are met. In order to achieve this, welfare economists focus research on two broad topics: efficiency and equity. Efficiency relates to choosing options that maximise utility from marginal expenditures (i.e., by optimising the production process of health, for which health care is one of the inputs). Equity relates to the fair distribution of all aspects related to health across members in society (e.g., equal access to care). Clearly, there may exist a trade-off between efficiency and equity and giving priority to either of them is a normative issue that should be decided by social and political debate.

Vaccination is undoubtedly one of the major contributors to health improvements in the last three centuries. During this period, the impact of vaccination on longevity is undeniable, despite the fact that its partial contribution is difficult to distinguish from that of improved hygienic conditions and nutrition, and the discovery of penicillin [3, 4]. All of these combined provided the basis for the so-called "epidemiological transition"[1] in industrialised countries. At the same time, infectious diseases remain the main cause of death in many developing countries. Despite the continuing expansion of the vaccine portfolio, implementing financially sustainable basic vaccination programs in poor countries remains problematic. Though this is not so much an economic as a financial aspect, we will return to this issue in the section "Financing vaccines".

Peculiarities of vaccination and the vaccine market

A number of peculiar characteristics set vaccination apart from other interventions in health care [5]: (1) Since vaccination is (usually) a form of primary prevention, it intervenes in people (often children) who are generally in good health. But unlike most other prevention programs, the interven-

1 Epidemiological transition: transition from infectious and parasitic diseases (in children) as the main causes of death to chronic and degenerative diseases of adulthood. This transition evolved parallel to the demographic transition: transition from high fertility and death rates to low fertility and death rates.

tion itself can cause harm to the vaccine recipient, because in rare cases vaccine-associated adverse events (VAAE) occur. This means that people make trade-offs between risks of vaccine-preventable disease and risks of VAAE. The perception of these risks is quintessential to the individual demand for vaccines (if left to free-market mechanisms), and dominates the influence of other factors such as price [6]. (2) Vaccination not only protects vaccine recipients, but it also reduces exposure of unvaccinated people, due to the reduced circulation of the infectious agent (if the transmission of infection occurs from human to human). This is not always beneficial for public health as the reduced risk of transmission leads to an increased average age at infection (with many "childhood" infections being more severe if contracted in adulthood) [7, 8]. Together with the first characteristic, this means that people generally have an interest in having everyone else vaccinated, but not themselves (or their children). (3) A number of infections can be eradicated in the long run if vaccination efforts are sustained at sufficiently high coverage levels around the world. In other words, sometimes vaccination has the potential of making itself redundant. Choices about eradication are closely linked to the welfare of future generations and societal time preference (see also below) [5, 9].

Since the perceptions outlined above are usually distorted by insufficient or biased information, government intervention (in the form of subsidies, or coercion) is desirable to ensure that vaccine uptake remains optimal. Indeed, as uptake increases the risk of VAAE remains constant, but individuals may perceive it to increase. At the same time the absence of vaccine-preventable disease may create a false sense of security, and lure people into believing that their risk of disease has reduced to zero as well, while this is highly dependent on historical and future rates of exposure and vaccination in the rest of the population.

The vaccine market represents only 1.5% of the global pharmaceutical market, but has high growth potential (estimated at 10–20% per year by various sources, mainly due to new combination, new prophylactic and new therapeutic vaccines) [10]. For a manufacturer, the contribution margins of vaccines are low compared to those of other products in both the developing and industrialised world (due to price and licensing regulations). The few suppliers of vaccines now aim to limit production to the projected global needs in any given year (UNICEF bought about 90% of "traditional" vaccine supply in 2003, compared to about 25% in 1997). Thus the market is very vulnerable to capacity problems: a problem with a single batch of vaccines by a single producer can have severe knock-on effects across the globe. This may also explain why, for some of the old vaccines, the price fluctuates, and has had the tendency to rise over the last 5 years. Close co-operation between demanders (governments or agencies) and suppliers is essential to ensure continued availability at the right time.

Vaccines are supplied under a tiered price system, with 88% of sales volume in developing countries and countries in transition, but 75% of sales revenue in industrialised countries [10]. It is therefore not surprising that global vaccine manufacturers (with three big producers (GlaxoSmithKline, Aventis and Merck) occupying 77% of the global market) tend to focus on products for the industrialised world.

It is to be expected that more combination vaccines will become available and existing combinations extended. Examples of this include the hexavalent diphteria-tetanus-pertussis-inactivated polio virus – *Haemophilus influenza* type b – hepatitis B (DTP–IPV-Hib–HepB) vaccine, and the quadrivalent measles-mumps-rubella-varicella-zoster (MMRVZ) vaccine. The research and development costs for these vaccines are high due to technical and regulatory complexity. The technicality, the multiple patents and requirements in terms of clinical trials (all demanding great time and money investments) increase barriers to enter the vaccine market. This may lead to more monopolistic behaviour, with risks to supply, choice and price. Clearly, the benefits of combination vaccines are many. For instance, reductions in the number of injections and associated administration costs (including reduced money, time and pain costs for children and their parents), and reduced transmission by contaminated needles benefit recipients and the public health bodies. Free-rider effects (important and not-so-important vaccines can hook up with established vaccines, irrespective of how recipients perceive their importance) and economies of scope[2] benefit manufacturers and perhaps public health bodies. These benefits will have to be traded off *versus* the higher price of combination vaccines.

Because governments, health insurers or agencies (UNICEF, PAHO) typically buy vaccines directly from producers, there is also little diversity on the demand side of the market. All of this implies that there is little competition on both sides of the market and that global societal goals (development and supply of affordable vaccines for poor countries as well as rich countries) are unlikely to be met by relying entirely on free-market mechanisms (particularly since these are hampered by (necessary) regulation with regards to quality control and licensing).

Economic evaluation as an aid to decision-making

Concept

By using economic evaluation we are essentially trying to answer the following questions [5]:

2 Economies of scope are similar to economies of scale, but rather than referring to efficiencies of changes to the scale of the output of a single product, economies of scope refer to efficiencies of changes to the scope of marketing and distributing a range of products (combination vaccines are an example of product building).

1) Is the vaccination program under study worth doing compared to alternative ways of using the same resources? In other words: should the (health care) resources be spent on such a vaccination program, and not on something else?
2) More specifically, if we are deciding to vaccinate against a particular disease, whom should we vaccinate, at which age, with which vaccine and how should the vaccine be delivered and administered in order to deploy our scarce resources in the most efficient way?

Most economic evaluations of vaccination are model-based, because the alternative, empirical analysis, is usually impractical, very time-consuming (for most vaccines it takes decades for the full effects to unfold), very expensive and potentially unethical.

A complete economic evaluation should compare different options for an intervention, in terms of economic costs as well as health consequences. There may be several options to prevent an infectious disease, some of which are mutually exclusive, while others are complementary. The relevant costs and benefits need to be collected for each option, and calculated relative (incremental) to another option. The choice of the reference strategy against which the other options are evaluated can be highly influential for the results of the evaluation. Unless it is a cost-ineffective strategy, current practice is the preferred strategy of reference. When a new vaccine is introduced, the reference strategy is often referred to as "doing nothing" (no vaccination), although in this case "doing nothing" usually means the treatment of cases as they arise, with the corresponding public health measures.

Perspective: costs and benefits for whom?

A generalised distinction between the costs and benefits of vaccination is presented in Table 1. The intervention costs dominate the cost side. These are the costs necessary to implement the vaccination program. Additionally there are costs incurred to receive the vaccine. The benefits of vaccination are the gains in health and the avoided costs. Direct costs can be avoided because less treatment is needed for curing or nursing the disease against which the vaccination program is aimed. Additionally indirect costs can be avoided because vaccination may partly prevent people having to interrupt their normal activities in society because of their illness or the illness of their relatives.

From the health-care payer's point of view, only direct medical costs need to be taken into account. However, from society's viewpoint, indirect non-medical costs are also relevant. Other viewpoints can be those of patients, hospitals, travel clinics, insurance companies, employers, etc. (see Fig. 1). For each of these perspectives different costs and benefits may be

Table 1 – Main costs and benefits of vaccination

Costs	Benefits
Direct costs (mainly intervention costs) Indirect costs (mainly time lost to receive vaccination)	Avoided direct costs (mainly treatment costs) Avoided indirect costs (mainly time gained by avoiding illness)
	Health gains (physical and psychological)

Source: [5]

relevant. This implies that it is possible for an intervention to be relatively cost-effective for one party involved, while it is not for another.

Different cost categories are listed in Table 2. The listings *in italics* are often not taken into account, because they can be relatively small in comparison to the other costs and/or because they are difficult to estimate. Sometimes their inclusion is not relevant to express the viewpoint of the analysis. However, if they are relevant for the viewpoint of the analysis, their impact on the results could be tested in a sensitivity analysis and their existence should be mentioned when the results are presented.

Some diseases affect expectations and behaviour beyond one degree of separation from the pathogen. For instance the global impact of the SARS outbreak in 2003 was modest in disease burden (8098 probable cases, 774 deaths) and associated health-care costs, but it had an impressive impact on the global economy (US$30–100 bn, or $3–10m per case) in macro-economic terms (when the impact on consumption and investments are considered) [11, 12]. A similar situation could arise for pandemic influenza, or any other disease that affects risk perceptions of consumers and investors (e.g., variant Creutzfeld Jacobs Disease). However, for most currently vaccine-preventable diseases, micro-economic evaluation would provide an appropriate analytical framework, preferably adopting a societal perspective. In reality, decisions about universal vaccination are often taken from the perspective of the National Health Service (NHS) or the Ministry of Health and at best from the health-care payer's perspective (which in addition to the NHS costs also includes direct co-insurance and co-payments by the patient). Indeed, decision-makers in health care tend to focus primarily on direct costs since these are most indicative of their immediate budgets, even if their decision has bearings on society at large.

Opportunity, average and marginal costs

When it comes to estimating unit costs or prices, it should be noted that costs in an economic sense are opportunity costs: they represent a sacrifice of the next best alternative application [13]. This entails that costs in an eco-

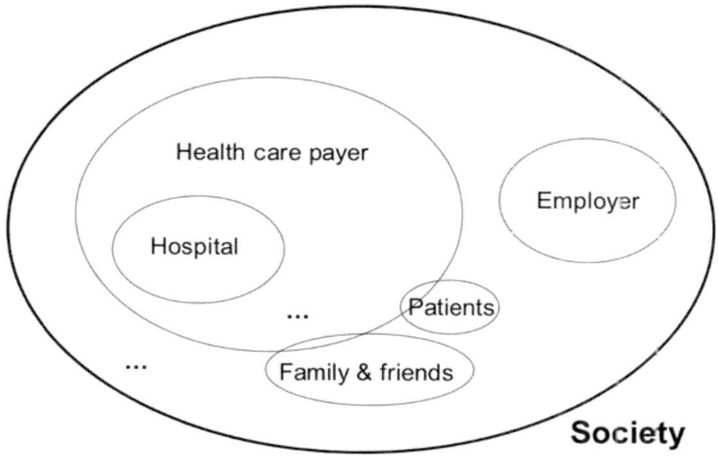

Figure 1. Perspective: different costs (and effects) may be relevant for different analytical viewpoints

nomic sense are not necessarily the same as financial expenditures, and that they can also represent goods and services that are not expressed in monetary terms. However, market prices are often used as a proxy. If particular goods and services are not traded on a market, ("shadow -") prices of a similar activity can be used instead. For example, work of volunteers can be approximated by wages of unskilled labour. Similarly, patients' leisure time could be based on average earnings or average overtime earnings. Average costs per unit of output are the total costs of producing a quantity divided by that quantity. Marginal costs constitute the additional costs of producing one additional unit of output. Since decisions are made at the margin, marginal costs should be used where they are substantially different from average costs [13]. For vaccination, this distinction is most relevant for estimating the costs of the program [5]. The costs of adding a particular vaccine to the existing program depends on how well the schedule of the new vaccine fits in with the other schedules, whether specific precautions need to be taken, whether potential vaccinees need to be screened prior to vaccination or whether a specific target group is envisaged. The costs that are most heavily affected by adding a new vaccine to the existing program are the variable costs of the program (time spent per vaccinee, number of vaccines bought, etc.), whereas the influence on the fixed intervention costs (buildings, general equipment, etc.) is usually small (unless a new vaccine requires a substantially different infrastructure in terms of storage and transport). A good example of this is provided by Hall et al. who examined the immunisation program in The Gambia (more recently these results were confirmed by a similar analysis in Addis Ababa, Ethiopia) [14, 15]. They found that the additional costs of adding hepatitis B vaccine to the existing Expanded

Table 2. Cost categories in an economic evaluation of a vaccination programme

Direct costs:	- Treatment costs directly related to medical consumption (consultations, medication, diagnostic tests, surgery, etc.) for diagnosis and treatment of the diseases against which the vaccine offers protection. - Intervention costs, directly related to the implementation of the vaccination program. These consist of administration costs (consultations, needles, syringes, screening, information campaign, cold chain, infrastructure (buildings, vehicles, etc.), training, etc.) and vaccine purchasing costs (based on the number of required doses, including wastage). Treatment costs for vaccine associated adverse events (VAAE) are often also included here. - *Personal direct costs (transport, home treatment, special education, etc.)*
Indirect costs:	- Costs of time losses (unpaid and paid productive time (and arguably leisure time) of patients and their caretakers) - *Unrelated future health care costs (future health care costs incurred during prolonged lifetime)* - *Unrelated future non-health care costs (future costs of living borne by society during prolonged lifetime)*
Intangible costs:	- *Costs of anxiety, pain and suffering*

Source: [5]

Program on Immunisation (EPI) vaccines (measles, polio, DTP and Bacille Calmette-Guérin (BCG)), would be for 94% recurrent costs (of which 87% for purchasing hepatitis B vaccine (hepB)). Still, the introduction of a new expensive vaccine could more than double the costs of the program in some countries because of its sheer price compared to other vaccines in the program.

Valuing health outcomes: different types of economic evaluations

The main objective of vaccination is to prevent disease. The most important benefits from a public health point of view are therefore the health gains (see Tab. 1). These are both physical (avoiding illness, suffering, mortality, etc.), and psychological (avoiding distress, anxiety, etc.). Specific vaccine-related psychological health gains include the general feeling of well-being and security of vaccine recipients from knowing that they are protected against disease. This could evidently lead to behavioural changes (e.g., a vaccine against HIV/AIDS could have a large influence upon the sexual behaviour of vaccine recipients).

The valuation of health outcomes has far-reaching consequences for the methodology and study design of applied analyses. Generally, a distinction is made between four different methods, depending on the way in which health gains are measured [13].

A cost-minimisation analysis compares the costs of equally effective alternatives, without quantifying the health gains. It differs from a pure cost analysis in that there is always more than one option analysed and that the effectiveness of the different alternatives is known to be equal.

In a cost-effectiveness analysis, health gains are measured in one-dimensional natural units (e.g., infections prevented, hospitalisations prevented, deaths averted, life-years gained…), implying that only one aspect of effectiveness is considered (e.g., postponing the time of death) and other related aspects are not (e.g., the quality of life). The results of cost-effectiveness analyses (CEA) are usually presented as a ratio. A Cost-Effectiveness Ratio (CER) is a measure of the incremental costs, which are necessary to obtain one unit of a health gain by implementing a strategy j instead of a strategy i (expressed in incremental costs per life-year gained, incremental costs per infection prevented, etc.).

$$\text{CER} = \frac{\text{Costs with strategy j} - \text{Costs with strategy i}}{\text{Effects with strategy j} - \text{Effects with strategy i}}$$

The lower the ratio, the more efficiently strategy j gains health compared to strategy i.

The units in which health gains are expressed should represent the final results or clinical endpoints of an intervention as adequately as possible, in order to enable comparison between different interventions [16]. If, hypothetically, the cost-effectiveness of hepatitis B vaccination were $50 per infection prevented, whereas Hib vaccination is estimated at $50,000 per infection prevented, it is wrong to conclude that hepatitis B vaccination is more cost-effective (because it is less costly to prevent one infection). To make that judgement, the avoided effects would need to be expressed in a more comparable endpoint, like life-years saved. To make the comparison even more relevant, different health states should be weighed by their quality (scaled from 0 (meaning death) to 1 (meaning perfect health)). This approach is used in cost-utility analysis (CUA), where health gains are measured in Quality-Adjusted Life-Years (QALYs) saved or another combined measure of morbidity and mortality (e.g., Disability-Adjusted Life-Years (DALY)). A Cost-Utility Ratio (CUR) is similar to a CER, except that the denominator contains the difference in QALYs (or DALYs), instead of the difference in natural units, such as cases avoided or life-years gained. The main advantage of CUA over CEA is that it allows comparison of very different health-care interventions, for instance, those that predominantly extend lives (e.g., flu vaccination of the elderly) with those that improve the quality of life (e.g., drugs against erectile dysfunction).

In Cost-Benefit Analysis (CBA), the health gains are converted into monetary units, which, in theory, allows the many dimensions that are associated with an improvement in health status (over and above the length and health-related quality of life) to be included. There are benefits beyond the health outcomes such as information, caring, regret, anxiety reduction, communication and process utility (benefits from health-care use). Furthermore, option value (i.e., benefits derived from needing care in the future) and non-use value (i.e., externalities related to caring for the health of others) can also be (potentially) elicited [17]. The results of a CBA can be presented as the difference between costs and benefits (the net costs (or net savings)) or as a ratio. The benefit-cost ratio (BCR) expresses to which extent an investment in an intervention can be recovered by the consequences of that intervention (expressed as a unitless number or a %).

Cost-benefit analysis allows for comparisons between totally different projects in society (e.g., comparing a vaccination campaign with the construction of a new bridge). When budgets are very limited and many urgent interventions compete, as in developing countries, such cross-sector comparisons may actually be used in practice. Clearly, the potential of CBA to make such comparisons possible is a major advantage to aid decision-making.

The strength of CBA in theory, i.e., the explicit monetary valuation of health gains, has up till now been also its weakness in practical decision-making. In theory it seems preferable that the valuation of health gains (and of life) is done in an explicit, transparent and representative way as in CBA, instead of the implicit, inconsistent and arbitrary way it is often done in today's decision-making. However, in a health-care environment the monetary valuation of health (and particularly of life) is often rejected on an emotional basis[3] [18]. Additionally, economists have few credible arguments to counter these objections, as the current methods which place a monetary value on health (human-capital and willingness-to-pay methods) can hardly be called consistent and reliable in practice [19–21]. In view of this, most economic evaluations in health care are based on CEA or CUA. The literature on these has increased exponentially since the 1980s, for vaccines at least as much as for other interventions in health care, underlining the importance of a sound theoretical framework for these analyses [17].

Time preference

Individuals (and societies), in general, prefer to receive benefits as early as possible and incur costs as late as possible. This so-called time preference means that the same amount of wealth or health would have a different value to a decision-maker in the present, if this amount is gained at different points in time. Note that time preference has nothing to do with inflation. A vaccination program is an investment made in the present (i.e., the costs of buying and administering vaccines) to gain benefits spread out over the future (i.e., avoided costs of treatment, avoided morbidity and mortali-

3 As noted by Mooney [18]: "To be trained in medicine, nursing or one of the other 'sharp end' disciplines and then be faced with some hard-nosed, cold-blooded economist placing money values on human life and suffering is anathema to many."

ty). Discounting is a technique by which future events (e.g., costs and health outcomes) are valued less the further in the future they arise. The degree to which they are valued less is determined by the discount rate (frequently assumed to be constant through time): the higher the rate the less future benefits and costs are valued. Although there is general agreement on the discounting of costs, the arguments for discounting non-monetised health outcomes are contradictory [5]. Discounting costs without discounting benefits leads, amongst others, to the paradoxical situation that any eradication program will yield infinite benefits [13]. This would imply that all current resources should be spent on research of eradicable diseases, and the implementation of eradication programs, and not a single penny on cure. Such paradoxes, and the observation that individuals generally have a positive discount rate for health, clearly indicates that health too should be discounted at a positive rate. But there is no general agreement on how the discount rate for health should compare to that of wealth. There are arguments to apply an equal discount rate to both costs and health effects [22, 23]. The underpinnings and relevance of these are questionable, so that a lower discount rate for health effects than for costs has also been proposed [24, 25]. Because of the very long time spans over which benefits accrue, the analysis of most vaccination programs is very sensitive to discounting (of costs as well as health effects). Nonetheless, this is no cause for a different approach to discounting for vaccination. Still, further empirical research is needed to strengthen or to change the basis for conventional discount rates (mostly 3%, or 5%) and discount models (mostly stationary) [5]. A slight decrease in discount rate (from, say, 5% to 3%) could change the cost-effectiveness of some vaccination programs from unattractive to attractive. Also, it is likely that time preference in developing countries is substantially different (i.e., higher) from that in industrialised countries, particularly for those countries that have decreasing health (e.g., life-expectancy due to HIV/AIDS) or wealth (e.g., real GDP) expectations [5].

Decision-making: are vaccines a good buy?

In theory, decisions are made by interpreting the results of economic evaluation as follows. In Figure 2 a new program is plotted in terms of costs and effectiveness *versus* the reference strategy in the origin. If the new program is less costly and more effective than the reference, then the new program (a "dominant" strategy) should be implemented. Likewise, if the new program is more costly and less effective than the reference, it should be rejected. In the other quadrants the decision is more complex, because it depends on a value judgement. If the incremental CER (or CUR) is smaller than a given willingness to pay (or threshold cost-effectiveness criterion), "K", it would be acceptable. The question then is, how to determine K? This could be determined by social debate or by comparing it to what is widely accept-

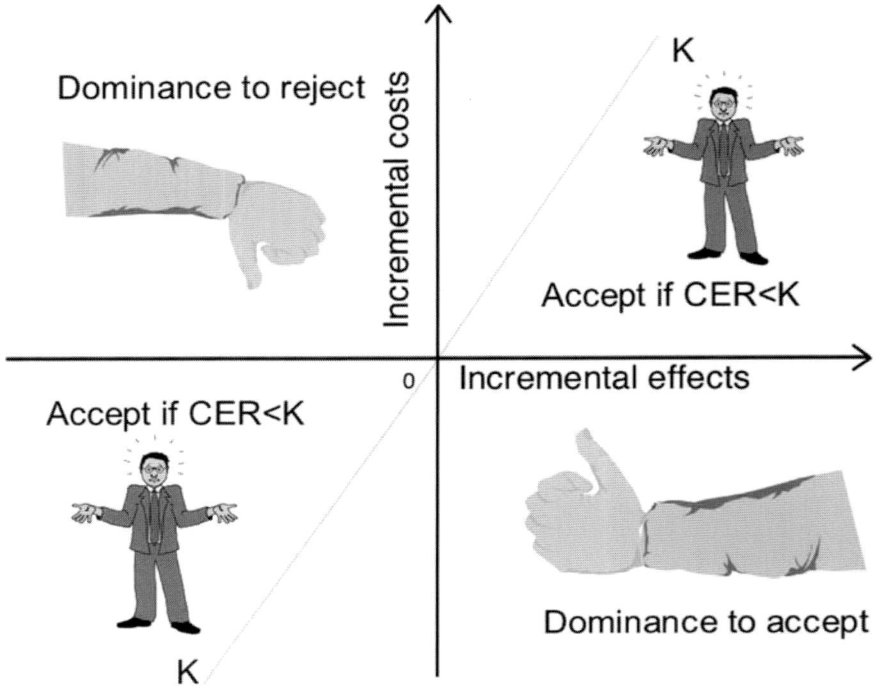

Figure 2. The cost-effectiveness plane. CER: Cost-effectiveness ratio, i.e., incremental costs divided by incremental effects; K = willingness to pay, or a cost-effectiveness ratio of acceptable magnitude. All points on a line in this plane have identical cost-effectiveness ratios.

ed in practice. The most widely cited K in industrialised countries is $50,000 per QALY gained. There may also be a grey zone for K in which some interventions are implemented and others are not (e.g., between $40,000 per QALY gained and $100,000 per QALY gained), whereas under and above that grey zone all and none of the interventions are implemented, respectively. However, the greater the analytical uncertainty and the burden of disease, the more decisions are likely to deviate from such clear cut-off practices [26]. Different societies should have a different willingness to pay, though there are few instances in which societies (or their decision-makers) have tried to determine what the appropriate value of K is. The World Bank has suggested using GNP per capita as a benchmark for K. Note that in CBA, K has already been given an explicit value.

In league tables, many vaccination programs rank with the most cost-effective interventions in health care in industrialised countries [5, 27–29]. It is tempting to try and estimate the global historical value of vaccination. However, due to scarcity of data in most parts of the world such an exercise

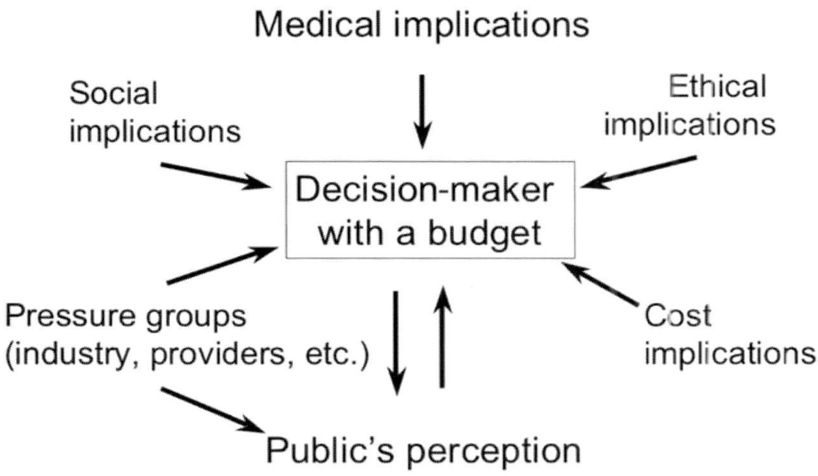

Figure 3. Factors influencing decision-making in practice

would be, by necessity, extremely crude. It seems clear, though, that the smallpox eradication program and the establishment of the EPI have generated enormous benefits, not only by directly protecting against important vaccine-preventable diseases, but also by providing opportunities for health education and infrastructure in developing countries [30]. Yet the associated disease reduction in smallpox, measles and tetanus alone is bound to have been a cost-saving enterprise around the world (i.e., in the lower right quadrant of Fig. 2), currently averting over 8 million deaths *per annum*, compared to a "never having vaccinations" situation. However, when we are making choices today, we have to consider what additional benefits we will achieve by making additional investments, and this is bound to vary between countries at different stages of economic development, different epidemiologies of disease, and different historical vaccine-uptake levels. Hence data from one country cannot always be simply extrapolated to another.

In practice, there are many factors that come into play when decisions are made about new health-care interventions (see Fig. 3). In a democracy, a decision-maker receives a temporary, renewable mandate from the public to allocate a given budget. That person is well aware of the public perceptions of public health problems, and the impact of decisions thereon. At the same time, pressure groups may try to influence decision-makers or the public's perception. These pressure groups have vested interests in the decisions (be it as sellers of vaccines, or sellers of services for the cure of vaccine-preventable diseases). Societal goals with regards to the decision can only be met by considering its medical, social, ethical and cost implications. The theoretical foundation of economic evaluation (so-called "Pareto optimality") addresses efficiency, without concern for distributional aspects (equity). Therefore, economic evaluation combines the medical/epidemiological and cost implications, but does not consider the social and ethical implications depicted in Figure 3 (though in CBA these aspects could theoretically be included, if a willingness-to-pay approach is used, and it is possible to weight quality-of-life gains to help achieve equity goals, as is commonly performed in DALYs). Therefore economic evaluation should be seen as an additional type of analysis that cannot stand on its own in its current form (it is an aid to decision-making, not a decision-maker in itself). At the same time, ideally, the influence of pressure groups, and the public's perceptions (rather than the public's true preferences) should be minimised in this process. It is noteworthy that most vaccination programs are likely to be equitable according to prevailing theories of justice [5]. Indeed, an analysis for Bangladesh indicated that socio-economic inequalities in mortality of under-5-year-olds were eliminated by measles vaccination [31].

Financing vaccines

In the past, vaccination interests of poor and wealthy nations seemed more in tune than today. Moreover, the research and development costs of the new generation of vaccines, based on biotechnology, are greater and the regulatory hurdles higher, meaning that new vaccines are much more expensive than the basic package of "traditional" vaccines. The first new expensive vaccine for global use was the hepatitis B vaccine, which became available in 1981. The main reason why it was not immediately included in universal vaccination programs was its price, because initially the hepatitis B vaccine cost more than the other six EPI vaccines put together.

With the advent of more expensive vaccines, the introduction of a new vaccine is not as straightforward as it used to be in the industrialised world. In contrast to some of the "older" vaccines (e.g., measles, pertussis), newer vaccines may not result in net savings to the health-care system. Nonetheless, if considered desirable, industrialised countries have no difficulty in financing the introduction of new vaccines, and ensuring the continuing uptake of old ones. For developing countries, the main difficulty is not so much to determine whether it would be cost-effective to introduce a vaccine, but to ensure that the introduction is financially sustainable. When external donors sponsor vaccination programs the sustainability takes the form of a partnership with shared responsibility and the promise by the receiver of the financing to create the conditions to become self-sufficient in the long run, either alone or by attracting further external funding.

Global immunisation efforts came under pressure as the EPI, which was launched in the 1970s as a way of building on the success of the smallpox eradication program, lost its momentum in the 1990s, and failed to attain the year 2000 goal of 90% global vaccination coverage. Indeed, global childhood immunisation coverage against the six main target diseases (polio, DTP, measles and tuberculosis), which was less than 5% in 1974, decreased from about 80% in 1990 to 75% in 2000 [32]. Coverage for the complete schedule of DTP remains well below 75% in tens of developing countries, mostly in sub-Saharan Africa. These countries are traditionally bottlenecks in the EPI because of great financial constraints, the evolution of the HIV epidemic, logistical difficulties, poor governance and general socio-economic conditions (sometimes aggravated by war). As these factors evolved unfavourably in the 1990s, international alliances shifted their efforts from reducing general global inequalities in health ("Health for All") to more selective strategies, like the polio eradication program and the introduction of new and improved vaccines.

The discrepancy between the developing and the industrialised world is likely to become greater, as private vaccine development focuses primarily on diseases that affect the wealthy. Indeed, only about 1% of world drug sales is for African countries. It has been estimated that of all expenditures on health research (over $70 billion per year), 90% is for diseases that affect 10% of the world's population [33].

Using recent examples, Kaddar et al. assert that financing vaccination should be affordable by all countries, at least for the basic vaccines [34]. The cost of fully immunizing a child with the basic vaccines is $5 to $25, which typically represents 5% to 10% of public health expenditures, <$0.4 *per capita* or about 0.1% of GDP. Most vaccination costs are fixed costs of personnel and infrastructure, and the marginal costs of an additional vaccine may often be bearable for the domestic budget (though still highly dependent on vaccine price). As the 20th century drew to a close, the landscape of external vaccine financing underwent dramatic changes with the inception of the Global Alliance for Vaccines and Immunization (GAVI) and the Vaccine Fund, with the aims to stimulate research and development for developing world problems, strengthen immunization systems, and promote and support the introduction of new and underused vaccines GAVI is an alliance of financiers (development banks, aid agencies, foundations), agencies (UNICEF, WHO), vaccine developers and manufacturers, as well as developing country governments, whereas the Vaccine Fund manages private financial resources, such as those from the Bill &Melinda Gates Foundation, and public contributions from a small number of wealthy countries.

Conclusion

The first generation of vaccines, such as measles and oral polio vaccines, was used against common and serious childhood diseases afflicting all countries in the world. Few of these vaccination programs were subject to economic analysis before introduction, and for good reason: the benefits were obvious and the costs low. Indeed, they were probably amongst the most effective and cost-effective public health programs of the 20th century. This is no longer necessarily the case with new vaccine introductions. New vaccines are generally higher priced and unlikely to fall in price to the level of the first generation of vaccines. Furthermore, they are often aimed at less common or less serious diseases (particularly in the industrialised world). Thus, whether these vaccines are worth introducing is less clear. Vaccine financing has recently changed with important initiatives stimulating development and use of vaccines for the developing world. These are to be welcomed as they may further alleviate the disease burden in developing countries at affordable cost, correct market imperfections with regard to research and development, and reduce inequalities in health. Nonetheless, the introduction of new vaccines demands cautious planning. If it comes at the expense of the uptake of the first generation of vaccines, it may have a detrimental influence on the effectiveness and cost-effectiveness of the whole program. In view of all these developments, the role of economic evaluation in vaccine program design is only likely to increase in the future.

Acknowledgements
The author is grateful to Dr John Edmunds (Health Protection Agency, UK) for constructive comments on an earlier version, and to the Flemish Fund for Scientific Research (FWO G.0023.01) and the European Union funded project POLYMOD (EU FP6) for financial support.

References

1 World Bank (2004) World Development Indicators, online publication available on CD ROM and at http://publications.worldbank.org/ecommerce/catalog/product?item_id=631625
2 WHO (2001) Commission on Macroeconomics and Health: investing in health for economic development. Available at http://www.cid.harvard.edu/cidcmh/CMHReport.pdf
3 Razzell PE (1977) *The conquest of smallpox*. Caliban Books, Firle (UK)
4 McKeown T, Record RG, Brown RG (1972) An interpretation of the modern rise of population in Europe. *Population Studies* 26: 345–382
5 Beutels P (2002) *Economic evaluation of vaccination programmes in humans: a methodological exploration with applications to hepatitis B, varicella-zoster, measles, pertussis, hepatitis A and pneumococcal vaccination*. University of Antwerp, Antwerp
6 Philipson T (2000) Economic epidemiology and infectious disease. In: Newhouse J, Culyer T (eds): *Handbook of health economics*. North-Holland, New York, 1761–1797

7 Anderson RM, May RM (1991) *Infectious diseases of humans – dynamics and control.* Oxford University Press, Oxford
8 Panagiotopoulos T, Antoniadou I, Valassi-Adam E (1999) Increase in congenital rubella occurrence after immunisation in Greece: retrospective survey and systematic review. *Brit Med J* 319 (7223): 1462–1467
9 Barrett S (2004) Economics of eradication vs control of infectious diseases. *Bull WHO* 82 (9): 639–718
10 Kaddar M (2004) Lecture at the advanced course in vaccinology, International Vaccine Institute, Seoul, 2004. Data based on Frost & Sullivan, Datamonitor, Theta reports and Genesis
11 Smith RD, Sommers T (2003) Assessing the economic impact of communicable disease outbreaks: the case of SARS. Working paper WHO, July 2003
12 Lee JW, McKibbin W (2004) Globalization and Disease: The Case of SARS. *Asian Economic Papers* 3 (1)*; in press*
13 Drummond M, O'Brien B, Stoddart G, Torrance G (1997) Methods for the economic evaluation of health care programmes (second ed.). Oxford University Press, Oxford
14 Edmunds WJ, Dejene A, Mekonnen Y, Haile M, Alemnu W, Nokes DJ (2000) The cost of integrating hepatitis B virus vaccine into national immunization programmes: a case study from Addis Ababa. *Health Policy and Planning* 15(4): 408–416
15 Hall AJ, Robertson RL, Crivelli PE, Lowe Y, Inskip H, Snow SK, Whittle H (1993) Cost-effectiveness of hepatitis B vaccine in The Gambia. *Trans Roy Soc Trop Med Hyg* 87: 333–336
16 Drummond M (1991) Output measurement for resource allocation decisions in health care. In: McGuire A, Fenn P, Mayhew K (eds): *Providing health care. The economics of alternative systems of finance and delivery.* University Press, Oxford, 99–119
17 Beutels P, Van Doorslaer E, Van Damme P, Hall J (2003) Methodological issues and new developments in the economic evaluation of vaccines. *Exp Rev Vacc* 2(5): 89–100
18 Mooney G (1992) *The economics of health and medicine.* Wheatsheaf, Brighton
19 Luce BR, Manning WG, Siegel JE, Lipscomb J (1996) Estimating costs in cost-effectiveness analysis. In: Gold MR, Siegel JE, Russel LB, Weinstein MC (eds): *Cost-effectiveness in health and medicine.* Oxford University Press, New York, 176–213
20 Mishan EJ (1971) Evaluation of life and limb: a theoretical approach. *Journal of Political Economy* 79: 687–706
21 Olsen JA, Smith RD (2001) Theory versus practice: a review of 'willingness to pay" in health and health care. *Health Econ* 10: 39–52
22 Keeler J, Cretin S (1983) Discounting of life saving and other non-monetary effects. *Management Science* 29(3): 300–306
23 Weinstein MC, Stason WB (1977) Foundations of cost-effectiveness analysis for health and medical practices. *N Engl J Med* 296: 716–721

24 van Hout BA (1998) Discounting costs and effects: a reconsideration. *Health Econ* 7(7): 581–594
25 Gravelle H, Smith D (2001) Discounting for health effects in cost-benefit and cost-effectiveness analysis. *Health Econ* 10(7): 587–599
26 Devlin N, Parkin D (2004) Does NICE have a cost-effectiveness threshold and what other factors influence its decisions? A binary choice analysis. *Health Econ* 13(5): 437–452
27 George B, Harris A, Mitchell A (2001) Cost-effectiveness analysis and the consistency of decision making: evidence from pharmaceutical reimbursement in Australia (1991 to 1996). *Pharmacoeconomics* 19(11): 1103–1109
28 Chapman RH, Stone PW, Sandberg EA, Bell C, Neumann PJ (2000) A comprehensive league table of cost-utility ratios and a sub-table of "panel-worthy" studies. *Med Decis Making* 20(4): 451–467
29 Tengs TO, Adams ME, Pliskin JS, Safran DG, Siegel JE, Weinstein MC, Graham JD (1995) Fivehundred life-saving interventions and their cost-effectiveness. *Risk Anal* 15(3): 369–390
30 Shearley AE (1999) The societal value of vaccination in developing countries. *Vaccine* 17 (Suppl 3): S109–S112
31 Bishai D, Koenig M, Ali Khan M (2003) Measles vaccination improves the equity of health outcomes: evidence from Bangladesh. *Health Econ* 12(5): 415–419
32 UNICEF (2001) The State of the World's Children. Early childhood. Available at www.unicef.org/SOWC01
33 Global Forum for Health Research (2004) The 10/90 gap report 2004. Available at http://www.globalforumhealth.org/pages/index.asp?ThePage=page1_419.asp
34 Kaddar M, Lydon P, Levine R (2004) Financial challenges of immunization: a look at GAVI. Bull WHO 82 (9): 697–702

Private hand

The Grand Challenge for the Future
ed. by Stefan H.E. Kaufmann and Paul-Henri Lambert

How and why vaccines are made

Stanley A. Plotkin[1] and James M. Robinson[2]

[1]*Emeritus Professor of Pediatrics, University of Pennsylvania, Medical and Scientific Advisor, Sanofi Pasteur, 4650 Wismer Road, Doylestown, PA 18901, USA; and* [2]*Vice President, Industrial Operations, Sanofi Pasteur, Inc., Discovery Drive, Swiftwater, PA 18370, USA*

Introduction

Vaccines to prevent disease remain the ultimate goals of medicine, following the proverb that says in many languages "Better to prevent than to cure." Certainly, the record of vaccines has been one of exemplary success in reducing, eliminating and even eradicating infectious diseases. Yet there is not a general appreciation of the difficulties that attend the development of vaccines, difficulties that increase with each passing year. This chapter attempts to give a perspective on the process of vaccine development: why a target is chosen, how the vaccine is developed for licensure, and what is involved in the modern production of a biological vaccine for use in humans.

Aside from the medical and humanitarian advantages of vaccination, the cost-benefit ratio is extremely favorable, as shown in Figure 1 [1].

The vaccine industry

Manufacture of vaccines is highly concentrated from an economic point of view, with five companies accounting for more than 80% of the market: Aventis Pasteur, Chiron, Glaxo SmithKline, Merck and Wyeth (Chryssomalis G, Hardy C, Sanofi Pasteur, personal communication; Fig. 2). These five manufacturers, and indeed most of the manufacturers in the second rank, are based in industrialized countries. However, there are many other manufacturers supplying limited ranges of vaccines or having sales in limited regions (Tab. 1). The largest part of the vaccine market is in North America, with Europe second and the rest of the world only accounting for about 15%. However, in terms of numbers of doses used, manufacturers from the developing world play a major role, particularly the Serum Institute of India in recent years.

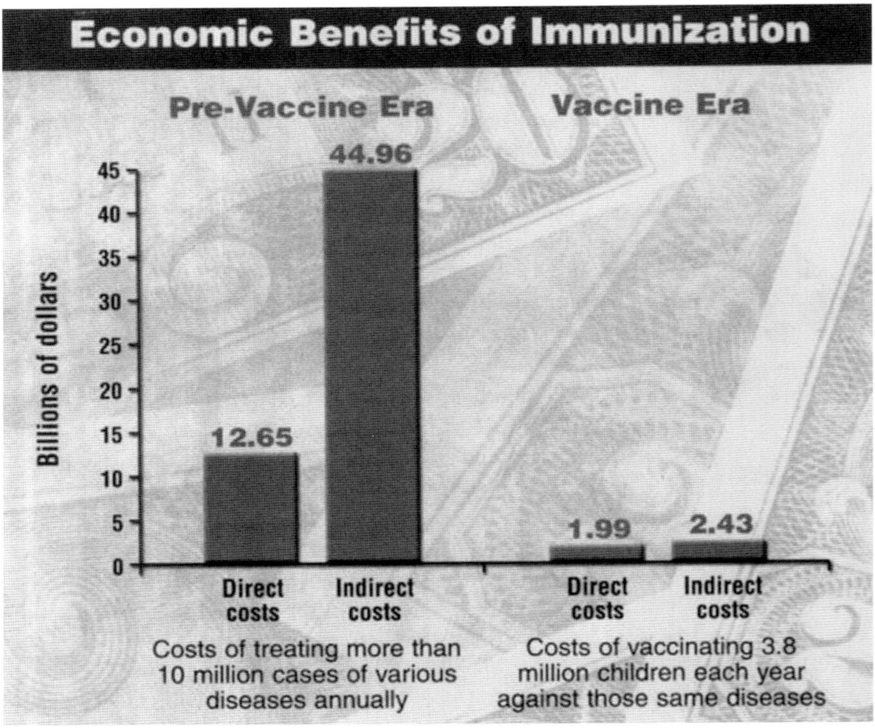

Figure 1. If there were no immunization in the United States, 33,494 deaths and 10,541,569 cases of diphtheria, tetanus, pertussis, polio, measles, mumps, rubella, congenital rubella syndrome, Hib and hepatitis B infection could be expected each year.

Although all of the major vaccine manufacturers are part of larger pharmaceutical corporations, vaccines are not the same as drugs. Vaccines are given to healthy people rather than to ill people, low efficacy is much less acceptable, infants are the primary targets, and they are given only a few times in life. Moreover, they are supposed to be cheap, which is inconsistent with modern quality control. The latter point is all the more problematic as the total vaccine market is only about 1% of the pharmaceutical market, and thus not attractive to investors.

The main products that generate income are Hepatitis A and B, MMR and flu vaccines. Flu vaccines are profitable because of high volume, whereas the hepatitis vaccines and MMR elicit high prices in industrialized countries. More recently, pneumococcal conjugate vaccine has turned into a "blockbuster". As newer vaccines are much more costly than older ones, for reasons that will be made clear below, it is likely that future vaccines will not be cheap.

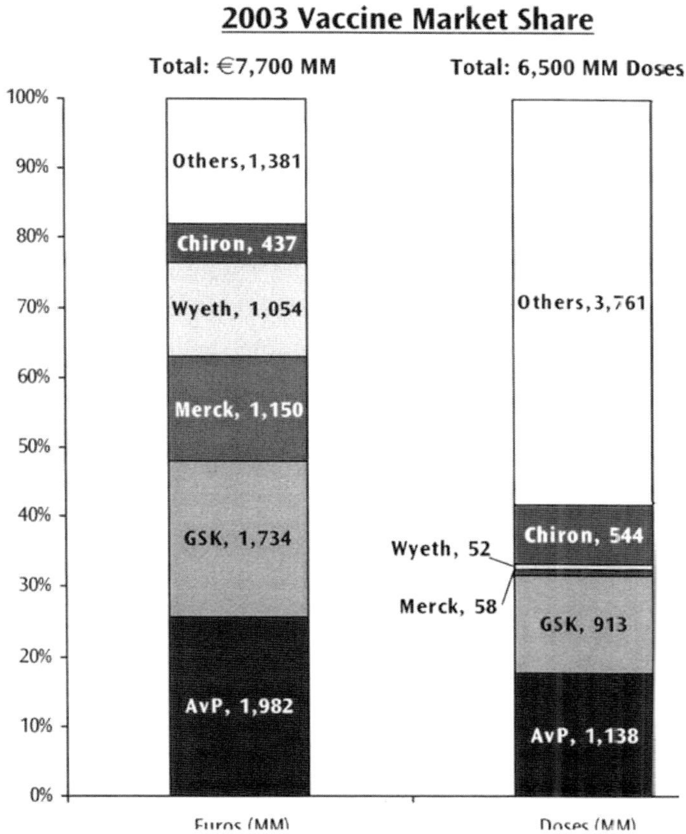

Figure 2. The vaccine market analyzed by income generated (million Euros) and by number of doses sold (million doses). GSK, GlaxoSmithKline, AvP, Aventis Pasteur, now Sanofi Pasteur.

Why does industry develop certain vaccines?

The selection by industry of which vaccines to develop is a complex one, involving many different factors, listed in Table 2. As industry must make a profit in order to satisfy investors, the size of a potential market is a key factor. Table 3 lists the often imprecise means by which market size is gauged. Demand from consumers is of course important, but difficult to measure. It was assumed that a high demand for a Lyme disease vaccine existed in the Northeast United States, but when the vaccine actually was commercialized, demand was feeble. In contrast, consumer demand propelled the development of less reactogenic acellular pertussis vaccines.

Demand from governmental authorities is more reliable, as ultimately they must pay for a vaccine. The request from United Kingdom authorities

Table 1. Vaccine manufacturers

Large market share:	Sanofi Pasteur (France, Canada, USA) Chiron (Italy, Germany, USA) GlaxoSmithKline (Belgium, USA) Merck (USA) Wyeth-Lederle (USA)
Smaller market share:	Baxter (Austria) Berna (Switzerland) Commonwealth Serum Labs (Australia) Serum Institute of India
Limited range:	Bioport (USA) Dynport (USA) Korean Green Cross Medimmune (USA) North American Biologicals (USA) RIVM (Netherlands) Powderject (UK) Shires (Canada) Solvay Statens Serum Institute (DK) Swedish Bact. Lab Acambis (UK, USA) Vaxgen (USA)
Regional:	Brazil China Cuba India Indonesia Iran Japan Russia South Africa Thailand

for a conjugated meningococcal vaccine drove several companies to develop one.

Epidemiological data, such as those collected on invasive pneumococcal infections, were a great stimulus for the development of protein-conjugated polysaccharide vaccines for infants. Epidemiological data are also often the basis for expert opinion. Experts serve as "champions" for particular vaccines. For example, it is unlikely a live mumps vaccine would have been developed if Maurice Hilleman at Merck had not insisted on it.

Finally, there is a good deal of guesswork involved in marketing predictions. Few would have imagined that hepatitis B vaccine would become a standard pediatric vaccine at the time when homosexuals and recipients of blood transfusions were considered the primary targets.

However, market size is far from the only consideration. Vaccine manufacturers respond to public health need, although unfortunately they some-

Table 2. Reasons why vaccine manufacturers launch a development program

1	Market
2	Public health interest
3	Technical feasibility
4	Intellectual property
5	Fit with other vaccines

Table 3. How market is determined

1	Demand from consumers in developed countries; e.g., Lyme disease, acellular pertussis
2	Demand from authorities in developed countries; e.g., Meningitis C
3	Epidemiological data; e.g., pneumococcal conjugate
4	Expert opinion; e.g., mumps
5	Guesses, buttressed by precise but inaccurate data; e.g., hepatitis B

times fail to receive useful advice from public health authorities. On the other hand, documents such as the Institute of Medicine's priority classification for the development of new vaccines are very helpful.

A key factor in the choice of vaccines for development is technical feasibility. By and large, the vaccine industry does not do basic research, but rather develops findings made in academic or biotech laboratories. If the latter have not provided a practical means of making a vaccine, manufacturers are loath to embark on a costly vaccine development effort. Moreover, academicians frequently do not understand how an idea that works in their laboratories on a small scale must be developed in a practical way, which at times may be impossible. The problem is usually scale-up, a process fraught with difficulties. Also, an experiment that works in mice may fail in humans, or as is sometimes said, "mice lie, or at least exaggerate."

Availability of intellectual property is another important factor, and unfortunately is still a quagmire [2]. Patent protection blocked the production of hepatitis B vaccine by multiple manufacturers for many years. On the other hand, the licensure of the Lyme disease OspA vaccine was made possible by a royalty agreement between two manufacturers who both held important intellectual property.

Lastly, a company may decide for or against a vaccine based on its fit with other vaccines the company produces. This becomes most obvious with regard to combinations: for example, if a company has no access to a pneumococcal conjugate vaccine, it may not wish to develop an Hib vaccine to prevent meningitis.

The strategies of vaccine development

Vaccine development has evolved greatly in recent years. Attenuation of living pathogens has been a major strategy, and continues to be so.

Table 4. Some newer strategies for vaccine development starting from information on the microbial genome (DNA, cDNA, or RNA)

Strategy	Examples
Recombinant protein production	Hepatitis B S_{Ag}, pertussis toxin, Lyme outer-surface-protein A
Live recombinants	Dengue, parainfluenza, tuberculosis
Replication – defective particles	Human papilloma virus, herpes simplex virus
Alpha virus replicons	Human immunodeficiency virus, hemorrhagic fevers
"Naked" DNA Plasmid	Hepatitis B
Recombinant vectors	Cytomegalovirus, human immunodeficiency virus
Prime boost using DNA and/or vectors	HIV, malaria
Reverse genetics	Influenza, parainfluenza, respiratory syncytial virus

Similarly, inactivation of whole bacteria or viruses remains a useful technique in certain cases, but recently the tendency has been to break down the organism to extract the protective antigen. Thus, the use of purified bacterial capsular polysaccharides, protein subunits, and detoxified toxins is seen. Reassortment of genome segments by coinfection with wild and attenuated viruses in tissue culture has been used for some time in the development of killed influenza vaccine, and more recently for the development of live influenza and live rotavirus vaccines.

With the advent of genetic engineering, many new strategies have become available, listed in Table 4 [3–5]. They have not only made vaccine development more feasible, but in a sense they have changed the definition of a vaccine. In 2004, a vaccine might be defined as a protein, polysaccharide, nucleic acid, living vector or infectious agent, that when inoculated or administered to the mucosa, induces antibodies and/or cellular immune responses specific to a pathogen that protect against the pathogen or suppress its chronic replication.

Recombinants of yeast, bacteria or animal cells are now used to produce proteins of many descriptions, most notably the hepatitis B surface antigen. Living recombinants themselves serve to carry genes from multiple related viruses, such as the envelope genes for four dengue serotypes, all carried on one attenuated dengue serotype. Replication-defective particles carrying no RNA or DNA can often be constructed from one or a few viral proteins. Alphavirus replicons are a special case of pseudoparticles, in that expression of foreign antigens during abortive replication can immunize a host. "Naked" DNA plasmids stimulate immune responses when injected, particularly cellular responses.

A major field in vaccinology is currently the use of vectors, which are attenuated bacteria or viruses into the genome of which are inserted genes that code for vaccine antigens. Examples of vectors are poxviruses like vaccinia, adenoviruses, and BCG. The expression of the inserted gene is often sufficient to stimulate both antibody and cellular responses, particularly the latter. Although vectors may be useful in themselves, they are frequently employed as primes or boosts in a so-called prime-boost configuration. For example, a vaccinee may be primed with a DNA plasmid and boosted with an adenovirus vector, both carrying the same genes from a pathogen.

Reverse genetics refers to the directed mutation of microbial genomes with subsequent examination of phenotype, which allows for rapid attenuation and identification of desirable mutations.

The process of vaccine development

The road to vaccine development is outlined in Table 5. As stated above, the basic ideas are likely to come from outside of industry, but at a certain point a vaccine can only advance with the help of industry scientists. Once a vaccine lot is produced for clinical trials, it can pass from the preclinical phase, which is conducted in animals and *in vitro* (Tab. 6); to phase 1, in which basic safety and immunogenicity are studied (Tab. 7); to phase 2, in which the dose, schedule and other properties of the vaccine are defined (Tab. 8); to phase 3, which defines safety, efficacy and consistency of manufacture (Tab. 9); and finally to phase 4, which measures safety and effectiveness after licensure by observation of large numbers of vaccinees.

Table 5. The road to vaccine development

Academic/biotech	
1	Identify the mechanism of natural protection against a pathogen
2	Isolate the antigen(s) responsible for the protection
3	Show in animals that the vaccine protects
4	Find the best method to present the antigen (live, killed, subunit)
Industry	
5	Increase yield and purity
6	Develop a process for large-scale production
7	Show the safety of the antigen in animals
8	Produce a lot under GMP
9	Proceed to clinical development

Table 6. Preclinical development

1	Define vaccine characteristics: (nature, chemical definition)
2	Follow good manufacturing practices:
	Write clear definition of a reproducible process
	Quality control: Show homogeneity from batch to batch.
	Show microbiological sterility
3	Animal tests
	Safety
	Immunogenicity
	Efficacy, if animal model is available

Table 7. Phase I Clinical development

- Safety in healthy adult volunteers (safe = absence of serious or unexpected effects)
- Usually fewer than 50 subjects not exposed to the natural disease
- Verify immunogenicity in volunteers
- Open uncontrolled study or randomized controlled study
- Maximal dose
- One or several dose vaccination schedules

Table 8. Phase II Clinical development

- Randomized, double-blind, controlled studies (control = reference vaccine or placebo) 100–200 subjects per group
- Cascade of studies to determine:
  - optimal dose (dose-response)
  - administration route
  - vaccination schedule (including the need for booster dose)
  - possible association with other vaccines (lack of interference, no acceptable increase of side-effects)
  - response in presence of pre-existing antibodies (natural or maternal antibodies)
  - safety: tolerability (incidence, duration and severity of side-effects)
  - immunogenicity: antibody response by standardized tests (geometric mean titer, AB kinetics and persistence, rate of responders, seroconversion rate, AB functionality)

Phase 2b (optional)
Efficacy study in high-risk population – small numbers, low statistical power

The preclinical phase includes the definition of the potential vaccine and the demonstration of likely safety and immunogenicity in animals. If there is an adequate animal model, efficacy will also be studied. A clinical lot is then produced under Good Manufacturing Processes.

Phase 1 involves demonstration of basic safety and immunogenicity in a limited number of healthy adult volunteers. A small number of control subjects may also be included. Dosage may also be studied in this phase, although more usually that occurs in phase 2.

Phase 2 comprises an enlargement of data on safety and immunogenicity, definition of optimal dose and schedule, and a variety of intense immunological tests of antibody and cellular responses. If the attack rate of the disease for which the vaccine is being developed is high enough, a phase 2b efficacy study may be organized. This is an effort to verify that the vaccine is likely to be efficacious in more extensive tests, although the statistical power of the phase 2b demonstration will be low.

Phase 3 involves three important considerations: verification of safety in 10,000 to 50,000 individuals, efficacy in a double-blind, placebo-controlled, randomized study with good statistical power, and demonstration of consistency between lots. The latter usually involves clinical tests of at least three lots for statistically similar immunogenicity.

Table 9. Phase III Clinical development

- Population: target population (susceptible, exposed)
- Safety profile in large numbers (10–50,000)
- Measurement of the protective effect of the vaccine
  - randomized, double-blind and controlled study for "absolute" efficacy; when controlled with a reference vaccine, obtain "relative" efficacy
  - main evaluation criterion: case of disease

Consistency studies
  - test 3 serial lots for equivalent
    - safety
    - immunogenicity
    - stability

Table 10. Phase IV Clinical development (post-licensing)

- Safety in large numbers (millions) of unselected vaccinees
- Effectiveness in actual use (vs un-randomized non-vaccinated)
- Duration of protection

Not surprisingly, the total process is long. The average time from conception to licensing of a vaccine was formerly about 10 years. At this point, 15 years is a more realistic figure.

Nevertheless, the process does not finish there. Phase 4 post-licensing studies are now mandatory. They confirm extent and duration of effectiveness in actual use, but also enable collection of more extensive information on adverse reactions (Tab. 10).

Vaccine production

The modern production of vaccines is a complex and tedious process. Regulatory bodies demand that biological vaccines come as close as possible to drugs with regard to purity and consistency, which is a tall order. Safety becomes a paramount concern, and quality control procedures are designed to exclude chemical or microbial contamination.

Traditional (non-recombinant) vaccine production begins with growth of the bacteria or viruses that cause the disease, followed by inactivation of the organism and/or detoxification of the bacterial toxins (e.g., tetanus), and purification of the cell or a component of the cell. Early vaccines were simply grown on media that supported good growth of the bacterium or propagation of the virus. Complex media including ingredients such as meat extracts and yeast extracts were common components and yielded good bacterial growth. Embryonated chicken eggs still prove to be a productive method for growing a number of viruses, including most importantly influenza virus. However, most viral vaccines are made in cell culture.

As drug guidelines were applied increasingly to vaccines, better characterization of the vaccines followed. The complex media used in early vaccines were not well defined, as the natural variations in meat, yeast, etc., translated into variable media composition, and hence variable yield and potency. These variations proved to be critical, causing vaccine manufacturers to screen multiple lots of the media ingredients to find some appropriate for manufacturing. Without clear definition of the nutritional requirements for each organism, the appropriate media composition was often difficult to develop. Likewise, for some vaccines whole bacterial cells were replaced by including only the cell components that were linked to protection (e.g., acellular pertussis vaccines are replacing whole-cell vaccines). These were considered new vaccines as new disruption/purification processes were developed and therefore they were submitted to clinical tests for safety and efficacy.

The current manufacture of influenza vaccine proves to be an interesting exercise in logistics. Each year, based on epidemiology of circulating strains, various health organizations worldwide select the virus strains thought to be the greatest threat for the coming year. Generally between February to April in the Northern hemisphere, these strains are identified and manufacturers then race to develop virus seeds from these strains and quickly inoculate many hundred thousand eggs per day to produce sufficient vaccine by the immunization season that fall. Earlier selection of strains could risk a poor choice for the vaccine, while a later choice would jeopardize a sufficient supply. Some firms make educated guesses and begin to manufacture before the official selection of the strains as they know they cannot manufacture enough product otherwise. A poor choice of strains by the manufacturer could have a serious financial impact.

The logistics of influenza production include management of the chicken farms to produce sufficient quantities of hens and cockerels to produce the embryonated eggs. As these eggs will be used in manufacture of a sterile vaccine, control of the farms, incubators, and delivery network is paramount. The entire process must also be protected by numerous security measures to prevent loss of the flock to circulating avian influenza strains. Once a quality egg supply is secured, the eggs are inoculated with virus, the virus is incubated for a few days in the embryo, the allantoic fluid is harvested from the egg, and the virus is purified, inactivated, sterile filtered, and tested for potency. When all three strains have been produced, they are combined in a tri-valent vaccine, filled into vials, labeled, tested, released, and distributed to physicians throughout the world. Serious challenges have arisen when poor yielding strains greatly reduced the number of doses that could be made in a given production campaign. Likewise, the inactivation and purification process may be modified for a campaign to suit the particular vaccine strain. These challenges have proven to be too great for many firms and the number of large-scale producers has dwindled in the last 5 years.

The final challenge to the task of providing flu vaccine to the customer is the filling process. This challenge will become even greater in the near future. Based on the logistics of when strains are selected (new strains require production of new test reagents to calibrate potency among manufacturers) and are ready for release, and the need for physicians to immunize before the flu season, manufacturing firms generally have just 15–17 weeks to fill sufficient vaccine to satisfy the demand for vaccine. Sterile filling and inspection of the product is often the rate-limiting step in the manufacturing process. The majority of influenza vaccine in many markets today is delivered in multi-dose vials. Increased demand for individual doses of product promises to put a tremendous strain on manufacturing capacity in the coming years.

For viral vaccines, replacing the embryonated egg or primary cell culture from animal organs has also been a challenge. For some viral vaccines, a mammalian cell line has been developed, optimized, and industrialized to produce a more consistent vaccine (e.g., poliovirus vaccines made on VERO cells). In the case of influenza, where the strains of virus change annually, the appropriate cell line for growth of multiple different viruses has been more elusive, although a number of new developments has brought promise of a new process in the next decade.

Inactivated poliovirus vaccine production was produced in primary mammalian cells from a new living animal for each lot of vaccine. To eliminate inconsistency, a cell line was developed from vervet monkey kidney and fully tested for safety (adventitious agents, etc.) and productivity (VERO cells). The VERO cell line was frozen in multiple aliquots for future production. The cell culture is grown from a frozen master seed and working seed was then produced in a quantity sufficient for future needs. Thawing of ampoules of working seed allow production of large quantities of cells (several thousand liters) in progressive stages. Once at production scale, these viable cells are infected with poliovirus (three unique strains are used) and the virus is harvested, purified, and inactivated. Similar to flu vaccine, three strains are combined in a final formulation and filled for distribution.

The use of cell lines for production has major benefits in process reliability, consistency, and robustness. Having a certified cell line for production eliminates the need to qualify new supplies of cells as must be done for influenza production in eggs, and also reduces the risks of extraneous agents and variability in the production process. VERO cells have the added benefit of growing in suspension, whereas many cell lines require attachment to a surface (micro-carrier) during growth, further complicating scale-up. Creation of a certified cell line involves tracing the history of the specific specimen used to create the master seed, and extensive testing for adventitious agents, as well as testing the ability to support viral propagation.

Recombinant vaccines have been successfully launched to prevent a number of bacterial (Lyme) and viral (Hepatitis B) diseases. This approach to manufacturing has many benefits over traditional approaches. Rather than growing the organism that is responsible for the disease, one can grow a harmless substrate into which the gene for a protein antigen that elicits a protective response in people has been inserted.

Choice of the host organism can be bacteria (*E. coli* for Lyme), yeast (Hepatitis B), or even a mammalian cell line. With proper choice of the host cell, tremendous manufacturing capabilities can be realized. Avoiding the direct handling of a pathogenic organism at large scale is a key benefit. One can also produce a modified protein through manipulation of the gene sequence (e.g., non-toxic pertussis toxin). Multiple gene copies can be inserted to further increase productivity. Using this technique, vaccines of very high purity have been developed. By avoiding the many contaminating proteins one might get from using the native organism, the capability of characterizing the product is improved. This enhances product licensing.

The challenges that recombinant vaccines present are the need to eliminate the host cell contaminants in the purification process as well as stability of the genome and the host cell itself in preparation of master seeds. The possession of intellectual property for the genes of protective antigens also presents a significant hurdle when implementing this approach.

An example of the steps in modern vaccine manufacture is given in Table 11, which concerns inactivated influenza vaccine.

Current problems

Three major problems for the future of vaccine manufacture are safety, cost, and adequacy of supply. A risk-adverse society demands from regulatory authorities and industry more guarantees of safety, however illusory. There is less and less tolerance of reactions, real or supposed. Legal liability in developed countries extorts heavier financial burdens, and they are just as heavy for false claims as for real ones.

There are multiple factors contributing to vaccine cost. Elaborate safety tests in animals and more elaborate observations in phase 3 trials are the two major ones, and it is estimated that the cost of development of a single vaccine varies between $300 million and $800 million. The manufacturer must then recoup its costs in developed countries before time and competition turn the vaccine into a commodity. Developing countries must then wait until market forces drive the price down or a donor decides to buy the vaccine for their use.

One cannot be against increased safety of vaccines, but the effort to achieve it results in a reduction of the number of vaccines available, as there is only a limited amount of funds for vaccine development. The public demand for safety encourages greater regulatory demands, which then aug-

Table 11. Steps in the manufacture of influenza vaccine

Steps
Choice of strain
Preparation of attenuated reassortant
Preparation of seed virus
Acquisition of million of SPF eggs
Incubation for 11 days
Inoculation with monovalent virus (regulated time, temperature, humidity)
Sterile harvest
Clarify
Add formalin (regulated time, temperature)
Ultracentrifuge
Sucrose gradient purification
Dilution
Add detergent
Pool three strains
Test sterility, inactivation, potency endotoxin, protein, stabilizer, pH, salt concentration, animal safety
Sterile filling of vials

ment manufacturing costs, but which governments are unwilling to pay. Reduced profits discourage private investors from providing capital, which in turn results in less production, ultimately compromising public health.

Vaccine supply is inadequate because of the high costs of vaccine production facilities and also because of the limited number of manufacturers. Only the appearance of new manufacturers in developing countries, or alliances between manufacturers in developed and developing countries can solve this problem, which could become disastrous in the event of a pandemic of a new infectious disease.

Conclusion

The development and production of vaccines is a difficult process. Manufacturers must make difficult choices of how to spend limited resources. The process of development itself is fraught with failure, for biological entities do not obey the same invariable rules as chemical entities. Moreover, the process is a "delicate fabric" [6, 7] that could easily tear in the near future if more attention and resources are not invested in this activity. Nevertheless, the many successes of vaccines encourage manufacturers to continue to develop new ones.

References

1 Anonymous (2003) *Infectious diseases in children.* Slack Inc., Thorofare, NJ, August, 19

2 Mahoney RT, Pablos-Mendez A, Ramachandran S (2004) The introduction of

new vaccines into developing countries. III. The role of intellectual property. *Vaccine* 22: 786–792

3 Ellis RW (2001) Technologies for the design, discovery, formulation and administration of vaccines. *Vaccine* 19: 2681–2687

4 Plotkin SA (2003) Vaccines, vaccination, and vaccinology. *J Infect Dis* 187: 1349–1359

5 Plotkin SA (2005) Six revolutions in vaccinology. *Pediatric Inf Dis J* 24: 1–9

6 Marcuse EK (1998) United States vaccine research: a delicate fabric of public and private collaboration. *Pediatrics* 102: 1002–1003

7 Douglas RG (1996) Fostering partnerships for vaccine development: a delicate fabric. *Bull NY Acad Med* 73: 113–123

The Grand Challenge for the Future
ed. by Stefan H.E. Kaufmann and Paul-Henri Lambert

How can the industrial world help to implement new vaccines against poverty-related diseases?

Ole F. Olesen and Arnd Hoeveler

European Commission, Unit for Poverty-related Diseases, DG Research, European Commission, 1050 Brussels, Belgium

Introduction

Communicable diseases are both a consequence and a cause of poverty. The most disadvantaged in society are subject to more social risk factors for contracting infections such as HIV, TB and malaria. By destroying human capital, these diseases reduce the potential for economic growth and fuel a vicious cycle of poverty at the individual, national and regional level. Contrary to common belief, however, the majority of diseases affecting the developing countries can be effectively treated using existing medicines. The Essential Drugs List [1] from the World Health Organization (WHO) contains safe, effective treatments for the infectious and chronic diseases which affect the vast majority of the world's population. The excessive mortality rate of many infectious diseases in developing countries is, therefore, mainly caused by limited access to drugs, unavailability of health services and failure to use prevention strategies [2].

The greatest successes in combating infectious diseases in tropical countries have all been vaccine-driven. Vaccination has resulted in the eradication of smallpox, the imminent eradication of polio, and a dramatic reduction in the prevalence of many other infectious diseases. Given the poor infrastructure and incomplete health-care systems in many developing countries, vaccines are, in fact, often the only pharmaceutical product that can make a substantial impact on public health.

There are, however, still a number of major infectious diseases for which an effective vaccine does not exist. The number of people affected by, infected with and dying from HIV/AIDS, TB and malaria continues to rise, and these diseases continue to evade immunisation efforts. In 2003, almost 3 million people died of AIDS, and there were about 5 million new HIV infections [3]. TB kills about 2 million people every year [4], whilst malaria kills more than one million people annually. New vaccines to combat these poverty-related diseases (PRD) are therefore urgently needed.

The political mandate

The genomic revolution of recent years has provided some tremendous advances in molecular biology and scientists of today are better equipped than ever to design effective vaccines. With recombinant technologies and production methods, vaccines can, in principle, be designed to be safer, more potent and even cheaper than traditional vaccines. Development of vaccines for many tropical diseases has nevertheless proven to be particularly challenging, as exemplified by HIV/AIDS and malaria. There are still major scientific hurdles to overcome before many communicable diseases can be efficiently tackled; this will need ample financial resources as well as leadership and determination among all the stakeholders.

The governments of G8 countries have on several occasions acknowledged the importance of increasing R&D investment in new vaccines to fight communicable diseases in the developing world. The Evian Communiqué of 2003 urged member governments to increase incentives, as well as to establish suitable regulatory capacity and support for ethical clinical trials. The Sea Island Communiqué issued in June 2004 specifically called for expanded involvement of both the private and public sectors in AIDS vaccine development. In addition, the World Bank as well as the US, French and UK governments have all been active in advocating increased spending and incentives. President Clinton announced in 1997 that finding an HIV vaccine within ten years was a national goal for the USA. In 2001, the US National Institute of Allergy and Infectious Diseases (NIAID) published a Global Health Research Plan for HIV/AIDS, Malaria, and Tuberculosis. The plan identified vaccine research as an important priority, and outlined the Institute's plans for fighting infectious diseases by building sustained research capability domestically and internationally and enhancing international partnerships. Within the European Union (EU), a strong commitment to combat PRD was provided in the "Programme for Action on HIV/AIDS, malaria and TB" [5], which promised a multi-sectorial approach to increase the affordability, accessibility and availability of new interventions for PRD. This massive support has resulted in renewed interest for vaccine research by the public sector, and vaccine development is now supported through specific programmes of the European Commission (EC), the U.S. government, the Australian government, and the WHO.

Public sector failure

The public sector harbours a significant pool of knowledge and experience in vaccinology, but resources are often uncoordinated and used ineffectively due to structural problems. Immunological research is a key discipline at all medical universities, and many countries have one or more specialised institutions that are dedicated to research in immunology, epidemiology or communicable disease control. Most of these are fully or predominantly publicly funded, while others, including such prominent institutions as the Pasteur Institute in Paris, are non-profit private institutions that operate on similar principles as public research centres. With few exceptions, however, the public sector is characterised by national priorities and human resources that are too scattered to make a significant impact.

Many of the institutions were established and developed to improve and protect the public health situation in their home country. Their main objective was to address the national research and health agenda, and they did so successfully in most of the 20th century.

Increased human migration means that threats to public health are increasingly found outside national borders, and many institutions will need to revise their objectives towards achieving a global health agenda. At the same time, the increased complexity of the pharmaceutical development process means that public institutions can no longer provide the critical mass to undertake a vaccine development programme on their own. The ability of the public sector to develop new vaccines has consequently been slowly eroded during the last 2–3 decades.

Reinventing translational research

Europe has historically had a dominant role in vaccine research ever since the BCG vaccine was discovered at the Pasteur Institute in Lille in 1921. Europe has the largest vaccine production in the world, and constitutes the largest single vaccine market. Europe is also the main vaccine producer for developing countries, supplying nearly 70% of their vaccines. Europe should therefore have a strong scientific and moral impetus to spearhead the development of new vaccines for PRD.

From 1998 to 2002, the European Commission provided funding to a broad range of PRD research activities through the 5th Framework Programme for research (FP5). A total of 77 collaborative research projects were supported with 109 M Euro. More than 60 M Euro (corresponding to 55% of the total budget) was allocated specifically to vaccine research, confirming the renewed focus on this field in combating PRD.

A major achievement during the course of FP5 was the creation of a common "European Research Area" concept for interventions against PRD. Previously small, fragmented efforts by individual research teams became part of a dense network of numerous trans-national collaborations. The projects in FP5 thus involved more than 500 research groups, representing 21 European countries as well as 40 countries outside Europe.

The integration of European research continues in the 6th Framework Programme (FP6, 2002–2006), which also represents a substantial increase in public funding. Compared to FP5, the indicative budget for PRD in FP6 is nearly 4 times higher, amounting to a total of 400 M Euro, much of which

Table 1: Europe's current portfolio of large integrated projects for PRD vaccine development. The European Commission presently supports three large-scale research consortia on translational research of new vaccine candidates for PRD, namely MUCVAPRED (Mucosal Vaccines for Poverty Related Diseases), TBVAC (Tuberculosis Vaccine Development) and AVIP (AIDS Vaccine Integrated Project). Additional project consortia are planned for development of HIV/AIDS and malaria vaccine candidates.

	MUVAPRED	TBVAC	AVIP
Disease focus	HIV/AIDS, TB	TB	HIV/AIDS
Total budget	€ 18 M	€ 21 M	€ 15 M
EU contribution	€ 15 M	€ 17 M	€ 10 M
No of participating research groups	24	30	15

will go to research on vaccines. FP6 includes two new instruments that will be used to further integrate European vaccine research in PRD: the discovery and development of new vaccine candidates are supported through Integrated Projects (IP), whereas clinical trials of promising candidate vaccines will be supported through the European and Developing Countries Clinical Trials Partnership (EDCTP).

IPs are organised as large-scale collaborative projects, which should bring together a critical mass of partners, private as well as public, to undertake "translational" research. Project consortia must have the capacity to develop new vaccine candidates from the bench into products that can be tested on humans. Two years after the launch of FP6, 3 such vaccine consortia have been launched with financial support from the European Commission (Tab. 1) while another 2 consortia are planned. All consortia have established genuine partnerships between academic scientists, industrial vaccinologists and research teams from disease-endemic countries. The aim is to create synergy between academic expertise and the applied research of the pharmaceutical industry, thereby strengthening the translational vaccine research. The challenge ahead for European vaccine research will be to align the IPs into a single pipeline with a balanced and broad portfolio of new vaccine candidates, ranging from early discovery to clinical trials.

The EDCTP is an ambitious attempt to integrate the national programmes of 15 European countries in the area of clinical trials for PRD. It aims at establishing harmonised approaches and joint implementation of clinical activities among the participating countries. The EDCTP was established in autumn 2003, and has a target budget of 600 M Euro for its first 4 years of operation. The European Commission has allocated 200 M Euro to this initiative, while another 200 M Euro come from the 15 participating European countries. The remaining 200 M Euro will be sought from private sources, the R&D industry, foundations, charities and development funds. The EDCTP will fund phase II and III clinical trials from both the private and public sectors, including industry, non-profit organisations and individuals from Europe, developing countries and elsewhere. A further aim of the

EDCTP is to support capacity-building at clinical sites in Africa, thereby creating a long-term research partnership between developed and developing countries in the fight against PRD.

Market failure

The incompleteness of the public sector, as mentioned above, is aggravated by an evident research gap in PRD in the private sector. The routine use of vaccines saves millions of lives every year, but the economic value associated with them is negligible in comparison with the total pharmaceutical market. In most countries, vaccines are distributed by the public sector and once a pharmaceutical company has developed a new vaccine, governments will often use their powers as regulators and dominant purchasers to keep prices low. In spite of a very large sales volume, the world-wide annual turnover of vaccines therefore only constitutes approximately 2% of the total pharmaceutical market.

In today's pharmaceutical market, candidate products must have a high potential return-of-investment as well as a manageable risk profile. New development projects are therefore selected in strong inter- and intra-company competition. This will often eliminate vaccines, which generally have a low price level combined with relatively high manufacturing costs. Many pharmaceutical manufacturers have therefore replaced their vaccine research by drug development projects, and the number of vaccine companies in Europe and the US has steadily declined during the last 30 years. This situation is particularly pronounced for new vaccines aimed at PRD. During the last decade, vaccine shortage has thus become a serious problem affecting even developed countries.

Two recent studies concluded that the cost of developing a new pharmaceutical product is around US$ 800 million [6]. This figure includes the costs of failure and opportunity cost of capital in developed countries, but controversy surrounds the actual cost of developing a new vaccine for use in developing countries. The costs may be relatively low according to studies by International AIDS Vaccine Initiative (IAVI) and the global alliance for TB drug development [7], while others have argued that development of new vaccines could be difficult and costly if clinical testing were to be carried out locally in low-income countries with poor infrastructure and no, or insufficient, capacity for undertaking clinical trials.

In high-income countries, effective intellectual property protection enables inventors to recoup R&D investments by ensuring a limited period of exclusive marketing rights for a new product. The combination of a market with sufficient purchasing power and enforced intellectual property rights is therefore the basis for generating profit from private investments in pharmaceutical R&D. In this equation, vaccines for poor countries are obviously less profitable for the innovating company than would be drugs destined for developed countries. Weak intellectual property protection in many parts of the developing world may further discourage private enterprises from focusing on PRD. The traditional business model for R&D investment is therefore challenged by the economic reality in developing countries, where a true domestic market for pharmaceutical products is either non-existent or at best unpredictable. Local financing for vaccines or medicines has been largely unavailable while external funding and donations have been random and unsustainable.

A number of non-economic factors may encourage a pharmaceutical company to pursue a PRD vaccine project. Most important would be the desire to demonstrate corporate social responsibility, but a new vaccine programme could also be part of a company's internal research capacity-building, or its strategy to expand its product range or geographical market. Private investment in PRD vaccine research has nevertheless remained negligible in recent years, and this situation is unlikely to change unless new motivating factors appear.

Accelerating clinical testing

The majority of R&D costs for new drugs and vaccines can be attributed to late-stage clinical trials. This is particularly true for new prophylactic vaccines that may have relatively low costs in the preclinical stages, but require very large clinical trials involving thousands of individuals. The cost of clinical development is also influenced by the dynamics of the target disease. For diseases such as HIV/AIDS and TB, several years of clinical trials in very large cohorts are necessary before a new vaccine can be released. Clinical trials of such an extensive nature consume huge resources and costs can be highly prohibitive for an otherwise cost-efficient R&D project.

A number of countries provide grants for clinical trials of new vaccines through their national research programmes. National institutions supporting clinical vaccine research include the US National Institute of Health (NIH), the French Agence Nationale de Recherche sur le SIDA (ANRS), and the U.K.'s Medical Research Council (MRC), but none of these initiatives have so far established a mechanism to provide sustainable support for full clinical programmes.

Some countries have further introduced special tax incentives to encourage private vaccine research in specific disease areas. In 2003, the UK government enacted the Vaccine Research Relief tax incentive for research and development related to AIDS, TB and malaria. In the US, tax credits are granted for costs derived from clinical testing of pharmaceuticals with orphan drug status, which would also include PRD vaccines.

Public-private partnerships (PPP) have recently become the most popular set-up for financial risk-sharing of R&D costs in the field of PRD (Tab. 2). Most of these ventures are established as separate legal entities

Table 2. Major product development public-private partnerships that are actively engaged in development of vaccines for PRD. Information about total funding originates mainly from the database of the Initiative for Public Private Partnerships for Health (www.ippph.org), while information about principal financial donors mainly originates from the websites of the respective PPPs. Public sector donors are indicated by country of origin or name of international organisation.

Disease focus	HIV/AIDS		Malaria		TB	HIV/AIDS, Malaria, TB
Public-Private Partnership (PPP)	International AIDS Vaccine Initiative (IAVI)	South African AIDS Vaccine Initiative (SAAVI)	European Malaria Vaccine Initiative (EMVI)	Malaria Vaccine Initiative (MVI)	AEREAS	European Developing Countries Clinical Trials Partnership (EDCTP)
Total funding	> 270 M US$	> 25 M US$	N/A	> 150 M US$	> 100 M US$	400 M Eur
Established	1996	1999	1998	1999	1997	2003
Major private charity donors	B&M Gates, Crusaid, Elton John, JM. Lloyd Mercury-Phoenix, MacArthur, Pendleton, Perls, Rockefeller, Sloan, Starr, Vanderbilt			B&M Gates, Rockefeller	B&M Gates	
Public sector donors	CA, DK, EU, GB, IE, NL, NO, SE, UNAIDS, US World Bank	EU, US, ZA	DK, EU, IE, NL, NO, SE		US	AT, BE, DE, DK, EU, ES, FR, GR, IE, IT, LU, NL, NO, PT, SE, UK
Pharma and healthcare industry	Becton, Dickinson & Company, GlaxoSmith Kline					
Other industry	Angel Music Ltd, DHL, MSN, Real-Networks, Yahoo, Viacom	Eskom, Implats, Transnet				

with relatively lean organisations, and with an objective to bridge the gap between preclinical research and early clinical trials. The PPPs involve collaboration between industry, academic institutes, and researchers in disease-endemic countries to develop new products for PRD. They operate by extensive outsourcing, which gives them the flexibility to quickly adapt to new circumstances, while their status as separate entities give them the freedom to attract funding from different sources. Roughly US$ 2 billion have been collected by drug and vaccine PPPs in the last 5 years, but additional financing required through 2007 is estimated to exceed US$ 1 billion [8].

Most of the vaccine PPPs focus their interest on a single disease, and the most mature of these ventures have built up sizeable portfolios of vaccine candidates that are entering the clinical testing stage. However, none of the PPPs have yet been able to bring a product to market, and the lack of success may be partly attributed to a limited involvement of industry. When the first PPPs were launched, it was generally expected that industry would contribute with active participation and direct funding, but this has only happened to a limited extent.

The vast majority of funding has so far come from philanthropic organisations such as the Bill and Melinda Gates Foundation or the Rockefeller Foundation, which is a pioneer in this area. European governments and the USA are the second largest group of donors, while multilateral donors such as the EU, UN and the World Bank have provided relatively small amounts. Industry have mainly contributed with "in-kind" donations such as staff, technical know-how and access to testing facilities.

Compared to the disease-specific PPPs mentioned above, the EDCTP initiative has a broader scope, as it addresses all of the three major PRDs. The EDCTP is unique in having started as a purely publicly funded initiative (PFI), although the active participation of private stakeholders is encouraged. The EDCTP is also unique in focusing on late-stage clinical trials, where the need for both financial and structural support becomes evident. An important aspect of the EDCTP is therefore to support capacity-building at clinical sites in Africa, thereby creating a research partnership between developed and developing countries that can accelerate the clinical testing of new disease interventions.

Given adequate coordination, the disease-specific PPPs and the EDCTP may effectively interact to support the full clinical development of new vaccine candidates (Fig. 1). With sufficient financial backing, PPPs could fill a crucial gap in the development pipeline by moving promising new vaccines from preclinical through early clinical phases. The EDCTP may then provide support through late-stage clinical trials and up to the regulatory phase.

Jumping the regulatory hurdles

Before a new pharmaceutical product can reach the market, it needs to be

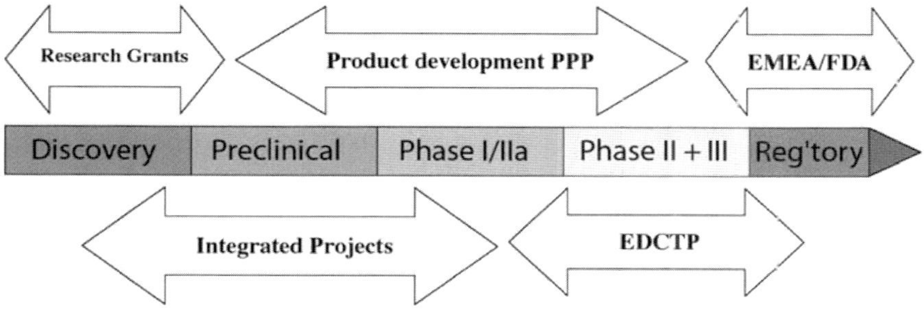

Figure 1. Simplified overview of the different steps for developing a new vaccine, and indication where existing support mechanisms have their primary intervention.

examined and approved by the relevant regulatory authorities. Provisions to facilitate the regulatory process exist in many countries for rare or orphan diseases. In 1983, the US Congress introduced the Orphan Drug Act for diseases affecting fewer than 200,000 persons in the United States. Vaccines for PRD would therefore technically fulfil the US orphan definition. Incentives include a 50% deduction tax credit for clinical trial expenses, formal protocol assistance and a market exclusivity of seven years. More than 200 orphan products have already been brought to market under the Orphan Drug Act [9]. As of 2000, however, only 8 candidate vaccines had been designated to have orphan status, and none of these had reached the market. The same is true for the EU, where an orphan drug regulation was introduced in 2000 with 10 years market exclusivity as the most important element. The US and EU experiences show that existing orphan regulations fail to stimulate vaccine development for PRD, mainly because market exclusivity in the US and/or EU is virtually irrelevant for PRD products. Vaccines for developing countries could thus be defined as "economically orphan" due to small markets rather than prevalence or burden of disease, and special incentives should be considered to facilitate their regulatory approval.

Using existing flexibility to reduce regulatory barriers to innovation is of current interest for the European Medicines Agency (EMEA), the US Food and Drug Administration (FDA) and a number of national authorities, and this possibility should be fully exploited to push the approval of new vaccines. A specific regulation for economically orphan products could introduce a number of additional facilities, including fast-track procedures, waiving of registration fees, scientific advice to develop medicines for resource-poor settings, and advice leading to Good Manufacturing Practice (GMP) and Good Clinical Practice (GCP) certification. Regulatory agencies could also assist with protocols for clinical trials and compilation of the regulatory dossier from an early stage. This may further be combined with special provisions for granting extended marketing exclusivity beyond the expiry of standard intellectual property rights.

The regulatory process in developing countries should also be facilitated. An important step could be to replace the individual national approvals of new products in developing countries with regional procedures of a type similar to those of EMEA in Europe. The recent revision of the EU pharmaceutical legislation enabled the EMEA to give a scientific opinion for the evaluation of medicines to be marketed outside the EU [10]. This procedure allows EMEA to review new products intended exclusively for use in developing countries. This could be the first step towards establishing regional approval procedures in parts of the world other than Europe, with support and guidance from EMEA.

New incentives to encourage R&D investments

Reduced regulatory requirements can surely save development costs and speed up approvals, but additional and innovative incentives will be necessary to boost private investments in PRD vaccines (Tab. 3). Incentives to encourage the development of new products can be broadly divided into push mechanisms, which finance research input, or pull mechanisms, which reward innovators for actually bringing a new product to the market. As summarised above, several ambitious push mechanisms have been established in recent years to predominantly support vaccine research within the public sector, but the vaccine manufacturers have often stated that the most attractive incentives for them are pull mechanisms.

Purchase funds

The optimal pull mechanism would be the creation of a stable, sustainable market for vaccines in the least developed countries. This cannot be realised in the short or medium term unless the developed countries finance it through purchase mechanisms established by public organisations or private charities. The Vaccine Fund under the Global Alliance for Vaccines & Immunization (GAVI) and The Global Fund to fight AIDS, TB and malaria (GFATM) are reflections of this idea, but the historic underfunding of purchase funds, the unpredictability of support from developed countries and the tendency to purchase existing rather than future products has so far made this option ineffective as an R&D incentive. To act with full impact, funding would have to be dedicated to new products rather than existing ones, and an appropriate legal framework as well as a credible and long-term funding mechanism would have to be secured. One way to structure a scheme for advance purchase of vaccines would be that potential sponsors such as governments, international organisations or private charity foundations make a legally binding commitment to pay a guaranteed price for a specified number of doses of a new vaccine with defined characteristics. If a commitment failed to produce an effective vaccine, no donor funds would be spent, making this a potentially cost-effective mechanism to stimulate R&D on vaccines. Given the complexity of vaccine development, purchase funds would nevertheless have to be very large to serve as a real incentive for private R&D investments. A recent study by Kremer and Glennerster [11] concluded that an advance purchase system could work with a guaranteed price of US$ 15–20 per treatment for the first 200 million individuals vaccinated, and the rest of the vaccine supply being priced at a modest mark-up over manufacturing cost. In the foreseeable future, it appears unlikely that potential sponsors will be prepared to make firm, legally binding promises to such financial commitments that amount to more than US$ 3 bn. Even if it happens, the individual vaccine developer will have to be convinced that funders or their successors will not try to avoid such commitments when they arise, given the huge rewards at stake and any potentially conflicting interests between sponsors and vaccine companies.

Transferable exclusivity rights

The possibility of transferring exclusivity or special privileges from one product to another can potentially be a very powerful incentive. Transferable market exclusivity covers the principle of granting extended market exclusivity for a pharmaceutical product in Europe and/or the US, as a reward for developing a new (but entirely different) vaccine for treatment of PRD. In exchange for such exclusive benefits, it would be reasonable to require that the company should also commit to produce and sell the PRD vaccine at a low price in developing countries. The prospect of extending the market exclusivity of a highly profitable, yet unrelated pharmaceutical product could create a strong incentive for vaccine development, but it may stimulate R&D at a high and unevenly distributed cost. The annual sales of a pharmaceutical blockbuster product is around 250 million Euro in Europe (more in the US), and the buyers of such pharmaceutical products would carry the entire burden of financing new vaccines for PRD. Most health-care expenditure in Europe is funded through public health insurance or welfare schemes, but health-care budget deficits are widening in many countries and extensions of marketing exclusivity will therefore be seen as an unwelcome increase in drug-related costs.

To make the incentive attractive to smaller companies without "blockbuster products" that could receive the extended exclusivity rights, such rights would have to be tradable between companies (e.g., though auctioning). An additional problem relates to the impact of new vaccines and how to evaluate them. Should all new vaccines elicit the same exclusivity extension or should the length of extension be related to the efficacy, safety, manufacturing costs, etc.? If a special committee or agency is supposed to rule on such matters, it will be an essential but difficult task to establish its credibility and independence. Given the large financial rewards at stake, the committee should be detached from stakeholders in both the private and public sector.

A more manageable and less controversial system could be envisaged by limiting the transferable privileges to a fast-track regulatory procedure. In such a scheme, development of a PRD vaccine would elicit a right to process another, unrelated product through a fast-track regulatory approval. The other product, which could be a potential blockbuster, may thus reach the market earlier than expected. This would enable a company to generate profit sooner and for a longer period. In a highly competitive situation, it could also equip the innovating company with a "first-on-the-market" advantage. If the gain in market time is sufficiently high, such a scheme could be attractive as an incentive and at the same time manageable through the existing regulatory procedures. Fast-track provisions already exist in both the US and EU pharmaceutical legislation, and flexible use of these mechanisms could allow the introduction of a transferable fast-track privilege system without the need to pass new legislation.

Cash premiums

Cash premiums can be seen as a simple mechanism to reward research results in PRD vaccinology, either on its own or in combination with other incentives. Once a new vaccine has reached the market, the cash premium would be awarded to the innovating company. The risk of development would be borne entirely by the industry, but a predefined reward would be paid out in case of success. On a stand-alone basis, the premium for developing a new vaccine would have to be substantial and probably be at least equal to the average development costs of a new vaccine. The actual size of the premium could also be made dependent on the therapeutic potential of the new product. In its most elaborate version, cash premiums thus share many similarities with advance purchase commitments, including many of the same weaknesses. However, cash premiums could also be set up in a simplified version as an international award that would elicit a substantial financial reward to the innovating company as well as prestige and world-wide recognition to the scientists involved. The financing of such an award can be envisaged through different mechanisms, either directly by the public sector through tax revenues, by private sponsors or charity foundations. Part of the reward money could also be accumulated from regula-

Table 3. A comprehensive summary of existing (marked with *) and proposed incentives. Incentives are grouped according to their phase of intervention in relation to the vaccine development pipeline

Basic research & discovery - Publicly funded R&D* – e.g., core research at public universities and research institutions - Research grants* – financial support to specific research projects from public, private or charity sources.
Early development/translational research - Large-scale collaborative projects* – e.g., EC-supported integrated projects - Public-private partnerships* – e.g., disease-specific PPPs with focus on translational research - Offsetting taxation against R&D expenditure* – e.g., UK regulation
Clinical development - Publicly funded initiatives for late stage clinical trial* – e.g., EDCTP - Government indemnification of damages caused by side-effects (e.g., for vaccines) - Clinical trial protocol support – simplified clinical requirements - Low-cost loans for clinical trials and establishment of manufacturing facilities
Regulatory - Existing orphan drug procedures* – e.g., the orphan drug regulations of FDA and EMEA - Special regulatory processing for economically orphan products – e.g., including fast-track procedures, waiving of registration fees, scientific advice to develop medicines for resource-poor settings, and advice leading to GMP/GCP certification. - Regulatory review by EMEA of products for use in developing countries*
Market related - Increased market exclusivity for economically orphan products – e.g., as in the orphan drug provisions - International IPR extensions – longer IP for relevant new products - Transferable market exclusivity as reward for developing a new PRD vaccine - Transferable fast track as reward for developing a new PRD vaccine - Advance commitments to purchase new vaccines - Cash premiums - International Awards – worldwide recognition - Tax credits for sales or donations to developing countries* – e.g., the US regulation

tory fees paid by the pharmaceutical industry for approval of pharmaceutical products for the developed part of the world. Interestingly, this type of risk-reward model seems to be working for another high-risk, high-cost programme, namely the commercial space travel enterprise (the X-Prize foundation will reward a cash prize of 10 M USD to the first team that privately finance, build and launch a spaceship that can carry 3 people into space.).

A global research policy for PRD is needed

In recent years a substantial increase in resources has become available to combat PRD in developing countries. This is most noticeable in the case of

Table 4. The average annual EC financial contribution to fight HIV/AIDS, malaria and tuberculosis in developing countries in the period 2003–2006 compared to 1994–2002 (in million Euro). Total and research contributions are indicated.

	HIV/AIDS		Malaria		TB		Total		Annual average	
	1994–2002	2003–2006	1994–2002	2003–2006	1994–2002	2003–2006	1994–2002	2003–2006	1994–2002	2003–2006
R&D	93,1	200,0	55,4	100,0	59,2	100,0	207,7	400,0	23,1	100,0
Total	494,2	674,5	159,4	264,0	77,2	216,5	730,8	1178,0	81,2	294,5

HIV/AIDS, where the official development assistance to fight HIV/AIDS increased by 15-fold – from US$300 million in 1996 to almost US$5 billion in 2003. The intensified fight against PRD has been accompanied by an even steeper mobilisation of public and private funds for research projects, including vaccine-oriented development. Within the European Union, the EC has increased its contribution to PRD research almost 5-fold since 2002, while the overall contribution to combat PRD increased less than 4-fold (Tab. 4). The improved funding for vaccine research has also been accompanied by improved research structures for preclinical vaccine development, as exemplified by the large-scale IPs that have been formed across Europe.

It is noteworthy that large financial contributions to vaccine research in the public sector is increasingly coming from private non-profit organisations such as the Wellcome Trust, the Rockefeller Foundation and in particular the Bill and Melinda Gates Foundation, which has donated over US$1 billion to research, development and distribution of vaccines since it was established in 2000. The global increase in funding for PRD has made it possible to launch a number of new initiatives that can support vaccine development. Each of these initiatives may play an important role by filling different niches of the vaccine development process. This could provide an important momentum to the translational research, which is necessary to move any new vaccine candidates from discovery to early stages of clinical testing. The challenge ahead will be to integrate the many initiatives correctly, so they supplement each other rather than duplicate or compete for the same resources. A global approach is therefore needed, and stakeholders at all levels, industry and the public sector, developed and developing countries must coordinate their efforts. Global health should be made a national priority in developed countries and development of new vaccines should be supported according to their global public health values. Developing countries, for their part, should engage more actively in the R&D process as part of their national research and health agendas. Governments in developing countries must acknowledge the value of research as a long-term solution to public health problems. Developed and developing countries should work together on lowering regulatory entry barriers for new vaccines.

The failures of both the private and public sector must be remedied to stimulate research in new vaccines against PRD. This will require sufficient funding, but will also require the creation of a suitable international framework, where private and public stakeholders are mutually motivated to develop new vaccines. In the area of HIV/AIDS, the recently launched Global HIV Vaccine Enterprise (GVE) is attempting to catalyse this process. The GVE is a virtual consortium to accelerate HIV vaccine development by enhancing coordination, information sharing, and collaboration globally. The concept was originally proposed by an international group of scientists [12] and took inspiration from the successful alliance and strategic plan that characterized the human genome project. The GVE was endorsed by G-8 governments at the Sea Island summit in June 2004, and was asked to develop a strategic plan for coordination of global vaccine development efforts and alignment of existing and new resources for this purpose.

On the political level, national policy-makers and health authorities in both developed and developing countries should therefore increasingly consolidate and coordinate their research priorities towards the global health needs. In this context, federal or transnational institutions like the WHO, European Commission, NIH and Japan's National Institute of Infectious Diseases (NIID) can play key roles by setting priorities, deliver organisational leadership and distribute funding. At the same time, new and more powerful incentives will have to be introduced to stimulate private investment in PRD vaccine research. Predictability and long-term commitment from the public sector in rich as well as poor countries are necessary to translate PRD research into new vaccines with societal value for disease-endemic countries. With sufficient funding and commitment from all stakeholders, the existing roadblocks for developing new effective vaccines can eventually be removed.

Acknowledgements

We would like to thank Dr. Timothy Hall for valuable comments and input to this paper, and to Evelyne Bastin and Peter Levy for preparing and typing the manuscript.

References

1 The World Health Organization Model List of Essential Medicines (revised April 2003), available on: www.who.int/medicines/rationale

2 WHO (1999) Removing obstacles to healthy development: World Health Organization report on infectious disease

3 Steinbrook R (2004) The AIDS Epidemic in 2004. *N Engl J Med* 351: 2
4 WHO Fact Sheet N°104 (Revised March 2004) "Basic Facts on TB"
5 Communication from the European Commission to the Council and the European Parliament (2001) Programme for Action: Accelerated action on HIV/AIDS, malaria and tuberculosis in the context of poverty reduction. *COM* 96.
6 DiMasi J, Hansen RW, Grabowski HG (2003) The price of innovation: new estimates of drug development costs. *J Health Econ* 22: 151–185
7 Global Alliance for TB drug development (2001) *The Economics of TB Drug Development*. New York
8 Estimate by the Initiative for Public Private Partnerships for Health (IPPPH): www.ippph.org
9 US Food and Drug Administration, Office of Orphan Products Development. www.fda.gov/orphan/
10 Regulation (EC) No 726/2004 of the European Parliament and of the Council (31 March 2004), Article 58, OJ L 136, 30.4.2004, p. 1
11 Kremer M, Glennerster R (2004) *Strong medicine: Creating incentives for Pharmaceutical Research on Neglected Diseases*. Princeton University Press, pp 86–96
12 Klausner RD, Fauci AS, Corey L, Nabel GJ, Gayle H, Berkley S, Haynes BF, Baltimore D, Collins C, Douglas RG et al (2003) The need for a global HIV vaccine enterprise. *Science* 300: 2036–2039

Public-private partnerships

The Grand Challenge for the Future
ed. by Stefan H.E. Kaufmann and Paul-Henri Lambert

New approaches towards development, production and use of developing-country market vaccines in developing countries

Luis Jodar and John D. Clemens

International Vaccine Institute, SNU Research Park, San 4-8 Bongcheon-7-dong, Kwanak-gu, Seoul, Korea 151-818

Background

Inequity in access to existing and newly licensed vaccines has increased over the past two decades as new vaccines have become available at prices that most low-income countries are unable to afford. From the time of introduction of a new vaccine in Europe or the US, it usually takes a decade or more for the adoption of these vaccines in developing countries. For example, *Haemophilus influenzae* type b (Hib) conjugate vaccine has been used routinely in North America, most European countries and some Latin American countries for more than a decade with dramatic reduction of disease incidence [1–3]. Although this vaccine has also been demonstrated to be highly effective in preventing disease in developing countries, with few exceptions vaccine uptake in these countries has been slow [4]. Several factors have contributed to the slow introduction of these vaccines in the developing world. In many countries, policymakers may still have uncertainties about whether an adequate case can be made for introducing the vaccine into real-life public health programs in their countries. This is because they either have insufficient data on the local disease burden, the evidence provided by pre-licensure evaluations fails to address many of the practical questions about implementing a new vaccine in real-life programs, or they lack the capacity and infrastructure to deliver these vaccines [5]. However, the principal obstacle to introducing new vaccines has been their cost [6]. When Hib conjugate vaccines were first marketed, their prices were affordable only in industrialized countries. As manufacturing production capacity increased and competing products entered the marketplace, prices gradually declined. Eventually, prices became tiered, with sales of vaccine in developing countries set at a lower price than those in developed countries [4, 7, 8]. However, even with tiered pricing, these vaccines were still unaffordable for the majority of the poorest countries in the world [4] . The failure to introduce these vaccines in countries with a GDP/*capita* below $1,000 is particularly notable. More recently, a 7-valent pneumococcal conjugate vaccine was licensed in the United States [9]. However, this vaccine is selling at a price of over US$50 per dose, which obviously restricts its use to affluent countries. Hib and pneumococcal diseases were important causes of disease in industrialized as well as developing countries. The pharmaceutical industry, therefore, was highly motivated to invest large sums of money in the development and licensure of these vaccines because of the high return on investment they could expect from sales of a high-priced vaccine in industrialized countries.

The recent availability of increased funding from international donors such as the Bill and Melinda Gates Foundation and the inception of the Global Alliance for Vaccines and Immunization (GAVI) and the Vaccine Fund [10] have opened new opportunities for the expanded use of Hib vaccines and the accelerated introduction of pneumococcal vaccines in developing countries. However, it is yet to be seen whether these funds will be enough to substantially accelerate the introduction of these vaccines, increase the limited capacity that currently exists for some of these vaccines in established vaccine manufacturers, and ensure their sustainable use in the poorest countries where the disease burden is highest [11].

In contrast with the examples above, there are a number of diseases that affect almost exclusively developing-country populations and pose little if any risk for individuals in industrialized countries unless they travel to disease-endemic areas. Historically, vaccines developed against these diseases have been termed “orphan” or “developing-market” vaccines [12, 13]. In the remainder of this paper the term “developing-market” vaccines will be used.

In general, the private sector has little financial incentive to produce developing-market vaccines since the returns on the investment needed for research and development, manufacturing capacity, conducting clinical trials and other activities needed for vaccine licensure are low, and these projects almost certainly compete with other high-value projects.

Developing-market vaccines can broadly be divided in two major groups. The first group consists of those vaccines against diseases prevalent in the developing world for which major R&D gaps still exist. Vaccines against dengue fever, malaria and TB belong to this group. For each of these diseases, science is a limiting factor for the development of effective vaccines. A combination of dearth of information about the pathogenesis of these diseases, technical hurdles, complex intellectual property rights and unattractive market potential has long made vaccine manufacturers very reluctant to invest large sums in R&D against these diseases. Only recently there appears to be glimpses of hope. The Bill and Melinda Gates Foundation has launched new programs focusing on the development and testing of new vaccine candidates against dengue, TB and malaria, through the Pediatric Dengue Vaccine Initiative at the International Vaccine

Institute, the Aeras Global Tuberculosis Foundation and the Malaria Vaccine Initiative at the Program for Appropriate Technology for Health (PATH) [14, 15]. These programs operate primarily through partnerships with academia, government, and biotech and pharmaceutical companies and aim at overcoming technical and financial hurdles to the development and clinical testing of promising vaccine candidates. They are also addressing potential barriers to eventual dengue, malaria and TB vaccine introduction, including market-related, intellectual property, and financing issues. While some programmatic, economic or ethical issues may be extrapolated from one disease to another, most of the scientific and technical barriers are disease-specific, and therefore would require a single chapter devoted to each of them.

There is a second group of developing-market vaccines that comprises diseases that constitute a major public health problem in developing countries, for which the technology for the development of effective vaccines already exists, but that are not developed by large vaccine manufacturers due to the lack of market opportunities. Bacterial enteric diseases (typhoid and paratyphoid fever, shigellosis, pathogenic *E. coli* and cholera), which kill around 2 million children per year, belong to this group. Even for vaccines that are of interest to populations in industrialized and less-developed countries alike, such as Hib, meningococcal or pneumococcal diseases, the situation is further complicated by the fact that for these vaccines, the industrialized and developing-country vaccine markets are diverging and differentiating. Factors including epidemiological variations by geographic region (circulating serotypes, carriage, co-infections), differences in cost-benefit ratios, characteristics of preferred formulations because of production and cold chain capacity may result in the development of vaccines that although suitable for industrialized countries might not be the most appropriate for developing-country populations. For example, certain formulations of pneumococcal conjugate vaccines may cover only serotypes prevalent in industrialized countries [16] and monodose thiomersal-free meningococcal vaccines may not be the most appropriate for mass immunization campaigns in the African meningitis belt [17].

For all of these pathogens, surface polysaccharides, in the form of capsule or lipopolysaccharide, are both essential virulence factors and protective antigens. Serum antibody to the surface polysaccharide confers protection against disease by activating complement-mediated bacteriolysis and/or opsonization. Parenteral polysaccharide vaccines against these diseases are safe and elicit protective serum IgG capsular antibody responses in adults or children older than 2 years of age, but are generally not immunogenic in younger children and infants. Because purified capsular polysaccharide acts like a T-lymphocyte-independent antigen, the serum antibody response cannot be readily boosted by administration of additional doses of the polysaccharide and do not induce immunological memory [18–22].

Glycoconjugate vaccines obtained by coupling these pathogens' polysaccharides with a carrier protein can overcome the limitations of existing polysaccharide vaccines against this group of developing-market diseases. However, Big Pharma is not likely to make a large investment in these vaccines for markets that are very unattractive. Thus, in order to guarantee a sustainable supply of these vaccines at affordable prices to programs for the poor in developing countries, alternative models for the development and large-scale production of conjugate vaccines need to be envisaged.

The remainder of this chapter aims at 1) demonstrating that conjugate vaccines are an essential platform technology for developing-market vaccines; 2) establishing the rational basis for the production of conjugate vaccines by a number of qualified local producers; 3) discussing the different models for transferring this technology to local producers for the accelerated introduction into and use of these vaccines by public health programs of developing countries.

Polysaccharide-protein conjugate vaccines are an important platform technology for developing-market vaccines against enteric and encapsulated respiratory bacteria

Polysaccharide-protein conjugate vaccines elicit immunological responses in infants and children

The development of polysaccharide-conjugate technology has been one of the most important developments in vaccinology and has allowed the production of several important vaccines such as those against Hib, meningococcal and pneumococcal diseases [23–25]. These vaccines are based on the observation that the immunogenicity of polysaccharides can be improved through chemical conjugation to a protein carrier, thereby eliciting a T-cell-dependent anti-saccharide antibody response [26, 27]. The resulting polysaccharide-protein conjugate vaccines are safe, immunogenic in young infants and induce long-term protection. For some pathogens, immunization with conjugate vaccines also decreases nasopharyngeal carriage and transmission of the organism. Vaccines with these properties are suitable for introduction into the Expanded Program on Immunization (EPI)

The public health impact of conjugate vaccines has been impressive. Vaccination with Hib conjugate vaccines has nearly eliminated Hib disease in affluent and middle-income countries [1–4]. In addition, a polysaccharide-protein conjugate vaccine against *S. pneumoniae*, recently licensed in the U.S. and Europe, was highly effective for the prevention of pneumococcal bacteremia and meningitis in clinical trials [9]. Widespread use of this vaccine is expected to eliminate invasive disease caused by the seven strains contained in the current vaccine (responsible for the majority of cases in infants and children). Finally, a group C meningococcal conjugate vaccine is part of the routine infant vaccination program in the UK and has resulted in a marked reduction in meningococcal disease [28]. Other countries, including Spain, Germany and the Republic of Ireland, have also introduced this vaccine into their routine infant immunization programs.

Polysaccharide-protein conjugate vaccines against enteric and respiratory bacteria have the potential to prevent at least three million deaths a year in the developing world

Hib and pneumococcal conjugate vaccines can prevent at least half of pneumonia cases. In the future, conjugate vaccines could virtually eliminate bacterial meningitis. Besides conjugate vaccines against Hib, pneumococcus and group C meningococcus, vaccine manufacturers are currently developing conjugate vaccine combinations incorporating groups A, C, Y and W-135 meningococcal polysaccharides [24]. In addition, a N-propionylated polysialic acid from *Escherichia coli* K1 polysaccharide capsule coupled to purified recombinant PorB outer membrane protein as a carrier is being tested in humans against group B meningococcus [29]. Finally, prototypes against group B streptococci [30] have also been developed and clinically evaluated. For all these vaccines, a variety of formulations and presentations not currently considered by large vaccine manufacturers either as stand-alone products or in combination with other antigens, may be required to accommodate the needs of individual countries or regions in the developing world

Furthermore, conjugate vaccines could also potentially drastically reduce mortality caused by enteric bacteria, such as *S. typhi* and *S. paratyphi*, *Shigellae*, *E. coli*, *V. cholerae O1* and *O139*. Conjugate prototype vaccines against typhoid fever, paratyphoid fever, *E. coli* O18 and shigellosis [31–34] have been shown to be safe and effective in proof-of-principle trials. Furthermore, prototypes against *V. cholerae* spp have been developed in the laboratory [35, 36] (Tab. 1).

Big Pharma will not likely be a source of most polysaccharide-protein conjugate vaccines for developing-country populations

Big Pharma is unlikely to give priority to developing a new generation of developing-market conjugate vaccines because it will not be able to obtain an adequate return on investment. Public sector attempts to induce industry to produce these vaccines by offering to offset the direct costs are unlikely to succeed because of the opportunity costs involved.

The public sector has attempted to influence the decisions of the research-based industry to develop new vaccines for use in the poorest

Table 1. Estimated deaths caused by pathogens against which conjugate vaccines are or could be developed

Pathogen	Estimated deaths/year
S. pneumoniae	1,000,000 [37]
H. influenzae type b	300,000–500,000 [38]
N. meningitides	30,000–60,000 [39]
Group B streptococci	Unknown
Non-typeable *H. influenzae*	Unknown
Shigella	1,100,000 [40]
Enterotoxigenic *E.coli*	380,000 [41]
V. cholerae	120,000 [42]
S. typhi and *S. paratyphi*	600,000 [43]

countries by a variety of means. Overall the results have been disappointing. Appealing to corporate altruism or provision of incentives ("push strategies") such as supporting the cost of clinical trials, strengthening of field sites in developing countries, R&D tax credits and small business grants, fast-track regulatory reviews, standardizing serological assays, and developing international recommendations for quality control and production, while useful in themselves, are rarely sufficient to influence the decisions of major manufacturers.

Notwithstanding the new funding opportunities that have emerged recently, public sector alliances with established manufacturers for the development of vaccines that largely target developing-country populations have proven to be difficult. Group A meningococcal conjugate vaccine is a revealing example [17].

In May 2001, the Bill and Melinda Gates Foundation awarded a US$70 million, 10-year grant to WHO and PATH to support the Meningitis Vaccine Project (MVP), with the goal of eliminating meningococcal epidemics in Sub-Saharan Africa. Meetings were held with major vaccine manufacturers to discuss ways to stimulate commercial development of a low-priced group A meningococcal conjugate vaccine. Possible incentives included providing capital investment in the form of a low-interest loan for increasing manufacturing plant capacity; underwriting costs of process development, production of investigational vaccine lots and conduct of clinical trials; and forming a partnership for joint management of clinical, serology and regulatory activities. Although several vaccine manufacturers in the US and Europe with expertise in conjugate or meningococcal vaccines were approached, only two companies made formal proposals. The most important obstacle for all of the companies was the perceived opportunity costs of the project. Their business models were based on the development of innovative products with high potential returns on investment. Developing a low-cost group A meningococcal conjugate vaccine for the meningitis-belt countries in Africa, and expanding manufacturing capacity, were major undertakings that would directly compete with resources needed for other higher-value projects. Some of the manufacturers indicated that the opportunity costs of the project would likely result in loss of revenue, even if all the costs of development of the group A meningococcal conjugate vaccine were subsidized [17].

More critical than subsidizing the costs of vaccine development or the capital investment required for building manufacturing capacity was the assurance of a profitable future revenue stream that would represent a sufficient return on investment to offset the high opportunity costs of the project, such as the guaranteed purchase of a large number of doses at a profitable price: the so-called "pull mechanism". This purchase-precommitment approach has as its most attractive feature the fact that it only rewards successful outputs rather than supporting research that may not succeed [44]. However, the public sector has yet to develop effective mechanisms by which to guarantee long-term vaccine purchases, particularly for a vaccine that was not expected to be available for the next several years.

One may argue that the MVP focused on the poorest countries in the world where the possibility of tiered pricing is very limited. For other vaccines, the existence of middle-income country markets may somehow prove a greater incentive to get vaccine manufacturers involved. This is only partially true. Whereas, theoretically, countries in Asia and Latin America provide greater possibilities for profit for vaccine manufacturers, increased costs for R&D and stringent regulatory requirements have pushed vaccine corporations to look increasingly for "blockbuster" products with high potential returns on investment. Furthermore, even for vaccines against group A meningococcus, one could have argued that potential markets existed for Middle Eastern and several Asian countries, but these prospects clearly did not lure manufacturers to pursue the development of the vaccine. It is unrealistic to expect that for other vaccines the same reasoning would not apply.

The role of local producers in the production of conjugate vaccines against developing-market diseases

Background

In the last few years, a new group of qualified local producers has emerged in the developing world. This group has not only greatly improved their ability to produce high-quality vaccines, but has also established robust financial systems and a managerial structure with clear lines of responsibility, accountability and authority. Indeed, two-thirds of the traditional EPI vaccines supplied to UNICEF come from manufacturers located in the developing world (Tab. 2) that have been previously pre-qualified by WHO [45].

Table 2. Distribution by source of vaccines purchased through UNICEF tenders [45]

	UNICEF supply specific to Global Fund purchase (Hep B, Hib, DTP-HB, DTP-HB-Hib)	UNICEF supply for basic EPI vaccines excluding OPV
Established vaccine manufacturers	73%	36%
Developing-country vaccine manufacturers	27%	64%

The pre-qualification system [46] depends on effective regulatory oversight. For vaccines, regulatory oversight includes adequate review of pre-clinical and clinical data for licensing, including review of the product file and assurance that the proposed facility is constructed and run in accordance with principles of Good Manufacturing Practices (GMP). In addition, it includes activities carried out post-licensing: lot release, regular GMP inspections, monitoring for field impact (including investigation of adverse event reports), resolution of complaints, and review and approval of changes in the license.

Manufacturers in the developing world producing vaccines pre-qualified by WHO include the Serum Institute of India and Shantha Biotechnics, India; Biofarma, Indonesia; Biomanguinhos, Brazil; CIGB, Cuba; and the Pasteur Institute, Senegal.

Another group of manufacturers with the necessary regulatory environment for safety and quality that are not yet pre-qualified include Panacea Biotech, Biological E and Bharat Biotech International, India; Vabiotech, Vietnam; Instituto Finlay, Cuba; and Instituto Butantan, Brazil. Finally, a third group of manufacturers that have made demonstrable steps to upgrade their oversight for quality and safety include Birmex, Mexico; Vacsera, Egypt; the Pasteur Institute, Iran; and the Lanzhou Institute, Chengdu Institute, and Shenzen Kangtai, China.

Several of these institutions have already shown the ability to acquire new technologies to develop a new generation of vaccines.

Unfortunately, the market for more profitable vaccines, such as Hep B, Hib conjugates and especially their combinations, is still dominated by established vaccine manufacturers (Tab. 2). In the last few years, though, the situation has been gradually changing with more manufacturers producing high-quality Hep B vaccines. However, the ability of local producers in the developing world to produce conjugate vaccines is still very limited. Only a sustained program of technology transfer, technical assistance and training will speed up this process.

Big Pharma is increasingly focusing its R&D efforts on products aimed at lucrative markets. Thus, for vaccines against diseases affecting populations in the developing world, the possibility of establishing partnerships between the public sector and qualified local producers is becoming increasingly vital; for conjugate vaccines, these alliances are becoming even more important. From an economic point of view, such alliances make sense. What Big Pharma normally views as an opportunity cost, local manufacturers may view as a good opportunity for: 1) potential capital investment for vaccine production and up-grading of their facilities; 2) increased sales of vaccines at a low price according to Western standards but at a profitable price for them; and 3) acquisition of conjugate technology/know-how for the development of a broad range of products that could, in the future, be sold in more profitable markets.

Conjugate vaccines can be produced locally but the process is demanding

As a consequence, transfer of technology will only be practical for a small group of the best WHO qualified manufacturers. The manufacturing of conjugate vaccines has 4 elements:

Availability of a purified carrier protein

Among the different carrier proteins that can be used for conjugate vaccines, tetanus toxoid (TT) stands out as the most appropriate for local production of conjugates for two important reasons: cost and availability. The cost of TT, based on international quotations for bulk TT, is negligible. Using TT of good purity at 1,500 Lf/mgPN (WHO specification ≥ 1,000 Lf/mgPN [47], one dose of vaccine (20 µg protein) translates to about 5 Lf of TT, or assuming 50% yield, 10 Lf of TT consumption. The corresponding cost is between US$0.01–0.02/dose. With regard to availability, several institutes and manufacturers in the developed and developing world have TT in production, or have established an agreement with a manufacturer to acquire it.

Availability of purified polysaccharide

The preparation of the polysaccharide (PS) involves fermentation of the bacterial strain, extraction of the cell wall and purification. Guidelines for glycoconjugate vaccines require that the PS meet agreed specifications for PS, residual protein, nucleic acids and endotoxins [48]. Local producers can acquire it from contract manufacturers such as Synco Ltd [17], or they can establish the methods in house, which is the better long-term option. The latter will require the preparation of master and working cell banks, optimization of fermentation processes and setting up the purification technology in a GMP facility.

Availability of a conjugation facility

Conjugation requires a small dedicated facility consisting of a room equipped with an exhaust hood for activation chemistry, a chromatographic unit for conjugate purification, and a recipient class A area for sterile filtration of the conjugate. All these elements would be grouped together. The chemical processing room (6–8 sqm) and the chemicals warehouse have special requirements, as the process uses toxic and volatile chemicals.

Acquisition of conjugation technology

Several technologies that are used for the production of existing Hib conjugate vaccines may be considered by local producers for production of other conjugate vaccines.

The PRP-T approach offers a number of advantages to developing-world producers, including a simple, rapid and efficient process, the absence of patent restrictions (at least for its original form designed by NICHD/NIH) and accessibility of the carrier protein [48]. The conjugation and purification process of PRP-T type conjugates is illustrated in Figure 1.

Because of the relatively complex manufacturing process, sustainable production and manufacturing of conjugate vaccines requires a cadre of well-trained individuals. As conjugate vaccines are manufactured from purified components by a defined chemical process, there is a need for standard operating procedures, meticulous attention to detail, and testing at many stages of the process. Modern physicochemical methods allow biological pharmaceuticals to be characterized with a degree of precision not previously possible. These techniques are based on the structure of the active ingredient and are thus complementary to traditional bioassays used in the industry. The techniques for analysis of conjugate vaccines include optical spectroscopy (circular dichroism and fluorescence spectroscopy), size exclusion chromatography (especially when combined with light-scattering detection techniques) and mass spectrometry; whereas the saccharide component of glycoconjugates (comprised of protein-saccharide) can be characterized by NMR spectroscopy and composition analysis performed using the sensitive technique of high-performance anion-exchange chromatography. Furthermore, it is necessary to ensure that manufacturing consistency for vaccine lots used in the clinical trials is documented, that these lots adequately represent the formulation intended for marketing and that all assay procedures used for quality control of the conjugate vaccines and vaccine intermediates are validated [49].

The additional skills acquired by local manufacturers who develop conjugate technology are likely to result in improvements in the quality of other vaccines produced in their facility.

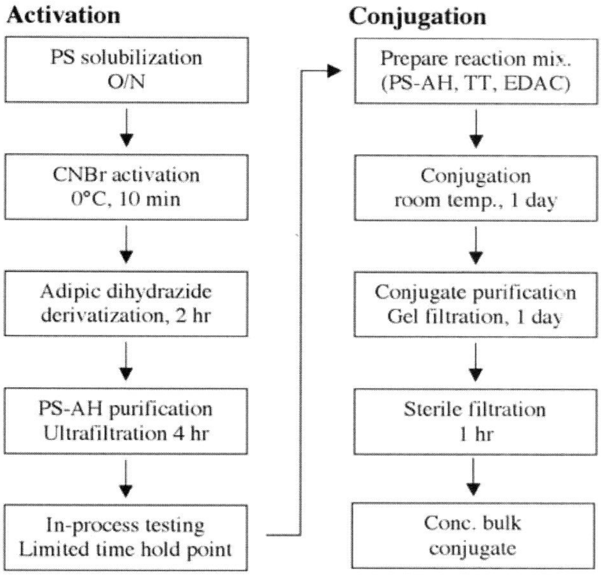

Figure 1. Conjugation and purification (PRP-T-like process)

Conjugate vaccines can be developed at reasonable cost for developing countries

The price of the vaccine is an important factor affecting its widespread use into EPI. A formal market study to assess the relationship between price and use has not been conducted, so the sensitivity of price to use cannot be formally assessed. Evidence from both WHO research and uptake of other new vaccines has repeatedly suggested that even with donor support, most developing countries struggle to finance immunization programs and have been reluctant to introduce the more expensive vaccines [4]. However, an early policymaker survey done by the International Vaccine Institute (unpublished document) revealed an unexpectedly high willingness to pay for typhoid and *Shigella* conjugate vaccines, both among the middle classes and the poor in developing countries of Asia, indicating that introduction of these vaccines through the private sector is viable, and could provide a platform for tiered pricing and provision of these vaccines to the poor at affordable prices.

A cost-of-goods analysis was undertaken by WHO in the year 2000 for the development of a group A meningococcal conjugate vaccine. In this analysis, the cost of goods (based on 2.5 million 10-dose vials) for a group A meningococcal conjugate vaccine was determined to be $0.15/dose. These numbers are based on theoretical yields since the final yields will be determined only through the experience of producing actual lots of vaccine in the manufacturing facility. What is important is that the cost of the antigen itself accounts for only $0.04 of the final costs. Thus even if the yields were only 50% of what is expected, the cost per dose would not rise appreciably. This is a fairly simplistic analysis of costs of manufacture because some of the costs, e.g. quality control (QC) release, are related to the number of lot failures. Using the analysis of manufacturing costs of group A meningococcal conjugate, a ceiling price of $US 0.40 per dose in lyophilized ten-dose vials was set for discussions with potential partners [17].

Models for transfer of technology to local producers

The availability of affordable conjugate vaccines for developing-market diseases is more likely if more than one qualified local producer enters the market. For this to occur, selected local producers must acquire the technology and the expertise to produce conjugate vaccines, be prepared to invest in facilities to allow large-scale production and be capable of sustaining high-quality production over time.

There are several models that could potentially be used by local producers to acquire the needed technology. This section describes these models, their advantages and disadvantages.

The private sector (Big Pharma, Small Pharma and Biotech companies)

The most efficient method for local producers to acquire technology and know-how for production of conjugate vaccines would be to form an alliance with an established vaccine manufacturer with a proven track record in developing and licensing these products and a strong IP position. Big Pharma has rarely exercised this option partly because of the difficulties in obtaining a return on investment, partly because of the difficulties of working in developing countries and partly because of their insistence that the resulting products meet current (or future) FDA or EMEA standards. Where relationships have developed they largely relate to filling and finishing product/s produced in Europe and the USA.

It is most unlikely that Big Pharma would either provide a license of its technology to developing-country manufacturers for production of conjugate-based developing-market vaccines intended for local use, or, given the increasing influence of the World Trade Organization (WTO), that local producers would be prepared to use "pirated" technology.

Even when transfer of technology is contemplated, such as GlaxoSmithKline's (GSK) agreement with Biomanguinhos for production of DTP-HepB-Hib combinations for Latin America, the local producer is constrained from producing developing-world products based on the parent companies' IP-protected technology.

Although useful, especially for conjugate vaccines targeting global diseases, this model is not likely to result in widespread diffusion of conjugate vaccines for the poor. At best, this pattern of collaboration will be *ad hoc* and poorly suited for ensuring a global supply of needed products. Moreover, this strategy will be employed primarily for products targeted at countries in which there is a middle-class market for profitable sales, a situation that clearly excludes most of the GAVI countries. Small Pharma or Biotech companies with a proven track record for conjugate technology, but with limited capacity for production, may also consider transferring the technology to local producers to enlarge their production capacity, allowing them to become global players. But again, the same limitations cited for alliances with Big Pharma will also be applicable to these partnerships.

Public-sector institutions

In the past, government-funded in-country producers, such as the Nordic Public Health Laboratories, have attempted to produce vaccines targeting developing country populations and to transfer the technology to local producers. Because these institutions were under-resourced and lacked the capacity to scale up operations, the results have been disappointing.

Some years ago, The National Institute for Public Health and the Environment (RIVM) in the Netherlands started a Hib conjugate project that is now idle as the organization has been privatized. RIVM's technical package has been made available to several institutes which are attempting to develop the product. These institutions include BioFarma in Indonesia, Birmex in Mexico and Biological-e in India. Although work has been in progress for several years, in the absence of dedicated experienced support, none of these organizations has yet been able to develop and license a product.

It is important to analyze these efforts so that critical success factors can be identified. There are several reasons to explain why these attempts have, for the most part, failed to materialize: firstly, their priorities were almost entirely dictated by in-country needs; secondly, their small additional capacity and resources limited their flexibility to adapt their development portfolio to products targeting the developing world; thirdly, there was a lack of sustained resources for long-term technical assistance and training; and fourthly, major investments were needed at the local producer level in the developing world to make this technology transfer a success. Furthermore, increased production costs have made small-scale production unprofitable and governments have started to question the viability of such institutions. Given the current trend to privatize or close down these institutions, it is improbable that they could fulfill this function, even if dedicated resources were provided.

Academic laboratories have also attempted to transfer the technology produced at laboratory level to producers in the developing world. The University of Gothenborg, with help from NIH and WHO, transferred the technology to produce a killed O1 oral cholera vaccine to the National Institute of Hygiene and Epidemiology (NIHE) in Vietnam [50]. The Laboratory of Developmental and Molecular Immunity at NICHD/NIH has transferred the technology for Vi conjugate and shigella conjugate vaccines to the Lanzhou and Chengdu Institutes in China, and has transferred Vi technology to Biofarma in Indonesia and the National Institute of Vaccine and Biological Substances (IVAC) in Vietnam. Unfortunately, academic institutions have limited capacity to conduct or to transfer the critical skills in in-process research and production necessary to assure successful transfer of technology for production of conjugate products for public health programs.

The dedicated not-for-profit and virtual company approaches

One way of developing vaccines against diseases that primarily occur in poor countries (where traditional market forces are insufficient to stimulate private investment) is establishing a not-for-profit (NFP) company, funded by the public sector [13]. The NFP company would be dedicated to production and licensure of one or a small number of products and not be distracted by competing projects of higher priority. A second advantage is that the NFP company would be free to design the product specifically for use in a developing-country setting, rather than adapt a product originally designed for industrialized countries. The disadvantages of this model are the need to construct and equip a dedicated facility and to recruit and retain staff with skills in all aspects of the development and production process and to establish a product pipeline which justifies the investment. As facilities are expensive and take a long time to construct and validate, and skilled staff are in scarce supply, it seems prudent to invest in manufacturers with existing facilities and staff rather than start from scratch.

Another alternative is to attempt to produce vaccines through a virtual company model as is being attempted by the International AIDS Vaccine Initiative (IAVI) [51] and the Malaria Vaccine Initiative (MVI) [15].

The MVP took a further step by attempting to develop a group A meningococcal conjugate vaccine in partnership with a developing-country vaccine manufacturer with financing, technical assistance, and coordination by the MVP. The MVP is also working with accredited National Control Laboratories (NCLs) for characterization of the vaccine and lot release, and has developed clinical and regulatory plans needed for licensure of the vaccine in the developing country where the vaccine will be manufactured. The MVP works as both funder and project manager. It is expected that a vaccine against group A meningococcus will be available by the epidemic season of 2007–2008 [17].

It is important to note that the management of virtual organizations is very complex and that contracting out all aspects of the development process increases the risk that something will go wrong. An added risk exists when some of the partners are governmental organizations, whose priorities may be affected by external factors, such as the recent focus on bioterrorism, leading to unexpected delays. Most partner institutions with skills in serology, physicochemical characterization or lot-to-lot release are governmental institutions that prioritize national vaccine programs over international work. After September 11th, national security interests have become an urgent priority and research on conventional vaccines has shifted dramatically to research on bio-terrorism [52].

It is not surprising that the most successful models for vaccine production (e.g., Merck, Sharpe, Dohme (MSD) in the 1960–80s, GSK since the late 1980s) have brought as many of the elements of vaccine production as possible (research, development, manufacturing, clinical and regulatory affairs) under central control.

A potential solution: The IVI Center for Developing-Market Conjugate Vaccines

This paper has argued that the development of conjugate vaccines will be essential to effectively combat a wide range of bacterial diseases that account for more than three million deaths a year. It is becoming increasingly evident that additional development, production and sustainable cost-competitive supply of conjugate vaccines will only be achieved if a number of highly qualified producers in Asia and Latin America can: 1) acquire this technology; 2) produce enough numbers of doses; and 3) be appropriately trained in production, quality control/quality assurance (QC/QA) and regulatory processes. For this to happen, there are different models that can potentially be followed, ranging from an alliance with established vaccine manufactures to a complex series of partnerships with developers and subcontractors. In the long run, none of these models will achieve sustainability of affordable production of conjugates against a broad spectrum of diseases. There is a dearth of institutions with the capacity to provide transfer of conjugate technology and/or PS fermentation/purification and continuous assistance in process research, physicochemical characterization, QC/QA and lot-to-lot release to local producers. The International Vaccine Institute (IVI), an international research organization located in the Republic of Korea, with its new research laboratories occupying 211,713 ft^2 of floor space, can become such an institution. The IVI Center for

Developing-Market Conjugate Vaccines aims to combine the best practices of successful manufacturers for the production of lots of a novel vaccine and to work closely with a small number of local manufacturers to successfully transfer the technology to mass production.

The critical elements of the program are (i) a laboratory-based program of process development, where IVI scientists, overseas experts and staff from developing-country manufacturers can work together to establish production technology and transfer it to the eventual production facility (or facilities) (ii) a complementary clinical trials program to assess the safety, efficacy and effectiveness of these vaccines and (iii) support for training programs to upgrade the skills from National Regulatory Authorities and NCLs from developing countries.

To achieve these goals, long-term financial and political commitment is needed. The GAVI and the public sector at large have an extraordinary opportunity to leverage the considerable resources and personnel already invested in the IVI to establish an operational arm at the IVI to accelerate the development and introduction of new-generation conjugate vaccines for developing-country populations.

References

1 Murphy TV, White KE, Pastor P, Gabriel L, Medley F, Granoff DM, Osterholm MT (1993) Declining incidence of Haemophilus influenzae type b disease since introduction of vaccination. *JAMA* 269: 246–248

2 Adams WG, Deaver KA, Cochi SL, Plikaytis BD, Zell ER, Broome CV, Wenger JD (1993) Decline of childhood Haemophilus influenzae type b (Hib) disease in the Hib vaccine era. *JAMA* 269: 221–226

3 Landaverde M, Di Fabio JL, Ruocco G, Leal I, de Quadros C (1999) Introduction of a conjugate vaccine against Hib in Chile and Uruguay. *Rev Panam Salud Publica* 5: 200–206

4 Wenger JD, DiFabio J, Landaverde JM, Levine OS, Gaafar T (1999) Introduction of Hib conjugate vaccines in the non-industrialized world: experience in four "newly adopting" countries. *Vaccine* 18: 736–742

5 Clemens JD, Jodar L (2004) Translational research to assist policy decisions about introducing new vaccines into developing countries. *J Health Popul Nutr* 22: 223–231

6 Wenger J (2001) Vaccines for the developing world: current status and future directions. *Vaccine* 19: 1588–1591

7 Pan American Health Organization (2000) PAHO's Revolving Fund Vaccine Prices for 2000. *EPI Newsletter* 22: 8

8 Batson A (1998) Win-win interactions between the public and private sectors. *Nature Medicine, Vaccine Supplement* 4: 487–491

9 Shinefield HR, Black S (2000) Efficacy of pneumococcal conjugate vaccines in large scale field trials. *Pediatr Infect Dis J* 19: 394–397

10 Martin JF, Marshall J (2003) New tendencies and strategies in international immunisation: GAVI and The Vaccine Fund. *Vaccine* 21: 587–592

11 Murasin W (2004) The global alliance for vaccines and immunization: is it a new model for effective public-private cooperation in international public health? *Am J Public Health* 94: 1922–1925

12 Plotkin SA (2002) Conclusions to the conference on orphan vaccines. *Dev Biol* 110: 167–169

13 Assessing the global needs for vaccine research and development. WHO/V&B/00.18 (available from WHO upon request)

14 Halstead SB, Deen J (2002) The future of dengue vaccines. *Lancet* 360: 1243–1245

15 Rabinovich NR (2002) Are we there yet? The road to a malaria vaccine. *West J Med* 176: 82–84

16 Hausdorff WP, Bryant J, Paradiso PR, Siber GR (2000) Which pneumococcal serogroups cause the most invasive disease: implications for conjugate vaccine formulation and use, part I. *Clin Infect Dis* 30: 100–121

17 Jódar L, LaForce FM, Ceccarini C, Aguado T, Granoff DM (2003) Meningococcal conjugate vaccine for Africa: A model for developing new vaccines for the poorest countries. *Lancet* 361: 1902–1904

18 Finkelstein RA (1984) Cholera. In Germanier R (ed): *Bacterial vaccines*. Academic Press, Inc, New York, NY, 107–129

19 Robbins JB, Chu CY, Schneerson R (1992) Hypothesis for vaccine development: protective immunity to enteric diseases caused by nontyphoidal salmonellae and shigellae may be conferred by serum IgG antibodies to the O-specific polysaccharide of their lipopolysaccharides. *Clin Infect Dis* 15: 346–361

20 Keitel WA, Bond NL, Zahradnik JM, Cramton TA, Robbins JB (1994) Clinical and serological responses following primary and booster immunization with *Salmonella typhi* Vi capsular polysaccharide vaccines. *Vaccine* 12: 195–199

21 Coughlin RT, Fattom A, Chu C, White AC, Winston S (1995) Adjuvant activity of QS-21 for experimental E. coli 018 polysaccharide vaccines. *Vaccine* 13: 17–21

22 Gold R, Lepow ML, Goldschneider I, Draper TF, Gotshlich EC (1979) Kinetics of antibody production to group A and group C meningococcal polysaccharide vaccines administered during the first six years of life: prospects for routine immunization of infants and children. *J Infect Dis* 140: 690–697

23 Frasch CE (1994) Regulatory perspectives in vaccine licensure. In: Ellis RW, Granoff DM (eds): *Development and clinical uses of Haemophilus influenzae type b conjugate vaccines*. New York: Marcel Dekker, 435–453

24 Jodar L, Feavers IM, Salisbury D, Granoff DM (2002) Development of vaccines against meningococcal disease. *Lancet* 359: 1499–1450

25 Jodar L , Butler J, Carlone G, Dagan R , Frasch C, Goldblatt D, Kahty H, Klugman K, Plykaytis B, Siber G et al (2003) Serological criteria for evaluation and licensure of new pneumococcal conjugate vaccine formulations for use in infants. *Vaccine* 21: 3265–3272

26 Robbins JB, Schneerson R, Szu SC, Fattom A, Yang Y, Lagergard T, Chu C, Sorensen US (1989) Prevention of invasive bacterial diseases by immunization with polysaccharide-protein conjugates. *Curr Top Microbiol Immunol* 146: 169–180

27 Goldblatt D (1998) Immunisation and the maturation of infant immune responses. *Dev Biol Stand* 95: 125–132

28 Ramsay ME, Andrews N, Kaczmarski EB, Miller E (2001) Efficacy of meningococcal serogroup C conjugate vaccine in teenagers and toddlers in England. *Lancet* 357: 195–196

29 Bruge J, Bouveret-Le Cam N, Danve B, Rougon G, Schulz D (2004) Clinical evaluation of a group B meningococcal N-propionylated polysaccharide conjugate vaccine in adult, male volunteers. *Vaccine* 22: 1087–1096

30 Paoletti LC, Kasper DL (2002) Conjugate vaccines against group B *Streptococcus* types IV and VII. *J Infect Dis* 186: 123–126

31 Lin FY, Ho VA, Khiem HB, Trach DD, Bay PV, Thanh TC, Kossaczka Z, Bryla DA, Shiloach J, Robbins J et al (2001) The efficacy of a *Salmonella typhi* Vi conjugate vaccine in two- to five-year old children. *N Engl J Med* 344: 1263–1269

32 Konadu EY, Lin FY, Ho VA, Thuy NT, Van Bay P, Thanh TC, Khiem HB, Trach DD, Karpas AB et al (2000) Phase 1 and phase 2 studies of *Salmonella enterica* serovar paratyphi A O-specific polysaccharide-tetanus toxoid conjugates in adults, teenagers, and 2- to 4-year-old children in Vietnam. *Infect Immun* 68: 1529–1534

33 Cryz SJ Jr, Cross AS, Sadoff JC, Wegmann A, Que JU, Furer E (1991) Safety and immunogenicity of *Escherichia coli* O18 O-specific polysaccharide (O-PS)-toxin A and O-PS-cholera toxin conjugate vaccines in humans. *J Infect Dis* 163: 1040–1045

34 Passwell JH, Harlev E, Ashkenazi S, Chu C, Miron D, Ramon R, Farzan N, Shiloach J, Bryla DA, Majadly F et al (2001) Safety and immunogenicity of improved Shigella O-specific polysaccharide-protein conjugate vaccines in adults in Israel. *Infect Immun* 69: 1351–1357

35 Kossaczka Z, Shiloach J, Johnson V, Taylor DN, Finkelstein RA, Robbins JB, Szu SC (2000) *Vibrio cholerae* O139 conjugate vaccines: synthesis and immunogenicity of *V. cholerae* O139 capsular polysaccharide conjugates with recombinant diphtheria toxin mutant in mice. *Infect Immun* 68: 5037–5043

36 Chernyak A, Kondo S, Wade TK, Meeks MD, Alzari PM, Fournier JM, Taylor RK, Kovac P, Wade WF (2002) Induction of protective immunity by synthetic *Vibrio cholerae* hexasaccharide derived from *V. cholerae* O1 Ogawa lipopolysaccharide bound to a protein carrier. *J Infect Dis* 185: 950–962

37 WHO (1999) Pneumococcal vaccines. WHO position paper. *Weekly Epidemiological Record* 74: 177–183

38 WHO (1998) Hib vaccines. WHO position paper. *Weekly Epidemiological Record* 73: 64–71

39 WHO (1999) Meningococcal A and C vaccines. WHO position paper. *Weekly Epidemiological Record* 74: 297–304

40 Kotloff KL, Winickoff JP, Ivanoff B, Clemens JD, Swerdlow DL, Sansonetti PJ, Adak GK, Levine MM (1999) Global burden of Shigella infections: implications for vaccine development and implementation of control strategies. *Bull World Health Organ* 77: 651–666
41 Black RE (1988) Overview of diarrheal diseases and strategies for their control. In: Holmgren J, Sack D (eds): *New prospects for vaccines against diarrheal diseases*. Swedish International Agency for Cooperation with Developing Countries, Stockholm, 47–59
42 WHO (2001) Cholera vaccines. WHO position paper. *Weekly Epidemiological Record* 76: 117–124
43 Ivanoff BN, Levine MM, Lambert PH (1994) Vaccination against typhoid fever: present status. *Bull WHO* 72: 957–971
44 Webber D, Kremer M (2001) Perspectives on stimulating industrial research and development for neglected infectious diseases. *Bull World Health Organ* 79: 735–741
45 Herrera L (2001) Developing Country Manufacturers Network, GAVI Board Meeting, London (unpublished document)
46 Procedure for assessing the acceptability in principle of vaccines for purchase by United Nations agencies (WHO/VSQ/97.06)
47 The World Health Organization (1990) Requirements for diphtheria, tetanus, pertussis and combined vaccines. Technical report series, No. 500. Geneva 88–167
48 The World Health Organization (2000) Recommendations for the production and control of Hib conjugate vaccines. Technical report series, No. 897. Geneva 27–56
49 Jodar L, Griffiths E, Feavers I (2004) Scientific challenges for the quality control and production of group C meningococcal conjugate vaccines. *Vaccine* 22: 1047–1053
50 Trach DD (1990) The problem of cholera vaccination in Vietnam. In: Sack D, Freij L (eds): *Prospects for public health benefits in developing countries from new vaccines against enteric infections*. SAREC Documentation, Stockholm, Conference Report 2, 217–218
51 AIDS vaccines (2000) IAVI issues blueprint to assure global access. *AIDS Wkly* 31: 23–25
52 Smith LA (2004) Bioterrorism: what level is the threat and are vaccines the answer? *Expert Rev Vaccines* 3: 493–495

Bench

The Grand Challenge for the Future
ed. by Stefan H.E. Kaufmann and Paul-Henri Lambert

Novel vaccination strategies

Maria Lattanzi and Rino Rappuoli

Chiron Vaccines, Via Fiorentina 1, 53100 Siena, Italy

Introduction

Vaccination is one of the most significant public health interventions ever made, sparing millions of people from infectious diseases. It has been calculated that use of currently available vaccines saves more than eight million lives annually, which corresponds to one person saved every five seconds. These remarkable results have been achieved in 200 years of vaccination history, which are largely based on two basic, simple technologies: the inactivation of toxins and pathogens with formaldehyde treatment (first performed by Glenny and Hopkins in 1923 and Ramon in 1924) [1–3], and the stable attenuation of pathogens by serial passage *in vitro*.

From 1920 to 1980, these now "easy technologies" were applied to develop vaccines that have been used worldwide to control or even eradicate many infectious diseases. One of the most brilliant successes of vaccination is the eradication of smallpox virus in 1977. It has been estimated that to date, smallpox eradication has spared the global community of some 350 million new smallpox victims and about 40 million deaths from the disease. The annual savings as a result of vaccination being stopped and hospitals being able to be converted to other uses is estimated to be in excess of US$ 2000 million each year [4].

Vaccination has also resulted in the elimination of poliovirus from the Americas in 1994, Western Pacific in 2000 and Europe in June 2002. The goal of the WHO Global Polio Eradication Initiative is to interrupt transmission of wild poliovirus by end-2004 leading to global certification by 2008. Overall, since the Initiative was launched in 1988, the number of cases has fallen by over 99%, from an estimated 350,000 cases to the 89 cases reported in the first three months of 2004. In the same period, the number of polio-infected countries was reduced from 125 to 6 [5].

Moreover, the incidence of seven other frightening diseases (diphtheria, measles, rubella, mumps, pertussis, *Haemophilus influenzae* type b – Hib –, and tetanus) has fallen by more than 98% in those states where the related vaccines have been introduced (see Tab. 1).

Table 1. Universal routine vaccination reduced by more than 98% the incidence of nine harmful diseases from the US and eradicated two of them (smallpox and polio).

Disease	Max number of cases (year)	Number of cases in 2002	Reduction (%)
Smallpox	48,164 (1901–1904)	0	100
Poliomyelitis	21,269 (1952)	0	100
Diphtheria	206,939 (1921)	1	99.99
Measles	894,134 (1941)	44	99.9
Rubella	57,686 (1969)	18	99.78
Mumps	152,209 (1968)	270	99.86
Pertussis	265,269 (1934)	9771	98.20
H. influenzae type b	20,000 (1992)	<100	98.79
Tetanus	1,560 (1923)	25	98.44

Source: CDC (1998) Impact of vaccines universally recommended for children – US, 1990–98. *MMWR* 48: 577-581; modified) [94].

Novel strategies for novel vaccines

The historical technologies for vaccine production have achieved remarkable successes, but the battle against infectious diseases has not been won. During the last several million years of existence on earth, microorganisms have learnt how to escape the surveillance of our immune system, either hiding themselves from host responses, or developing the capacity of infecting different hosts. These two main mechanisms of pathogen defense explain why vaccines against several pathogens such as HIV, HCV, *Streptococcus pyogenes*, *Staphylococcus aureus*, *Plasmodium falciparum*, *Schistosoma* spp. and others are difficult to develop and are not yet available.

Moreover, during the last 25 years, there has been a big revolution in microbial ecology: pathogens that have circulated since many years, but whose existence was ignored were discovered (HCV, MetaPneumoVirus, etc.); old pathogens have changed their geographical habitat and have been introduced into new areas where they have become endemic (e.g. West Nile Virus in North America); completely new pathogens have emerged and pose a serious threat to human health (HIV, SARS Coronavirus, etc); pathogens thought to be controlled have re-emerged (*Mycobacterium tuberculosis*, etc.) (Tab. 2).

It was soon clear that the old vaccine strategies were unable to face with the new challenges posed by infectious diseases, and modern approaches were needed. Therefore, from the beginning of the 1980s, taking advantage of the better understanding of the immune system and the emergence of the recombinant DNA technologies, new vaccines were developed (Tab. 3). Moreover, nowadays the range of technologies and strategies available for vaccine development is extremely broad. The availability of the whole genomic sequences of many pathogens is considered a real revolution and

Table 2. New and emerging pathogens identified in the last 25 years

Period	Pathogen
1980–1990	HTLV HIV *Escherichia coli* O157H7 *Borrelia burgdorferi* *Helicobacter pylori* Human herpesvirus type 6 *Ehrlichia chalffeensis*
1990–2004	HCV *Vibrio cholerae* O139 *Bartonella* spp. Hantavirus Nipah virus West Nile virus TT virus Meta Pneumo virus SARS Coronavirus

a start of a new era in the vaccine field. Genomics, proteomics, molecular biology, recombinant DNA, and advanced immunology have removed most of the technical barriers that formerly limited vaccine development approaches to prevent and not only treat infectious diseases, but eventually also cancer, allergies, and other chronic conditions.

Conjugate vaccines

It is now common knowledge that the capsular polysaccharide of many important bacterial pathogens is their major virulence factor and that vaccination using purified polysaccharides could protect people from those diseases. Polysaccharide vaccines have been developed against *Neisseria meningitidis* serogroup A (MenA), group C (Men C), group Y (MenY), and group W135 (Men W135) in the late 1960s [6, 7], against *H. influenzae* type b in the 1980s [8], against 23 types of *Streptococcus pneumoniae* in the early 1990s [9], and against *Salmonella typhi* in the mid 1990s [10]. However, the use of all these vaccines is inadequate. Polysaccharides are T-independent antigens: their immunogenicity and efficacy is very poor or absent in infants, so that they are unsuitable to be included in the infant routine immunization schedule.

The solution was found by covalently linking the sugar to a carrier protein (conjugation). This procedure converts T-independent antigens into T-dependent ones by providing a source of appropriate T-cell epitopes (present in the carrier protein). Conjugation technology is one of the biggest achievements of the novel vaccination strategies. The capacity of transforming poor immunogens such as polysaccharides into excellent immuno-

Table 3. Vaccines licensed after 1980

Disease	Year
Hepatitis B (HBV)	1986
Haemophilus influenzae type b, conjugate	1990
Salmonella typhi (live attenuated, capsular polysaccharide)	1991
Hepatitis A (HAV)	1994
Varicella	1995
Acellular pertussis (aP)	1996
Influenza (adjuvanted)	1997
Lyme disease	1998
Neisseria meningitidis group C conjugated	2000
Streptococcus pneumoniae 7 valent conjugated	2000

gens such as the protein-sugar complex has provided outstanding tools for the fight against infectious diseases.

Haemophilus influenzae type b (Hib)

The first conjugate vaccine developed was the one against *Haemophilus influenzae* type b (Hib) [11]. Hib is a respiratory pathogen that causes a wide spectrum of human infections. Before the availability of the Hib conjugate vaccine, Hib was the leading cause of bacterial meningitis, especially in infants, in most developed and developing countries worldwide, resulting in substantial morbidity and mortality. The first Hib conjugated vaccine was introduced in the US in December 1987 for children 18 months of age and older; subsequently, more immunogenic vaccines were introduced, in US as well as in many other countries, in the early 1990s, for the use in infants from the age of two months.

Within a few years, the effectiveness and public impact of Hib conjugate vaccines on Hib disease has been demonstrated in all those countries that have introduced the vaccination [12]. In the US, the annual cases of Hib invasive disease among children under five years of age decreased from more than 20,000 of the pre-vaccination era [13], to less than 50 in 2002 [14].

In general, the decrease in incidence of disease has exceeded that predicted on the basis of estimated proportion of the population that is completely immunized, suggesting that the vaccine use is able to generate herd immunity. On this topic, many studies have shown that Hib conjugated vaccines are able to reduce nasopharyngeal carriage [15–18], which gives a major contribution to herd immunity. Precisely how Hib conjugate immunization reduces nasopharyngeal colonization, whether this impact is due to decreased acquisition or decreased duration of carriage is not clear. Additional work on the immunology and microbiology of transmission and carriage is needed to clarify this issue. On the other hand, reduction of Hib carriage may open ecological niches for *H. influenzae* non-type b strains and therefore potentially increase the risk of colonization and invasive disease by other dangerous strains, for which a vaccine is not available [19–21]. However, so far, widespread vaccination against Hib has not caused this problem: strains recovered from vaccinated children are indistinguishable from those recovered from unvaccinated ones [22].

Streptococcus pneumoniae

The first conjugate vaccine licensed for human use, initially in US in February 2000, and subsequently in Europe, contains capsular polysaccharides of seven serotypes (4, 6B, 9V, 14, 18C, 19F and 23F) conjugated to the CRM197 as carrier protein by reductive amination. Other vaccines under evaluation cover nine and 11 serotypes. However, due to practical and economic reasons, only a limited number of serotypes could be included in conjugate vaccine formulations [23]. The choice of the strains should be based to target the serotypes that most commonly cause diseases among population and the geographic region to be vaccinated [24]. The seven serotypes in the first licensed conjugate vaccine account for >80% of isolates from blood and cerebrospinal fluid of children aged <2 years in the US, compared with <60% of isolates from older children and adults in US, and with <60% of isolates from young children in Latin America and Asia [25, 26].

The seven-valent conjugate pneumococcal vaccine has been recommended in US for all infants as three primary doses (approximately at 2, 4, and 6 months of age) and one booster dose at the ages of 12 and 15 months [27]. This vaccine repeated the successes of the Hib conjugate vaccine, showing high efficacy in preventing meningitis and efficacy, although to less extent, in preventing pneumonia [28] and acute otitis media [29] due to the vaccine serotypes. Moreover, several studies have established that the conjugate vaccine is effective also in reducing nasopharyngeal carriage of the serotypes covered by the vaccine, potentially extending the benefits beyond those children who are vaccinated. Post licensure evaluation of the efficacy of the seven-valent conjugated vaccine found that the reduction in disease was greater than the percentage of children who have been vaccinated, with evidence of herd immunity [30].

Neisseria meningitidis serogroup C

Neisseria meningitis group C conjugate vaccines began clinical development at the end of the 1980s, and, after extensive clinical studies during the 1990s, were proved to be safe and capable of inducing highly bactericidal and boostable immune responses in infants and children [31–39]. These vaccines were first introduced in the United Kingdom in late 1999, to be used for a countrywide vaccination initiative. Population-based active surveillance monitored age-specific and capsular group-specific incidence of disease and estimated vaccine coverage [40]. The results were impressive: within 18 months of vaccine introduction, the cases of MenC diseases almost disappeared in the vaccinated population, with an estimated vaccine efficacy of 90%, or above, in all targeted age groups [41]. According to a large carriage study performed in the United Kingdom, the vaccine induced also a 66% decrease in the carriage of MenC strain, with no evidence of any increase in carriage of MenB isolates or other capsular groups [42]. Moreover, the vaccine provides some evidence of herd immunity, as there is also a reduction of MenC disease in unvaccinated individuals ranging from 34 percent (9–14 years old) to 61 percent (15–17 years old) [43].

Since 1999, the MenC conjugate vaccine has been licensed in many European countries and also in Canada and Australia, either as routine infant immunization, or for catch-up programs of varying forms.

Multivalent meningococcal conjugate vaccines containing groups A, C, Y, and W135 are in clinical development. Introduction of these vaccines into routine infant and/or toddler immunization programs could have a substantial effect on the incidence of meningococcal disease [44, 45].

Recombinant DNA for subunit vaccines: HBV example

In the 1970s it was discovered that protection towards hepatitis B is correlated to the presence of antibodies against the surface antigen of the virus (HBsAg), which circulates in the bloodstream of infected subjects in large quantities. These discoveries led to the development of first generation, plasma-derived HBsAg subunit vaccines, first licensed in the US in 1982 [46]. Concerns about safety of blood products and the advances of recombinant DNA technology conducted to the development of second-generation recombinant subunit vaccines produced in yeast or in mammalian cells [47], which were first licensed in US in 1986. The application of the recombinant DNA technology has the advantage to produce safer vaccines than the plasma- derived ones and in unlimited supplies. This recombinant HBV vaccine is highly effective: a standard course of three doses induces protective levels of anti-HBs (i.e. >10 mIU/ml) in over 95% of healthy infants, children and adolescents and in more than 90% of healthy adults younger than 40 years. After the age of 40, immunogenicity drops below 90%: however, and by the age of 60 years, 65 to 75% of vaccinees develop protective anti HBs titers [48–50]. Moreover, the vaccine prevents development of chronic hepatitis in at least 75% of early-vaccinated infants born from HBeAg-positive mothers [51].

Cost-benefit analyses have strongly supported the introduction of universal immunization against HBV to newborns [52]. Since 1992, the WHO has called for all countries to add hepatitis B vaccine into their national childhood immunization schedules, and substantial progress has been made in implementing this recommendation: by the end of 2003 more than 160 countries worldwide will have introduced the vaccine [53]. Substantial help in achieving this goal has been given by the Global Alliance for Vaccines and Immunization (GAVI) and the Vaccine Fund, which since 2000 began to provide technical and financial support to introduce routine HBV immunization into 71 of the world's poorest countries [54].

The effectiveness of routine infant HBV immunization in significantly reducing or eliminating the prevalence of chronic HBV infection has been demonstrated in a variety of countries and settings. The experience in Taiwan is particularly impressive. Universal vaccination decreased the prevalence of HBsAg carriage in children younger than 15 years of age from 9.8% in 1984 to 0.7% in 1999 [55]. Moreover, rates of hepatocellular carcinoma (HCC) among cohorts of children born after routine infant immunization have started in the mid 1980s declined by greater than 50% [56]. These results clearly show that the HBV vaccine is the first successful anti-cancer vaccine, opening the way to other anti-cancer vaccines like vaccines against human papilloma virus (HPV) that causes cervical cancer [57], or *Helicobacter pylori*, responsible for many gastric cancers [58].

Genetically detoxified vaccines

The first example of a vaccine developed with a new rational strategic design, taking advantage of the power of the molecular biology and genomic technologies is the recombinant acellular pertussis vaccine.

A vaccine composed of the whole, killed *Bordetella pertussis* cells has been available for mass vaccination since the late 1940s [59]. This vaccine is very efficacious in preventing the disease, but the presence of severe adverse reactions, although no proof exists of their having been caused by the vaccine, brought about a drop in vaccine compliance in the 1970s and stressed the need for a new safer vaccine.

A considerable amount of work was initially required to identify the bacterial antigens responsible for the induction of protection. Pertussis toxin (PT) was then identified as a major protective antigen, while other antigens, such as adenylate cyclase, filamentous haemagglutinin (FHA), pertactin and the fimbriae, were found to provide some help in protective immunity. Several researchers developed acellular pertussis vaccines containing purified PT inactivated by the old classical chemical treatment with formaldehyde and glutaraldehyde. However, it is recognized that this treatment of PT may be associated with significant reversion rates [60].

To overcome these problems, the pertussis toxin was detoxified by using the powerful tools of molecular biology to make stable changes, by site-directed mutagenesis, to the amino acids responsible for the toxicity of pertussis toxin. This molecular approach allowed the development of a naturally nontoxic molecule, inactivated by a rational design that did not need a denaturing chemical treatment [61].

The genetically detoxified PT had successfully shown its safety and immunogenicity in clinical trials, both in adult volunteers and in infants and children, either as a monovalent mutant PT alone [62, 63], or in association with FHA and pertactin [64, 65], and also with FHA and pertactin in association with diphtheria and tetanus toxoids (DTaP) [66, 67]. These trials showed that the different acellular vaccine formulations containing the non-toxic PT mutant were extremely safe, and much safer than the whole-cell pertussis vaccines. Furthermore, all formulations induced high titers of anti-PT neutralizing antibodies and very strong antigen-specific T-cell proliferative responses. Interestingly enough, five to six years after the primary immunization schedule, this vaccine still exhibited an efficacy of about 80%, and both antigen-specific antibody and $CD4^+$ T-cell responses were still detectable at significant levels [68, 69].

The new strategy used to develop this genetically detoxified acellular pertussis vaccine shows that this approach can provide tremendous advantages, eliciting very high, protective immune responses with very low amounts of antigen.

The genomic approach: reverse vaccinology

Despite the introduction of these new strategies (conjugation, recombinant DNA etc.), one of the major issues for the development of new vaccines is the identification of protective antigens from a microorganism. Biochemical, immunological and microbiological methods have been successful in many cases, but they require the pathogen to be grown in laboratory conditions, are time-consuming and allow for the identification only of the most abundant antigens, which can be purified in quantities suitable for vaccine testing. Unfortunately, in many instances the most abundant proteins could not be good vaccine candidates. Moreover, the antigens expressed *in vivo* during the infection could not be expressed *in vitro* to the same extent. Furthermore, when dealing with non-cultivable pathogens, there is no approach to vaccine development.

The availability of the complete genome sequence of a free-living organism (*H. influenzae*) [70] marked the beginning of the "genomic era" that opened novel strategies in vaccine design. The possibility of determining the whole sequence of a genome (bacterial, viral or parasitic) led to the idea of using the genomic information to discover novel antigens that have been missed by conventional vaccinology. This approach, called "reverse vaccinology", involves the computer (*in silico*) analysis of the microbial genome sequence and predicts those antigens that are most likely to be vaccine candidates [71, 72]. The success of genomic-based strategies for vaccine development is highly dependent on the criteria used for the *in silico* selection of the potential antigens, which are usually secreted or extracellular proteins, more easily accessible to antibodies than intracellular ones. Several approaches can be used to mine genomic sequences, and the appropriate combination of various algorithms and the critical evaluation of the information generated are essential for the proper selection of the antigens.

The *in silico* approach results in the selection of a large number of genes. Therefore, it is necessary to use simple procedures that allow large numbers of genes to be cloned and expressed, like robotics and PCR. The product of each PCR reaction is cloned and screened for expression in a heterologous system. Successful expression depends on the predicted localization of the protein. Integral transmembrane proteins have proven to be particularly difficult to produce by recombinant techniques in *E. coli*.

Once purified, the recombinant proteins are used to immunize mice and the post-immunization sera are analyzed to verify the computer-predicted surface localization of each polypeptide and their ability to elicit a quantitative and qualitative immune, protective response.

The genomic approach has many novel features and advantages. There is no need to cultivate the pathogen. As the whole process starts *in silico*, it could be equally applied to cultivable and non-cultivable microorganisms. Pathogens dangerous to handle can be studied as easily as commensals. Virtually all protein antigens encoded by the pathogen's genome could become vaccine candidates, regardless whether they are expressed *in vitro* or *in vivo*, abundant or scarce. This process allows the identification of all the antigens seen by the conventional methods and the discovery of novel antigens that work on a totally different paradigm.

Unfortunately, reverse vaccinology suffers from limitations related to our incomplete knowledge of vaccine immunology: a rate-limiting step of the process is linked to the rarity (or, more often, absence) of widely accepted correlates of protection and reliable animal models of infection. The other constraint of this approach is the inability to identify non-protein antigens such as polysaccharides, and CD-1 restricted antigens such as glycolipids, which represent new promising vaccine candidates.

Meningococcus B

Meningococcus B represents the first example of the application of the genomic approach and the demonstration of the power of this novel strategy for target antigen identification [73]. Conventional approaches to MenB vaccine development have been ineffective for more than 40 years. A capsular polysaccharide-based approach, which has been extremely successful for other major meningococcal serogroups, cannot be used for this strain, because the MenB capsular polysaccharide is identical to a widely distributed human carbohydrate (α(2–8)N-acetyl neuraminic acid, or polysialic acid). This condition not only makes the polysaccharide a poor immunogen for humans, but also a potential generator of autoantibodies. On the other hand, a protein-based approach, developed using surface-exposed proteins contained in outer membrane vesicles (OMVs), has shown to have efficacy in clinical trials only against homologous strains, especially in children below five years of age, because of the high sequence variability of the major protein antigens [74].

Using the reverse vaccinology, DNA fragments were screened by computer analysis while the *N. meningitidis* sequencing project was in progress. The screening was aimed to select proteins predicted to be on the surface of the bacterium or to have homologies to known bacterial factors involved in pathogenesis and virulence. After clearance of cytoplasmic proteins and known *Neisseria* antigens, 570 genes predicted to code for surface-exposed or membrane-associated proteins were recognized. Successful cloning in *E. coli* and expression was achieved for 350 proteins, which were then purified and tested for localization, immunogenicity and protective efficacy in animal models. Of the 85 proteins found to be surface exposed, 22 were able to induce complement-mediated bactericidal antibody response, which is the most convincing indication of the capability of inducing protective immunity. In addition, to test the appropriateness of these proteins as candidate antigens for conferring protection against heterologous strains, the proteins were evaluated for gene presence, phase variation and sequence conservation in a panel of genetically diverse MenB strains representative of the global diversity of the natural *N. meningitidis* population. Most of the selected antigens were able to induce cross-protection against heterologous strains, demonstrating that these new antigens are good candidates for the clinical development of a vaccine against MenB [73, 75].

It is impressive to notice that within only 18 months the genomic approach allowed the discovery of more potential vaccine candidates than the previous 40 years of conventional research.

The success of the MenB project, together with the availability of an increasing number of genomic sequences and the faster and faster development of bioinformatics tools, has encouraged the application of the reverse vaccinology approach to many other pathogens. Nowadays, this approach is widely used to develop vaccine candidates against those pathogens for which conventional approaches have failed so far. The potential of the genomic approach is so extensive that it could be used not only for bacteria, but also for viruses and parasites.

Streptococcus pneumoniae

Despite the successes of the conjugate vaccine against *Streptococcus pneumoniae* (see above), the absence of cross protection between the different serotypes, with the threat of serotype replacement by strains that are not represented in the vaccine composition, makes it unsuitable for universal use [20]. To identify more appropriate vaccine candidates, the whole genome sequence of *S. pneumoniae* was scanned and 130 potential ORFs with significant homology to surface proteins and virulence factors of other bacteria were identified [76]. 108 of these proteins were effectively expressed in *E. coli* and used to immunize mice; six of them were able to confer protection against pneumococcal challenge in a mouse sepsis model. Flow cytometry confirmed the surface localization of these new proteins. Furthermore, each of the six protective antigens showed a high degree of cross reactivity against the majority of capsular antigens that are expressed *in vivo* and are immunogenic during human infection, providing a good base for the development of improved vaccines against *S. pneumoniae*.

Streptococcus agalactiae

Streptococcus agalactiae, or group B streptococcus, is the leading cause of bacterial sepsis, pneumonia, and meningitis in neonates in US and Europe [77]. As for *S. pneumoniae*, the capsular polysaccharide is the major protective antigen, but at least nine different seroptypes exist with little or no cross protection [78]. Therefore, a protein-based vaccine is required to overcome serotype differences.

The complete genome of a serotype V strain of *S. agalactiae* was determined and analyzed [79]. The genome is predicted to code for 2175 ORFs of which 650 were predicted to be exposed on the surface of the bacteria. Approximately 350 of these ORFs were successfully expressed in *E. coli* and used to immunize mice. Using the sera in ELISA and flow cytometric analysis against intact bacteria, it has been demonstrated that 55 of these proteins are in fact measurably expressed on the surface of the bacterium. These new antigens are now being evaluated in *in vitro* and *in vivo* models for their capacity to protect against invasive infection by group B streptococcus.

Staphylococcus aureus

To identify vaccine candidates for *Staphylococcus aureus*, an approach based on genomic peptide libraries and well-characterized human sera was developed [80]. *S. aureus* peptides were displayed on the surface of *E. coli via* fusion to one or two outer membrane proteins (LamB and FhuA) and probed with sera selected for high antibody titers and opsonic activity. The exhaustive screening of the two different peptide expression libraries by the application of MACS technology (magnetic cell sorting) enabled the profile of antigens that are expressed *in vivo* and that are able to elicit an immune response in humans to be identified. A total of 60 antigenic proteins were identified, most of which were predicted to be secreted, or located on the surface of the bacterium, and their antibody-binding sites were mapped. These antigens represent promising vaccine candidates for further evaluation.

Porphyromonas gingivalis

A process very similar to the one used to develop a vaccine against MenB was used also for *Porphyromonas gingivalis*, a pathogen implicated in the etiology of chronic adult periodontitis [81]. From a genomic sequence of 2000 genes, 120 were selected using a series of bioinformatics tools. The selected genes were cloned for expression in *E. coli* and screened by Western blotting using sera from human periodontitis patients and animal antisera. This subset of 40 recombinant proteins were then purified and used to immunize mice, which were subsequently challenged with live bacteria in a subcutaneous abscess model. Two of these recombinant proteins (showing homology to *Pseudomonas* sp. OprF protein) demonstrated significant protection in the animal model and therefore could represent potential vaccine candidates [82].

Chlamydia pneumoniae

Chlamydia pneumoniae is an obligate intracellular parasite with a complex biphasic lifecycle: an extracellular infectious phase characterized by a spore-like form, the elementary bodies (EB), and an intracellular replicating stage characterized by the reticular bodies (RB). The pathogen is a common cause of community-acquired acute respiratory infections and more recently has also been associated with atherosclerotic cardiovascular disease [83].

Because of the technical difficulties in working with *C. pneumoniae* and the absence of reliable tools for genetic manipulation, not much is known about the cell surface composition of the EB. To define the surface protein organization of *C. pneumoniae*, a systematic genomic and proteomic approach was used [84]. The approach is based on six main experimental steps: (i) *in silico* analysis of the *C. pneumoniae* genome sequence to identify genes potentially encoding surface proteins (including outer and inner membrane and periplasmic proteins); (ii) cloning, expression, and purification of selected candidates; (iii) use of purified antigens to generate mouse immune sera; (iv) analysis of sera specificity by Western blotting of total EB extracts; (v) assessment of antigen localization by FACS analysis on whole EBs; and (vi) identification of FACS-positive antigens on bidimensional electrophoresis (2DE) maps of *C. pneumoniae* EB proteins. The results of this systematic genome-proteome approach represent the first successful attempt to define surface protein organization of *C. pneumoniae* and raise the possibility to find suitable candidates for a purified vaccine.

Reverse vaccinology for bioterrorism-associated agents: Bacillus anthracis and Yersinia pestis

Currently licensed anthrax vaccines have been developed during the 1960s and are based on cell-free filtrates containing mainly the Protective Antigen (PA). PA is the common cell-binding domain capable of interacting with two different domains, the lethal and the edema factors, which elicit cell damage. These vaccines, originally licensed for selected veterinary personnel, textile workers and abattoir workers, have been widely used for the first time for the US military during the 1990–91 Desert Storm campaign. However, this extended use has raised issues and controversies regarding safety, efficacy, and an unsatisfactory dosing regimen, as the vaccine requires 6-dose series of injections and annual boosters [85, 86].

Therefore, identification of novel antigens is essential for the development of second-generation *B. anthracis* vaccines. ORF products similar to proteins involved in bacterial pathogenesis, and secreted and surface exposed proteins are the focus of the research. Using functional genomic analysis, 11 candidates were selected. In this case, a simple method that relied on the *in vitro* translation of the linear full-length DNA of the selected ORFs was used. Polypeptides obtained *in vitro* were then evaluated for immunogenicity by analysis of their reactivity with hyperimmune anti-*B. anthracis* antisera. The combination of bioinformatic genomic analysis and an efficient and fast screening facilitated the identification of unknown antigenic proteins, three of which appear to be similar to immunogenic PA. These new proteins could represent parts of a second-generation anthrax vaccine [87].

Old plague vaccines are based on killed whole cell preparations [86, 88]. Although they appeared to be effective against endemic plague, they were not considered to be protective against respiratory plague, which is the form of most concern in case of biological attack. Moreover, these vaccines have high rates of reactions, both systemic and local, especially with successive doses and suffer from short duration of protection, requiring biannual boosters. A live-attenuated vaccine (EV76 strain) also existed. While this vaccine seemed to be effective, it retained some virulence and in most countries it was considered not suitable for human use.

In a search for novel attenuated vaccine candidates for use against *Y. pestis*, a signature-tagged mutagenesis (STM) strategy was used [89]. A library of tagged mutants of the virulent *Y. pestis* Kimberley53 strain was generated. Screening of 300 mutants through two consecutive cycles resulted in selection of 16 mutant strains. Characterization of the phenotypes and genotypes of the selected mutants led to identification of virulence-associated genes coding for factors involved in global bacterial physiology (e.g., *purH*, *purK*, *dnaE*, and *greA*) or for hypothetical polypeptides, as well as for the virulence regulator gene *lcrF*. One of the avirulent mutant strains was found to be disrupted in the *pcm* locus, which is presumably involved in the bacterial response to environmental stress. This Kimberley*53pcm* mutant was superior to the EV76 live vaccine strain in an animal model in which mice were infected subcutaneously with the virulent *Y. pestis* Kimberley53 strain, either because the mutant induced 10- to 100-fold-higher antibody titers to the protective V and F1 antigens and because it conferred efficacious protective immunity. These results indicate that mutants with mutations in the *pcm* locus can serve as a platform for generation of a novel live vaccine with more promise for inducing efficacious protective immunity to virulent *Y. pestis* strains than previously suggested mutants.

New strategies for new diseases: SARS example

The SARS epidemic has been the first infectious disease outbreak to fully benefit from the revolutionary technologies of the post-genomic era. Thanks to an unprecedented collaboration effort between scientists from many countries, coordinated by WHO and including clinical, epidemiological and laboratory investigations, within 15 days from the issue of the global alert, the causative agent of the new disease was discovered [90]. In less than a month after the initial identification of a new coronavirus (called SARS-CoV) as the infectious agent of SARS, two independent genome sequences of the virus had been obtained [91, 92]. Within three months, the genome sequences of 20 independent clinical isolates were made available in the GenBank database. The rapid availability of the genomic sequence of the new virus has been very important from the public health perspective, giving prompt answers to a number of critical questions. It was clear that the agent was a natural (and not a laboratory-fabricated) coronavirus, diagnostic kits were set up, and possible drug and vaccine targets identified.

Today, some of these vaccines, based on a killed virus, are already being tested in pre-clinical and even in clinical trials, but their efficacy needs to be shown. Moreover, in addition to the traditional approach, a number of newer strategies are being used. These include subunit vaccines containing recombinant spike protein expressed in mammalian cells or yeast, either alone or in combination with other SARS-CoV antigens. Alternatively, these antigens could be delivered by DNA immunization by non-replicating viruses, or viral vectors that are based on adenovirus, canarypox, modified vaccinia virus Ankara (MVA) or alphavirus. In particular, the development of non-replicating coronavirus-like particles that mimic the structure of native virions could prove promising in the search for a successful vaccine as they display a large repertoire of antigenic sites and discontinuous epitopes [93].

It is crucial to remember that none of these approaches would have been possible in such a way and with such a speed without the knowledge of the complete genomic sequence of the virus. To make a comparison, the last time mankind faced the appearance of a new pandemic was in the early 1980s, with the appearance of HIV: at that time, only 20 years ago, it took two years to identify the etiologic agent of the infection, and a safe and effective vaccine is still lacking.

Conclusion

When Edward Jenner gave birth to the concept of vaccination little could he know that after more than 200 years mankind would still be battling against emerging and re-emerging infectious diseases. However, contemporary society is lucky in that science is constantly offering more effective tools to combat and control infectious diseases. The question is whether the many social, political, cultural, and economic barriers that still exist *vis-à-vis* vaccines will be eventually overcome, thus recognizing the real value of vaccination.

References

1 Glenny AT, Hopkins BE (1923) Diphtheria toxoid as an immunizing agent. *Br J Exp Pathol* 4: 283–288

2 Ramon G (1923) Sur le pouvoir floculant et sur les propriétés immunisantes d'une toxine diphthérique rendue anatoxique (anatoxine). *CR Acad Sci (Paris)* 177: 1338–1340

3 Ramon G (1925) Sur la production des antitoxins. *CR Acad Sci (Paris)* 181: 157–159

4 Ehreth J (2003) The global value of vaccination. *Vaccine* 21: 596–600

5 World Health Organization, Fact sheet N.114, Poliomyelitis, revised April 2003, accessed May 2004: http://www.who.int/mediacentre/factsheets/fs114/en/

6 Jodar L, Feavers IM, Salisbury D, Granoff DM (2002) Development of vaccines against meningococcal disease. *Lancet* 359: 1499–1508

7 Morley SL, Pollard AJ (2002) Vaccine prevention of meningococcal disease, coming soon? *Vaccine* 20: 666–687

8 Wenger JD, Ward JI (2004) Haemophilus influenzae vaccine. In: SA Plotkin, WA Orenstein (eds): *Vaccines*. Fourth Edition, Saunders, Philadelphia, 229–268

9 Wuorimaa T, Kayhty H (2002) Current state of pneumococcal vaccines. *Scand J Immunol* 56: 111–129

10 Plotkin SA, Bouveret-Le Cam N (1995) A new typhoid vaccine composed of the Vi capsular polysaccharide. *Arch Intern Med* 155: 2293–2299

11 Wenger J, Campbell H, Miller E., Salisbury D (2004) The postlicensure impact of Haemophilus influenzae type b and serogroup C *Neisseria meningitidis* conjugate vaccines. In: MM Levine, JB Kaper, R Rappuoli, MA Liu, MF Good (eds): *New generation vaccines*. Third Edition. Marcel Dekker, New York, 427–441

12 Peltola H (2000) Worldwide Haemophilus influenzae type b disease at the beginning of the 21st century: global analysis of the disease burden 25 years after the use of the polysaccharide vaccine and a decade after the advent of conjugates. *Clin Microbiol Rev* 13: 302–317

13 Cochi SL, Broome CV, Hightower AW (1985) Immunization of US children with Haemophilus influenzae type b polysaccharide vaccine: a cost-effectiveness model of strategy assessment. *JAMA* 253: 521–529

14 CDC (2004) Summary of notifiable diseases, United States, 2002. MMWR, Published April 30, 2004 for 2002 51(53): 8

15 Takala AK, Eskola J, Leinonen M, Kayhty H, Nissinen A, Pekkanen E, Makela PH (1991) Reduction of oropharyngeal carriage of *Haemophilus influenzae* type b (Hib) in children immunized with an Hib conjugate vaccine. *J Infect Dis* 164: 982–986

16 Murphy TV, Pastor P, Medley F, Osterholm MT, Granoff DM (1993) Decreased *Haemophilus* colonization in children vaccinated with *Haemophilus influenzae* type b conjugate vaccine. *J Pediatr* 122: 517–523

17 Barbour ML, Mayon-White RT, Coles C, Crook DW, Moxon ER (1995) The impact of conjugate vaccine on carriage of *Haemophilus influenzae* type b. *J Infect Dis* 171: 93–98

18 Forleo-Neto E, de Oliveira CF, Maluf EM, Bataglin C, Araujo JM, Kunz LF Jr, Pustai AK, Vieira VS, Zanella RC, Brandileone MC et al (1999) Decreased point prevalence of *Haemophilus influenzae* type b (Hib) oropharyngeal colonization by mass immunization of Brazilian children less than 5 years old with Hib polyribosylribitol phosphate polysaccharide-tetanus toxoid conjugate vaccine in combination with diphtheria-tetanus toxoids-pertussis vaccine. *J Infect Dis* 180: 1153–1158

19 Lipsitch M (1997) Vaccination against colonizing bacteria with multiple serotypes. *Proc Natl Acad Sci USA* 94: 6571–6576

20 Lipsitch M (1999) Bacterial vaccines and serotype replacement: lessons from Haemophilus influenzae and prospects for *Streptococcus pneumoniae*. *Emerg Infect Dis* 5: 336–345

21 Ribeiro GS, Reis JN, Cordeiro SM, Lima JB, Gouveia EL, Petersen M, Salgado K, Silva HR, Zanella RC, Almeida SC et al (2003) Prevention of *Haemophilus influenzae* type b (Hib) meningitis and emergence of serotype replacement with type a strains after introduction of Hib immunization in Brazil. *J Infect Dis* 187: 1109–1116

22 Lucher LA, Reeves M, Hennessy T, Levine OS, Popovic T, Rosenstein N, Parkinson AJ (2002) Reemergence, in Southwestern Alaska, of invasive *Haemophilus influenzae* type b disease due to strains indistinguishable from those isolated from vaccinated children. *J Infect Dis* 187: 958–965

23 Siber GR (1994) Pneumococcal disease: prospects for a new generation of vaccines. *Science* 265: 1385–1387

24 Levine O, Klein DL, Butler JC (2004) Pneumococcal protein-polysaccharide conjugate vaccines. In: MM Levine, JB Kaper, R Rappuoli, MA Liu, MF Good

(eds): *New generation vaccines*. Third edition. Marcel Dekker, New York, 443–457

25 Robinson KA, Baughman W, Rothrock G, Barrett NL, Pass M, Lexau C, Damaske B, Stefonek K, Barnes B, Patterson J et al (2001) Epidemiology of invasive *Streptococcus pneumoniae* infections in the United States, 1995–1998: opportunities for prevention in the conjugate vaccine era. *JAMA* 285: 1729–1735

26 Hausdorff WP, Bryant J, Paradiso PR, Siber GR (2000) Which pneumococcal serogroups cause the most invasive disease: implications for conjugate vaccine formulation and use, Part I. *Clin Infect Dis* 30: 100–121

27 CDC (2000) Prevention of pneumococcal disease among infants and young children using a pneumococcal conjugate vaccine. Recommendations of the Advisory Committee on Immunization Practices (ACIP). *MMWR* 49 (RR-9): 1–35

28 Black S, Shinefield H, Fireman B, Lewis E, Ray P, Hansen JR, Elvin L, Ensor KM, Hackell J, Siber G et al (2000) Efficacy, safety, and immunogenicity of heptavalent pneumococcal conjugate vaccine in children. Northern California Kaiser Permanente Vaccine Study Center Group. *Pediatr Infect Dis J* 19: 187–195

29 Eskola J, Kilpi T, Palmu A, Jokinen J, Haapakoski J, Herva E, Takala A, Kayhty H, Karma P, Kohberger R et al (2001) Efficacy of a pneumococcal conjugate vaccine against acute otitis media. *N Engl J Med* 344: 403–409

30 Eskola J, Black S, Shinefield H (2004) Pneumococcal conjugate vaccines. In: SA Plotkin, WA Orenstein (eds): *Vaccines*. Fourth edition, Saunders, Philadelphia, 589–624

31 Costantino P, Viti S, Podda A, Velmonte MA, Nencioni L, Rappuoli R (1992) Development and phase I clinical testing of a conjugate vaccine against meningococcus A and C. *Vaccine* 10 (10): 691–698

32 Anderson EL, Bowers T, Mink CM, Kennedy DJ, Belshe RB, Harakeh H, Pais L, Holder P, Carlone GM (1994) Safety and immunogenicity of meningococcal A and C polysaccharide conjugate vaccine in adults. *Infect Immun* 62(8): 3391–3395

33 Twumasi PA Jr, Kumah S, Leach A, O'Dempsey TJ, Ceesay SJ, Todd J, Broome CV, Carlone GM, Pais LB, Holder PK et al (1995) A trial of a group A plus group C meningococcal polysaccharide-protein conjugate vaccine in African infants. *J Infect Dis* 171(3): 632–638

34 Lieberman JM, Chiu SS, Wong VK, Partidge S, Chang SJ, Chiu CY, Gheesling LL, Carlone GM, Ward JI (1996) Safety and immunogenicity of a serogroups A:C *Neisseria meningitidis* oligosaccharide-protein conjugate vaccine in young children. A randomized controlled trial. *JAMA* 275(19): 1499–1503

35 Fairley CK, Begg N, Borrow R, Fox AJ, Jones DM, Cartwright K (1996) Conjugate meningococcal serogroup A and C vaccine: reactogenicity and immunogenicity in United Kingdom infants. *J Infect Dis* 174(6): 1360–1363

36 Leach A, Twumasi PA, Kumah S, Banya WS, Jaffar S, Forrest BD, Granoff DM, LiButti DE, Carlone GM, Pais LB et al (1997) Induction of immunologic mem-

ory in Gambian children by vaccination in infancy with a group A plus group C meningococcal polysacchairde-protein conjugate vaccine. *J Infect Dis* 175(1): 200–204

37 MacDonald NE, Halperin SA, Law BJ, Forrest B, Danzig LE, Granoff DM et al (1998) Induction of immunologic mamory by conjugated vs plain meningococcal C polysaccharide vaccines in toddlers: a randomized controlled trial. *JAMA* 280: 1685–1689

38 Richmond P, Borrow R, Miller E, Clark S, Sadler F, Fox A, Begg N, Morris R, Cartwright K et al (1999) Meningococcal group C conjugate vaccine is immunogenic in infancy and primes for memory. *J Infect Dis* 179: 1569–1572

39 Borrow R, Fox AJ, Richmond PC, Clark S, Sadler F, Findlow J, Morris R, Begg NT, Cartwright KA et al (2000) Induction of immunological memory in UK infants by a meningococcal AC conjugate vaccine. *Epidemiol Infect* 124(3): 427–432

40 Miller E, Salisbury D, Ramsay M (2001) Planning, registration, and implementation of an immunization campaign against meningococcal serogroup C disease in the UK: a success story. *Vaccine* 20 (Suppl. 1): S58–S67

41 Ramsay M, Andrews N, Kacmarski EB, Miller E (2001) Efficacy of meningococcal serogroup C conjugate vaccine in teenagers and toddlers in England. Lancet 357: 195–196

42 Maiden MC, Stuart JM, UK Meningococcal Carriage Group (2002) Reduced carriage of serogroup C meningococci in teenagers one year after the introduction of meningococcal C conjugate vaccine in the United Kingdom. *Lancet* 359: 1829–1831

43 Balmer P, Borrow R, Miller E (2002) Impact of meningococcal C conjugate vaccine in the UK. *J Med Microbiol* 51: 717–722

44 Granoff DM, Feavers IM, Borrow R (2004) Meningococcal vaccines. In: SA Plotkin, WA Orenstein (eds): *Vaccines*. Fourth edition, Saunders, Philadelphia, 959–987

45 Rappuoli R, Pollard AJ, Moxon R (2004) Meningococcal conjugate and protein-based vaccines. In: MM Levine, JB Kaper, R Rappuoli, MA Liu, MF Good (eds): *New generation vaccines*. Third edition. Marcel Dekker, New York, 421–426

46 Szmuness W, Stevens CE, Harley EJ, Zang EA, Oleszko WR, William DC, Sadovsky R, Morrison JM, Kellner A (1980) Hepatitis B vaccine: demonstration of efficacy in a controlled clinical trial in a high risk population in the US. *N Engl J Med* 303: 833–841

47 Valenzuela P, Medina A, Rutter WJ, Ammerer G, Hall BD (1982) Synthesis and assembly of hepatitis B virus surface antigen particles in yeast. *Nature* 298: 347–350

48 Coates T, Wilson R, Patrick G, Andre F, Watson V (2001) Hepatitis B vaccines: assessment of the seroprotective efficacy of two recombinant DNA vaccines. *Clin Ther* 23: 392–403

49 Andre FE (1990) Overview of a 5-year clinical experience with a yeast-derived hepatitis B vaccine. *Vaccine* 8 (Suppl): S74–S78

50 Clements ML, Miskovsky E, Davidson M, Cupps T, Kumwenda N, Sandman LA, West D, Hesley T, Ioli V, Miller W et al (1994) Effect of age on the immunogenicity of yeast recombinant hepatitis B vaccines containing surface antigen S or PreS2 + S antigens. *J Infect Dis* 170: 510–516

51 Poovorawan Y, Sanpavat S, Pongpunglert W, Chumdermpadetsuk S, Sentrakul P, Vandepapeliere P, Safary A (1992) Long term efficacy of hepatitis B vaccine in infants born to hepatitis B e antigen-positive mothers. *Pediatr Infect Dis J* 11: 816–821

52 Arevalo JA, Washington E (1988) Cost effectiveness of perinatal screening and immunization for hepatitis B virus. *JAMA* 259: 365–369

53 World Health Organization (1992) Expanded program on immunization global advisory group. *Wk Epidemiol Rec* 3: 11–16

54 Mast E, Mahoney F, Kane M, Margolis H (2004) Hepatitis B vaccine. In: SA Plotkin, WA Orenstein (eds): *Vaccines*. Fourth edition, Saunders, Philadelphia, 299–337

55 Lin YC, Chang MH, Ni YH, Hsu HY, Chen DS (2003) Long-term immunogenicity and efficacy of universal hepatitis B virus vaccination in Taiwan. *J Infect Dis* 187: 134–138

56 Chang MH, Chen CJ, Lai MS, Hsu HM, Wu TC, Kong MS, Liang DC, Shau WY, Chen DS (1997) Universal hepatitis B vaccination in Taiwan and the incidence of hepatocellular carcinoma in children. Taiwan Childhood Hepatoma Study Group. *N Engl J Med* 336: 1855–1859

57 Koutsky LA, Ault KA, Wheeler CM, Brown DR, Barr E, Alvarez FB, Chiacchierini LM, Jansen KU, Proof of Principle Study Investigators (2002) A controlled trial of a human papillomavirus type 16 vaccine. *N Engl J Med* 347(21): 1645–1651

58 Del Giudice G, Covacci A, Telford J, Montecucco C, Rappuoli R (2001) The design of vaccines against *Helicobacter pylori* and their development. *Annu Rev Immunol* 19: 523–563

59 Kendrick PL, Eldering G, Dixon MK (1947) Mouse protection tests in the study of pertussis vaccine: a comparative study using intracerebral route for challenge. *Am J Publ Health* 37: 803

60 National Bacteriological Laboratory, Sweden (1988) A clinical trial of acellular pertussis vaccine in Sweden. Technical Report 1988, Stockholm.

61 Pizza M, Covacci A, Bartoloni A, Perugini M, Nencioni L, De Magistris MT, Villa L, Nucci D, Manetti R, Bugnoli M et al (1989) Mutants of pertussis toxin suitable for vaccine development. *Science* 246: 497–500

62 Podda A, Nencioni L, De Magistris MT, Di Tommaso A, Bossu P, Nuti S, Pileri P, Peppoloni S, Bugnoli M, Ruggiero P et al (1990) Metabolic, humoral, and cellular responses in adult volunteers immunized with the genetically inactivated pertussis toxin mutant PT-9K/ 129G. *J Exp Med* 172: 861–868

63 Podda A, De Luca EC, Titone L, Casadei AM, Cascio A, Peppoloni S, Volpini G, Marsili I, Nencioni L, Rappuoli R (1992) Acellular pertussis vaccine composed of genetically inactivated pertussis toxin: safety and immunogenicity in 12- to 24- and 2- to 4-month-old children. *J Pediatr* 120: 680–685

64 Podda A, Nencioni L, Marsili I, Peppoloni S, Volpini G, Donati D, Di Tommaso A, De Magistris MT, Rappuoli R (1991) Phase I clinical trial of an acellular pertussis vaccine composed of genetically detoxified pertussis toxin combined with FHA and 69 kDa. *Vaccine* 9: 741–745

65 Podda A, Carapella De Luca E, Titone L, Casadei AM, Cascio A, Bartalini M, Volpini G, Marsili I, Nencioni L, Rappuoli R (1993) Immunogenicity of an acellular pertussis vaccine composed of genetically inactivated pertussis toxin combined with filamentous hemagglutinin and pertactin in infants and children. *J Pediatr* 123: 81–84

66 Greco D, Salmaso S, Mastrantonio P, Giuliano M, Tozzi AE, Anemona A, Ciofi degli Atti ML, Giammanco A, Panei P, Blackwelder WC et al (1996) A controlled trial of two acellular vaccines and one whole-cell vaccine against pertussis. Progetto Pertosse Working Group. *N Engl J Med* 334(6): 341–348

67 Olin P, Rasmussen F, Gustafsson L, Hallander HO, Heijbel H (1997) Randomised controlled trial of two-component, three-component, and five-component acellular pertussis vaccines compared with whole-cell pertussis vaccine. Ad Hoc Group for the Study of Pertussis Vaccines. *Lancet* 350(9091): 1569–1577

68 Di Tommaso A, Bartalini M, Peppoloni S, Podda A, Rappuoli R, De Magistris MT (1997) Acellular pertussis vaccines containing genetically detoxified pertussis toxin induce long-lasting humoral and cellular responses in adults. *Vaccine* 15: 1218–1224

69 Salmaso S, Mastrantonio P, Tozzi AE, Stefanelli P, Anemona A, Ciofi degli Atti ML, Giammanco A, Stage III Working Group (2001) Sustained efficacy during the first 6 years of life of 3-component acellular pertussis vaccines administered in infancy: the Italian experience. *Pediatrics* 108, E81

70 Fleischmann RD, Adams MD, White O, Clayton RA, Kirkness EF, Kerlavage AR, Bult CJ, Tomb JF, Dougherty BA, Merrick JM et al (1995) Whole-genome random sequencing and assembly of *Haemophilus influenzae* Rd. *Science* 269: 496–512

71 Rappuoli R (2001) Reverse vaccinology, a genome-based approach to vaccine development. *Vaccine* 19: 2688–2691

72 Mora M, Veggi D, Santini L, Pizza M (2003) Reverse vaccinology. *Drug Discovery Today* 8(10): 459–464

73 Pizza M, Scarlato V, Masignani V, Giuliani MM, Aricò B, Comanducci M, Jennings GT, Baldi L, Bartolini E, Capecchi B et al (2000) Whole genome sequencing to identify vaccine candidates against serogroup B meningococcus. *Science* 287: 1816–1820

74 Tappero JW, Lagos R, Ballesteros AM, Plikaytis B, Williams D, Dykes J, Gheesling LL, Carlone GM, Hoiby EA, Holst J et al (1999) Immunogenicity of 2 serogroup B outer-membrane protein meningococcal vaccines: A randomised controlled trial in Chile. *JAMA* 281: 1520–1527

75 Adu-Bobie J, Capecchi B, Serruto D (2003) Two years into reverse vaccinology. *Vaccine* 21: 605–610

76 Wizemann TM, Heinrichs JH, Adamou JE, Erwin AL, Kunsch C, Choi GH,

Barash SC, Rosen CA, Masure HR, Tuomanen E et al (2001) Use of a whole genome approach to identify vaccine molecules affording protection against *Streptococcus pneumoniae* infection. *Infect Immun* 69: 1593–1598
77 Schuchat A (1999) Group B streptococcus. *Lancet* 353: 51–56
78 Paoletti LC, Kasper DL (2002) Conjugate vaccines against group B *Streptococcus* types IV and VII. *J Infect Dis* 186(1): 123–126
79 Tettelin H, Masignani V, Cieslewicz MJ, Eisen JA, Peterson S, Wessels MR, Paulsen IT, Nelson KE, Margarit I, Read TD et al (2002) Complete genome sequence and comparative genomic analysis of an emerging human pathogen, serotype V Streptococcus agalactiae. *Proc Natl Acad Sci USA* 99: 12391–12396
80 Etz H, Minh DB, Henics T, Dryla A, Winkler B, Triska C, Boyd AP, Sollner J, Schmidt W, von Ahsen U et al (2002) Identification of *in vivo* expressed vaccine candidate antigens from *Staphylococcus aureus*. *Proc Natl Acad Sci USA* 99(10): 6573–6578
81 The American Academy of Periodontology (1999) The pathogenesis of periodontal diseases. *J Periodontol* 70: 457–470
82 Ross BC, Czajkowski L, Hocking D, Margetts M, Webb E, Rothel L, Patterson M, Agius C, Camuglia S, Reynolds E et al (2001) Identification of vaccine candidate antigens from a genomic analysis of *Porphyromonas gingivalis*. *Vaccine* 19(30): 4135–4142
83 Grayston JT (2000) Background and current knowledge of *Chlamydia pneumoniae* and atherosclerosis. *J Infect Dis* 181(Suppl 3): S402–S410
84 Montigiani S, Falugi F, Scarselli M, Finco O, Petracca R, Galli G, Mariani M, Manetti R, Agnusdei M, Cevenini R et al (2002) Genomic approach for analysis of surface proteins in *Chlamydia pneumoniae*. *Infect Immun* 70(1): 368–379
85 Brachman PS, Friedlander AM, Grabenstein JD (2004) Anthrax vaccine. In: SA Plotkin, WA Orenstein (eds): *Vaccines*. Fourth edition, Saunders, Philadelphia, 887–903
86 Cieslak TJ, Kortepeter MG, Eitzen EM (2004) Vaccines against agents of bioterrorism. In: MM Levine, JB Kaper, R Rappuoli, MA Liu, MB Good (eds): *New generation vaccines*. Third edition. Marcel Dekker, New York, 1067–1079
87 Ariel N, Zvi A, Grosfeld H, Gat O, Inbar Y, Velan B, Cohen S, Shafferman A (2002) Search for potential vaccine candidate open reading frames in the *Bacillus anthracis* virulence plasmid pXO1: *in silico* and *in vitro* screening. *Infect Immun* 70: 6817–6827
88 Titball RW, Williamson ED, Dennis DT (2004) Plague. In: SA Plotkin, WA Orenstein (eds): *Vaccines*. Fourth edition, Saunders, Philadelphia, 999–1010
89 Flashner Y, Mamroud E, Tidhar A, Ber R, Aftalion M, Gur D, Lazar S, Zvi A, Bino T, Ariel N et al (2004) Generation of *Yersinia pestis* attenuated strains by signature-tagged mutagenesis in search of novel vaccine candidates. *Infect Immun* 72(2): 908–915
90 Peiris JS, Phil D, Yuen KY (2003) The severe acute respiratory syndrome. *N Engl J Med* 349: 2431–2441
91 Rota PA, Oberste MS, Monroe SS, Nix WA, Campagnoli R, Icenogle JP, Penaranda S, Bankamp B, Maher K, Chen MH et al (2003) Characterization of

a novel coronavirus associated with severe acute respiratory syndrome. *Science* 300: 1394–1399

92 Marra MA, Jones SJ, Astell CR, Holt RA, Brooks-Wilson A, Butterfield YS, Khattra J, Asano JK, Barber SA, Chan SY et al (2003) The genome sequence of the SARS-associated coronavirus. *Science* 300: 1399–1404

93 Stadler K, Masignani V, Eickmann M, Becker S, Abrignani S, Klenk HD, Rappuoli R (2003) Sars – beginning to understand a new virus. *Nat Rev Microbiol* 1: 209–218

94 CDC (1998) Impact of vaccines universally recommended for children – US, 1990–98. *MMWR* 48: 577–581

Design and selection of vaccine adjuvants: principles and practice

Carl R. Alving and Gary R. Matyas

Department of Vaccine Production and Delivery, Division of Retrovirology, Walter Reed Army Institute of Research, U.S. Military HIV Research Program, 1600 East Gude Drive, Rockville, MD 20850, USA

The requirement for vaccine adjuvants

Experience has shown that the initiation, quality, and magnitude of the immune response to a vaccine antigen can be influenced by numerous factors. These include the type and dose of the antigen, the timing of immunization and boosting, the route of immunization, and even the age and general health of the vaccinee.

Addition of an adjuvant to the vaccine formulation to enhance the immune response in a safe and nonspecific manner has also been a strategy that has been successfully employed for many vaccines. In past years, and even to the present, this has been accomplished mainly through adsorption of the antigen to an aluminum salt [1–3]. However, it should be noted that aluminum salts generally perform only weakly as adjuvants, particularly for booster immunizations, even though they do have a relatively good record of safety.

Modern research has demonstrated that different adjuvants can have profound effects not only on the magnitude of the immune response, but also on the qualitative type of immune response. Two illustrative examples of this are given below. In the first example, among many that could be cited, differences in protection against *Mycobacterium tuberculosis* challenge in mice were induced by different adjuvant formulations [4]. In this study it was found that injection of recombinant mycobacterial 65 kDa heat shock protein (hsp65) as an antigen by itself was unable to protect mice, even with Freund's incomplete adjuvant. However, when the antigen was administered as a DNA vaccine or as a recombinant protein entrapped in cationic liposomes, protection was observed. In contrast, when hsp65 was encapsulated in polymeric microspheres for sustained release of antigen, high levels of specific antibody were observed but the mice were not protected after challenge. As the authors stated, the vaccine adjuvant "makes the difference." In another illustrative example of differences induced by different combinations of adjuvants, it was shown that interleukin-12 (IL-12) together with granulocyte-macrophage colony-stimulating factor (GM-CSF) or tumor necrosis factor-alpha emulsified in Freund's adjuvant could be used to steer immune responses to induction of cytotoxic T lymphocytes [5]. GM-CSF alone gave mixed Th1 and Th2 responses, while GM-CSF plus IL-7 gave predominantly a Th2 response in BALB/c mice.

Inclusion of an adjuvant is not always necessary in order to achieve a successful vaccine effect. Sometimes a highly purified vaccine antigen by itself has inherent adjuvant activity. Cholera toxin (CT) from *Vibrio cholerae* or heat-labile enterotoxin (LT) from *Escherichia coli* are examples of purified antigens that can exhibit both antigenic and adjuvant activity [6–9], and CT directly activates dendritic cells [10]. More commonly, however, particularly in the past, a partly purified vaccine antigen has been used that also contains a contaminating adjuvant compound or that has adjuvant activity that has not been removed by further purification. The original smallpox vaccine, containing pus from cow pox sores, represents a quintessential example of utilization of a crude semi-purified viral antigen surrounded by its own contaminating adjuvant materials. Among other examples of crude antigen preparations are included parenterally-injected killed inactivated whole cell bacterial vaccines, such as inactivated whole cell *Bordetella pertussis*, *Salmonella typhi*, or *Vibrio cholerae* vaccines, which may be contaminated with bacterial endotoxin [11]. Endotoxin is a compound that can have strong natural adjuvant activity, and all of the adjuvant activity of endotoxin is due to the lipid A moiety of the bacterial surface lipopolysaccharide.

New generations of highly purified or synthetic antigens rarely have any inherent adjuvant activity, and the low immunogenicity of most highly purified antigens has highlighted the need to include adjuvants in vaccine formulations. It may be important for certain vaccines, particularly those that address difficult diseases, such as malaria or HIV infection, to include modern adjuvants that are much stronger than the weak adjuvant activity obtained from simple adsorption of antigen to aluminum salts.

Historical adjuvants

Freund's adjuvant

Perhaps the most famous adjuvant formulations are the water-in-oil emulsions devised by Jules Freund which are commonly designated as either complete or incomplete Freund's adjuvant [12, 13]. Although complete Freund's, containing mycobacteria, is universally regarded as too toxic for human use, incomplete Freund's (lacking mycobacteria) has been used as a potent adjuvant formulation for a diversity of vaccines in more than a million people [12, 14, 15]. It is currently being developed for certain human and veterinary vaccines [13].

Unfortunately, incomplete Freund's adjuvant has a widespread, albeit mainly undeserved, reputation for toxicity in humans [13, 14]. The reputation of incomplete Freund's adjuvant for toxicity is probably largely undeserved because it is based mainly on faulty animal models that do not reflect or translate to expression of human toxicity [15, 16]. Nonetheless, acceptance of vaccines is greatly dependent on the positive or negative perceptions that exist among potential recipients of vaccines, and because of fears of toxicity of Freund's adjuvant new generations of oil-in-water (rather than water-in-oil) vaccines have been devised that retain adjuvant activity but have essentially no toxicity in humans [17–19].

Complete Freund's adjuvant is also notable for having the dubious distinction of having created an unwarranted public fear that adjuvants might cause arthritis in humans. Adjuvant-induced arthritis, also often called adjuvant arthritis, is a condition that is uniquely associated with rodents, and is produced mainly after injection of complete Freund's adjuvant [20, 21]. The pathogenesis of the arthritogenic effects in rodents is strongly associated with a mycobacterial 65-kDa heat shock protein (Bhsp65) [22]. However, certain rodents can be so sensitive to the arthritogenic effects of Freund's adjuvant that arthritis can be induced even by painting the oil of incomplete Freund's adjuvant on the skin of genetically susceptible rats [23].

Although the rodent adjuvant arthritis model is interesting and has proven to be a boon to researchers interested in experimental rheumatology and in autoimmunity models in rodents, and is widely viewed as a model that illustrates the characteristics of rheumatoid arthritis in humans, and even for autoimmune disease in general [22], the induction of arthritis by adjuvants occurs only in rodents. Adjuvant-induced arthritis has never been recognized as an established pathological condition in humans and it therefore does not exist as a recognized human syndrome or disease entity. In a famous study in 1951–1953 Jonas Salk injected 18,000 American soldiers with an influenza vaccine that contained incomplete Freund's adjuvant, along with 26,000 control soldiers who did not receive adjuvant [24]. As reviewed earlier [15, 16], because the continuing health records of these Korean War veteran cohorts were available due to the excellent continuity of the military and veterans' medical health care system, extensive follow-up analyses after 9 years [25], 16–18 years [26], and >35 years [27] were undertaken. When records were examined for: mortality; separation or retirement from the military for disability; and for hospitalization and morbidity, no statistically significant evidence of increased incidence of any of 74 different diagnostic disease categories was found in the adjuvant cohort, including autoimmune diseases, connective tissue diseases, arthritis, or cancer. As previously concluded [16], the relative lack of toxicity of incomplete Freund's adjuvant in humans illustrates the pitfall of relying on evidence obtained only in rodents.

Aluminum salts

Aluminum salts, first introduced in 1926, are currently the most commonly used adjuvants for vaccines. Although the adjuvant activity of an aluminum salt is often relatively weak, adsorption of multiple antigens to aluminum salts does serve the function of formulating combination vaccines, such as diphtheria-pertussis-tetanus (DPT), DPT-haemophilis influenzae, or hepatitis B-haemophilus influenzae vaccines [28]. In addition, adsorption to alum salt might have the interesting benefit of stabilizing and retarding the degradation of an antigen that degrades with a pH-dependent mechanism [29].

The literature on aluminum adjuvants is quite extensive, and recent research on mechanisms suggests that the adjuvant mechanisms of aluminum and calcium salts may be complex. Excellent reviews have covered the literature and technical characteristics of these adjuvants, and regulatory issues [2, 3, 28, 30]. The commonly used aluminum salt adjuvants include various physical forms of aluminum phosphate, aluminum hydroxide, and aluminum-precipitates of protein [32]. These compounds are currently so widely referred to informally as a group by the term alum that this term has become an accepted generic shorthand in the vaccine field for aluminum salt adjuvants even though the name alum was originally given to potassium aluminum sulfate, a chemical entity that is not actually being used as an adjuvant [3].

Certain vaccines can be created by precipitation of protein with an aluminum salt, but currently the most common method of using aluminum is by simple adsorption, and this is accomplished by mixing of antigen with pre-formed aluminum gel. As noted earlier, even at their best, aluminum salts have only modest adjuvant activity, and they are often inconsistent in their ability to serve as adjuvants for widely used protein antigens, particularly for booster immunization [2, 28]. Different lots or different brands of the same type of aluminum salt can be inconsistent in adsorptive capacity [33]. Despite the deceptive ease of adsorption by bringing protein antigen and aluminum salt together, considerable difficulty in adjuvant reproducibility may be encountered because of the huge complexity of aluminum-protein interactions, an area particularly explored in detailed physicochemical studies by Stanley Hem [34]. This complexity extends not only to the adsorption of antigen during vaccine manufacture, but also due to potential exchange of protein antigen with interstitial proteins and other constituents of interstitial fluids after injection [35–37]. Likewise, it is through the mechanism of cycles of disaggregation and reaggregation of aluminum hydroxide adjuvant that homogeneous mixing of multiple antigens occurs on aluminum adjuvant particles in combination vaccines containing more that one antigen [38].

The adsorptive binding of proteins to aluminum is often due to electrostatic interactions, and adsorption can be strongly affected by the age of the gel [39], the charge of the gel, the charge of the adsorbed protein, by the physical structure of the aluminum compound, and by the pH and other characteristics of the buffer that is used ([29, 40–42], reviewed in [3]). It is possible to manipulate the electrostatic adsorption in certain cases. Aluminum hydroxide gel is positively charged at pH 7.4 and it adsorbs negatively charged proteins. However, pretreatment of aluminum hydroxide with buffer containing phosphate can lower, or even reverse, the positive charge, even allowing the electrostatic adsorption of cationic protein [43].

Many other mechanisms also play a role in the adsorptive process, including hydrophobic interactions, van der Waals forces, and hydrogen bonding (reviewed in [3]). Recently it was suggested that ligand exchange between the phosphate groups of phospholipids in the hepatitis B surface antigen with the hydroxyl groups of aluminum hydroxide provides a mechanism of high affinity binding [44]. Presumably this mechanism could also account for the binding of phospholipid liposomes containing monophosphoryl lipid A to aluminum hydroxide adjuvant [33, 45].

The dose of aluminum adjuvant is an important consideration. It is important to understand that there may be an optimal level of aluminum for a given vaccine antigen, with decreased immune response at higher levels of aluminum [3]. Although it has been stated that aluminum remains at the site of injection for a long period [3], aluminum salts are known to be removed from the body with time [46]. The acceptable dose of aluminum in adjuvants ranges up to 1.25 mg both by U.S. and by WHO regulations, but currently licensed US vaccines have a range of only 0.125 to 0.85 mg [28]. The latter reference can also be consulted for a list of all licensed US vaccines containing aluminum and the aluminum content of each.

Side-effects of widely used human adjuvants

It is well known that immunostimulators in general, and adjuvants in particular, can sometimes be double-edged swords. Side-effects and toxicities of adjuvants can be widespread and commonplace and the toxicity and reactogenicity of a given adjuvant is often cited as having equal or greater importance than the potency as a criterion to be considered in the selection of an adjuvant [11, 47]. It is the introduction of side-effects or toxicities that are produced in otherwise healthy persons that are the most troubling aspects of vaccine- and adjuvant-induced side-effects, and this is particularly true for pediatric vaccines.

Some local effects, such as local ulceration induced by live Vaccinia organisms that are used for smallpox or the bacillus Calmette-Guérin (BCG) organism that is widely used around the world as a tuberculosis vaccine, and the familiar local redness and swelling at the site of injection induced by aluminum salts [31], are usually tolerated as levels of toxicity that are generally not so stressful as to preclude the use of the offending materials. It is generally believed that the local inflammation associated with intramuscular injection of aluminum salts is due to the escape of adjuvant along the injection track into the subcutaneous space [12]. Pain after injection and the occurrence of painless nodules after multiple injections of aluminum adjuvanted vaccines are associated with the subcutaneous route of injection [48, 49].

Systemic effects of various adjuvant materials sometimes can be more serious, and these can include: nausea and vomiting that are associated with a small fraction of vaccinated cohorts; pyrogenic effects due to endotoxin that are almost universally found with crude vaccines containing endotoxin; or even uveitis, a rare occurrence that may be associated with certain adjuvants.

Sometimes the adjuvant can even produce a set of symptoms that partly mimics the disease against which the vaccine is directed. Such is the case of orally administered CT or LT, each of which can induce diarrhea similar to that found in cholera or in *E. coli* diarrhea. However, a much more dramatic and dangerous example of toxicity of LT was recently discovered in a licensed Swiss vaccine that was administered intranasally [50, 51]. When LT was included in a liposomal (virosome) vaccine containing hemagglutinin and neuraminidase surface antigens of influenza virus, intranasal administration of the vaccine resulted in a strong association with an increased risk of facial nerve paralysis (Bell's palsy). The increased risk was highest at 31–60 days after vaccination and the toxic effect resulted in withdrawal of the vaccine from the market.

It is known that ganglioside GM1 serves as a high affinity receptor for LT and CT and, although the natural targets for CT and LT are the cells of the intestine, GM1 is widely distributed in many other tissues, including neural tissues [52]. Thus, although the mechanism of the induction of Bell's palsy was not completely clear, it would seem likely that the interaction of LT with GM1 on the olfactory nerve played an important role [51]. This unfortunate neurological toxicity involving the facial nerve was probably uniquely related to the intranasal administration of enterotoxin. Fear of facial nerve toxicity should not have a negative impact on the use of native or modified enterotoxin vaccine adjuvants when given by other routes for immunomodulation and adjuvant effects. Furthermore, there is no reason to suspect that the virosome itself exhibited any toxicity independent of its role as a carrier of LT.

Because of the use of crude antigenic materials contaminated with endotoxin, or even because of the local granulomatous inflammation caused by aluminum salts, the impression has arisen that the function of many adjuvants is mainly to cause an inflammatory reaction and that the toxic effects of the reaction are critical contributors to adjuvant activity. It is true that local inflammation can often enhance the immunogenicity of an antigen, mainly because inflammatory cells contain a large fraction of phagocytes and lymphocytes that may serve as antigen presenting cells. However, it is not true that toxic effects are necessarily required for adjuvant activity. Quite the opposite: modern adjuvants strive to enhance immunogenicity in a focused manner that minimizes or avoids local adverse reactions or systemic toxicity.

Elimination of the toxicity of Gram-negative bacterial endotoxin, a potent classic adjuvant, while retaining the adjuvant effects provided by the endotoxin, is a dramatic example of the lack of reliance of an adjuvant on toxicity for expression of adjuvant effect. Essentially all of the toxic effects of endotoxin, including pyrogenicity, are due to the lipid A moiety of the lipopolysaccharide that is present on the surface of Gram-negative bacteria [53]. Because of this, the terms endotoxin and lipid A are often used interchangeably, but the toxic effects of purified lipid A are greatly reduced, and the entire adjuvant effect is retained, by utilization of monophosphoryl lipid A instead of the complete diphosphoryl lipid A molecule [54]. Monophosphoryl lipid A still retains some toxicity at high doses, but the residual toxicity, including pyrogenicity, of monophosphoryl lipid A can be completely eliminated by incorporation of monophosphoryl lipid A into liposomes [55]. The complete detoxification of monophosphoryl lipid A by liposomes allows the potential safe use of even higher doses of monophosphoryl lipid A with still higher adjuvant activity, if higher adjuvant activity is indeed required [55, 56].

Lessons from historical adjuvants

Certain types of adjuvant formulations that have been widely used in the past could serve as useful practical starting points for adjuvant selection for many vaccines. Among such materials are included: aluminum salts; lipid A or monophosphoryl lipid A; and a variety of emulsions, including water-in-oil or oil-in-water emulsions. Lipid A is the constituent of Gram-negative bacterial endotoxin that has given particular potency to certain whole cell bacterial vaccines. Each of these adjuvants has advantages and disadvantages involving availability, potency, safety, cost, or ease of manufacture. Improvements on these, such as by the use of liposomes with lipid A, can introduce additional factors or complications.

Improvements on other historical adjuvants that were previously not easily available or not acceptable because of toxicity or other factors, include introduction of cytokines either directly or through the use of DNA coding [57, 58]; highly purified less toxic derivatives of saponin-like materials [19]; and nontoxic analogs of toxins such as analogs of CT and LT. The latter compounds in their native forms as CT or LT are highly toxic as oral mucosal adjuvants, and generally induce diarrhea, but newer derivatives of CT and LT have been introduced that have reduced, or completely lack, toxicity [59]. Even the native forms of CT and LT lack systemic or mucosal toxicity when applied directly to the skin as adjuvants for induction of transcutaneous immunization [8, 9, 60]. A fascinating discovery has been made that when either native CT or LT is used as an adjuvant with co-administered antigen on the surface of the hydrated skin for transcutaneous immunization, the combined adjuvant formulation can induce both systemic (IgG) immunity [8, 9, 60], cytotoxic T lymphocytes [61], and even mucosal immunity [9, 60, 62] both in animal models and in humans.

Selection of vaccine adjuvants

After a useful and extensive textbook review of the history of adjuvants and of the status of research on current and new generations of vaccine adjuvants, Professor G. J. V. Nossal recorded the following conclusion: "The reader will by now have gathered that the field of adjuvants is not too rich in simplifying or overarching paradigms. It seems likely that empirical research will continue to dominate for some time." [63]. While it is true that this conclusion might seem somewhat grim, it is the same conclusion that could be made of vaccine research in general, and, indeed, for many areas of medical research. However, modern adjuvant research is beginning to identify the hint of useful general paradigms, or at least beginnings of rational explanations of certain adjuvant activities, based on the understanding of dendritic cells as "Nature's adjuvants" that modulate immune responses through activities of pathogen recognition receptors (PRRs), Toll-like receptors (TLRs) and C-type lectins [64].

The field of vaccines is by history and by nature fraught with difficulties, and adjuvants by themselves do not serve as a transforming principle for creating simplicity out of complexity. They also do not necessarily serve as a means for illuminating predictable paths to overcome all of the difficult and diverse obstacles that microorganisms have created against immune attack that allow them to beset humans and other mammals with disease burdens. It is undoubtedly for the reason that combinations of vaccine components are unpredictable with respect to stability, efficacy, and safety, that the U.S. Food and Drug Administration, and many other national regulatory agencies, have not licensed adjuvants as stand-alone products but only as constituents of complete vaccine formulations [65, 66].

Adjuvant mechanisms

Mechanisms of adjuvant expression exist on several levels. At a macro level, a slowly dispersed depot, such as aluminum salt, oil emulsion deposits, or other particulate scaffolding materials may serve either as a slow release mechanism, or as a concentration of antigen and adjuvant that attracts antigen presenting cells that ingest the depot through phagocytosis or endocytosis over a long period of time. At a cellular level, dendritic cells exert activities through the aforementioned PRRs, TLRs, and C-type lectins, leading to steering of the immune response through complicated signaling processes and so-called conversations between cells that are mediated by cytokines, chemokines, and other mediators. Other mechanisms of innate immunity, such as complement activation, can also play an important, or even critical, role in the evolution of the immune response. Mechanisms involving targeting of the antigen to a desired cell, or local delivery of the antigen to a desired location, such as for oral, intranasal, or transcutaneous delivery, can be viewed as a useful adjuvant-like strategy. This also holds true for altering the dose of adjuvant and the timing of vaccination. It seems obvious that if an adjuvant exerts a strong depot effect, it would provide little benefit to provide a booster immunization at the site of the depot before the earlier depot material had been depleted. Discussions of numerous adjuvant mechanisms and available adjuvants have been provided in various reviews [11, 47, 63, 64, 67].

The process of optimization of vaccine adjuvants generally employs multiple mechanisms, which may require putting together groups of adjuvants that exhibit both macro and cellular, and perhaps even targeting, mechanisms. The evolution of understanding of TLRs and PRRs has given some recent useful insights into the rationale of using certain combinations of adjuvants. For example, CpG DNA acts on TLR 9 to trigger both IL-12 and IFN-alpha to induce strong Th1 and cytotoxic T lymphocyte (CTL) responses, while *E. coli* LPS acts on TLR 4 to trigger mainly IL-12 plus a little IFN-alpha and Th1 responses [64]. While it is true that this information could provide a possible rationale for combining adjuvants such as these together, it would be naive to believe that such responses could be easily predicted for any given human vaccine, and it would be naive to believe that true optimization of immune responses could be achieved without providing other mechanisms of targeting or scaffolding.

Commercial adjuvants

There are numerous success stories in the adjuvant field that can allow the selection of useful adjuvants that could be employed for practical success in the creation of important vaccines. A plethora of reviews on adjuvants provides a rich selection of adjuvant candidates that can be examined [11, 12, 47, 63, 67]. A useful compendium of a large number of available vaccine adjuvants can also be accessed electronically on the website of the Division of AIDS at NIAID at the U.S. National Institutes of Health [http://www.niaid.nih.gov/daids/vaccine/pdf/compendium.pdf]. But the huge variety of potential adjuvants that are available also presents the further problem that the adjuvant or adjuvant combination for a given vaccine must be additionally selected based on criteria such as ease of manufacture, cost, potency, and risk/benefit ratio. As Professor Nossal accurately observed: "…each commercial firm interested in the field has simply gone its own way, with little collaboration between the groups." [63]. Many of the best known and best studied adjuvants have been invented through commercial research and are therefore restricted for exclusive use by individual companies. The holding of proprietary adjuvants for their own exclusive use by companies should not be viewed as a serious impediment for many vaccines because the basic reasons for success or failures of most commercially developed adjuvants are well known and it is often not too difficult to create similar generic alternatives.

A more difficult problem is that the use of a particular adjuvant or adjuvant strategy by a company does not necessarily imply that the adjuvant selected by the company is the most effective one that could be employed; indeed, compromises in adjuvant selection are often made by companies based largely on issues of profitability. While this is not necessarily a bad strategy in itself for the company or even the consumer, it might not always be the best initial route for conducting research to attack huge and difficult international diseases, such as HIV/AIDS or malaria, or other important diseases for which potent and safe vaccines have not yet been developed or licensed.

Many of the commercial adjuvants that have been proposed or are being developed appear to have excellent potential for future use, and some have enjoyed success as constituents of licensed vaccines. Although in the U.S. aluminum salts are still the only adjuvants that have been used in any licensed vaccine to date, new types of adjuvants are now in advanced stages of clinical testing for licensing. In several other countries, a variety of novel new aluminum-free commercial adjuvants have already been included in licensed vaccines as described below.

An oil-in-water emulsion (MF59) has been developed and manufactured by Chiron that is used in a licensed influenza vaccine in Europe [17, 18]. Prior to the 2004–2005 influenza season, more than 11 million doses had been administered and the vaccine has proved to be remarkably safe. It is reported to be particularly effective for inducing effective immunity to influenza in elderly vaccinees [17].

A liposome (virosome) containing hepatitis A antigen has been developed by Berna for use as a licensed hepatitis A vaccine in Switzerland [68]. The vaccine appears to be safe, effective, and competitive in the commercial market.

A melanoma vaccine containing an oily dispersion having monophosphoryl lipid A and mycobacterial cell as constituents has been developed by Corixa Corp [69] and licensed in Canada [http://www.corixa.com/default.asp?pid=release_detail&year=2001&ID=19].

While these licensed vaccines serve as examples, and even as inspirations, numerous other adjuvant formulations are working through commercial pipelines toward eventual applications for new-generation vaccines.

A clinical algorithm for selection of vaccine adjuvants

As noted earlier, hundreds of adjuvants and adjuvant formulations have been proposed as immunostimulants for various purposes for vaccines. When combined with a variety of options for route of delivery of the vaccine, the selection process for adjuvant choice presents a maze of complexities. It is therefore not surprising that animal models have often been employed for simplification of the process. Unfortunately, considerable experience with numerous animal models has demonstrated that in many cases conclusions from such models do not accurately predict adjuvant-enhanced immunogenicity or protection against the infection or disease being modeled, and may not even correctly predict the safety profile of the adjuvant [16]. In certain instances animal disease models that might be used for adjuvant selection do not even exist.

One such example that lacked a suitable animal model involved the development of an immunotherapeutic vaccine against prostate cancer. When faced with this latter difficulty, we took it as an opportunity to create an interesting and useful clinical experimental algorithm for rational selection of adjuvants. The challenge in this algorithm had the following parameters. An immunotherapeutic vaccine, utilizing recombinant prostate-specific antigen (PSA), was to be developed for treatment of advanced metastatic prostate cancer under circumstances in which the patients had previously exhausted essentially all available conventional therapeutic options. This situation was particularly challenging because the patients were elderly, extremely ill, and highly immunosuppressed because of cancer. In addition, the difficulty was compounded both by the requirement to overcome immunological tolerance against PSA, a circulating self antigen, and the further requirement to induce cellular immunity, in essence to induce cellular autoimmunity against PSA.

To address this situation, our strategy was to conduct multiple sequential small (5–10 patient) phase I safety and immunogenicity trials with recombinant PSA in which changes and improvements in the adjuvant formulation and route of immunization would be devised based on the results from the previous trial. Liposomes containing encapsulated rPSA and monophosphoryl lipid A (MPL) (Walter Reed liposomes) [33, 45] were selected as a core adjuvant platform technology. These types of liposomes had been shown to induce potent immune responses in previous comparative adjuvant trials in humans for experimental vaccines to malaria [56, 70] and HIV [71].

As summarized in Table 1, six sequential trials were conducted with rationally selected adjuvant formulations [16, 72]. The trials, the rationales for adjuvant formulation, and a summary of the results, are described below. In the first two trials, consisting of intramuscular (i.m.) and intravenous (i.v.) immunization, respectively, with Walter Reed liposomes containing lipid A and rPSA, only 2 of 10 patients exhibited either antibodies

Table 1. Immunization regimens of prostate cancer patients

Trial	Route of immunization	Number of patients*	Dose**	Immunization schedule (days)	Additional adjuvants
1	Intramuscular	6/5	1 ml	0, 30, 60	None
2	Intravenous	6/5	1 ml	0, 30, 60	None
3	Subcutaneous	11/10	1 ml	0, 30, 60	GM-CSF, 125 mg injected subcutaneously into the vaccine site on the day of immunization and for 4 days thereafter
4	Intradermal	5/5	0.25 ml to 4 sites	0, 1, 2, 15, 30	Cyclophosphamide, 300 mg/m^2 intravenously on days –3 and 27; BCG, 0.01 ml of a 1:10 dilution injected into the vaccine sites on Study Days 0, 15, and 30
5	Intramuscular	9/8	0.9 ml	0, 30, 60	Vaccine emulsified in oil-in-water (o/w) emulsion in light mineral oil
6	Subcutaneous	5/5	1 ml	0, 30, 60	Cyclophosphamide, 300 mg/m^2 intravenously 3 days before each immunization; GM-CSF, 125 mg injected subcutaneously into the vaccine site on the day of immunization and for 4 days thereafter; IL-2 self-administered subcutaneously by the patient in a dose of 3 million IU/m^2 daily on days 7–13, 37–43, and 67–73

* Number of patients available for evaluation for safety/immunologic responses.
** Liposomes containing recombinant PSA, 100 mg/ml and lipid A, 200 mg/ml.

or DTH responses to PSA. The i.v. route was selected in order to increase delivery of the vaccine to the lymphocytes in the spleen, but this strategy failed to induce any detectable immune response. We concluded that although the liposomes by themselves had previously proved quite potent, they still did not have sufficient potency for this unique challenge.

The next two trials were conducted simultaneously. In trial 3, GM-CSF was added to the core liposome formulation containing rPSA and MPL because it had been shown to enhance maturation of dendritic cells and macrophages [73] and to increase antigen presentation of protein and peptide-based vaccines [74–77]. GM-CSF was injected subcutaneously at the vaccine injection site on the day of immunization and four days after immunization. This strategy finally worked – immune responses were measured in 100% of the patients. Nine of 10 had antibodies to PSA and 7 of 10,

Table 2. Immune responses following immunization with liposomal PSA containing lipid A

Trial	Route of immunization	Additional adjuvants	Antibodies to PSA*	Lymphocyte proliferation**	DTH*** (induration)
1	Intramuscular	None	1/5	0/5	1/5
2	Intravenous	None	0/5	0/5	0/5
3	Subcutaneous	GM-CSF	9/10	4/10	7/10
4	Intradermal	Cyclophosphamide, BCG	4/5	3/5	2/5
5	Intramuscular	Liposomal oil-in-water emulsion	7/8	6/8	7/8
6	Subcutaneous	Cyclophosphamide, GM-CSF, IL-2	3/5	5/5	2/5

* Number of patients/total number patients immunized having serum antibody titers to PSA >6,400.

** Number of patients/total number patients immunized having positive proliferative responses to PSA. Data are normalized to the response obtained from PBMC obtained prior to immunization.

*** Number of patients/total number patients immunized having induration >10 mm following skin challenge with PSA.

including the patient who did not develop antibodies to PSA, had >10 mm induration upon challenge with PSA in a skin test (Tab. 2) [78]. Four patients also had lymphocyte proliferative responses to PSA.

In trial 4, cyclophosphamide was administered 3 days prior to immunization with the liposome formulation because cyclophosphamide had been reported to augment delayed-type hypersensitivity responses to antigens [79, 80]. BCG was used because it had been shown to be effective for prophylaxis and therapy of cancer [81, 82]. Four of 5 patients developed antibodies to PSA following immunization, but only 2 patients had induration after skin test challenge with PSA. One patient had no demonstrable immune responses following vaccination. Three patients also had lymphocyte proliferation responses to PSA.

Trial 5 used a novel liposome-stabilized oil-in-water liposomal emulsion [83, 84]. The liposomes containing lipid A and rPSA were used as a stabilizer for emulsifying light mineral oil. During the emulsification process some of the liposomes were degraded and coated the oil droplets, and this had the effect of stabilizing the emulsion. Seven of 8 patients immunized with the emulsion developed antibodies to PSA. Seven of 8 patients had induration after a skin test with PSA [78] and 6 of 8 were positive for PSA-induced lymphocyte proliferation (Tab. 2).

The last formulation tested (Trial 6) consisted of cyclophosphamide pretreatment prior to immunization, injection of GM-CSF at the injection site and interleukin 2 (IL-2) subcutaneous administration every day for one week starting a week after vaccination. IL-2 was included because it has been shown to enhance immune response in patients undergoing vaccine therapy by expanding cells with antigen-induced high affinity receptors [85] and up-regulating T-cell cytokines [86]. Three of 5 patients had antibodies to PSA and 2 of those patients had induration reactions following skin challenge with PSA. All of the patients had PSA-induced lymphocyte proliferative responses (Tab. 2).

The PBMC from patients immunized in trials 3 and 5 were further analyzed for PSA-induced interferon-γ (INF-γ) secretion by ELISPOT analysis [87]. CD4 and/or CD8 PSA-responding cells were observed in samples from both trials. In addition, vaccination decreased the percentage of zeta-negative $CD3^+$ cells routinely observed in cancer patients and increased the percentage of IL-10-secreting cells [78].

Based on the immune responses, the formulations that utilized GM-CSF or emulsion were judged to be superior to the other formulations. The liposome-stabilized emulsion was further tested in colon cancer patients using liposome-encapsulated recombinant KSA, a formulation also manufactured at Walter Reed [88]. Antibody responses and cellular immune responses to KSA, as measured by lymphocyte proliferation, DTH and INF-γ ELISPOT responses, were induced in this latter study following immunization with the emulsion. By using our clinical algorithm strategy of employing successive small clinical trials, we were able to identify a unique new liposomal oil-in-water emulsion as a potent new vaccine adjuvant formulation.

From this successful experience we believe that a similar clinical research algorithm could be used with almost any antigen as a cost-effective method to optimize the immunogenicity of the antigen with competing formulations of rationally selected adjuvant candidates and routes of delivery. In those instances involving chronic or difficult diseases, such as HIV/AIDS, malaria or cancer, where successful creation of a protective vaccine has encountered considerable barriers Draconian measures may be required involving extremely potent adjuvants. The clinical research algorithm described above may therefore have general utility as a means to provide rational guidance for adjuvant selection.

References

1 Glenny AT, Pope CG, Waddington H, Wallace U (1926) Immunological Notes. XVII–XXIV. *J Pathol Bacteriol* 29: 31–40

2 Aprile MA, Wardlaw, AC (1966) Aluminium compounds as adjuvants for vaccines and toxoids in man: A review. *Can J Publ Hlth* 57: 343–354

3 Gupta RK (1998) Aluminum compounds as vaccine adjuvants. *Adv Drug Delivery Rev* 32: 155–172

4 Lima KM, dos Santos SA, Rodrigues Jr JM, Silva CL (2004) Vaccine adjuvant: it makes the difference. *Vaccine* 22: 2374–2379

5 Ahlers JD, Dunlop N, Alling DW, Nara PL, Berzofsky JA (1997) Cytokine-in-

adjuvant steering of the immune response phenotype to HIV-1 vaccine constructs. Granulocyte-macrophage colony-stimulating factor and TNF-α synergize with IL-12 to enhance induction of cytotoxic t lymphocytes. *J Immunol* 158: 3947–3958
6 Elson CO, Ealding W (1984) Cholera toxin feeding did not induce oral tolerance in mice and abrogated oral tolerance to an unrelated protein antigen. *J Immunol* 133: 2892–2897
7 Snider DP (1995) The mucosal adjuvant activities of ADP-ribosylating bacterial enterotoxins. *Crit Rev Immunol* 15: 317–348
8 Glenn GM, Rao M, Matyas GR, Alving CR (1998) Skin immunization made possible by cholera toxin. *Nature* 391: 851
9 Glenn GM, Scharton-Kersten T, Vassell R, Matyas GR, Alving CR (1999) Transcutaneous immunization with bacterial ADP-ribosylating exotoxins as antigens and adjuvants. *Infect Immun* 67: 1100–1106
10 Kawamura YI, Kawashima R, Shirai Y, Kato R, Hambata T, Yamamoto M, Furukawa K, Fujihashi K, McGhee JR, Hayashi H et al (2003) Cholera toxin activates dendritic cells through dependence on GM1-ganglioside which is mediated by NF-κB translocation. *Eur J Immunol* 33: 3205–3212
11 Gupta RK, Relyveld EH, Lindblad EB, Bizzini B, Ben-Efraim S, Gupta CK (1993) Adjuvants – a balance between toxicity and adjuvanticity. *Vaccine* 11: 293–306
12 Edelman R (1980) Vaccine adjuvants. *Rev Infect Dis* 2: 370–383
13 Chang JCC, Diveley JP, Savary JR, Jensen FC (1998) Adjuvant activity of incomplete Freund's adjuvant. *Adv Drug Deliv Rev* 32: 173–186
14 Davenport FM (1968) Seventeen years' experience with mineral oil adjuvant influenza virus vaccines. *Ann Allergy* 26: 288–292
15 Stuart-Harris CH (1969) Adjuvant influenza vaccines. Bull WHO 41: 617–621
16 Alving CR (2002) Design and selection of vaccine adjuvants: animal models and human trials. *Vaccine* 20: S56–S64
17 Podda A (2001) The adjuvanted influenza vaccines with novel adjuvants: experience with the MF59-adjuvanted vaccine. *Vaccine* 19: 2673–2680
18 Frey S, Poland G, Percell S, Podda A (2003) Comparison of the safety, tolerability, and immunogenicity of a MF59-adjuvanted influenza vaccine and a non-adjuvanted influenza vaccine in non-elderly adults. *Vaccine* 21: 4234–4237
19 Alonso PL, Sacarlal J, Aponte JJ, Leach A, Macete E, Milman J, Mandomando I, Spiessens B, Guinovart C, Espasa M et al (2004) Efficacy of the RTS.S/AS02A vaccine against P*lasmodium falciparum* infection and disease in young African children: randomised controlled trial. *Lancet* 364: 1411–1429
20 Pearson CM (1956) Development of arthritis, periarthritis and periostitis in rats given adjuvants. *Proc Soc Exp Biol Med* 91: 95–101
21 Taurog JD, Argentieri DC, McReynolds RA (1988) Adjuvant arthritis. *Meth Enzymol* 162: 339–355
22 Durai M, Kim HR, Moudgil KD (2004) The regulatory C-terminal determinants within mycobacterial heat shock protein 65 are cryptic and cross-reactive

with the dominant self homologs: Implications for the pathogenesis of autoimmune arthritis. *J Immunol* 173: 181–188

23 Kleinau S, Erlandsson H, Klareskog L (1994) Percutaneous exposure of adjuvant oil causes arthritis in DA rats. *Clin Exp Immunol* 96: 281–284

24 Salk JE, Contakos M, Laurent AM, Sorensen M, Rapalski AJ, Simmons IH, Sandberg H (1953) Use of adjuvants in studies on influenza immunization. 3. Degree of persistence of antibody in human subjects two years after vaccination. *J Am Med Assn* 151: 1169–1175

25 Beebe GW, Simon AH, Vivona S (1964) Follow-up study on army personnel who received adjuvant influenza virus vaccine 1951–1953. *Am J Med Sci* 247: 385–407

26 Beebe GW, Simon AH, Vivona S (1972) Long-term mortality follow-up of army recruits who received adjuvant influenza virus vaccine in 1951–1953. *Am J Epidemiol* 95: 337–346

27 Page WF, Norman JE, Benenson AS (1993) Long-term followup of army recruits immunized with Freund's incomplete adjuvanted vaccine. *Vaccine Res* 2: 141–149

28 Baylor NW, Egan W, Richman P (2002) Aluminum salts in vaccines – US perspective. *Vaccine* 20: S18–S23

29 Wittayanukulluk A, Jiang D, Regnier FE, Hem SL (2004) Effect of microenvironment pH of aluminum hydroxide adjuvant on the chemical stability of adsorbed antigen. *Vaccine* 22: 1172–1176

30 Gupta RK, Rost BE, Relyveld E, Siber GR (1995) Adjuvant properties of aluminum and calcium compounds. In: Powell MF, Newman MJ (eds): *Vaccine design, the subunit and adjuvant approach.* New York: Plenum Press, 229–248

31 Jefferson T, Rudin M, Di Pietrantonj C (2004) Adverse events after immunisation with aluminium-containing DTP vaccines: systematic review of the evidence. *Lancet Infect Dis* 4: 84–90

32 Shirodkar S, Hutchinson RL, Perry DL, White JL, Hem SL (1990) Aluminum compounds used as adjuvants in vaccines. *Pharmaceut Res* 7: 1282–1288

33 Wassef NM, Alving CR, Richards RL (1994) Liposomes as carriers for vaccines. *Immunomethods* 4: 217–222

34 Hem SL, White JL (1995) Structure and properties of aluminum-containing adjuvants. *Pharm Biotech* 6: 249–276

35 Seeber SJ, White JL, Hem SL (1991) Solubilization of aluminum-containing adjuvants by constituents of interstitial fluid. *J Parenteral Sci Technol* 45: 156–159

36 Heimlich JM, Regnier FE, White JL, Hem SL (1999) The *in vitro* displacement of adsorbed model antigens from aluminium-containing adjuvants by interstitial proteins. *Pharm Biotech* 17: 2873–2881

37 Iyer S, HogenEsch H, Hem SL (2003) Relationship between the degree of antigen adsorption to aluminum hydroxide adjuvant in interstitial fluid and antibody production. *Vaccine* 21: 1219–1223

38 Morefield GL, HogenEsch H, Robinson JP, Hem SL (2004) Distribution of

adsorbed antigen in mono-valent and combination vaccines. *Vaccine* 22: 1973–1984

39 Burrell LS, White JL, Hem SL (2000) Stability of aluminium-containing adjuvants during aging at room temperature. *Vaccine* 18: 2188–2192

40 Seeber SJ, White JL, Hem SL (1991) Predicting the adsorption of proteins by aluminium-containing adjuvants. *Vaccine* 9: 201–203

41 Callahan PM, Shorter AL, Hem SL (1991) The importance of surface charge in the optimization of antigen-adjuvant interactions. *J Pharmaceut Res* 8: 851–858

42 Feldkamp JR, Shah DN, Meyer SL, White JL, Hem SL (1981) Effect of adsorbed carbonate on surface charge characteristics and physical properties of aluminum hydroxide gel. *J Pharmaceut Sci* 70: 638–640

43 Rinella Jr JV, White JL, Hem SL (1996) Treatment of aluminium hydroxide adjuvant to optimize the adsorption of basic proteins. *Vaccine* 14: 298–300

44 Iyer S, Robinett RSR, HogenEsch H, Hem SL (2004) Mechanism of adsorption of hepatitis B surface antigen by aluminum hydroxide adjuvant. *Vaccine* 22: 1475–1479

45 Alving CR, Shichijo S, Mattsby-Baltzer I, Richards RL, Wassef NM (1993) Preparation and use of liposomes in immunological studies. In: Gregoriadis G (ed): *Liposome technology,* 2nd edition, *Vol III, Interactions of liposomes with the biological milieu*. Boca Raton: CRC Press, 317–343

46 Hem SL (2002) Elimination of aluminum adjuvants. *Vaccine* 20 (Suppl 3): S40–S43

47 Gupta RK, Siber GR (1995) Adjuvants for human vaccines – current status, problems and future prospects. *Vaccine* 13: 1263–1276

48 Frost L, Johansen P, Pedersen S, Veien N, Østergaard PA, Nielsen MH (1985) Persistent subcutaneous nodules in children hyposensitized with aluminium-containing allergen extracts. *Allergy* 40: 368–372

49 Pittman PR (2002) Aluminum-containing vaccine associated adverse events: role of route of administration and gender. *Vaccine* 20: S48–S50

50 Mutsch M, Zhou W, Rhodes P, Bopp M, Chen RT, Linder T, Spyr C, Steffen R (2004) Use of the inactivated intranasal influenza vaccine and the risk of Bell's palsy in Switzerland. *N Engl J Med* 350: 896–903

51 Couch RB (2004) Nasal vaccination, *Escherichia coli* enterotoxin, and Bell's palsy. *N Engl J Med* 350: 860–861

52 Eidels L, Proia RL, Hart DA (1983) Membrane receptors for bacterial toxins. *Microbiol Rev* 47: 596–620

53 Takada H, Kotani S (1989) Structural requirements of lipid A for endotoxicity and other biological activities. *CRC Crit Rev Microbiol* 16: 477–523

54 Alving CR (1993) Lipopolysaccharide, lipid A, and liposomes containing lipid A as immunologic adjuvants. *Immunobiol* 187: 430–446

55 Richards RL, Swartz Jr GM, Schultz C, Hayre MD, Ward GS, Ballou WR, Chulay JD, Hockmeyer WT, Berman SL, Alving CR (1989) Immunogenicity of liposomal malaria sporozoite antigen in monkeys: adjuvant effects of aluminum hydroxide and nonpyrogenic liposomal lipid A. *Vaccine* 7: 506–512

56 Fries LF, Gordon DM, Richards RL, Egan JE, Hollingdale MR, Gross M,

Silverman C, Alving CR (1992) Liposomal malaria vaccine in humans: a safe and potent adjuvant strategy. *Proc Natl Acad Sci USA* 89: 358–362

57 Calarota SA, Weiner DB (2004) Enhancement of human immunodeficiency virus type 1-DNA vaccine potency through incorporation of T-helper 1 molecular adjuvants. *Immunol Rev* 199: 84–99

58 Toka FN, Pack CD, Rouse BT (2004) Molecular adjuvants for mucosal immunity. *Immunol Rev* 199: 100–112

59 Pizza M, Giuliani MM, Fontana MR, Monaci E, Douce G, Dougan G, Mills KHG, Rappuoli R, Del Giudice G (2001) Mucosal vaccines: non-toxic derivatives of LT and CT as mucosal adjuvants. *Vaccine* 19: 2534–2541

60 Glenn GM, Taylor DN, Li X, Frankel S, Montemarano A, Alving CR (2000) Transcutaneous immunization: A human vaccine delivery strategy using a patch. *Nature Med* 6: 1403–1406

61 Belyakov IM, Hammond SA, Ahlers JD, Glenn GM, Berzofsky JA (2004) Transcutaneous immunization induces mucosal CTLs and protective immunity by migration of primed skin dendritic cells. *J Clin Invest* 113: 998–1007

62 Güereña-Burgueño F, Hall ER, Taylor DN, Cassels FJ, Scott DA, Wolf MK, Roberts ZJ, Nesterova GV, Alving CR, Glenn GM (2002) Safety and immunogenicity of a prototype enterotoxigenic *Escherichia coli* vaccine administered transcutaneously. *Infect Immun* 70: 1874–1880

63 Nossal GJV (1999) Vaccines. In: Paul WE (ed): *Fundamental immunology*. Philadelphia: Lippincott-Raven, 1387–1425

64 Pulendran B (2004) Modulating vaccine responses with dendritic cells and Toll-like receptors. *Immunol Rev* 199: 227–250

65 Goldenthal KL, Cavagnaro JA, Alving CR, Vogel FR (1993) Safety evaluation of vaccine adjuvants: National Cooperative Vaccine Development Meeting Working Group. *AIDS Res Hum Retrovir* 9 (Suppl 1): S47–S51

66 Sesardic D, Dobbelaer R (2004) European union regulatory developments for new vaccine adjuvants and delivery systems. *Vaccine* 22: 2452–2456

67 Kenney RT, Edelman R (2004) Adjuvants for the future. In: Levine MM, Kaper JB, Rappuoli R, Liu MA, Good MF (eds): *New generation vaccines*, 3rd edition. New York: Marcel Dekker, 213–223

68 Glück R, Mischler R, Finkel B, Que JU, Scarpa B, Cryz Jr SJ (1994) Immunogenicity of new virosome influenza vaccine in elderly people. *Lancet* 344: 160–163

69 Sondak VK, Sosman JA (2003) Results of clinical trials with an allogenic melanoma tumor lysate vaccine: Melacine. *Semin Cancer Biol* 13: 409–415

70 Heppner DG, Gordon DM, Gross M, Wellde B, Leitner W, Krzych U, Schneider I, Wirtz RA, Richards RL, Trofa A et al (1996) Safety, immunogenicity and efficacy of plasmodium falciparum repeatless circumsporozoite protein vaccine encapsulated in liposomes. *J Inf Dis* 174: 361–366

71 McElrath MJ (1995) Selection of potent immunological adjuvants for vaccine construction. *Sem Cancer Biol* 6: 375–385

72 Harris DT, Matyas GR, Gomella LG, Taylor E, Winship MD, Spitler LE,

Mastrangelo MJ (1999) Immunologic approaches to the treatment of prostate cancer. *Sem Oncol* 26: 439–447

73 Reid CDL, Stackpole A, Meager A, Tikerpae J (1992) Interactions of tumor necrosis factor with granulocyte-macrophage colony-stimulating factor and other cytokines in the regulation of dendritic cell growth *in vitro* from early bipotent CD34+ progenitors in human bone marrow. *J Immunol* 149: 2681–2688

74 Dranoff G, Jaffee E, Lazenby A, Golumbek P, Levitsky H, Brose K, Jackson V, Hamada H, Pardoll D, Mulligan RC (1993) Vaccination with irradiated tumor cells engineered to secrete murine granulocyte-macrophage colony-stimulating factor stimulates potent, specific, and long-lasting anti-tumor immunity. *Proc Natl Acad Sci USA* 90: 3539–3543

75 Samanci A, Yi Q, Fagerberg J, Strigård K, Smith G, Rudén U, Wahren B, Mellsted H (1998) Pharmacological administration of granulocyte/macrophage-colony stimulating factor is of significant importance for the induction of a strong humoral and cellular response in patients immunized with recombinant carcinoembryonic antigen. *Cancer Immunol Immunother* 47: 131–142

76 Disis ML, Bernhard H, Shiota FM, Hand SL, Gralow JR, Huseby ES, Gillis S, Cheever MA (1996) Granulocyte-macrophage colony-stimulating factor: an effective adjuvant for protein and peptide-based vaccines. *Blood* 88: 202–210

77 Ragnhammar P, Fagerberg J, Frödin JE, Wersäll P, Hansson LO, Mellstedt H (1995) Granulocyte/macrophage-colony-stimulating factor augments the induction of antibodies, especially anti-idiotypic antibodies, to therapeutic monoclonal antibodies. *Cancer Immunol Immunother* 40: 367–375

78 Meidenbauer N, Gooding W, Spitler L, Harris D, Whiteside TL (2002) Recovery of zeta-chain expression and changes in spontaneous IL-10 production after PSA-based vaccines in patients with prostate cancer. *Br J Cancer* 86: 168–178

79 Berd D, Mastrangelo MJ, Engstrom PF, Paul A, Maguire H (1982) Augmentation of the human immune response by cyclophosphamide. *Cancer Res* 42: 4862–4866

80 Berd D, Maguire Jr HC, Mastrangelo MJ (1986) Induction of cell-mediated immunity to autologous melanoma cells and regression of metastases after treatment with a melanoma cell baccine preceded by cyclophosphamie. *Cancer Res* 46: 2572–2577

81 Hanna MG Jr, Peters LC, Hoover HC Jr (1989) Fundamentals of active specific immunotherapy of cancer using BCG-tumor cell vaccines. *Prog Clin Biol Res* 310: 51–65

82 Leong SP, Enders-Zohr P, Zhou YM, Stuntebeck S, Habib FA, Allen RE Jr, Sagebiel RW, Glassberf AB, Lowenberg DW, Hayes FA (1999) Recombinant human granulocyte macrophage-colony stimulating factor (rhGM-CSF) and autologous melanoma vaccine mediate tumor regression in patients with metastatic melanoma. *J Immunother* 22: 166–174

83 Muderhwa JM, Matyas GR, Spitler LE, Alving CR (1999) Oil-in-water liposo-

mal emulsions: characterization and potential use in vaccine delivery. *J Pharm Sci* 88: 1332–1339

84 Matyas GR, Muderhwa JM, Alving CR (2003) Oil-in-water liposomal emulsions for vaccine delivery. *Meth Enzymol* 373: 34–50

85 Lotze MT, Rosenberg SA (1991) Interleukin-2: clinical applications. In: DeVita J, Hellman S, Rosenberg SA (eds): *Biologic therapy of cancer.* JD Lippencott, Philadelphia, 159–177

86 Hladik F, Tratkiewicz JA, Tilg H, Vogel W, Schwulera V, Krönke M, Aulitzky WE, Huber C (1999) Biologic activity of low dosage IL-2 treatment *in vivo.* Molecular assessment of cytokine network interaction. *J Immunol* 153: 1449–1454

87 Meidenbauer N, Harris DT, Spitler LE, Whiteside TL (2000) Generation of PSA-reactive effector cells after vaccination with a PSA-based vaccine in patients with prostate cancer. *The Prostate* 43: 88–100

88 Neidhart J, Allen KO, Barlow DL, Carpenter M, Shaw DR, Triozzi PL, Conry RM (2004) Immunization of colorectal cancer patients with recombinant baculovirus-drived KSA (Ep-CAM) formulated with monophosphoryl lipid A in liposomal emulsion, with and without granulocyte-macrophage colony factor. *Vaccine* 22: 773–780

The Grand Challenge for the Future
ed. by Stefan H.E. Kaufmann and Paul-Henri Lambert

Vaccination in the context of immunological immaturity

Ann M. Arvin and David B. Lewis

Departments of Pediatrics and Microbiology & Immunology, Stanford University School of Medicine, Stanford, CA 94305-5164, USA

Introduction

Neonates, infants, and young children are at higher risk of infection and are more susceptible to serious consequences of infections than adults. This susceptibility results from limitations of both innate and adaptive (antigen-specific) immunity. All major lineages of hematopoietic cells that are part of the immune system are present in the human by the beginning of the second trimester, but their state of differentiation and their functional capacity may limit the immune response. In this chapter, we review general information about phenotypic and functional studies of antigen-presenting cells (APCs), T cells and B cells in the human neonate, infant, and young child, including responses to specific infectious agents and vaccines. To illustrate recent insights into the acquisition of antigen-specific immunity in the context of the developing immune system after the neonatal period, we summarize our recent investigations of immune responses in infants and young children with post-natally acquired human cytomegalovirus (CMV) infection and infants given live attenuated measles vaccine at six, nine or twelve months of age.

Antigen presentation and dendritic cells

CD8 T cells usually recognize foreign peptide antigens presented by major histocompatibility complex (MHC) class I molecules, which consist of HLA-A, -B, and -C in humans. MHC class I expression is almost ubiquitous. Most MHC class I-bound peptides are 8–10 amino acids in length and are derived from proteins recently synthesized *de novo* within host cells [1]. CD4 T cells usually recognize peptide antigens presented by MHC class II molecules, which consist of HLA-DR, -DP, and -DQ in humans. MHC class II antigen is usually expressed on professional APCs, which include dendritic cells, mononuclear phagocytes, and B cells. Most MHC class II peptides are from 14–18 amino acids in length, and mostly derived from phagocytosis or endocytosis of soluble or membrane-bound protein. MHC class I and class II molecule expression by human fetal tissues is evident by 12 weeks of gestation [2, 3]. MHC class I expression by neonatal lymphocytes is lower than on adult cells [4], but the significance of this difference is not known. Importantly, relatively normal levels of basal MHC surface expression do not exclude subtle deficiencies in antigen presentation in the neonate and young infant, particularly under conditions that more stringently test APC function. Infection with herpesviruses, such as herpes simplex virus (HSV) that can inhibit peptide loading of MHC class I, is an example [5, 6]. The amount of MHC class II expression per cell on neonatal monocytes or B cells is similar or greater than that of adult cells [4], but fewer neonatal monocytes may express HLA-DR [7]. Whether this decreased expression is functionally significant and continues beyond the neonatal period is unknown.

Myeloid dendritic cells (DCs), which are also known as DC1-lineage cells, play an essential role in antigen presentation to naïve CD4 and CD8 T cells and the initiation of the primary immune response. DC1s in uninflamed tissues are referred to as immature because they express only moderate levels of MHC class I and class II molecules. Immature DC1s are also found in the blood, and are likely to be in transit to the tissues from sites of production in the bone marrow. After exposure of immature DC1s to inflammatory stimuli, such as cytokines or microbial pathogen-derived ligands that bind their Toll-like receptors (TLRs) [8], further antigen uptake ceases. As part of maturation, antigenic peptides derived from previously internalized particles are displayed on cell surfaces in the groove of MHC class I and II molecules. Increased surface expression of the CCR7 chemokine receptor during maturation facilitates DC migration *via* the lymphatics into T-cell-rich areas of secondary lymphoid organs that express the CCR7 ligand chemokines, CCL19 and CCL21 [9].

Mature DC1s express high levels of peptide-MHC complexes and molecules that act as costimulatory signals for T-cell activation, such as CD80 (B7-1) and CD86 (B7-2). These features make them highly efficient APCs for the activation of naïve CD4 and CD8 T cells [10]. DCs are unique among APCs in being able to present antigenic peptides on MHC class I molecules by cross-presentation, in which extracellular proteins that are taken up as large particles (phagocytosis), small particles (macropinocytosis), or in soluble form (micropinocytosis) are transferred from endocytic vesicles to the cytoplasm and then onto MHC class I molecules [11]. Cross-presentation is essential for the activation of naïve CD8 T cells by antigenic peptides from pathogens that do not directly infect DCs. DCs also influence the quality of the T-cell response by directing the differentiation of naive CD4 T cells into Th1 (capable of producing IFN-γ but not IL-4, IL-5, or IL-13) or Th2 (capable of producing IL-4, IL-5, or IL-13 but not IFN-γ) effector T cells. For example, the production of IL-12 by DCs skews differentiation towards the Th1 pathway [12–14].

DC2-lineage cells, also known as plasmacytoid DCs, are a distinct DC subtype that have an important role in immunity by secretion of high levels of cytokines, particularly type I interferon (IFN-αs and IFN-β), in response to certain pathogens or pathogen-derived products. The secretion of type I interferon may not only provide a systemic anti-viral effect but also enhance the ability of myeloid DCs to present exogenous acquired antigens to CD8 T cells by cross-presentation [15]. Most DC2-lineage cells circulate as pre-DC2 precursors that lack cytoplasmic protrusions characteristic of immature or mature DC1s and have a limited capacity to present antigen. Although mature DC2s can present antigen to T cells, at least *in vitro*, their importance for antigen presentation to T cells *in vivo* is less clear.

Because most T-cell responses in the neonate and young infant are to neoantigens, any quantitative or qualitative differences in DC function would be expected to limit T-cell responses. Epidermal Langerhans cells and dermal DCs are found in the fetal skin by 16 weeks of gestation [16], and immature DC1 lineage cells are found in the interstitium of solid organs by this age [17]. Cells with the features of pre-DC2s are found in fetal lymph nodes between 19–21 weeks of gestation [18]; they have an immature phenotype and are not recent emigrants from inflamed tissues. In normal adults, circulating DCs represent about 0.5% of circulating blood mononuclear cells and consist usually of immature DC1s and pre-DC2s. In the neonatal circulation, pre-DC2s with a HLA-DR^{mid}CD11c-CD33-CD123$^{mid\text{-}hi}$ surface phenotype and lacking markers for other cell lineages (Lin$^-$) predominate in early infancy. They constitute about 75% of circulating DCs and ~0.75% of total blood mononuclear cells [19–22]. The remaining 25% of circulating DCs have an HLA-DR^{hi}CD11c$^+$CD33$^+$CD123^{lo} surface phenotype that is similar to that of circulating adult DC1s, except that CD83 expression is absent [20]. The number of circulating DC2-lineage cells appears to decline with increasing post-natal age, whereas the number of circulating DC1s does not. The predominance of DC2 lineage cells in the neonatal and infant circulation may reflect their high rate of colonization of newly formed lymphoid tissue, which undergoes rapid expansion at this age.

Circulating DC1s and pre-DC2s from adults and neonates are similar in their basal expression of HLA-DR and costimulatory molecules that are important in T-cell activation, such as CD40, which binds to CD40-ligand on T cells, and CD80 and CD86, which bind to CD28 on T cells [19, 23]. Stimulation of neonatal DC1s with lipopolysaccharide (LPS), a ligand for TLR4, and poly I:C, which is a surrogate for double-stranded RNA, a ligand for TLR3, increases their expression of HLA-DR and CD86 to adult DC1 levels. However, these stimuli are less effective for increasing CD40 and CD80 on neonatal DC1s [23]. Stimulation of neonatal and adult pre-DC2s with unmethylated CpG DNA (a ligand for TLR9 that is a component of DNA from bacteria or herpesviruses) increases their expression of HLA-DR similarly; however, CD40, CD80 and CD86 are increased to a lesser extent for neonatal pre-DC2s. In contrast to adult DC1s, neonatal DC1s do not upregulate expression of HLA-DR, CD80, and CD86 in response to pertussis toxin [24].

Circulating DCs from cord blood can allogeneically stimulate cord blood T cells *in vitro* [20, 25, 26], but their efficiency has not been directly compared with adult DCs. Virtually all of this allostimulatory activity is mediated by DC1s rather than pre-DC2s [20], which raises the possibility that neonatal DC1 function may be normal on a per cell basis. A *caveat* is that the activation of allogeneic T cells does not require uptake, processing and presentation of exogenous antigens, and is not as stringent a test of DC1 function as activation of foreign antigen-specific T cells.

The influence of DCs on Th1 *versus* Th2 phenotype is dependent on the type of DC and the particular activation conditions [27–30]. Antigen presentation by pre-DC2 favors Th2 differentiation unless these cells have been activated by viruses or unmethylated CpG DNA that cause them to release type I IFN or IL-12 that drive Th1 polarization [28]. The predominance of pre-DC2s in the fetus, neonate, and young infant might limit their response to intracellular pathogens, if this applies to the tissues. Neonatal DCs also appear to produce less type I IFN and IL-12 compared to DCs from adults, as inferred from studies using peripheral blood mononuclear cells (PBMCs) or whole blood, and assuming that DCs are the dominant source of these cytokines. For example, type I IFN production or the frequency of IFN-α-producing cells in response to HSV [31], parainfluenzae virus [32], and unmethylated DNA [19] was lower in assays using neonatal blood compared to adult blood. In the case of the response to unmethylated DNA, this decreased production is accounted for by differences between neonatal and adult pre-DC2 cells [19]. Neonatal blood cells also produce less IFN-α than adult cells in response to poly I:C, a stimulus that most likely acts on DC1s *via* TLR3 [23]. In aggregate, these studies suggest that neonatal DC1 and DC2 lineage cells produce ~10–30% as much type I IFN as analogous adult cells.

Circulating DC1s appear to be the major source of IL-12 in assays using PBMCs or whole blood. LPS induces less IL-12 production by neonatal blood mononuclear cells than by adult cells. Cord blood monocyte-derived DCs, which serve as a model of DC1 cells, also have a low capacity to produce IL-12 in response to LPS, engagement of CD40, or treatment with poly I:C [33]. Since IL-12 plays a key role in directing naïve T cells towards Th1 differentiation, this might account for limitations in adaptive immunity to LPS-containing pathogens, such as *Salmonella*. In contrast, neonatal and adult blood mononuclear cells stimulated with *Staphylococcus aureus*, other Gram-positive and Gram-negative bacterial cells, or meningococcal outer membrane proteins produce equivalent amounts of IL-12, suggesting that decreased IL-12 production is relatively stimulus-specific [34–37].

T cells

T cells mainly originate in the thymus and play a central role in antigen-specific immunity by directly mediating cellular immune responses and by facilitating antigen-specific humoral immune responses by B cells. Most T cells in the blood and peripheral lymphoid organs express antigen-specific T-cell receptors (TCR) that are heterodimeric molecules composed of TCR-α and TCR-β chains [38], with the amino-terminal portion of these chains being variable and involved in antigen recognition. The highly variable nature of this portion of the TCR is generated by intrathymic TCR gene rearrangement of variable (V), diversity (D), and joining (J) segments for TCR-β and V and J segments for TCR-α. Additional diversity of the TCR is provided by the random addition of nucleotides (referred to as N-nucleotides) to V, D, and J segments during the joining process by the enzyme terminal deoxytransferase (TdT). The TCR on the cell surface is invariably associated with the nonpolymorphic complex of CD3 proteins, which serve as docking sites for intracellular tyrosine kinases that transduce activation signals to the interior of the cell after the TCR has been engaged by antigen [39].

T-cell production, TCR repertoire, and surface phenotype

The production of peripheral T cells is established by the second trimester of pregnancy, with the concentration of circulating CD4 and CD8 T cells found at birth being substantially higher than in adults [40]. The αβ-TCR repertoire of cord blood T cells that is expressed on the cell surface has a diversity of TCR-β usage and a distribution of complementarity determining region 3 (CDR3) lengths that are similar to those of antigenically-naïve T cells in adults and infants. The CDR3 region is the most important source of TCR diversity and is formed by the junction of V segments with D and J segments. Thus, the functional pre-immune repertoire is fully formed by birth [41–43].

Circulating T cells of the healthy neonate typically lack markers for memory T cells, such as the CD45R0 isoform, β1 integrins (e.g., VLA-4), and, in the case of CD8 T cells, killer inhibitory receptors [44] and CD11b [45, 46]. This is consistent with a predominance of an antigenically-naïve population due to limited prenatal exposure to foreign antigens. The proportion of circulating T cells with a memory/effector phenotype, i.e., $CD45R0^{hi}$ surface expression, increases gradually with post-natal age [40, 47], presumably due to cumulative post-natal antigenic exposure.

CD38, an ectoenzyme that generates cyclic ADP-ribose, is expressed on most thymocytes, and some activated peripheral blood T cells and B cells, plasma cells, and DCs. Unlike adult naïve T cells, virtually all peripheral fetal and neonatal T cells express the CD38 molecule [48-51], suggesting that peripheral T cells in the fetus and neonate may represent a thymocyte-like immature transitional population. Neonatal CD4 T cells lose expression of CD38 after *in vitro* culture with IL-7 for 10 days [52], which suggests that loss of CD38 may occur with further maturation independently of engagement of the αβ-TCR/CD3 complex.

T-cell proliferation and IL-2 production

Most early studies comparing neonatal and adult T-cell activation used unfractionated T cells or unpurified circulating mononuclear cells. However, memory T cells typically have more robust signaling and activation-induced gene expression than naïve T cells [53–57], and naïve T cells may be more dependent on co-stimulation *via* engagement of CD28 [58]. This discussion will focus on more recent studies in which neonatal T cells, either unfractionated or purified based on high expression of the CD45RA marker, were compared with naïve T cells from adults since these are more likely to be informative for *bona fide* ontogenetically-related differences in activation or effector function.

Compared to adult naïve CD4 T cells, neonatal naïve CD4 T cells produce less IL-2 mRNA and express fewer high-affinity IL-2 receptors in response to stimulation with anti-CD2 monoclonal antibody (mAb) [59–61]. These differences were abrogated when phorbol ester, which bypasses proximal signaling pathways by activating Ras proteins and protein kinase C, was included [59]. This suggests a relatively inefficient generation of proximal signals after T-cell activation. Similarly, the production of IL-2 by neonatal naïve CD4 T cells is reduced compared to adult naïve ($CD45RA^{hi}$) CD4 T cells after allogeneic stimulation with adult monocyte-derived DCs (D. Lewis, unpublished data), again arguing that neonatal cells may be intrinsically limited in their ability to be physiologically activated for IL-2 production.

The ability of activated T cells to efficiently divide in response to IL-2 depends on the expression of the high-affinity IL-2 receptor, which consists of CD25 (IL-2 receptor alpha chain), the beta chain (shared with the IL-15 receptor), and the γc cytokine receptor (a chain shared with multiple other cytokine receptors). Neonatal T cells express similar or higher amounts of CD25 after stimulation with anti-CD3 mAb [62]. Although basal expression of the γc cytokine receptor is lower by neonatal T cells than by either adult naïve ($CD45RA^{hi}$) or memory ($CD45R0^{hi}$) T cells [63], the importance of this finding is unclear since activated neonatal T cells appear to proliferate in response to exogenous IL-2 as well as or better than adult T cells [62].

Two *in vitro* studies suggest that neonatal T cells may be less able to differentiate into effector cells in response to neoantigen. One study using newborns who were not infected with CMV found that the frequency of neonatal T cells proliferating to whole inactivated CMV antigen was significantly less than that of adult T cells from uninfected adults [64]. A pitfall of this study is that it used a complex antigen preparation, and one to which the T cells of adults might have previously been primed by infections other than CMV. Another study [65] found decreased antigen-specific T-cell proliferation and IL-2 production by PBMCs incubated with a protein neoantigen (keyhole limpet hemocyanin). Although these results require confirmation, they are consistent with the more limited ability of neonatal naïve CD4 T cells to produce IL-2 in response to allogeneic DCs than adult naïve cells (D. Lewis, unpublished data).

Production of other cytokines and chemokines

Many studies (reviewed in [66]), suggest that the CD4 T-cell subset or unfractionated T cells of the neonate have a reduced capacity to produce a wide range of cytokines, including IL-3, IL-4, IL-5, IL-6, IL-10, IL-13, IFN-γ and GM-CSF, compared to adult cells. However, since memory/effector T cells have a markedly greater capacity to produce these cytokines than naïve T cells, in most instances the apparent deficit of the neonatal T cells is accounted for by the lack of a circulating memory/effector cell population. However, we have found that highly purified naïve CD4 T cells from neonates have a substantially reduced capacity to produce IFN-γ *in vitro* compared to adult naïve CD4 T cells following 24–48 hours of stimulation with the same pool of monocyte-derived DCs from multiple unrelated blood donors [67]. This was demonstrable using cell culture supernatants as well as single-cell assays of CD4 T cells using intracellular cytokine staining [67]. The mechanism for this decreased expression of IFN-γ appears to involve decreased expression of CD40-ligand by neonatal T cells as well as decreased IL-12 production by the DCs, as both of these factors are important in this system for early Th1 differentiation (D. Lewis, unpublished data).

This strongly suggests that the capacity of neonatal naïve CD4 T cells to produce IFN-γ is intrinsically more limited, even when a potent, physiological APC population is used for antigen presentation. Reduced expression of IFN-γ by neonatal CD4 T cells is associated with greater methylation of DNA at a few sites in the IFN-γ gene locus in neonatal T cells compared to adult naïve T cells [68, 69]. Whether neonatal and adult naïve CD4 T cells differ at multiple other sites in their methylation of the IFN-γ gene or in other epigenetic modifications that may influence IFN-γ gene expression remains to be explored.

Highly purified neonatal naïve CD4 T cells have a limited increase in the intracellular concentration of free calcium ($[Ca^{2+}]_i$) following anti-CD3 mAb stimulation compared to identically treated adult naïve cells [70]. Although the mechanism for this reduced calcium response remains to be defined, it is likely to contribute not only to reduced production of cytokines, such as IFN-γ, but also of important cell surface molecules, such as CD40-ligand, since an elevated $[Ca^{2+}]_i$ is important for the *de novo* transcription of these genes. Neonatal naïve CD4 T cells also express reduced levels of certain transcription factors, such as NFATc2 [71, 72], which require increases in $[Ca^{2+}]_i$ for their function and that are a key factor for inducing multiple cytokine genes, including IFN-γ, and CD40-ligand. These intrinsic T-cell deficiencies, in conjunction with immature DC function may account for delayed production of IFN-γ by antigen-specific CD4 T cells following infection in early infancy.

Although cytokine production by neonatal CD8 T cells has not been as well characterized as for the CD4 T-cell subset, neonatal naïve CD8 T cells produce significantly more of the Th2 cytokine, IL-13, than adult naïve cells after stimulation with anti-CD3 and anti-CD28 mAbs and exogenous IL-2 [73]. Whether this unusual cytokine profile, which needs to be confirmed, applies to antigen-specific immune responses, such as to viral pathogens, is unclear.

Expression of TNF ligand family members

CD40-ligand (CD154), a member of the TNF ligand family, is expressed on the cell surface in high amounts by activated but not resting CD4 T cells. CD40-ligand engages CD40, a molecule expressed by APCs, including DCs, mononuclear phagocytes, and B cells. Cell-cell interactions involving CD40-ligand and CD40 are essential for many events in adaptive immunity, including the generation of memory CD4 Th1 cells, memory B cells, and, as discussed below, most immunoglobulin isotype switching [74]. In most studies, neonatal CD4 T cells, including purified naïve cells, have a much more limited capacity to express CD40-ligand and accumulate CD40-ligand mRNA than adult naïve CD4 T cells after pharmacological activation with calcium ionophore and phorbol ester [75–78]. Thus, this may represent a true developmental limitation in activation-induced gene expression. Human $CD4^{hi}CD8^{-}$ thymocytes, the immediate precursors of naïve CD4 T cells, also have a low capacity to express CD40-ligand [78, 79], suggesting that neonatal peripheral CD4 T cells have delayed post-thymic maturation of this function. However, use of a pharmacological stimulus might not accurately mimic physiological T-cell activation. Although we [70] and others [80] observed similar relative reductions in CD40-ligand surface expression by purified neonatal naïve CD4 T cells compared to adult naïve CD4 T cells using more physiological stimuli that engage the αβ-TCR/CD3 complex, this reduction was not observed in studies from two other laboratories [81, 82]. This suggests that the particular *in vitro* conditions employed may influence the outcome of the assay.

There are also conflicting results as to whether CD40-ligand expression by neonatal T cells is decreased after allogeneic stimulation. One study using irradiated adult monocyte-derived DCs as allogeneic stimulators, found that CD40-ligand expression by neonatal T cells was similar to that of adult T cells after 5 days of culture [83]. In contrast, we observed substantially lower levels of CD40-ligand expression by purified naïve CD4 T cells than adult naïve CD4 T cells after 24–48 hours of such allogeneic stimulation [67]. We favor a model in which limited initial expression of CD40-ligand by neonatal naïve CD4 T cells can be overcome with continued priming. Thus, the differentiation of neonatal naïve CD4 T cells into Th1 effector cells by CD40-ligand- and IL-12-dependent processes may both be limited during the early stages of T-cell differentiation. Although limitations in CD40-ligand production could contribute to decreased antigen-specific immunity in the neonate and young infant [74], little is known about the adequacy of CD40-ligand expression following activation of naïve CD4 T cells by antigen *in vivo*, which primarily occurs in the T-cell-rich regions of peripheral lymphoid tissue.

Fas ligand (CD95L), another member of the TNF ligand family, is important in inducing apoptotic cell death on target cells that express Fas on the surface, including lymphocytes, myeloid cells, and hepatocytes. Neonatal T cells have decreased Fas ligand expression after anti-CD3 and anti-CD28 mAb stimulation compared to unfractionated adult T cells [80], but it is unclear whether there is also a decrease relative to adult naïve cells.

Co-stimulation and anergy

Neonatal T cells produce IL-2 and proliferate as well as do adult T cells when optimal sources of CD28 co-stimulation are provided (e.g., transfectants expressing the CD28 ligands CD80 or CD86, or CD28 mAbs) [60, 61, 84]. However, neonatal CD4 T cells have a greater tendency than adult CD45RA^{hi} T cells to become anergic and functionally unresponsive when they are activated *in vitro via* the αβ-TCR/CD3 complex without concurrent optimal co-stimulation [85]. This anergic tendency may be relevant since newborns with toxic shock syndrome-like exanthematous disease, in which Vβ2-bearing T cells are markedly expanded *in vivo* by the Staphylococcal exotoxin, TSST-1, have a greater fraction of anergic Vβ2-bearing T cells than do adults with TSST-1-mediated disease [86].

Chemokine receptor expression

The differential expression of chemokine receptors by T cells is important in their selective trafficking to sites of antigen presentation *versus* inflamed tissues [87]. CCR7 expression by naïve T cells allows these cells to recirculate between the blood and uninflamed lymphoid organs. Naïve T cells of the adult express CCR1, CCR7, and CXCR4 on the cell surface, and have low to undetectable levels of CCR5. The role served by CCR1 and CXCR4 expression on naïve T cells is unclear, and CCR1 may be non-functional in this cell type [88]. Infant and adult naïve T cells have a similar phenotype, except that infant cells lack CCR1 surface expression and, unlike adult naïve T cells, they do not increase CXCR3 expression and decrease CCR7 expression after activation *via* anti-CD3 and anti-CD28 mAb [89, 90]. The increased expression of CXCR3 and decreased expression of CCR7 is important for allowing T cells to enter inflamed tissues that express chemokine ligands for CXCR3. The CCR7 expressed on neonatal T cells is functional and mediates chemotaxis of these cells in response to cognate chemokines [91]. Together, this suggests that activated neonatal T cells may be limited in their capacity to traffic to non-lymphoid tissue sites of inflammation and, instead, may continue to recirculate between the blood and peripheral lymphoid organs.

Memory T-cell subsets

Memory T cells are heterogeneous in their expression of CCR7 [92]. The $CCR7^{hi}$ population (putative central memory cells) appears to preferentially recirculate between the secondary lymph nodes and blood, have limited effector function, and may serve as a reservoir for the generation of additional memory cells. The $CCR7^{lo}$ cell population (putative effector memory cells), is enriched in memory cells that can rapidly induce effector functions, such as IFN-γ or IL-4 production or cytotoxin expression. The $CCR7^{lo}$ cell subset is also enriched in the expression of other chemokine receptors, which facilitates their preferential entry into inflamed or infected tissues [87]. Central memory cells may be intermediates between naïve T cells and effector memory T cells [93], although this remains highly controversial [94].

Our study of CMV-specific CD4 T-cell responses showed that the memory CD4 T-cell subset of infants and young children had a significantly higher ratio of central memory to effector memory CD4 T cells than adults [66]. This difference may reflect reduced activity of the IL-12/IL-23-dependent Th1 pathway, since effector memory CD4 T cells are markedly reduced in IL-12Rβ1 deficiency, which ablates IL-12 and IL-23 signaling [95]. Circulating monocytes in infants also have a reduced capacity to produce IL-12 compared to older children and adults that could contribute to this mechanism [96]. Although the numbers of circulating effector memory CD4 T cells may be reduced, this population appears to be functionally normal. For example, the frequency of effector memory CD4 T cells that produced IFN-γ and the amount of IFN-γ produced per cell in response to the *Staphylococcus aureus* toxin SEB was similar in the blood of infants and young children compared to adults [66].

T-cell cytotoxicity

Effector and memory CD8 T cells kill more efficiently than antigenically-naïve T cells after stimulation with lectins or anti-CD3 mAb [97] or after allogeneic sensitization [98-100]. Thus, the early reports of deficiency of neonatal CTL activity after *in vitro* activation or priming (reviewed in [66]) can be explained by the absence among neonatal CD8 T cells of effector and memory cells, as identified by their expression of CD45R0 and/or their lack of CD27 and CD28 [101]. Until recently, the capacity of fetal T cells to mediate cytotoxicity received little scrutiny. One recent study documented robust fetal effector CD8 T-cell responses, including clonal expansion, IFN-γ production, and perforin expression, in response to congenital CMV infection [102]. A robust fetal CD8 T-cell response also appears to occur in cases of congenital infection with the parasite *Trypanosoma cruzi*, the agent of Chagas disease [103]. Thus, the capacity to generate a functional CD8 T-cell effector population *in vivo* is established *in utero*, at least under conditions of chronic stimulation. These studies, as well as our studies of the CD8 T-cell response to primary CMV infection in infants and young children, which are discussed below, suggest that CD8 T-cell responses to persistent viral infection are similar to those of adults. However, it is unclear whether this applies to CD8 T-cell responses that occur more acutely, e.g., within one week, such as in response to respiratory viral infections.

Antigen-specific CD4 T-cell immunity

Infants between 6–12 months of age have lower IL-2 production in response to tetanus toxoid than older children and adults [104]. This suggests that either antigen-specific memory CD4 T-cell generation or function is decreased during early infancy. Whether this reflects limitations in antigen processing, T-cell activation and co-stimulation, or proliferation and differentiation remains unclear.

In contrast to inactivated vaccine antigens, BCG vaccination at birth *versus* 2 months or 4 months of age was equally effective in inducing CD4 T-cell proliferative and IFN-γ responses to purified protein derivative (PPD), extracellular *M. tuberculosis* antigens, and a *M. tuberculosis* intracellular extract [33, 105]. The responses were robust not only at 2 months following immunization but also at one year of age, and there was no skewing towards Th2 cytokine production [105], even by PPD-specific CD4 T-cell clones [33]. Thus, early post-natal administration of BCG vaccine does not result in decreased vaccine-specific Th1 responses, tolerance, or Th2 skewing. How these responses compare to older children and adult vaccinees is not known. Early BCG vaccination may also influence antigen-specific responses to unrelated vaccine antigens. BCG given at birth increased Th1- and Th2-specific responses and antibody titers to hepatitis B surface antigen (HBsAg) given simultaneously [106]. BCG vaccine given at birth did not enhance the Th1 response to tetanus toxoid given at 2 months of age, but did increase the Th2 response (IL-13 production). It is likely that BCG vaccination may accelerate DC maturation so that these cells can augment either Th1 or Th2 responses.

The T-cell-specific response to oral poliovirus vaccine (OPV), another live vaccine, suggests a decreased Th1 response. Neonates given OPV at birth, 1, 2, and 3 months of age, have lower OPV-specific CD4 T-cell proliferation, IFN-γ production, and the number of IFN-γ-positive cells than previously immunized (but not recently reimmunized) adults [107]. In contrast, their antibody titers were higher than those of adults, suggesting that CD4 T-cell help for B cells is not impaired. OPV may be less effective at inducing a Th1 response than BCG in neonates and young infants because of its limited replication, site of inoculation or ability to stimulate APC in a manner conducive to Th1 immunity, relative to BCG, which induces persistent infection in the recipient.

Although neonates and young infants have been suggested to have skewing of CD4 T-cell responses towards a Th2 cytokine profile, this may be an oversimplification. For example, the tetanus toxoid-specific response following vaccination indicates that both Th1 (IFN-γ) and Th2 (IL-5 and IL-13) memory responses occur, particularly following the third vaccine dose at 6 months of age [108]. The tetanus toxoid-specific Th1 response may decrease transiently by 12 months of age, while Th2 responses are not affected [108].

Antigen-specific CD8 T-cell immunity

CD8 T-cell responses to CMV infection acquired *in utero* [102] or during infancy and early childhood [109] are robust. Cytotoxic responses to human immunodeficiency virus (HIV) in perinatally infected infants suggest that CD8 T cells capable of mediating cytotoxicity have undergone clonal expansion *in vivo* as early as 4 months of age [110]. However, their cytotoxicity may be reduced and delayed in appearance compared to adults [111]. There is also decreased HIV-specific CD8 T-cell production of IFN-γ by young infants after perinatal HIV infection [112], and an inability to generate HIV-specific cytotoxic T cells following highly-active anti-retroviral therapy [113]. When evaluated beyond infancy, cytolytic activity directed to HIV envelope proteins was commonly detected, but cytolytic activity directed against gag or pol proteins was rarely detected [114], suggesting that the TCR repertoire of cytotoxic CD8 T cells was less diverse than in adults.

HIV-1 infection may inhibit antigen-specific immunity by depleting circulating DCs [115], impairing antigen presentation [116], decreasing the output of naïve T cells by the thymus [117], and promoting T-cell apoptosis [118]. In addition, maintenance of HIV-specific CD8 T cells with effector function depends on HIV-specific CD4 T cells, which may be selectively and severely impaired by the virus. Regardless of the precise mechanism, the suppressive effects of HIV-1 on cytotoxic responses may be relatively specific for HIV-1, since HIV-infected infants who lack HIV-specific cytotoxic T cells may maintain cytolytic T cells against Epstein Barr virus (EBV) and CMV [112, 113]. A surprising and poorly characterized effect of HIV-1 infection is to inhibit the responses of HIV-exposed but uninfected infants born to HIV-infected mothers [117, 119].

An early study found that respiratory syncytial virus (RSV)-specific cytotoxicity was more pronounced and frequent in infants 6-24 months of age than in younger infants [120]. Murine studies indicate that RSV infection suppresses CD8 T-cell-mediated effector activity (IFN-γ production and cytolytic activity) and that only transient memory CD8 T-cell responses occur following infection [121]. Longitudinal studies of CD8 T-cell immunity to RSV in children and adults following primary and secondary infection will be of interest to determine if this immunoevasive mechanism applies to humans.

In summary, T-cell function in the fetus, neonate, and likely the young infant, is impaired compared to adults. T-cell participation in T-cell help for B-cell differentiation is diminished. Selectively decreased expression of activation-dependent proteins by fetal and neonatal T cells, such as cytokines and CD40-ligand, may contribute to these deficits. The repertoire of αβ-TCR is probably adequate except in early fetal gestation. Following fetal or neonatal infection, the acquisition of CD4 T-cell antigen-specific responses may be typically delayed. *In vitro* studies suggest that deficiencies of DC function and intrinsic limitations in the activation and differentiation of antigenically-naïve CD4 T cells into memory/effector cells may be contributory, although the function of tissue-associated DCs is unknown. In contrast to diminished CD4 T-cell function, CD8 T-cell-mediated cytotoxicity and cytokine production in response to strong chronic stimuli, such as congenital CMV infection, appears to be intact in the fetus and neonate.

B cells

Mature B cells are identified by their expression of surface immunoglobulin (sIg). Immunoglobulin (Ig), which is synonymous with antibody, is a heterotetrameric protein consisting of two identical heavy chains and two identical light chains linked by disulfide bonds [122]. Like the TCR, the amino terminal portion of the antibody chains is highly variable as a consequence of the assembly of V, D, and J gene segments (Ig heavy chain) or V and J segments (Ig light chain). However, antibody molecules are distinct from the αβ-TCR in that they typically recognize antigens based on their three-dimensional structure, such as those found on intact proteins or on non-protein molecules, such as complex carbohydrates. The B-cell antigen receptor (BCR) is also distinct from the TCR in that Ig variants are generated in mature B cells by the process of somatic hypermutation, in which germinal center B cells accumulate apparently random point mutations within existing V, D, and J segments. These variants undergo a selection process favoring B cells that bear sIg with high affinity for antigen. As for T cells, B cells are activated to proliferate and differentiate after engagement of their sIg antigen-specific receptor. sIg is invariably associated with nonpolymorphic membrane proteins, Ig-α (CD79a) and Ig-β (CD79b), which are structural and functional homologues of the CD3 complex proteins, and are involved in the intracellular transmission of activating signals to the interior of the cell.

For B cells to be activated effectively and to produce antibody against protein antigens requires help from T cells in most cases. This help is in the form of soluble cytokines, such as IL-4 and IL-21 [123], and of cell surface–associated signals, such as CD40-ligand, which is transiently expressed on the surface of activated CD4 T cells. The engagement of CD40 on the B cell is also instrumental in inducing B cells to undergo Ig isotype switching, for example, from IgM to IgE, in which the constant region at the carboxy-terminus of the Ig heavy chain gene is replaced with another isotype-specific segment but the antigen-combining site at the amino-terminus is preserved. In cases in which the antigen has multiple and identical surface determinants (e.g., complex polysaccharides or certain viral proteins with repetitive motifs) and multiple sIg are cross linked, antigen binding alone may be sufficient to induce B-cell activation without cognate (direct cell-cell interaction) help from T cells. In this case, other signals derived from non–T cells or T cells, such as cytokines, or from microorganisms, such as bacterial lipoproteins or pathogen-derived DNA containing unmethylated CpG motifs, may enhance antibody responses [124]. Isotype switching, however, is much more limited in this context. As for T cells, B cells receive additional regulatory signals from the engagement of surface molecules other than the BCR that act as either co-stimulatory or inhibitory molecules. A B-cell co-stimulatory molecular complex consisting of CD19, CD21, and CD81 [125] binds the CD3d fragment of the C3 complement component. B-cell activation is suppressed when a surface receptor for the Fc (fragment crystallizable) portion of IgG, FcγRIIB, is engaged concurrently with the sIg by antigen-IgG complexes [126], and, as discussed below, this may be a mechanism by which maternal antibody inhibits the B-cell response of infants.

B-cell production, Ig repertoire, and surface phenotype

The proportion of B cells in the spleen, blood, and bone marrow is similar to that in the adult by 22 weeks of gestational age [127, 128]. Mature B cells circulate at higher concentration during the second and third trimesters than at birth, and concentrations decline further by adulthood [50, 129]. The Ig repertoire of peripheral B cells of the neonate and young infant is similar to that of the adult based on V and D segment usage. Certain segments (e.g., DH7-27) [130] may be over-represented in the neonate and certain V segments may be lacking [131, 132], but this is unlikely to limit the humoral immune response of the neonate and young infant. Other V segments, such as VH3, are present at a greater frequency in the pre-immune Ig repertoire of the neonate [132, 133], which allow antibody molecules to bind protein A of *Staphylococcus aureus*, perhaps providing some intrinsic protection during the perinatal period.

The CDR3 region is the most hypervariable portion of Igs, and is at the center of the antigen-binding pocket of the antibody [134]. Thus, reduced CDR3 diversity could limit the efficiency of the antibody response. The CDR3 region of the Ig heavy chain gene remains relatively short until the beginning of the third trimester due to a lack of activity of the TdT enzyme. Subsequently, the CDR3 length gradually increases in length so that by birth it is similar to that of adult B cells [130, 135–137]. A complete lack of nucleotide additions by TdT would be predicted to result in antibodies with combining sites that are relatively flat and potentially inefficient at combining with antigen [138], but the importance of shortened CDR3 regions by themselves in limiting antibody responses is doubtful: gene knockout mice lacking TdT produce normal antibody responses following immunization or infection [139]. A combination of a relative lack of TdT and limitations in V and D usage could limit the ability of the fetal B cells to recognize a full spectrum of foreign antigens, particularly prior to mid-gestation, but this is unlikely to occur in term neonates and young infants.

The B cells of neonates and young infants have increased surface levels of IgM compared to adult B cells [140, 141]. In flow cytometric studies in which non-specific binding is carefully excluded, <1% of circulating B cells of the neonate express surface IgG or IgA [142], indicating that isotype switching prior to birth is rare. Consistent with this finding, true germinal centers in the spleen and lymph nodes are absent during fetal life, but appear during the first months after postnatal antigenic stimulation [143].

A high frequency of circulating and lymphoid tissue-associated fetal and neonatal B cells express CD5, indicating that most belong to the B-1a subset [144–147]. These circulating CD5+ B cells are prominent at birth [40] and gradually decline with increasing postnatal age [145, 148, 149]. Like adult B-1a cells, newborn B-1a cells express IgM antibodies that are polyreactive, including with self antigens, such as DNA [145, 146, 150, 151]. Neonatal B cells also differ from adult B cells in expressing CD10 (CALLA), which typically is limited in the adult to immature B-lineage cells of the bone marrow. Thus, similar to the finding of a thymocyte marker, CD38, on neonatal T cells, CD10 expression by some neonatal B cells raises the possibility of a maturational arrest, although $CD10^{+}$ B cells are functionally mature based on their ability to undergo isotype switching. The small fraction of CD10$^+$ B cells found at birth gradually declines during infancy [152]. Neonatal B cells also have reduced expression of CD21, which is involved in co-stimulation of B cells by complement [153], and of the FcγRII receptor (CD32) [140, 154], which may render them less subject to the inhibitory effect of antigen/antibody complexes. Reduced expression by neonatal CD5$^-$ B cells of the adhesion molecules CD11a, CD44, CD54 (ICAM-1), and L-selectin has also been reported [155, 156], which might reduce their ability to traffic to tissues from the circulation compared to adult B cells.

T-cell-dependent Ig production and isotype switching

Most studies have found that neonatal or fetal B cells have similar capacity to adult naïve B cells to undergo isotype switching and produce IgM, the four subclasses of IgG, IgA, and IgE, if they are optimally activated using exogenous cytokines (e.g., IL-4 or IL-10) and by CD40 engagement (reviewed in [66]). However, neonatal B cells may produce substantially less IgA than do adult naïve B cells in the presence of adult T cells stimulated by anti-CD3 mAb (as a source of CD40-ligand) and IL-10 [157], suggesting intrinsic limitations of B-cell function, particularly when T-cell help may be limited. This decrease in isotype switching is not attributable to decreased neonatal B-cell activation or proliferation, since these cells proliferate like adult B cells after engagement of CD40 and/or surface IgM [141].

In systems in which neonatal B cells are dependent on neonatal T cells for a source of CD40-ligand, Ig production and isotype switching are reduced compared to when adult T cells are used [78]. However, as discussed above, it remains controversial whether CD40-ligand production by neonatal T cells limits immune responses *in vivo*. Whether decreased neonatal DC function also contributes to diminished B-cell responses has not been determined, but an increasing body of literature suggests that direct interactions between B cells and DCs may be important for regulation of B-cell immunity.

B-cell response to T-independent antigens

T-independent (TI)-type I antigens are those which bind to B cells and directly activate them *in vitro* to produce antibody without T cells or exogenous cytokines. In the human, one such TI-1 antigen is fixed *Brucella abortus*, which is likely to utilize TLRs for B-cell activation [158]. TI-type II antigens are mostly polysaccharides with multiple identical subunits, and certain proteins that contain multiple determinants of identical or similar antigenic specificity. Responses to these antigens are enhanced *in vitro* and *in vivo* by a variety of cytokines, including IL-6, IL-12, IFN-γ, and GM-CSF [159, 160–162]. NK cells, T cells, or macrophages may produce these cytokines *in vivo*. TI-type II responses are also enhanced by bacterially derived LPS, lipoproteins, porin proteins, or unmethylated CpG DNA [161, 163, 164]. This enhancement probably occurs primarily by engagement of TLRs on B cells [124]. The response to TI-type II antigens is characterized by the lack of B-cell memory or somatic hypermutation and is largely restricted to the IgM and IgG2 isotypes [153].

Antibody production by human neonatal B cells to a TI-type I antigen *in vitro* (*Brucella abortus*) is only modestly reduced [165]. This appears to be due to a decreased ability of antigen-activated B cells to proliferate rather than a decreased precursor frequency of antigen-specific clones [165]. The response to TI-type II antigens is the last to appear chronologically. This is likely to account, at least in part, for the susceptibility of the neonate and young infant to infection with encapsulated bacteria, e.g., such as group B streptococci [166, 167] and, as discussed in detail below, the poor response to bacterially derived polysaccharide antigens in vaccines until after 2 years of age. These poor antibody responses are associated with the lack of circulating memory ($CD27^{hi}$) B cells that express IgM and have not undergone isotype switching in children less than 2 years of age [168]. The reduction or absence of these IgM memory B cells in adult patients after splenectomy suggests that they may depend on the spleen microenvironment for their generation or long-term survival.

Whether the decreased response to TI-type II antigens of early childhood is an intrinsic B-cell immaturity and/or is due to decreased function of other cells such as APCs of the spleen, remains unclear. Decreased CD21 expression by infant B cells has been proposed as a possible mechanism for limitations in the TI-type II response. CD19 and CD21 together constitute the type 2 complement receptor, which serves to transduce B-cell activating signals after its engagement by C3 complement components and promote cell proliferation, and murine experiments support an important role for this receptor for antibody responses to pathogens, such as *Streptococcus pneumoniae* [169]. Studies using human splenic tissue suggest that TI–type II antigens activate complement and bind C3 and subsequently localize to the marginal zone splenic B cells expressing type 2 complement receptors [153, 170]. The acquisition of a capacity to respond to bacterial polysaccharides at approximately 2–3 years of age correlates with the appearance of B cells expressing CD21 in the marginal zone region of the spleen [171]. Although recent studies have not found decreased expression of CD21 by circulating neonatal B cells [140, 172], it remains possible that B cells that preferentially traffic to the marginal zone could have such decreased expression. Mechanisms for reduced responses to polysaccharides that involve APC populations of the splenic marginal zone have also not been excluded. Neonatal B cells appear to have intact pathways of activation *via*

TLR9 [156], suggesting that this does not account for the poor response to TI-type II antigens at this age.

B-cell response to T-dependent antigens

Most proteins are T-dependent antigens requiring cognate T-cell/B-cell interaction for production of antibodies (other than small amounts of IgM). Conjugation of polysaccharide antigens with protein carriers also results in responses to the polysaccharide moiety that is T-dependent. The antibody response to T-dependent antigens is characterized by the generation of memory B cells with somatically-mutated, high-affinity Ig and the potential for isotype switching. The production of CD40-ligand by CD4 T cells and the engagement of CD40 on B cells are critical for these B-cell responses.

The capacity of humans to respond to T-dependent antigens is well established at birth, and is only modestly reduced compared to the response of the adult. There are many potential mechanisms for this modest reduction including: decreased DC interactions or function with CD4 T cells or B cells; limitations in CD4 T-cell activation and expansion into a T helper-effector cell population; impaired cognate interactions between CD4 T cells and B cells; an intrinsic B-cell defect; or a combination of these factors. Another possibility is that T-dependent antigens preferentially upregulate CD22 on neonatal B cells compared to adult B cells, and which may raise the threshold for B-cell activation on neonatal compared to adult B cells [173]. Most studies of the neonatal immune response to T-dependent antigens have not evaluated antibody affinity, a reflection of somatic mutation, or isotype expression. Although such responses might be limited early in the immune response, e.g., because of decreased CD40-ligand expression by CD4 T cells [70, 75, 76, 78, 174], this has not been documented. Decreased CD40-ligand expression by antigen-specific T cells would also be expected to result in reduced memory B-cell development, but this has not been documented for B cells of the neonate and young infant responding to T-dependent antigens.

Antibody responses to vaccines

Immunization starting in the neonatal period, even within the first 48 hours after birth, usually elicits a protective response to T-dependent protein antigens, including tetanus and diphtheria toxoids [175], OPV [176], hepatitis B surface antigen (HBsAg) [177], and the experimental bacteriophage ϕX174 vaccine [178]. The response to some vaccines may be less vigorous in the neonate than in older children or adults. For example, this has occurred in the primary antibody response to recombinant HBsAg in term neonates lacking maternally-derived HBsAg antibody, compared to unimmunized older infants, children, and adults [177, 179]. Anti-HBsAg titers achieved in infants after the second and third doses are similar to those of older children, indicating that early immunization does not result in tolerance [177]. If initial immunization is delayed until one month of age, the antibody response to primary HBsAg vaccination is increased and nearly equivalent to older children, suggesting that the developmental limitations responsible for reduced antibody responses are transient [177, 180]. Similarly, although two-week-old infants immunized with a single dose of diphtheria or tetanus toxoid had delayed production of specific antibody compared to older infants, by two months of age their response was similar to that of six-month-old infants [181]. Isotype switching from IgM to IgG may also be delayed following neonatal vaccination for some vaccines, such as *Salmonella* H antigen [167] but not all antigens, e.g., bacteriophage ϕX174 [178]. Immunization of infants of HIV-infected mothers starting at birth with recombinant HIV-1 gp120 vaccine in MF59 adjuvant also elicited high antibody titers without evidence of tolerance [182].

In contrast to most inactivated vaccines, newborns given whole cell pertussis vaccination may not only have a poor initial antibody response, but a subsequently reduced antibody response to certain antigenic components, such as pertussis toxin, compared to infants first immunized at 1 month of age or older [183-185]. This suggests tolerance induction, which is relatively vaccine-specific.

The response to purified polysaccharide antigens, such as from *Haemophilus influenzae* type b or group B streptococci, is absent or severely blunted when these vaccines are given in the neonatal period. The response to some polysaccharide antigens, such as from *Neisseriae meningitidis* type A, can be demonstrated by 3 months of age, but the response to vaccination with polysaccharides from *H. influenzae* type b, *Neisseriae meningitidis* type C, or most pneumococcal serotypes, is poor until approximately 18–24 months [186]. As discussed above, this inability to respond to polysaccharides and other TI-type II antigens is not clearly understood, but does not appear to be due to limitations in expression of an appropriate antibody repertoire [187].

Coupling of the *H. influenzae* type b polysaccharide or other polysaccharides to a protein carrier converts a TI-type II antigen to a T-dependent antigen [188]. This is accompanied by an enhanced magnitude and higher avidity antibody response on subsequent boosting, presumably resulting from T-dependent memory B-cell generation and somatic hypermutation. Conjugation of *H. influenzae* type b capsular polysaccharide covalently to a protein carrier renders it immunogenic in infants as young as 2 months of age, and primes for an enhanced antibody response to unconjugated vaccine given at 12 months of age. Since this is an age when the response to the unconjugated vaccine is usually poor, the conjugate vaccine has induced polysaccharide-specific B-cell memory [189]. Conjugation of *H. influenzae* type b polysaccharide to tetanus or diphtheria toxoid does not change the repertoire of the anti-polysaccharide antibodies produced from that observed using vaccination with the free polysaccharide [187, 189]. Vaccination with protein-capsular polysaccharide conjugate vaccines containing polysaccharides of *Streptococcus pneumoniae* (types 4, 6B, 9V, 14, 18C, 19F, 23F) [190–192] and *N. meningitidis* (types A and C) [193] is immunogenic in infants as young as 2 months of age, and primes them for subsequent memory responses. Thus, the neonatal and young infant response to conjugate vaccines now mimics their response to other T-dependent antigens.

The administration of a single dose of *H. influenzae* type b polysaccharide-tetanus toxoid conjugate to term neonates as early as a few days of age may enhance the antibody response to unconjugated *H. influenzae* type b polysaccharide vaccine at 4 months of age [194]. However, this enhanced response is weak and does not occur when the neonate is primed with tetanus toxoid followed by immunization with conjugate vaccine at two months of age [195].

Inhibition of post-natal antibody responses by maternal antibodies

Maternal antibody can inhibit the production by the newborn or young infant of antibodies of the same specificity. The degree of inhibition varies with the maternal antibody titer, and the type and amount of antigen. For example, maternal antibody has been reported to markedly inhibit the response to measles and rubella vaccine, but not to mumps vaccine [196]. Inhibition of the response to live attenuated viral vaccines may result in part from reduced replication of vaccine virus in the recipient. Maternal antibodies may also inhibit the response to non-replicating "dead" vaccines such as whole cellular pertussis vaccine [185], diphtheria toxoids [197], *Salmonella* flagellar antigen [167] and inactivated poliovirus vaccine [198]. This inhibition may be due to masking of immunogenic epitopes by maternal antibody so that these cannot be bound to sIg on antigen-specific B cells. Another mechanism may involve the formation of antigen/maternal IgG antibody complexes that inhibit activation of B cells by simultaneous engagement of sIg and the inhibitory FcγRII receptor by the IgG component of the complex. Maternal antibody may also lead to more rapid clearance of vaccine antigen and decreased immunogenicity. Despite these multiple potential inhibitor mechanisms, for certain antigens, such as HBsAg, neither maternal antibodies nor hyperimmune IgG administration has a substantial inhibitory effect on the newborn immune response to HBsAg vaccination.

In summary, the inability of the neonate and young infant to produce antibodies in response to polysaccharides, particularly bacterial capsular polysaccharides, limits resistance to bacterial pathogens for up to 2 years of age. The basis for this defect remains unclear, but may reflect an intrinsic limitation of B-cell function or a deficiency in the anatomical microenvironment or APC function required for B cells to become activated and differentiate into plasma cells. In contrast, neonatal immunization with most T-dependent vaccines results in intact IgM responses and only slightly diminished IgG responses without evidence of tolerance, except possibly for pertussis vaccination. These modest differences between neonates and older infants in the magnitude of the antibody response to protein neoantigens rapidly resolves following birth, and may reflect transient limitations in T-cell function, such as reduced CD40-ligand production, as well as intrinsic limitations of B-cell maturation and function.

T-cell immunity to cytomegalovirus (CMV) infection in infants and young children

Early studies by our group at Stanford and at the University of Washington in Seattle showed that infection of neonates with HSV resulted in antigen-specific proliferation and cytokine (IL-2, IFN-γ, and TNF-α) production by CD4 T cells. However, these responses were reduced in magnitude and substantially delayed compared to adults with primary HSV infection [199, 200]. The postnatal age at which the kinetics of this response becomes similar to that of adults is not known, although clinically HSV rarely causes central nervous system or disseminated disease after the neonatal period.

Many infants and young children become infected with CMV by exposure to maternal CMV in cervical secretions or breast milk, or by close contact with infected children, e.g., in day care [201]. In recent studies, we compared the CD4 and CD8 T-cell immune responses to CMV in young children with post-natally acquired CMV infection to investigate possible developmental limitations in the immune response to this common herpesvirus. Although infected children are almost always asymptomatic, primary CMV infection of neonates and infants usually results in continuous or frequent viral shedding into the urine and saliva for up to several years [201, 202]. In contrast, limited studies have indicated that adults with primary CMV infection stop continual viral shedding by 9–12 months after acquisition, and have only infrequent recurrences of shedding thereafter [203, 204]. The reason for age-related differences in the duration of CMV shedding after primary viral acquisition is unknown but T-cell immunity appears to be important to maintain CMV in a latent state [205, 206]. Studies of murine CMV indicate that CD4 T cells producing IFN-γ, i.e., Th1 cells, are important for the control of CMV replication and shedding from epithelial sites, such as the salivary glands [207–209]. Our hypothesis was that differences in the duration of CMV shedding and the quantity of virus detected in urine by PCR assay between young children and adults would correlate with quantitative or qualitative differences in the T-cell-mediated immune response, as measured by flow cytometric analysis of whole blood specimens stimulated with CMV or CMV peptides.

Analyses of CMV-specific CD4 T-cell responses

In these studies, frequencies of CMV-specific CD4 T cells were assessed in 13 asymptomatic young children with primary CMV infection of approximately 8–29 months duration and 14 asymptomatic CMV-seropositive adults. Following the approach of Waldrop and Picker [210], we analyzed the frequency of IFN-γ^+ cells using intracellular cytokine staining, and only considered cells that were both IFN-γ^+ and CD69$^+$ to be true-positives for IFN-γ expression. In agreement with previous studies by others [210–212], adults had discrete subsets of CD4 and CD8 T cells that co-expressed IFN-γ and CD69, an activation-dependent protein, in response to either whole CMV antigen (CMV) or a mixture of CMV pp65 (UL83) peptides (pp65) [66]. A control antigen (mock-infected and lysed fibroblasts) and a control peptide pool derived from carcinoembryonic antigen (CEA) amino acid sequence, a self-antigen, resulted in a minimal response (<0.07% IFN-γ^+ cells) similar to incubation of cells without additive.

In contrast, young children had a markedly and significantly ($P<0.05$ by the two-tailed, unpaired Student's t-test) lower frequency of circulating CMV-specific CD4 T cells that produced IFN-γ compared to adults. Children also had a markedly and significantly reduced frequency of CD4 T cells that produced IFN-γ in response to the pp65 peptide mixture. Since activation of pp65-reactive CD4 or CD8 T cells by the peptide mixture requires only peptide binding to MHC surface molecules and not antigen uptake and processing by APCs [211, 213], these results indicated that the decreased CMV-specific CD4 T-cell response of children was not due to impaired APC function during the ex vivo stimulation. These significant decreases of CMV-specific CD4 T cells for young children were likely to apply to the absolute number of these cells. Although total lymphocyte counts per microliter were not determined as part of this study, we reanalyzed the data, assuming that the young children had on average a 2.0-fold greater absolute number of CD4 T cells than the adults, the largest difference reported in the literature [214], all of the differences that were significant for CMV-specific and pp65-specific CD4 T-cell frequency remained significant when expressed as cells/μl of blood.

CMV-specific CD4 T cells producing IFN-γ have been detected as early as 30 days following viral exposure in adults with primary CMV infection as a result of renal transplantation, and who receive potent immunosuppressive drugs to limit transplant rejection [215, 216]. However, it remained plausible that the reduced IFN-γ response by CD4 T cells of healthy CMV-infected young children reflected their shorter duration of CMV infection compared to the healthy adult group with presumed chronic infection. To exclude this, we compared the CMV-specific Th1 immune responses of 4 healthy adults with primary CMV infection of an estimated 12 to 15 months of duration with those of children for whom the estimated period of CMV infection was 12 to 29 months, i.e., it was equal to or greater than that of the adults. The CMV- and pp65-specific Th1 immune responses of adults with recent primary infection were similar to those of the adult chronic group and, again, were significantly greater than those of the children with primary infection of a similar duration ($P<0.05$). Thus, healthy young children had a markedly limited ability to mount a CMV-specific Th1 immune response for a year or more following viral acquisition, while this lag in anti-viral immunity was not observed in adults.

To assess whether the reduced CMV-specific Th1 response of young children reflected a generally limited ability to mount Th1 immune responses to antigens, we examined the phenotype of CMV-specific CD4 T cells that produced IFN-γ in adults and children. Previous studies have reported that IFN-γ production by adult CD4 T cells in response to protein antigens [217–219], including CMV [210] or SEB [95], is largely confined tothe $CD45RA^{lo}CD45R0^{hi}$ memory subset. We first verified that this applied to CMV-specific and SEB-induced IFN-γ production by CD4 T cells from adults with presumed chronic CMV infection or adults and children with documented recent primary infection.

Next, since memory CD4 T cells expressing low levels of CCR7 have been reported to be highly enriched in IFN-γ production after engagement of CD3 and CD28 [93, 95], we analyzed the relationship between CCR7 expression and Th1 responses for CMV-specific and SEB-activated memory CD4 T cells: we found that among adult and child memory CD4 T cells, more than 90% of cells that produced IFN-γ in response to either stimulation with CMV antigen, the pp65 peptide mixture, or SEB were $CCR7^{lo}$. Similar results were also observed for CD4 T cells from adults with documented recent primary CMV infection. These results suggested that Th1 responses after postnatal antigenic exposure, or at least to CMV-derived antigens, are largely restricted to a $CCR7^{lo}$ memory CD4 T-cell subset. The finding of this restriction of SEB-induced Th1 responses to the $CCR7^{lo}$ subset of memory CD4 T cells in children and adults suggests that this is likely to be a general feature of the CD4 T-cell response to most antigens.

Since the CMV-specific Th1 response was limited to the $CCR7^{lo}$ memory CD4 T-cell subset, we considered whether the reduced CMV-specific Th1 responses of children reflected a general tendency to accumulate fewer $CCR7^{lo}$ cells during memory CD4 T-cell generation. In fact, the fraction of memory CD4 T cells that were $CCR7^{lo}$ was modestly but significantly lower in children with documented recent primary CMV infection (about 50–60% of the adult value) compared to adults with chronic CMV infection [66]. A trend was also observed in a comparison of children and adults with primary CMV infection of similar duration. Although additional studies of other antigen-specific immune responses are needed, these results suggest that infants and young children may have a tendency to accumulate a lower fraction of CCR7^{lo} cells as part of memory CD4 T-cell responses than adults, and that this may contribute to reduced Th1 immunity to pathogens, such as CMV.

The ability of CCR7^{lo} memory CD4 T cells to produce IFN-γ was further compared between children and adults with documented primary CMV infection of similar duration. The CCR7^{lo} subset of memory CD4 T cells of children had a markedly and significantly ($P < 0.05$) lower frequency of IFN-γ-producing cells in response to whole CMV antigen or the pp65 peptide mixture than the same adult cell population. This was in agreement with the earlier results that analyzed all CD4 T cells or memory CD4 T cells. In contrast, after SEB stimulation, the child and adult CCR7^{lo} subsets of memory CD4 T cells contained a similar frequency of cells producing IFN-γ, and similar amounts of IFN-γ produced per cell, based on mean fluorescent intensity measurements. Thus, the decreased CMV-specific Th1 response by CCR7^{lo} cells in young children was relatively selective in that it did not apply to all Th1 immune responses.

As observed for IFN-γ, the frequency of CMV-specific CD4 T cells expressing IL-2 or CD40-ligand was substantially and significantly ($P<0.05$) lower for children compared to adults with similar duration of primary CMV infection. Interestingly, in contrast to IFN-γ expression, IL-2 and CD40-ligand were expressed by a small but detectable fraction of CMV-specific adult CCR7^{hi} memory CD4 T cells, although a greater fraction was found in the CCR7^{lo} subset. This is consistent with IL-2 and CD40 ligand expression not requiring Th1 differentiation for their effective expression. Nevertheless, the expression of IL-2 and CD40-ligand by the CD4 T cells of the children was essentially undetectable for either the CCR7^{lo} or the CCR7^{hi} subsets, indicating it generally applied to memory cell responses, and these differences were significant when compared with adult cells ($P<0.05$). CMV-specific CD4 T cells from children and adults were also analyzed for production of IL-4, IL-10, and IL-13 using intracellular cytokine staining, but we were unable to detect cells expressing these cytokines in any samples. This argues against developmentally related skewing of CMV-specific CD4 T-cell responses to produce Th2 or regulatory cytokines rather than Th1 cytokines.

Analysis of CMV-specific CD8 T-cell responses

In parallel with the CD4 T-cell studies, we analyzed the frequencies of CMV-specific CD8 T cells in 17 children, ages 17–41 months (median 24 months), who were shedding CMV in urine, and in 23 CMV-seropositive adults, who were presumed to have chronic infection for years to decades. Since CMV-specific CD8 T-cell frequencies may vary in chronically-infected adults [212], adult subjects were tested twice, at a one-year interval. The mean frequency of CMV-specific IFN-γ^+ CD8 T cells was 0.4% ± 0.1 (SE) in children tested at a median of 13 months after onset of CMV shedding in urine. The mean frequency in the adults was 0.7% ± 0.2 at the initial testing and 0.5% ± 0.1 after 12 months. Comparing CMV-specific CD8 T-cell responses in children compared to adults at the first time point suggested a difference (P=0.04), but not compared to the same adults tested at 12 months (P=0.2).

As for CD4 T cells, CD8 T-cell stimulation was also done with the peptide mixture for the CMV pp65 protein, which is known to be a major target for CMV-specific CD8-T cells [213, 220]. The mean IFN-γ^+ CD8 T-cell frequency after pp65 stimulation was 0.3% ±0.1 in children compared to 0.4% ± 0.1 in adults at initial testing (P=0.09) and 0.5% ±0.1 in adults at 12 months (P=0.01). Again, the CMV-specific CD8 T-cell frequencies in chronically-infected adults indicated a difference from children at one time point, but this was not confirmed by the second comparison.

CMV-specific CD8 T-cell frequencies were also determined in five HLA-A*0201 children and five HLA-A*0201 chronically-infected adults using a pp65-HLA-A*0201 tetramer [221, 222]. These experiments were done to assess CD8 T-cell numbers independently of the capacity to produce IFN-γ or other effector functions, which might be reduced in children. The range of tetramer positive CD8 T cells was 0.3–4.6% and did not differ between children and adults (P=0.5). Perforin expression by tetramer positive cells was also measured in order to determine whether CD8 T-cells had the functional capacity to mediate cytotoxicity, and a similar percentage of these cells were found in children (34%) as in adults (41%) (P=0.4). Since inadequate differentiation of virus-specific CD8-T cells could result in abnormal effector functions, the pp65-HLA-A*0201 tetramers were used for simultaneous assessment of CD28, which is downregulated during the later stages of CD8 T-cell differentiation [101]. All tetramer$^+$ CD8 T cells from one actively infected child were CD28$^-$ with most cells expressing perforin, as was observed in two chronically-infected adults. Thus, we found no evidence of a limitation in cytotoxic effector function or differentiation of CD8 T cells in infants and young children following primary CMV infection.

Relationship of CMV-specific CD4 and CD8 T-cell frequencies to viral shedding

Previous studies have documented prolonged urinary and salivary shedding of CMV in young children acquiring this infection in the daycare setting [202, 223]. This applied to the young children in our study based on measurements of CMV DNA levels in urine using a real-time PCR assay and viral culture of urine. All children were positive by both assays, indicating that viral shedding in the urine persisted for at least 12–29 months after acquisition of CMV. In contrast, CMV was not detected by either assay for urine from any adult with recent primary infection. To determine if this result was typical for adults with primary CMV infection, we also retrospectively analyzed data on a group of 30 healthy women with documented primary CMV infection. We found that 90% of these subjects ceased urinary shedding by 6 months after acquisition of virus. Together, these findings demonstrate a striking inverse correlation between viral shedding and a delay in the CD4 but not the CD8 T-cell CMV-specific immune response.

Since chronically-infected adults were likely to have been infected for many years, we compared four adults and 12 children with a similar duration of CMV infection. Three adults had CMV seroconversion within an estimated 12–16-month period but were not shedding virus when evaluated. One adult had primary infection documented by onset of CMV shedding in urine 12 months previously; this adult had a viral load of 1×10^4 copies/ml and stopped shedding after eight months. The 12 children had an estimated duration of infection of 12-28 months, with a mean of 16 months. All 12 children were actively shedding, with a mean of 1×10^4 copies/ml (range: 1×10^3–1×10^5 copies/ml) at the time their CD4 and CD8 T cells were analyzed. Despite these differences in shedding, the frequency of CMV-specific or pp65-specific CD8 T cells detected by CMV antigen stimulation was not different for actively infected children compared to adults. Further, CMV or pp65-specific CD8 T-cell frequencies did not significantly correlate with reduced CMV viral load in urine, which averaged $1\times10^{4.6}$ genome copies/ml (range: 1×10^2–-10^5 genome copies/ml). Thus, high viral loads were detected in some children with the highest CMV-specific CD8 T-cell frequencies, and conversely, low viral loads were observed in some children with the fewest CMV-specific CD8 T cells. In addition, CMV viral load was not related to duration of shedding in these children. Thus, these findings suggest that the circulating levels of CMV-specific CD8 T cells are not predictive of the control of urinary shedding following primary CMV infection in children.

Summary of CMV-specific studies

Previous studies have shown that healthy infants and young children who acquire CMV infection after birth have prolonged viral urinary and salivary shedding compared to adults [201, 202, 205, 224], but the mechanism of this prolonged viral shedding has until now remained unclear. Our results demonstrate a selective limitation in Th1 immunity in young children with postnatally acquired primary CMV infection. This is paralleled by a striking inverse correlation between viral shedding and the CMV-specific Th1 response. The importance of Th1 responses in control of CMV shedding is strongly supported by studies of murine CMV, in which CD4 T cells producing IFN-γ but not CD8 T cells were found to be critical for limiting CMV replication in acinar epithelial cells and consequent salivary shedding [207–209]. This is likely to apply to other epithelial sites of shedding, such as the kidney. In contrast, control of CMV replication at other tissue sites, such as the lung, depends critically on CD8 T cells but not CD4 Th1 cells [209]. We speculate that the limited consequence of reduced Th1 responses in these healthy children (i.e., asymptomatic but prolonged CMV shedding) is due to the fact that children develop reduced but detectable CMV-specific Th1 immunity and have robust CD8 T-cell responses. However, we cannot exclude that CMV-specific CD8 T cells of young children and infants might be limited in their ability to traffic to sites of viral replication, such as renal epithelium.

The decreased CMV-specific Th1 response of young children was mainly attributable to a lack of CMV-reactive Th1 cells among the CCR7^{lo} memory CD4 T-cell population. Thus, our results indicate that antigen-specific Th1 immune responses *in vivo* in humans, or at least those that are involved in anti-viral immunity, may be largely mediated cells that are CCR7^{lo}. Importantly, CCR7^{lo} memory CD4 T cells were present in substantial numbers in young children and had a similar capacity to produce IFN-γ after SEB simulation. SEB activates T cells based on Vβ segment usage by the αβ-TCR rather than peptide antigenic specificity [225]. Therefore, these IFN-γ^{+} T cells induced by SEB are likely to have undergone clonal expansion and Th1 differentiation in response to a diverse group of peptide antigens. This suggests that the reduced CMV-specific CD4 T-cell IFN-γ production of children is likely to be selective, and not due to a general inability of their CCR7^{lo} memory CD4 T cells to mediate Th1 effector function, or related to an inability to generate Th1 cells from naïve precursors. Further studies evaluating CCR7 restriction of the responses to other antigens will be of interest in young children compared to adults.

We observed that the proportion of circulating memory CD4 T cells that were CCR7^{lo} in young children was approximately 50–60% of that found in adults. This modest but statistically significant reduction could reflect a general tendency of young children to produce fewer CCR7^{lo} cells in response to antigenic stimuli. This possibility is consistent with the recent finding that circulating monocytes from healthy infants and young children have a reduced capacity to produce IL-12 [96]. Moreover, in our studies of a patient with a genetic deficiency of a component of the IL-12 receptor we have previously implicated IL-12 as being necessary for the accumulation of CCR7^{lo} memory CD4 T cells with Th1 function in humans [95]. An alternative and non-exclusive possibility is that the increased proportion of CCR7^{lo} memory CD4 T cells in adults reflects the greater proportion of immune stimulation coming from natural infections that are effective at driving Th1 immune responses rather than from currently used inactivated vaccines that include alum adjuvant, which is a relatively ineffective Th1 inducer.

The underlying mechanism of the reduced CMV-specific Th1 response in young immunocompetent children is unknown. The finding that CMV-specific IL-2 production and CD40-ligand expression by CCR7^{lo} or CCR7hi CD4 T cells of young children is reduced, suggests that it applies to early steps by which naïve CD4^{+} T cells expand and differentiate into memory CD4 T cells. This mechanism does not appear to be attributable to skewing of the CMV-specific CD4 T-cell response towards either Th2 or regulatory cytokine production. A major question is whether this poor Th1 immune response is unique to pathogens, such as CMV, which are known to encode several gene products that could potentially inhibit the generation of CD4^{+} T-cell immune responses *in vivo* [226]. If so, this would indicate that CD4 T cells and/or cells required for T-cell activation, such as DCs, may have an age-dependent susceptibility to viral immunoevasion or viral-mediated immunosuppression that is more evident in young children. We speculate that considerable evolutionary pressure may have favored human CMV to develop and maintain the capacity to avoid inducing Th1 responses in order to spread efficiently *via* secretions during early life, as occurs predominantly in less developed countries today [201]. Regardless of the precise mechanism, this developmental limitation in adaptive immunity will need to be considered in immunotherapeutic strategies to control CMV, such as vaccination.

Immunity to live attenuated measles vaccine during the first year of life

Measles virus is a highly contagious human pathogen [227]. Although measles vaccine campaigns have been quite effective in controlling the annual epidemics in most developed countries, an estimated 800,000 children continue to die from measles annually. Measles morbidity and mortality is highest among infants who become infected during the first year of life, in developed and in developing countries [228–231]. Periodic re-introduction of measles virus is of concern in developed countries because many women are protected from measles by childhood immunization. Measles antibody titers are lower in vaccinated women than in those who had natural infection. As a consequence, the infants of vaccinated women receive lower titers of transplacentally transferred, passive antibodies against measles than infants whose mothers had natural measles infection. Earlier loss of passive antibodies at 6–9 months results in a longer period of susceptibility before the primary measles vaccine dose is given at 12–15 months of age [232–235]. Thus, understanding the obstacles to inducing measles immunity in infants vaccinated at less than 12 months old is important. To address this issue, we have compared the acquisition of the measles-specific T-cell and antibody response of infants given measles vaccine at 6, 9 and 12 months of age [232, 236–238]. Immunity elicited by mumps vaccine was also assessed to determine whether observations about measles immunity were unique or characteristic of responses to live viral vaccines given during the first year of life.

Humoral and cell-mediated immune responses to measles and mumps vaccines given to infants at 6, 9 or 12 months of age

We found that infants in all three age groups after immunization had equivalent T-cell responses, as assessed by the cell proliferation and IFN-γ production by PBMCs to measles or mumps antigen, regardless of whether maternal antibody to the virus was present at the time of immunization [238]. A second important finding was that 6-month-old infants had relatively low measles or mumps geometric mean titers (GMTs) and seroconversion rates, but that this occurred even when no maternally-derived measles or mumps antibodies were detected at the time of vaccination. Measles-specific T-cell proliferation, as assessed by stimulation index (SI) after vaccination was > 3.0 in 72%, 69%, and 65% of 6-, 9-, and 12-month-old-infants. Mean SIs were equivalent in all three age groups. Measles-specific SIs after immunization did not differ for infants with or without measles-neutralizing antibodies when vaccinated: mean SIs were 7.3±0.9 vs 6.9±2.2 in 6 month olds and 5.6±0.8 vs 7.6±1.6 in 9 month old infants, with and without passive antibodies, respectively. Measles T-cell proliferative responses were also not affected by the amounts of measles-passive antibodies when infants were stratified by passive antibody titers >50 and <50 mIU/ml: Mean SIs were 8.2±1.9 in infants who had higher titers and 7.9±10.9 among those with lower titers. As observed after measles vaccination, mumps-specific T-cell proliferation responses were induced in infants vaccinated at 6, 9 or 12 months and were not affected by passive antibodies: mean SIs were 8.0±12.4 vs 8.7±1.6 for 6-month-old infants with and without passive antibodies, respectively, and 6.1±1.5 vs 7.1±1.1 for 9-month-old infants with and without passive antibodies, respectively (both not significantly different).

Concentrations of IFN-γ produced by PBMCs in infants given measles vaccine at 6, 9, or 12 months did not differ by age cohort. IFN-γ concentrations were 184±52 pg/ml, 349±95 pg/ml, and 115±26 pg/ml, in 6-, 9-, and 12-month-olds. IFN-γ concentrations were equivalent in infants with and without passive antibodies when immunized at 6 months of age (172±38 pg/ml vs. 273±83 pg/ml) (P=0.22), or at 9 months (188±58 pg/ml vs 326±86 pg/ml) (P=0.31). Mumps vaccination also induced IFN-γ-producing T cells in infants 6, 9 or 12 months of age. Mean IFN-γ concentrations were 239±77 pg/ml, 156±54 pg/ml, and 327±96 pg/ml, respectively. Mumps-specific IFN-γ production was not affected by passive antibodies at the time of immunization.

Although T-cell responses were not different by infant age group, measles and mumps-neutralizing antibody titers were lower after vaccination of 6-month-old infants. Measles GMTs were 120 mIU/ml (71–200 range) and 146 mIU/ml (44–490), in 6-month-olds with or without passive measles antibodies. Nine-month-old infants who had lost passive antibodies at the time of vaccination had measles GMTs of 744 mIU/ml (467–1183) compared to 180 mIU/ml (68–473) in those with passive antibodies when immunized ($P=0.01$). Measles GMT in 9-month-olds without passive antibodies did not differ from GMT of 1210 mIU/ml (774–1893) in 12-month-olds without passive antibodies. In the absence of passive antibodies, measles GMT were lower in 6-month-olds than GMTs in 9-month-old ($P=0.01$) or 12-month-old infants who had no passive antibodies ($P=0.0002$). Seroconversion rates were also lower in 6-month-olds than 9-month-olds (77% vs 97% in 9-month-olds ($P=0.02$) and in 12-month-olds (77% vs 96%) ($P=0.01$). Only 59% of 6-month-olds had measles titers >1:120 compared to 97% and 94% of 9- and 12-month-olds vaccinated in the absence of passive antibodies (6 vs 9, $P<0.0001$; 6 vs 12, $P=0.0001$). Passive antibody interference alone accounted for the difference in GMT between 9- and 12-month-olds ($P=0.003$). Six-month-olds immunized with mumps vaccine in the absence of passively acquired mumps-neutralizing antibodies also had lower GMTs than 12-month-olds; GMT were 18 (9–37), 35 (20–63), and 51 (28–89) at 6, 9, and 12 months (6 vs 12 months: $P=0.04$).

These studies indicated that 6-month-old infants had an intrinsic deficiency in humoral immunity elicited by each of these live attenuated paramyxovirus vaccines. However, lower responses were not due solely to inhibitory effects of passive antibodies. In contrast, cellular immunity, measured as measles- or mumps-specific T-cell proliferation and IFN-γ production, was equivalent in 6-, 9- and 12-month-olds. It is important to emphasize that antiviral T-cell immunity was induced by immunization with live attenuated viral vaccines during the first year, even when passive antibodies were present. Thus, assessing the induction of adaptive antiviral immunity by antibody titers only gives an inaccurate evaluation of the immune responses of infants given live attenuated viral vaccines. Therefore, to define primary vaccine failure as a failure to develop antiviral humoral immunity, does not consider the effect of priming of antiviral T-cell responses that occurs in infants immunized during the first year of life. In addition, the commonly accepted view that passive antibodies block the infant immune response by preventing the vaccine virus replication is likely to be incorrect. The low concentrations of viral antigens in measles and mumps vaccines are not adequate to elicit antiviral T-cell responses without viral replication to enhance the antigenic signal. Other mechanisms that probably affect measles or mumps antibody production in the presence of passive antibodies include formation of antigen-antibody complexes which undergo phagocytosis, facilitating presentation of viral peptides to naïve T cells but inhibiting B-cell sensitization, and masking of B-cell epitopes by pre-existing antibodies to these regions of viral protein antigens [239].

Interleukin-12, IFN-γ and T-cell proliferative responses to measles in immunized infants

Decreased IL-12 production could impair the acquisition of adaptive immunity to measles vaccination because IL-12 promotes the rapid induction of antigen-specific T cells of the Th1 type in the naïve host. A lack of IL-12 might also favor polarization of CD4 T cells towards a Th2 type of response. Measles-specific T-cell proliferation or IFN-γ production in infants vaccinated at 6, 9 or 12 months of age were lower compared to vaccinated adults. Since limited IL-12 might explain this difference, infants and adults who had vaccine-induced measles immunity were tested using assays for IL-12 production, T-cell proliferation and IFN-γ release by PBMCs stimulated with measles [14]. Our hypothesis was that a limited Th1-like response to measles in infants could contribute to a diminished measles-specific cellular immune response. IL-12 and IFN-γ production by measles-stimulated PBMCs was measured along with measles-specific CD4 T-cell proliferative responses before and after measles vaccination of infants. These experiments showed that both IL-12 and IFN-γ release by measles-stimulated PBMCs increased significantly following immunization of infants at 6, 9 or 12 months of age. Although there were no age-related differences in IL-12 and IFN-γ production in infants of varying ages, IL-12 release by PBMCs stimulated with measles antigen was significantly lower in the infants than in adults ($P = 0.04$). In addition, PBMC cultures were supplemented with exogenous recombinant human IL-12 during the period of stimulation with measles antigen in order to determine whether the infant deficiency in IFN-γ release was caused by limited production of IL-12 by infant monocytes. The addition of rhIL-12 enhanced IFN-γ production by infant PBMC, but even when IL-12 was provided, infant T cells still made significantly less IFN-γ than adult T cells in response to measles antigen. No differences were observed in measles-specific T-cell proliferation or in the concentrations of IFN-γ produced by PBMC stimulated with measles antigen when rhIL12 was added to PBMC cultures from infants with or without passive antibodies.

In summary, diminished IFN-γ and IL-12 production in response to measles antigens may limit cellular immunity to measles in infants compared to adults. If IL-12 production is deficient, IFN-γ concentrations may not support the optimal development of infant T cells of the Th1 type reactive with measles antigens after vaccination. If responses to natural infection are similarly limited, the increased susceptibility of infants to severe measles may be attributed in part to lower IL-12 responses compared to adults, along with an intrinsic limitation in the capacity of infant T cells to produce IFN-γ [15]. These differences were detected in infants in all three age groups, including those immunized at 12 months, irrespective of passive antibody status at the time of vaccination.

Measles-specific CD4 T-cell responses in infants

Flow cytometry-based, intracellular cytokine assays have been useful for evaluating CMV immunity in infants and young children [66]. We have applied similar methods to determine measles-specific CD4 T-cell frequencies and to assess up-regulation of CD4 T-cell activation markers, CD69 and CD40 ligand and cytokine production. In studies that are now in progress, the frequencies of CD4 T cells that express CD69 or CD40-ligand after stimulation of whole blood with measles antigen *in vitro*, were not different in infants who were vaccinated at 6, 9 or 12 months. Compared to vaccinated adults, infants had fewer CD40-ligand$^+$/IFN-γ^+ CD4 T cells after stimulation of PBMC with measles antigen. Age-related differences were not detected by measuring the numbers of measles-specific activated, IFN-γ-producing CD4 T cells in 6-month-olds compared to 12-month-olds after measles vaccination, but CD40 ligand$^+$/IFN-γ^+ CD4 T-cell frequencies appear to be somewhat lower ($P = 0.05$). As expected from proliferation assays, the presence of passive antibodies to measles at the time of immunization did not affect measles-specific CD4 T-cell frequencies in vaccinated infants. These observations suggest that CD4 T cells appear to respond to measles antigen by appropriate up-regulation of the activation markers, CD69 and CD40-ligand. However, as in previous assays, infant CD4 T cells have deficiencies in IFN-γ production. Even though these responses are lower, the flow cytometry experiments indicate that immunized infants develop measles-specific CD4 T cells and should be primed to respond to an exposure to measles or to a second vaccination.

Effects of a two-dose measles vaccine regimen

An important question about the infant immune response to measles vaccination is whether age-related deficiencies of antibody production will suppress responses to re-vaccination given at later ages. To address this question, we have evaluated humoral and cellular immune responses in infants who were immunized at 6 months and re-vaccinated with measles-mumps-rubella (MMR) vaccine at 12–15 months. Among these infants, the mean SIs were 8.9 ± 3.1 after the initial monovalent measles and 11.6 ± 2.4 after MMR. The SIs in 9-month-olds were 8.2 ± 2.7 after monovalent measles vaccine and 9.3 ± 2.8 after MMR. The measles-specific T-cell proliferation responses measured after MMR was given to infants who had received monovalent measles vaccine at 6 or 9 months of age were higher than those of 12-month-olds who had received MMR only (6 vs 12 months, $P = 0.008$; 9 vs 12 months, $P = 0.04$). In addition, the measles-neutralizing antibody responses increased after MMR to GMTs of 1487 mIU/ml (884–2497) in the 6-month-olds and 1994 mIU/ml (809–4920) in the 9-months-olds. All infants developed titers ≥120 mIU/ml after MMR. These studies showed that an early two-dose measles immunization regimen elicited measles-specific T-cell responses in infants as young as 6 months, which were associated with enhanced humoral responses after receiving MMR at 12 months of age. Further, seroconversion rates and measles GMTs after second doses of measles vaccine were not affected by initial interference from passive antibodies with the responses of 6- or 9-month-old infants to the first measles vaccine dose.

Summary

These studies of neutralizing antibody responses to measles and mumps vaccination of 6-month-old infants imply an intrinsic deficiency in humoral responses in this age group which are separate from the well-known effects of passive antibodies on initial seroconversion and GMTs. Importantly, measles- or mumps-specific T-cell proliferation or IFN-γ production showed no age-related differences when vaccines were given at 6, 9 or 12 months. Furthermore, passive antibodies had no effect on T-cell proliferation or cytokine production by PBMCs stimulated with measles or mumps antigens. Nevertheless, comparisons of responses in vaccinated infants and adults revealed significant differences, including lower measles-specific CD4 T-cell proliferation and IFN-γ and IL-12 production. Infants had also lower frequencies of $CD69^+$/IFN-γ^+ CD4 T cells and fewer $CD40L^+$/IFN-γ^+ CD4 T cells than adults after measles stimulation *in vitro*. Mechanisms that may account for less robust humoral immune responses in younger infants may include limited IFN-γ production by helper T cells, decreased measles-induced IL-12 production by APCs affecting induction of CD4 T cells and limited antigen-induced up-regulation of CD40-ligand which could restrict interactions of helper T cells and B cells. These analyses of infant responses to live attenuated viral vaccines suggest that concepts about antiviral immunity in the first year of life should be re-examined, e.g., passive antibody interference should be re-defined since antiviral CD4 T cells are elicited in the presence of passive antibodies with virus-neutralizing function. Neutralization of live viral vaccines by maternal antibodies appears to be an oversimplification of the biological events. Instead, specific mechanisms that modulate antibody production need to be identified, independently of the induction of antiviral T cells. Re-thinking the biology also requires considering an alternative paradigm in which inhibition of antibody production by passive antibodies is not "interference", but modulation to avoid antibody excess and immune-mediated disease in early infancy. As noted, priming of antigen-specific helper T cells occurred in some infants who did not develop measles or mumps antibodies, indicating a need to re-define primary vaccine failure since virus-specific T cells provide these infants with some measure of active, antiviral adaptive immunity. Induction of partial immunity may explain the clinical experiences in which early immunization has been associated with protection from severe measles disease and mortality despite the occurrence of breakthrough infections [240]. Although measles-specific responder CD4 T-cell frequencies, T-cell proliferation, and IFN-γ and IL-12 production were lower in infants than adults, a second dose of measles vaccine at 12–15 months increased antiviral T-cell responses to measles in infants who were vaccinated at 6 or 9 months, and resulted in equivalent seroconversion rates. Our hypothesis is that since T-cell immunity is induced under the "cover" of passive antibodies, repeated doses of live viral vaccines given during the first year of life constitute a "prime" and "boost" strategy that mimics the pattern of exposure and re-exposure to pathogens during infancy and early childhood, which was a common occurrence before live viral vaccines were introduced to protect against measles, mumps and other childhood infections.

Acknowledgments

CMV- and measles-specific immune studies were supported by grants from the National Institute of Allergy and Infectious Diseases (AI48212, A137127, AI53589, and AI050153) and the National Institute of Child Health and Human Development (HD01310 and HD33698). The authors thank our colleagues Corry Dekker, M.D., Hayley Gans, M.D., Wen-Wei Tu, M.D., Ph.D., Sharon Chen, M.D., and the many other post-doctoral fellows, students, and technicians who contributed to the studies of human CMV- and measles-specific immunity.

References

1 Yewdell JW, Reits E, Neefjes J (2003) Making sense of mass destruction: quantitating MHC class I antigen presentation. *Nat Rev Immunol* 3: 952–961

2 Hofman FM, Danilovs JA, Taylor CR (1984) HLA-DR (Ia)-positive dendritic-like cells in human fetal nonlymphoid tissues. *Transplantation* 37: 590–594

3 Oliver AM, Thomson AW, Sewell HF, Abramovich DR (1988) Major histocompatibility complex (MHC) class II antigen (HLA-DR, DQ, and DP) expression in human fetal endocrine organs and gut. *Scand J Immunol* 27: 731–737

4 Keever CA, Abu HM, Graf W, McFadden P, Prichard P, O'Brien J, Flomenberg N (1995) Characterization of the alloreactivity and anti-leukemia reactivity of cord blood mononuclear cells. *Bone Marrow Transplant* 15: 407–419

5 Vossen MT, Westerhout EM, Soderberg-Naucler C, Wiertz EJ (2002) Viral immune evasion: a masterpiece of evolution. *Immunogenetics* 54: 527–542

6 Arrode G, Boccaccio C, Lule J, Allart S, Moinard N, Abastado JP, Alam A, Davrinche C (2000) Incoming human cytomegalovirus pp65 (UL83) contained

in apoptotic infected fibroblasts is cross-presented to CD8(+) T cells by dendritic cells. *J Virol* 74: 10018–10024

7 Kanakoudi-Tsakalidou F, Debonera F, Drossou-Agakidou V, Sarafidis K, Tzimouli V, Taparkou A, Kremenopoulos G (2001) Flow cytometric measurement of HLA-DR expression on circulating monocytes in healthy and sick neonates using monocyte negative selection. *Clin Exp Immunol* 123: 402–407

8 Takeda K, Kaisho T, Akira S (2003) Toll-like receptors. *Annu Rev Immunol* 21: 335–376

9 Lanzavecchia A, Sallusto F (2001) Regulation of T cell immunity by dendritic cells. *Cell* 106: 263–266

10 Banchereau J, Briere F, Caux C, Davoust J, Lebecque S, Liu YJ, Pulendran B, Palucka K (2000) Immunobiology of dendritic cells. *Annu Rev Immunol* 18: 767–811

11 Larsson M, Fonteneau JF, Bhardwaj N (2001) Dendritic cells resurrect antigens from dead cells. *Trends Immunol* 22: 141–148

12 Farrar JD, Murphy KM (2000) Type I interferons and T helper development. *Immunol Today* 21: 484–489

13 Parronchi P, Mohapatra S, Sampognaro S, Giannarini L, Wahn U, Chong P, Maggi E, Renz H, Romagnani S (1996) Effects of interferon-alpha on cytokine profile, T cell receptor repertoire and peptide reactivity of human allergen-specific T cells. *Eur J Immunol* 26: 697–703

14 Rogge L, Barberis ML, Biffi M, Passini N, Presky DH, Gubler U, Sinigaglia F (1997) Selective expression of an interleukin-12 receptor component by human T helper 1 cells. *J Exp Med* 185: 825–831

15 Le Bon A, Etchart N, Rossmann C, Ashton M, Hou S, Gewert D, Borrow P, Tough DF (2003) Cross-priming of CD8+ T cells stimulated by virus-induced type I interferon. *Nat Immunol* 4: 1009–1015

16 Drijkoningen M, De Wolf-Peeters C, Van der Steen K, Moerman P, Desmet V (1987) Epidermal Langerhans' cells and dermal dendritic cells in human fetal and neonatal skin: an immunohistochemical study. *Pediatr Dermatol* 4: 11–17

17 Fossum S (1989) The life history of dendritic leukocytes (DL). *Curr Top Pathol* 79: 101–124

18 Olweus J, BitMansour A, Warnke R, Thompson PA, Carballido J, Picker LJ, Lund-Johansen F (1997) Dendritic cell ontogeny: a human dendritic cell lineage of myeloid origin. *Proc Natl Acad Sci USA* 94: 12551–12556

19 De Wit D, Olislagers V, Goriely S, Vermeulen F, Wagner H, Goldman M, Willems F (2004) Blood plasmacytoid dendritic cell responses to CpG oligodeoxynucleotides are impaired in human newborns. *Blood* 103: 1030–1032

20 Borras FE, Matthews NC, Lowdell MW, Navarrete CV (2001) Identification of both myeloid $CD11c^+$ and lymphoid $CD11c^-$ dendritic cell subsets in cord blood. *Br J Haematol* 113: 925–931

21 Teig N, Moses D, Gieseler S, Schauer U (2002) Age-related changes in human blood dendritic cell subpopulations. *Scand J Immunol* 55: 453–457

22 Hagendorens MM, Ebo DG, Schuerwegh AJ, Huybrechs A, Van Bever HP, Bridts CH, De Clerck LS, Stevens WJ (2003) Differences in circulating den-

dritic cell subtypes in cord blood and peripheral blood of healthy and allergic children. *Clin Exp Allergy* 33: 633–639

23 De Wit D, Tonon S, Olislagers V, Goriely S, Bourtriaux M, Goldman M, Willems F (2003) Impaired responses to toll-like receptor 4 and toll-like receptor 3 ligands in human cord blood. *J Autoimmun* 21: 277–281

24 Tonon S, Goriely S, Aksoy E, Pradier O, Del Giudice G, Trannoy E, Willems F, Goldman M, De Wit D (2002) *Bordetella pertussis* toxin induces the release of inflammatory cytokines and dendritic cell activation in whole blood: impaired responses in human newborns. *Eur J Immunol* 32: 3118–3125

25 Sorg RV, Kogler G, Wernet P (1998) Functional competence of dendritic cells in human umbilical cord blood. *Bone Marrow Transplant* 22 Suppl 1: S52–54

26 Sorg RV, Kogler G, Wernet P (1999) Identification of cord blood dendritic cells as an immature CD11c^{-} population. *Blood* 93: 2302–2307

27 Rissoan MC, Soumelis V, Kadowaki N, Grouard G, Briere F, de Waal Malefyt R, Liu YJ (1999) Reciprocal control of T helper cell and dendritic cell differentiation. *Science* 283: 1183–1186

28 Cella M, Facchetti F, Lanzavecchia A, Colonna M (2000) Plasmacytoid dendritic cells activated by influenza virus and CD40L drive a potent TH1 polarization. *Nat Immunol* 1: 305–310

29 Liu YJ (2001) Dendritic cell subsets and lineages, and their functions in innate and adaptive immunity. *Cell* 106: 259–262

30 Palucka K, Banchereau J (2002) How dendritic cells and microbes interact to elicit or subvert protective immune responses. *Curr Opin Immunol* 14: 420–431

31 Cederblad B, Riesenfeld T, Alm GV (1990) Deficient herpes simplex virus-induced interferon-alpha production by blood leukocytes of preterm and term newborn infants [published erratum appears in *Pediatr Res* (1990) 5: 507]. *Pediatr Res* 27: 7–10

32 Neustock P, Kruse A, Bein G, Nissen S, Kirchner H (1995) Failure to detect type 1 interferon production in human umbilical cord vein endothelial cells after viral exposure. *J Interferon Cytokine Res* 15: 129–135

33 Goriely S, Vincart B, Stordeur P, Vekemans J, Willems F, Goldman M, De Wit D (2001) Deficient IL-12(p35) gene expression by dendritic cells derived from neonatal monocytes. *J Immunol* 166: 2141–2146

34 Lee S, Suen Y, Chang L, Bruner V, Qian J, Indes J, Knoppel E, van de Ven C, Cairo MS (1996) Decreased interleukin-12 (IL-12) from activated cord blood *versus* adult peripheral blood mononuclear cells and upregulation of interferon-gamma, natural killer, and lymphokine-activated killer activity by IL-12 in cord blood mononuclear cells. *Blood* 88: 645–654

35 Scott ME, Kubin M, Kohl S (1997) High level interleukin-12 production, but diminished interferon-gamma production, by cord blood mononuclear cells. *Pediatr Res* 41: 547–553

36 Perez-Melgosa M, Ochs HD, Linsley PS, Laman JD, van Meurs M, Flavell RA, Ernst RK, Miller SI, Wilson CB (2001) Carrier-mediated enhancement of cognate T cell help: the basis for enhanced immunogenicity of meningococcal

outer membrane protein polysaccharide conjugate vaccine. *Eur J Immunol* 31: 2373–2381
37 Karlsson H, Hessle C, Rudin A (2002) Innate immune responses of human neonatal cells to bacteria from the normal gastrointestinal flora. *Infect Immun* 70: 6688–6696
38 Glusman G, Rowen L, Lee I, Boysen C, Roach JC, Smit AF, Wang K, Koop BF, Hood L (2001) Comparative genomics of the human and mouse T cell receptor loci. *Immunity* 15: 337–349
39 Pitcher LA, van Oers NS (2003) T-cell receptor signal transmission: who gives an ITAM? *Trends Immunol* 24: 554–560
40 Hannet I, Erkeller YF, Lydyard P, Deneys V, DeBruyere M (1992) Developmental and maturational changes in human blood lymphocyte subpopulations [see comments]. *Immunol Today* 13: 215, 218
41 Garderet L, Dulphy N, Douay C, Chalumeau N, Schaeffer V, Zilber MT, Lim A, Even J, Mooney N, Gelin C et al (1998) The umbilical cord blood alphabeta T-cell repertoire: characteristics of a polyclonal and naive but completely formed repertoire. *Blood* 91: 340–346
42 Kou ZC, Puhr JS, Rojas M, McCormack WT, Goodenow MM, Sleasman JW (2000) T-Cell receptor Vbeta repertoire CDR3 length diversity differs within CD45RA and CD45RO T-cell subsets in healthy and human immunodeficiency virus-infected children. *Clin Diagn Lab Immunol* 7: 953–959
43 van den Beemd R, Boor PP, van Lochem EG, Hop WC, Langerak AW, Wolvers-Tettero IL, Hooijkaas H, van Dongen JJ (2000) Flow cytometric analysis of the Vbeta repertoire in healthy controls. *Cytometry* 40: 336–345
44 D'Andrea A, Lanier LL (1998) Killer cell inhibitory receptor expression by T cells. *Curr Top Microbiol Immunol* 230: 25–39
45 Azuma M, Cayabyab M, Phillips JH, Lanier LL (1993) Requirements for CD28-dependent T cell-mediated cytotoxicity. *J Immunol* 150: 2091–2101
46 Azuma M, Phillips JH, Lanier LL (1993) $CD28^{-}$ T lymphocytes. Antigenic and functional properties. *J Immunol* 150: 1147–1159
47 Frenkel L, Bryson YJ (1987) Ontogeny of phytohemagglutinin-induced gamma interferon by leukocytes of healthy infants and children: evidence for decreased production in infants younger than 2 months of age. *J Pediatr* 111: 97–100
48 Wilson M, Rosen FS, Schlossman SF, Reinherz EL (1985) Ontogeny of human T and B lymphocytes during stressed and normal gestation: phenotypic analysis of umbilical cord lymphocytes from term and preterm infants. *Clin Immunol Immunopathol* 37: 1–12
49 Comans-Bitter WM, de Groot R, van den Beemd R, Neijens HJ, Hop WC, Groeneveld K, Hooijkaas H, van Dongen JJ (1997) Immunophenotyping of blood lymphocytes in childhood. Reference values for lymphocyte subpopulations. *J Pediatr* 130: 388–393
50 Carballido JM, Namikawa R, Carballido-Perrig N, Antonenko S, Roncarolo MG, de Vries JE (2000) Generation of primary antigen-specific human T- and B-cell responses in immunocompetent SCID-hu mice. *Nat Med* 6: 103–106

51 Tsegaye A, Wolday D, Otto S, Petros B, Assefa T, Alebachew T, Hailu E, Adugna F, Measho W, Dorigo W et al (2003) Immunophenotyping of blood lymphocytes at birth, during childhood, and during adulthood in HIV-1-uninfected Ethiopians. *Clin Immunol* 109: 338–346

52 Hassan J, Reen DJ (1998) IL-7 promotes the survival and maturation but not differentiation of human post-thymic CD4$^+$ T cells. *Eur J Immunol* 28: 3057–3065

53 Sanders ME, Makgoba MW, June CH, Young HA, Shaw S (1989) Enhanced responsiveness of human memory T cells to CD2 and CD3 receptor-mediated activation. *Eur J Immunol* 19: 803–808

54 Horgan KJ, Van Seventer GA, Shimizu Y, Shaw S (1990) Hyporesponsiveness of "naive" (CD45RA$^+$) human T cells to multiple receptor-mediated stimuli but augmentation of responses by co-stimuli. *Eur J Immunol* 20: 1111–1118

55 Kimachi K, Croft M, Grey HM (1997) The minimal number of antigen-major histocompatibility complex class II complexes required for activation of naive and primed T cells. *Eur J Immunol* 27: 3310–3317

56 Zaitseva MB, Lee S, Rabin RL, Tiffany HL, Farber JM, Peden KW, Murphy PM, Golding H (1998) CXCR4 and CCR5 on human thymocytes: biological function and role in HIV-1 infection. *J Immunol* 161: 3103–3113

57 Liu K, Li Y, Prabhu V, Young L, Becker KG, Munson PJ, Weng N (2001) Augmentation in expression of activation-induced genes differentiates memory from naive CD4$^+$ T cells and is a molecular mechanism for enhanced cellular response of memory CD4$^+$ T cells. *J Immunol* 166: 7335–7344

58 Woodside DG, Long DA, McIntyre BW (1999) Intracellular analysis of interleukin-2 induction provides direct evidence at the single cell level of differential coactivation requirements for CD45RA$^+$ and CD45RO$^+$ T cell subsets. *J Interferon Cytokine Res* 19: 769–779

59 Hassan J, O'Neill S, O'Neill LA, Pattison U, Reen DJ (1995) Signalling *via* CD28 of human naive neonatal T lymphocytes. *Clin Exp Immunol* 102: 192–198

60 Hassan J, Rainsford E, Reen DJ (1997) Linkage of protein kinase C-beta activation and intracellular interleukin-2 accumulation in human naive CD4 T cells. *Immunology* 92: 465–471

61 Hassan J, Reen DJ (1997) Cord blood CD4$^+$ CD45RA$^+$ T cells achieve a lower magnitude of activation when compared with their adult counterparts. *Immunology* 90: 397–401

62 Wilson CB, Westall J, Johnston L, Lewis DB, Dower SK, Alpert AR (1986) Decreased production of interferon-gamma by human neonatal cells. Intrinsic and regulatory deficiencies. *J Clin Invest* 77: 860–867

63 Saito S, Morii T, Umekage H, Makita K, Nishikawa K, Narita N, Ichijo M, Morikawa H, Ishii N, Nakamura M et al (1996) Expression of the interleukin-2 receptor gamma chain on cord blood mononuclear cells. *Blood* 87: 3344–3350

64 Chilmonczyk BA, Levin MJ, McDuffy R, Hayward AR (1985) Characterization of the human newborn response to herpesvirus antigen. *J Immunol* 134: 4184–4188

65 Hassan J, Reen DJ (1996) Reduced primary antigen-specific T-cell precursor frequencies in neonates is associated with deficient interleukin-2 production. *Immunology* 87: 604–608

66 Tu W, Chen S, Sharp M, Dekker C, Manganello AM, Tongson EC, Maecker HT, Holmes TH, Wang Z, Kemble G et al (2004) Persistent and selective deficiency of CD4$^+$ T cell immunity to cytomegalovirus in immunocompetent young children. *J Immunol* 172: 3260–3267

67 Chen L, Cleary AM, Lewis DB (2005) Impaired allogeneic activation and TH1 differentiation of human neonatal naive CD4 T cells. *Submitted for publication*

68 White GP, Watt PM, Holt BJ, Holt PG (2002) Differential patterns of methylation of the IFN-gamma promoter at CpG and non-CpG sites underlie differences in IFN-gamma gene expression between human neonatal and adult CD45RO$^-$ T cells. *J Immunol* 168: 2820–2827

69 Melvin AJ, McGurn ME, Bort SJ, Gibson C, Lewis DB (1995) Hypomethylation of the interferon-gamma gene correlates with its expression by primary T-lineage cells. *Eur J Immunol* 25: 426–430

70 Jullien P, Cron RQ, Dabbagh K, Cleary A, Chen L, Tran P, Stepick-Biek P, Lewis DB (2003) Decreased CD154 expression by neonatal CD4$^+$ T cells is due to limitations in both proximal and distal events of T cell activation. *Int Immunol* 15: 1461–1472

71 Kadereit S, Mohammad SF, Miller RE, Woods KD, Listrom CD, McKinnon K, Alali A, Bos LS, Iacobucci ML, Sramkoski MR et al (1999) Reduced NFAT1 protein expression in human umbilical cord blood T lymphocytes. *Blood* 94: 3101–3107

72 Kiani A, Garcia-Cozar FJ, Habermann I, Laforsch S, Aebischer T, Ehninger G, Rao A (2001) Regulation of interferon-gamma gene expression by nuclear factor of activated T cells. *Blood* 98: 1480–1488

73 Ribeiro-do-Couto LM, Boeije LC, Kroon JS, Hooibrink B, Breur-Vriesendorp BS, Aarden LA, Boog CJ (2001) High IL-13 production by human neonatal T cells: neonate immune system regulator? *Eur J Immunol* 31: 3394–3402

74 Schonbeck U, Libby P (2001) The CD40/CD154 receptor/ligand dyad. *Cell Mol Life Sci* 58: 4–43

75 Brugnoni D, Airo P, Graf D, Marconi M, Lebowitz M, Plebani A, Giliani S, Malacarne F, Cattaneo R, Ugazio AG (1994) Ineffective expression of CD40 ligand on cord blood T cells may. *Eur J Immunol* 24: 1919–1924

76 Fuleihan R, Ahern D, Geha RS (1994) Decreased expression of the ligand for CD40 in newborn lymphocytes. *Eur J Immunol* 24: 1925–1928

77 Durandy A, De-Saint-Basile G, Lisowska GB, Gauchat JF, Forveille M, Kroczek RA, Bonnefoy JY, Fischer A (1995) Undetectable CD40 ligand expression on T cells and low B cell responses to CD40 binding agonists in human newborns. *J Immunol* 154: 1560–1568

78 Nonoyama S, Penix LA, Edwards CP, Lewis DB, Ito S, Aruffo A, Wilson CB, Ochs HD (1995) Diminished expression of CD40 ligand by activated neonatal T cells. *J Clin Invest* 95: 66–75

79 Fuleihan R, Ahern D, Geha RS (1995) CD40 ligand expression is develop-

mentally regulated in human thymocytes. *Clin Immunol Immunopathol* 76: 52–58

80 Sato K, Nagayama H, Takahashi TA (1999) Aberrant CD3- and CD28-mediated signaling events in cord blood. *J Immunol* 162: 4464–4471

81 Splawski JB, Nishioka J, Nishioka Y, Lipsky PE (1996) CD40 ligand is expressed and functional on activated neonatal T cells. *J Immunol* 156: 119–127

82 Elliott SR, Roberton DM, Zola H, Macardle PJ (2000) Expression of the costimulator molecules, CD40 and CD154, on lymphocytes from neonates and young children. *Hum Immunol* 61: 378–388

83 Matthews NC, Wadhwa M, Bird C, Borras FE, Navarrete CV (2000) Sustained expression of CD154 (CD40L) and proinflammatory cytokine production by alloantigen-stimulated umbilical cord blood T cells. *J Immunol* 164: 6206–6212

84 Cayabyab M, Phillips JH, Lanier LL (1994) CD40 preferentially costimulates activation of CD4+ T lymphocytes. *J Immunol* 152: 1523–1531

85 Takahashi N, Imanishi K, Nishida H, Uchiyama T (1995) Evidence for immunologic immaturity of cord blood T cells. Cord blood T cells are susceptible to tolerance induction to *in vitro* stimulation with a superantigen. *J Immunol* 155: 5213–5219

86 Takahashi N, Kato H, Imanishi K, Miwa K, Yamanami S, Nishida H, Uchiyama T (2000) Immunopathophysiological aspects of an emerging neonatal infectious disease induced by a bacterial superantigen. *J Clin Invest* 106: 1409–1415

87 Langenkamp A, Messi M, Lanzavecchia A, Sallusto F (2000) Kinetics of dendritic cell activation: impact on priming of TH1, TH2 and nonpolarized T cells. *Nat Immunol* 1: 311–316

88 Sato K, Kawasaki H, Morimoto C, Yamashima N, Matsuyama T (2002) An abortive ligand-induced activation of CCR1-mediated downstream signaling event and a deficiency of CCR5 expression are associated with the hyporesponsiveness of human naive CD4+ T cells to CCL3 and CCL5. *J Immunol* 168: 6263–6272

89 Berkowitz RD, Beckerman KP, Schall TJ, McCune JM (1998) CXCR4 and CCR5 expression delineates targets for HIV-1 disruption of T cell differentiation. *J Immunol* 161: 3702–3710

90 Sato K, Kawasaki H, Nagayama H, Enomoto M, Morimoto C, Tadokoro K, Juji T, Takahashi T (2001) Chemokine receptor expressions and responsiveness of cord blood T cells. *J Immunol* 166: 1659–1666

91 Christopherson Kn, Brahmi Z, Hromas R (1999) Regulation of naive fetal T-cell migration by the chemokines Exodus-2 and Exodus-3. *Immunol Lett* 69: 269–273

92 Sallusto F, Kremmer E, Palermo B, Hoy A, Ponath P, Qin S, Forster R, Lipp M, Lanzavecchia A (1999) Switch in chemokine receptor expression upon TCR stimulation homing potential for recently activated T cells. *Eur J Immunol* 29: 2037–2045

93 Sallusto F, Lenig D, Forster R, Lipp M, Lanzavecchia A (1999) Two subsets of memory T lymphocytes with distinct homing potentials and effector functions [see comments]. *Nature* 401: 708–712

94 Baron V, Bouneaud C, Cumano A, Lim A, Arstila TP, Kourilsky P, Ferradini L, Pannetier C (2003) The repertoires of circulating human CD8(+) central and effector memory T cell subsets are largely distinct. *Immunity* 18: 193–204

95 Cleary AM, Tu W, Enright A, Giffon T, Dewaal-Malefyt R, Gutierrez K, Lewis DB (2003) Impaired accumulation and function of memory CD4 T cells in human IL-12 receptor beta 1 deficiency. *J Immunol* 170: 597–603

96 Upham JW, Lee PT, Holt BJ, Heaton T, Prescott SL, Sharp MJ, Sly PD, Holt PG (2002) Development of interleukin-12-producing capacity throughout childhood. *Infect Immun* 70: 6583–6588

97 de-Jong R, Brouwer M, Miedema F, van-Lier R-A (1991) Human CD8+ T lymphocytes can be divided into $CD45RA^+$ and $CD45RO^+$ cells with different requirements for activation and differentiation. *J Immunol* 146: 2088–2094

98 Akbar AN, Salmon M, Ivory K, Taki S, Pilling D, Janossy G (1991) Human $CD4^+CD45R0^+$ and $CD4^+CD45RA^+$ T cells synergize in response to alloantigens. *Eur J Immunol* 21: 2517–2522

99 Mescher MF (1995) Molecular interactions in the activation of effector and precursor cytotoxic T lymphocytes. *Immunol Rev* 146: 177–210

100 Hamann D, Baars PA, Rep MH, Hooibrink B, Kerkhof-Garde SR, Klein MR, van-Lier R-A (1997) Phenotypic and functional separation of memory and effector human $CD8^+$ T cells. *J Exp Med* 186: 1407–1418

101 Appay V, Dunbar PR, Callan M, Klenerman P, Gillespie GM, Papagno L, Ogg GS, King A, Lechner F, Spina CA et al (2002) Memory $CD8^+$ T cells vary in differentiation phenotype in different persistent virus infections. *Nat Med* 8: 379–385

102 Marchant A, Appay V, Van Der Sande M, Dulphy N, Liesnard C, Kidd M, Kaye S, Ojuola O, Gillespie GM, Vargas Cuero AL et al (2003) Mature CD8(+) T lymphocyte response to viral infection during fetal life. *J Clin Invest* 111: 1747–1755

103 Hermann E, Truyens C, Alonso-Vega C, Even J, Rodriguez P, Berthe A, Gonzalez-Merino E, Torrico F, Carlier Y (2002) Human fetuses are able to mount an adultlike CD8 T-cell response. *Blood* 100: 2153–2158

104 Clerici M, DePalma L, Roilides E, Baker R, Shearer GM (1993) Analysis of T helper and antigen-presenting cell functions in cord blood and peripheral blood leukocytes from healthy children of different ages. *J Clin Invest* 91: 2829–2836

105 Marchant A, Goetghebuer T, Ota MO, Wolfe I, Ceesay SJ, De Groote D, Corrah T, Bennett S, Wheeler J, Huygen K et al (1999) Newborns develop a Th1-type immune response to *Mycobacterium bovis* bacillus Calmette-Guerin vaccination. *J Immunol* 163: 2249–2255

106 Ota MO, Vekemans J, Schlegel-Haueter SE, Fielding K, Sanneh M, Kidd M, Newport MJ, Aaby P, Whittle H, Lambert PH et al (2002) Influence of Mycobacterium bovis bacillus Calmette-Guerin on antibody and cytokine responses to human neonatal vaccination. *J Immunol* 168: 919–925

107 Vekemans J, Ota MO, Wang EC, Kidd M, Borysiewicz LK, Whittle H, McAdam KP, Morgan G, Marchant A (2002) T cell responses to vaccines in infants:

defective IFNgamma production after oral polio vaccination. *Clin Exp Immunol* 127: 495–498
108 Rowe J, Macaubas C, Monger T, Holt BJ, Harvey J, Poolman JT, Loh R, Sly PD, Holt PG (2001) Heterogeneity in diphtheria-tetanus-acellular pertussis vaccine-specific cellular immunity during infancy: relationship to variations in the kinetics of postnatal maturation of systemic th1 function. *J Infect Dis* 184: 80–88
109 Gibson L, Piccinini G, Lilleri D, Revello MG, Wang Z, Markel S, Diamond DJ, Luzuriaga K (2004) Human cytomegalovirus proteins pp65 and immediate early protein 1 are common targets for CD8(+) T cell responses in children with congenital or postnatal human cytomegalovirus infection. *J Immunol* 172: 2256–2264
110 Riviere Y, Buseyne F (1998) Cytotoxic T lymphocytes generation capacity in early life with particular reference to HIV. *Vaccine* 16: 1420–1422
111 Pikora CA, Sullivan JL, Panicali D, Luzuriaga K (1997) Early HIV-1 envelope-specific cytotoxic T lymphocyte responses in vertically infected infants. *J Exp Med* 185: 1153–1161
112 Park AY, Scott P (2001) Il-12: keeping cell-mediated immunity alive. *Scand J Immunol* 53: 529–532
113 Luzuriaga K, McManus M, Catalina M, Mayack S, Sharkey M, Stevenson M, Sullivan JL (2000) Early therapy of vertical human immunodeficiency virus type 1 (HIV-1) infection: control of viral replication and absence of persistent HIV-1-specific immune responses. *J Virol* 74: 6984–6991
114 Luzuriaga K, Holmes D, Hereema A, Wong J, Panicali DL, Sullivan JL (1995) HIV-1-specific cytotoxic T lymphocyte responses in the first year of life. *J Immunol* 154: 433–443
115 Pacanowski J, Kahi S, Baillet M, Lebon P, Deveau C, Goujard C, Meyer L, Oksenhendler E, Sinet M, Hosmalin A (2001) Reduced blood $CD123^+$ (lymphoid) and $CD11c^+$ (myeloid) dendritic cell numbers in primary HIV-1 infection. *Blood* 98: 3016–3021
116 Stumptner-Cuvelette P, Morchoisne S, Dugast M, Le Gall S, Raposo G, Schwartz O, Benaroch P (2001) HIV-1 Nef impairs MHC class II antigen presentation and surface expression. *Proc Natl Acad Sci USA* 98: 12144–12149
117 Nielsen SD, Jeppesen DL, Kolte L, Clark DR, Sorensen TU, Dreves AM, Ersboll AK, Ryder LP, Valerius NH, Nielsen JO (2001) Impaired progenitor cell function in HIV-negative infants of HIV-positive mothers results in decreased thymic output and low CD4 counts. *Blood* 98: 398–404
118 Badley AD, Pilon AA, Landay A, Lynch DH (2000) Mechanisms of HIV-associated lymphocyte apoptosis. *Blood* 96: 2951–2964
119 Chougnet C, Kovacs A, Baker R, Mueller BU, Luban NL, Liewehr DJ, Steinberg SM, Thomas EK, Shearer GM (2000) Influence of human immunodeficiency virus-infected maternal environment on development of infant interleukin-12 production. *J Infect Dis* 181: 1590–1597
120 Chiba Y, Higashidate Y, Suga K, Honjo K, Tsutsumi H, Ogra PL (1989) Development of cell-mediated cytotoxic immunity to respiratory syncytial

virus in human infants following naturally acquired infection. *J Med Virol* 28: 133–139

121 Chang J, Braciale TJ (2002) Respiratory syncytial virus infection suppresses lung CD8+ T-cell effector activity and peripheral CD8$^+$ T-cell memory in the respiratory tract. *Nat Med* 8: 54–60

122 Rajewsky K (1996) Clonal selection and learning in the antibody system. *Nature* 381: 751–758

123 Ozaki K, Spolski R, Feng CG, Qi CF, Cheng J, Sher A, Morse HC, 3rd, Liu C, Schwartzberg PL, Leonard WJ (2002) A critical role for IL-21 in regulating immunoglobulin production. *Science* 298: 1630–1634

124 Vos Q, Lees A, Wu ZQ, Snapper CM, Mond JJ (2000) B-cell activation by T-cell-independent type 2 antigens as an integral part of the humoral immune response to pathogenic microorganisms. *Immunol Rev* 176: 154–170

125 Poe JC, Hasegawa M, Tedder TF (2001) CD19, CD21, and CD22: multifaceted response regulators of B lymphocyte signal transduction. *Int Rev Immunol* 20: 739–762

126 Ravetch JV, Bolland S (2001) IgG Fc receptors. *Annu Rev Immunol* 19: 275–290

127 Gupta S, Pahwa R, O'Reilly R, Good RA, Siegal FP (1976) Ontogeny of lymphocyte subpopulations in human fetal liver. *Proc Natl Acad Sci USA* 73: 919–922

128 Gathings WE, Lawton AR, Cooper MD (1977) Immunofluorescent studies of the development of pre-B cells, B lymphocytes and immunoglobulin isotype diversity in humans. *Eur J Immunol* 7: 804–810

129 Schultz C, Reiss I, Bucsky P, Gopel W, Gembruch U, Ziesenitz S, Gortner L (2000) Maturational changes of lymphocyte surface antigens in human blood: comparison between fetuses, neonates and adults. *Biol Neonate* 78: 77–82

130 Zemlin M, Schelonka RL, Bauer K, Schroeder HW, Jr (2002) Regulation and chance in the ontogeny of B and T cell antigen receptor repertoires. *Immunol Res* 26: 265–278

131 Sanz I (1991) Multiple mechanisms participate in the generation of diversity of human H chain CDR3 regions. *J Immunol* 147: 1720–1729

132 Mortari F, Newton JA, Wang JY, Schroeder HJ (1992) The human cord blood antibody repertoire. Frequent usage of the VH7 gene family. *Eur J Immunol* 22: 241–245

133 Silverman GJ, Sasano M, Wormsley SB (1993) Age-associated changes in binding of human B lymphocytes to a VH3-restricted unconventional bacterial antigen. *J Immunol* 151: 5840–5855

134 Padlan EA (1994) Anatomy of the antibody molecule. *Mol Immunol* 31: 169–217

135 Cuisinier AM, Fumoux F, Moinier D, Boubli L, Guigou V, Milili M, Schiff C, Fougereau M, Tonnelle C (1990) Rapid expansion of human immunoglobulin repertoire VH, V kappa, V lambda expressed in early fetal bone marrow. *New Biologist* 2: 689–699

136 Mortari F, Wang JY, Schroeder HJ (1993) Human cord blood antibody reper-

toire. Mixed population of VH gene segments and CDR3 distribution in the expressed C alpha and C gamma repertoires. *J Immunol* 150: 1348–1357

137 Villa A, Sobacchi C, Notarangelo LD, Bozzi F, Abinun M, Abrahamsen TG, Arkwright PD, Baniyash M, Brooks EG, Conley ME et al (2001) V(D)J recombination defects in lymphocytes due to RAG mutations: severe immunodeficiency with a spectrum of clinical presentations. *Blood* 97: 81–88

138 Schroeder HW, Jr, Ippolito GC, Shiokawa S (1998) Regulation of the antibody repertoire through control of HCDR3 diversity. *Vaccine* 16: 1383–1390

139 Gilfillan S, Bachmann M, Trembleau S, Adorini L, Kalinke U, Zinkernagel R, Benoist C, Mathis D (1995) Efficient immune responses in mice lacking N-region diversity. *Eur J Immunol* 25: 3115–3122

140 Macardle PJ, Weedon H, Fusco M, Nobbs S, Ridings J, Flego L, Roberton DM, Zola H (1997) The antigen receptor complex on cord B lymphocytes. *Immunology* 90: 376–382

141 Gagro A, McCloskey N, Challa A, Holder M, Grafton G, Pound JD, Gordon J (2000) CD5-positive and CD5-negative human B cells converge to an indistinguishable population on signalling through B-cell receptors and CD40. *Immunology* 101: 201–209

142 Wedgwood JF, Weinberger BI, Hatam L, Palmer R (1997) Umbilical cord blood lacks circulating B lymphocytes expressing surface IgG or IgA. *Clin Immunol Immunopathol* 84: 276–282

143 Zheng B, Kelsoe G, Han S (1996) Somatic diversification of antibody responses. *J Clin Immunol* 16: 1–11

144 Punnonen J, Aversa GG, Vandekerckhove B, Roncarolo MG, de-Vries J-E (1992) Induction of isotype switching and Ig production by $CD5^+$ and $CD10^+$ human fetal B cells. *J Immunol* 148: 3398–3404

145 Bhat NM, Kantor AB, Bieber MM, Stall AM, Herzenberg LA, Teng NN (1992) The ontogeny and functional characteristics of human B-1 CD5+ B cells. *Intern Immunol* 4: 243–252

146 Kipps TJ, Robbins BA, Carson DA (1990) Uniform high frequency expression of autoantibody-associated crossreactive idiotypes in the primary B cell follicles of human fetal spleen. *J Exp Med* 171: 189–196

147 Antin JH, Emerson SG, Martin P, Gadol N, Ault KA (1986) Leu-1^+ ($CD5^+$) B cells. A major lymphoid subpopulation in human fetal spleen: phenotypic and functional studies. *J Immunol* 136: 505–510

148 Griffiths CS, Patterson JA, Berger CL, Edelson RL, Chu AC (1984) Characterization of immature T cell subpopulations in neonatal blood. *Blood* 64: 296–300

149 Small TN, Keever C, Collins N, Dupont B, O'Reilly RJ, Flomenberg N (1989) Characterization of B cells in severe combined immunodeficiency disease. *Hum Immunol* 25: 181–193

150 Lydyard PM, Quartey PR, Broker B, Mackenzie L, Jouquan J, Blaschek MA, Steele J, Petrou M, Collins P, Isenberg D et al (1990) The antibody repertoire of early human B cells. I. High frequency of autoreactivity and polyreactivity. *Scand J Immunol* 31: 33–43

151 Chen ZJ, Wheeler CJ, Shi W, Wu AJ, Yarboro CH, Gallagher M, Notkins AL (1998) Polyreactive antigen-binding B cells are the predominant cell type in the newborn B cell repertoire. *Eur J Immunol* 28: 989–994
152 Calado RT, Garcia AB, Falcao RP (1999) Age-related changes of immunophenotypically immature lymphocytes in normal human peripheral blood. *Cytometry* 38: 133–137
153 Rijkers GT, Sanders EA, Breukels MA, Zegers BJ (1998) Infant B cell responses to polysaccharide determinants. *Vaccine* 16: 1396–1400
154 Jessup CF, Ridings J, Ho A, Nobbs S, Roberton DM, Macardle P, Zola H (2001) The Fc receptor for IgG (Fc gamma RII; CD32) on human neonatal B lymphocytes. *Hum Immunol* 62: 679–685
155 Parra C, Rold'an E, Brieva JA (1996) Deficient expression of adhesion molecules by human CD5– B lymphocytes both after bone marrow transplantation and during normal ontogeny. *Blood* 88: 1733–1740
156 Tasker L, Marshall-Clarke S (2003) Functional responses of human neonatal B lymphocytes to antigen receptor cross-linking and CpG DNA. *Clin Exp Immunol* 134: 409–419
157 Splawski J, Yamamoto K, Lipsky P (1998) Deficient interleukin-10 production by neonatal T cells does not expalin their ineffectiveness at promoting neonatal B cell differentiation. *Eur J Immunol* 28: 4248–4256
158 Huang LY, Aliberti J, Leifer CA, Segal DM, Sher A, Golenbock DT, Golding B (2003) Heat-killed *Brucella abortus* induces TNF and IL-12p40 by distinct MyD88-dependent pathways: TNF, unlike IL-12p40 secretion, is Toll-like receptor 2 dependent. *J Immunol* 171: 1441–1446
159 Ambrosino DM, Delaney NR, Shamberger RC (1990) Human polysaccharide-specific B cells are responsive to pokeweed mitogen and IL-6. *J Immunol* 144: 1221–1226
160 Peeters CC, Tenbergen-Meekes AM, Heijnen CJ, Poolman JT, Zegers JM, Rijkers GT (1992) Interferon-gamma and interleukin-6 augment the human *in vitro* antibody response to the Haemophilus influenzae type b polysaccharide. *J Infect Dis* 165 (Suppl 1): S161–S162
161 Snapper CM, Mond JJ (1996) A model for induction of T cell-independent humoral immunity in response to polysaccharide antigens. *J Immunol* 157: 2229–2233
162 Buchanan RM, Arulanandam BP, Metzger DW (1998) IL-12 enhances antibody responses to T-independent polysaccharide vaccines in the absence of T and NK cells. *J Immunol* 161: 5525–5533
163 Snapper CM, Rosas FR, Jin L, Wortham C, Kehry MR, Mond JJ (1995) Bacterial lipoproteins may substitute for cytokines in the humoral immune response to T cell-independent type II antigens. *J Immunol* 155: 5582–5589
164 Chelvarajan RL, Raithatha R, Venkataraman C, Kaul R, Han SS, Robertson DA, Bondada S (1999) CpG oligodeoxynucleotides overcome the unresponsiveness of neonatal B cells to stimulation with the thymus-independent stimuli anti-IgM and TNP-Ficoll. *Eur J Immunol* 29: 2808–2818
165 Golding B, Muchmore AV, Blaese RM (1984) Newborn and Wiskott-Aldrich

patient B cells can be activated by TNP-Brucella abortus: evidence that TNP-*Brucella abortus* behaves as a T-independent type 1 antigen in humans. *J Immunol* 133: 2966–2971

166 Fink C, Miller WE Jr, Dorward B, Lospalluto J (1962) The formation of macroglobulin antibodies II. Studies on neonatal infants and older children. *J Clin Invest* 41: 1422–1428

167 Smith R, Eitzman DV (1964) The development of the immune response. *Pediatrics* 33: 163–183

168 Kruetzmann S, Rosado MM, Weber H, Germing U, Tournilhac O, Peter HH, Berner R, Peters A, Boehm T, Plebani A et al (2003) Human immunoglobulin M memory B cells controlling Streptococcus pneumoniae infections are generated in the spleen. *J Exp Med* 197: 939–945

169 Haas KM, Hasegawa M, Steeber DA, Poe JC, Zabel MD, Bock CB, Karp DR, Briles DE, Weis JH, Tedder TF (2002) Complement receptors CD21/35 link innate and protective immunity during Streptococcus pneumoniae infection by regulating IgG3 antibody responses. *Immunity* 17: 713–723

170 Peset-Llopis MJ, Harms G, Hardonk MJ, Timens W (1996) Human immune response to pneumococcal polysaccharides: complement-mediated localization preferentially on CD21-positive splenic marginal zone B cells and follicular dendritic cells. *J Allergy Clin Immunol* 97: 1015–1024

171 Timens W, Rozeboom T, Poppema S (1987) Fetal and neonatal development of human spleen: an immunohistological study. *Immunology* 60: 603–609

172 Thornton CA, Holloway JA, Warner JO (2002) Expression of CD21 and CD23 during human fetal development. *Pediatr Res* 52: 245–250

173 Viemann D, Schlenke P, Hammers HJ, Kirchner H, Kruse A (2000) Differential expression of the B cell-restricted molecule CD22 B lymphocytes depending upon antigen stimulation. *Eur J Immunol* 30: 550–559

174 Durandy A, De Saint BG, Lisowska-Grospierre B, Gauchat JF, Forveille M, Kroczek RA, Bonnefoy JY, Fischer A (1995) Undetectable CD40 ligand expression on T cells and low B cell. *J Immunol* 154: 1560–1568

175 Dengrove J, Lee EJ, Heiner DC, St.Geme JJ, Leake R, Baraff LJ, Ward JI (1986) IgG and IgG subclass specific antibody responses to diphtheria and tetanus toxoids in newborns and infants given DTP immunization. *Pediatr Res* 20: 735–739

176 Smolen P, Bland R, Heiligenstein E, Lawless MR, Dillard R, Abramson J (1983) Antibody response to oral polio vaccine in premature infants. *J Pediatr* 103: 917–919

177 West DJ (1989) Clinical experience with hepatitis B vaccines. *Am J Infect Control* 17: 172–180

178 Uhr J, Dancis J, Franklin E, Finkelstein MS, Lewis EW (1962) The antibody response to bacteriophage in newborn premature infants. *J Clin Invest* 41: 1509–1513

179 Lee SS, Lo YC, Young BW, Wong KH, Lim WL (1995) A reduced dose approach to hepatitis B vaccination for low-risk newborns and preschool children. *Vaccine* 13: 373–376

180 Greenberg DP (1993) Pediatric experience with recombinant hepatitis B vaccines and relevant safety and immunogenicity studies. *Pediatr Infect Dis J* 12: 438–445
181 Dancis J, Osburn JJ, Kunz HW (1953) Studies of the immunology of the newborn infant. *Pediatrics* 12: 151–157
182 McFarland EJ, Borkowsky W, Fenton T, Wara D, McNamara J, Samson P, Kang M, Mofenson L, Cunningham C, Duliege AM et al (2001) Human immunodeficiency virus type 1 (HIV-1) gp120-specific antibodies in neonates receiving an HIV-1 recombinant gp120 vaccine. *J Infect Dis* 184: 1331–1335
183 Peterson J (1951) Immunization in the young infant. Response to combined vaccines: I–IV. *American Journal of Diseases of Children* 81: 484–491
184 Provenzano R, Wetterlow LH, Sullivan CL (1965) Immunization and antibody response in the newborn infant. *N Engl J Med* 273: 959–965
185 Baraff LJ, Leake RD, Burstyn DG, Payne T, Cody CL, Manclark CR, St.Geme JJ (1984) Immunologic response to early and routine DTP immunization in infants. *Pediatrics* 73: 37–42
186 Smith DH, Peter G, Ingram DL, Harding AL, Anderson P (1973) Responses of children immunized with the capsular polysaccharide of Hemophilus influenzae, type b. *Pediatrics* 52: 637–644
187 Adderson EE, Shackelford PG, Quinn A, Carroll WL (1991) Restricted Ig H chain V gene usage in the human antibody response to *Haemophilus influenzae* type b capsular polysaccharide. *J Immunol* 147: 1667–1674
188 Schlesinger Y, Granoff DM (1992) Avidity and bactericidal activity of antibody elicited by different *Haemophilus influenzae* type b conjugate vaccines. The Vaccine Study Group. *Jama* 267: 1489–1494
189 Granoff DM, Holmes SJ, Osterholm MT, McHugh JE, Lucas AH, Anderson EL, Belshe RB, Jacobs JL, Medley F, Murphy TV (1993) Induction of immunologic memory in infants primed with Haemophilus influenzae type b conjugate vaccines. *J Infect Dis* 168: 663–671
190 Siber G (1994) Pneumococcal disease: prospects for a new generation of vaccines. *Science* 265: 1385–1387
191 Anderson EL, Kennedy DJ, Geldmacher KM, Donnelly J, Mendelman PM (1996) Immunogenicity of heptavalent pneumococcal conjugate vaccine in infants. *J Pediatr* 128: 649–653
192 Daum RS, Hogerman D, Rennels MB, Bewley K, Malinoski F, Rothstein E, Reisinger K, Block S, Keyserling H, Steinhoff M (1997) Infant immunization with pneumococcal CRM197 vaccines: effect of saccharide size on immunogenicity and interactions with simultaneously administered vaccines. *J Infect Dis* 176: 445–455
193 Fairley CK, Begg N, Borrow R, Fox AJ, Jones DM, Cartwright K (1996) Conjugate meningococcal serogroup A and C vaccine: reactogenicity and immunogenicity in United Kingdom infants. *J Infect Dis* 174: 1360–1363
194 Eskola J, Kayhty H (1998) Early immunization with conjugate vaccines. *Vaccine* 16: 1433–1438
195 Lieberman JM, Greenberg DP, Wong VK, Partridge S, Chang SJ, Chiu CY,

Ward JI (1995) Effect of neonatal immunization with diphtheria and tetanus toxoids on antibody responses to *Haemophilus influenzae* type b conjugate vaccines. *J Pediatr* 126: 198–205

196 Sato H, Albrecht P, Reynolds DW, Stagno S, Ennis FA (1979) Transfer of measles, mumps, and rubella antibodies from mother to infant. Its effect on measles, mumps, and rubella immunization. *American Journal of Diseases of Children* 133: 1240–1243

197 Vahlquist B (1949) Response of infants to diphtheria immunization. *Lancet* 1: 16–18

198 Perkins F, Yetts R, Gaisfurd W (1959) Response of infants to a third dose of poliomelitis vaccine given 10 to 12 months after primary immunization. *Br Med J* 115: 680–682

199 Sullender WM, Miller JL, Yasukawa LL, Bradley JS, Black SB, Yeager AS, Arvin AM (1987) Humoral and cell-mediated immunity in neonates with herpes simplex virus infection. *J Infect Dis* 155: 28–37

200 Burchett SK, Corey L, Mohan KM, Westall J, Ashley R, Wilson CB (1992) Diminished interferon-gamma and lymphocyte proliferation in neonatal and postpartum primary herpes simplex virus infection. *J Infect Dis* 165: 813–818

201 Stagno S, Cloud GA (1994) Working parents: the impact of day care and breast-feeding on cytomegalovirus infections in offspring. *Proc Natl Acad Sci USA* 91: 2384–2389

202 Adler SP (1992) Cytomegalovirus transmission and child day care. *Adv Pediatr Infect Dis* 7: 109–122

203 Revello MG, Zavattoni M, Sarasini A, Percivalle E, Simoncini L, Gerna G (1998) Human cytomegalovirus in blood of immunocompetent persons during primary infection: prognostic implications for pregnancy. *J Infect Dis* 177: 1170–1175

204 Zanghellini F, Boppana SB, Emery VC, Griffiths PD, Pass RF (1999) Asymptomatic primary cytomegalovirus infection: virologic and immunologic features. *J Infect Dis* 180: 702–707

205 Pass R (2001) Cytomegalovirus. In: Knipe DM (ed): *Fields virology*. Lippincott Williams & Wilkins, Philadelphia, p. 2675

206 Riddell SR, Greenberg PD (2000) T-cell therapy of cytomegalovirus and human immunodeficiency virus infection. *J Antimicrob Chemother* 45 (Suppl) T3: 35–43

207 Jonjic S, Mutter W, Weiland F, Reddehase MJ, Koszinowski UH (1989) Site-restricted persistent cytomegalovirus infection after selective long-term depletion of $CD4^+$ T lymphocytes. *J Exp Med* 169: 1199–1212

208 Lucin P, Pavic I, Polic B, Jonjic S, Koszinowski UH (1992) Gamma interferon-dependent clearance of cytomegalovirus infection in salivary glands. *J Virol* 66: 1977–1984

209 Polic B, Hengel H, Krmpotic A, Trgovcich J, Pavic I, Luccaronin P, Jonjic S, Koszinowski UH (1998) Hierarchical and redundant lymphocyte subset con-

trol precludes cytomegalovirus replication during latent infection. *J Exp Med* 188: 1047–1054

210 Waldrop SL, Pitcher CJ, Peterson DM, Maino VC, Picker LJ (1997) Determination of antigen-specific memory/effector CD4$^+$ T cell frequencies by flow cytometry: evidence for a novel, antigen-specific homeostatic mechanism in HIV-associated immunodeficiency. *J Clin Invest* 99: 1739–1750

211 Maecker HT, Dunn HS, Suni MA, Khatamzas E, Pitcher CJ, Bunde T, Persaud N, Trigona W, Fu TM, Sinclair E et al (2001) Use of overlapping peptide mixtures as antigens for cytokine flow cytometry. *J Immunol Methods* 255: 27–40

212 Dunn HS, Haney DJ, Ghanekar SA, Stepick-Biek P, Lewis DB, Maecker HT (2002) Dynamics of CD4 and CD8 T cell responses to cytomegalovirus in healthy human donors. *J Infect Dis* 186: 15–22

213 Kern F, Bunde T, Faulhaber N, Kiecker F, Khatamzas E, Rudawski IM, Pruss A, Gratama JW, Volkmer-Engert R, Ewert R et al (2002) Cytomegalovirus (CMV) phosphoprotein 65 makes a large contribution to shaping the T cell repertoire in CMV-exposed individuals. *J Infect Dis* 185: 1709–1716

214 Erkeller-Yuksel FM, Deneys V, Yuksel B, Hannet I, Hulstaert F, Hamilton C, Mackinnon H, Stokes LT, Munhyeshuli V, Vanlangendonck F (1992) Age-related changes in human blood lymphocyte subpopulations. *J Pediatr* 120: 216–222

215 Rentenaar RJ, Gamadia LE, van DerHoek N, van Diepen FN, Boom R, Weel JF, Wertheim-van Dillen PM, van Lier RA, ten Berge IJ (2000) Development of virus-specific CD4(+) T cells during primary cytomegalovirus infection. *J Clin Invest* 105: 541–548

216 Gamadia LE, Remmerswaal EB, Weel JF, Bemelman F, van Lier RA, Ten Berge IJ (2003) Primary immune responses to human CMV: a critical role for IFN-gamma-producing CD4$^+$ T cells in protection against CMV disease. *Blood* 101: 2686–2692

217 Young JL, Ramage JM, Gaston JS, Beverley PC (1997) *In vitro* responses of human CD45R0brightRA- and CD45R0-RAbright T cell subsets and their relationship to memory and naive T cells. *Eur J Immunol* 27: 2383–2390

218 Picker LJ, Singh MK, Zdraveski Z, Treer JR, Waldrop SL, Bergstresser PR, Maino VC (1995) Direct demonstration of cytokine synthesis heterogeneity among human memory/effector T cells by flow cytometry. *Blood* 86: 1408–1419

219 Sanders ME, Makgoba MW, Sharrow SO, Stephany D, Springer TA, Young HA, Shaw S (1988) Human memory T lymphocytes express increased levels of three cell adhesion molecules (LFA-3, CD2, and LFA-1) and three other molecules (UCHL1, CDw29, and Pgp-1) and have enhanced IFN-gamma production. *J Immunol* 140: 1401–1407

220 Wills MR, Carmichael AJ, Mynard K, Jin X, Weekes MP, Plachter B, Sissons JG (1996) The human cytotoxic T-lymphocyte (CTL) response to cytomegalovirus is dominated by structural protein pp65: frequency, specificity, and T-cell receptor usage of pp65-specific CTL. *J Virol* 70: 7569–7579

221 Engstrand M, Tournay C, Peyrat MA, Eriksson BM, Wadstrom J, Wirgart BZ, Romagne F, Bonneville M, Totterman TH, Korsgren O (2000) Characterization of CMVpp65-specific CD8+ T lymphocytes using MHC tetramers in kidney transplant patients and healthy participants. *Transplantation* 69: 2243–2250

222 Altman JD, Moss PA, Goulder PJ, Barouch DH, McHeyzer-Williams MG, Bell JI, McMichael AJ, Davis MM (1996) Phenotypic analysis of antigen-specific T lymphocytes. *Science* 274: 94–96

223 Adler SP (1991) Molecular epidemiology of cytomegalovirus: a study of factors affecting transmission among children at three day-care centers. *Pediatr Infect Dis J* 10: 584–590

224 Adler SP (1985) The molecular epidemiology of cytomegalovirus transmission among children attending a day care center. *J Infect Dis* 152: 760–768

225 Marrack P, Kappler J (1990) The staphylococcal enterotoxins and their relatives. *Science* 248: 705–711

226 Mocarski ES, Jr (2002) Immunomodulation by cytomegaloviruses: manipulative strategies beyond evasion. *Trends Microbiol* 10: 332–339

227 Cherry JD (1997) Measles. In: Feigin R (ed): *Textbook of pediatric infectious diseases*, Vol. 2. Saunders, Philadelphia

228 Papania M, Baughman AL, Lee S, Cheek JE, Atkinson W, Redd SC, Spitalny K, Finelli L, Markowitz L (1999) Increased susceptibility to measles in infants in the United States. *Pediatrics* 104: e59

229 Hutchins S, Markowitz L, Atkinson W, Swint E, Hadler S (1996) Measles outbreaks in the United States, 1987 through 1990. *Pediatr Infect Dis J* 15: 31–38

230 Clements CJ, Cutts FT (1995) The epidemiology of measles: thirty years of vaccination. *Curr Top Microbiol Immunol* 191: 13–33

231 Aaby P, Clements J, Orinda V (1991) Mortality from measles: measuring the impact. *Expanded Programme on Immunization*, Geneva

232 Samb B, Aaby P, Whittle HC, Seck AM, Rahman S, Bennett J, Markowitz L, Simondon F (1995) Serologic status and measles attack rates among vaccinated and unvaccinated children in rural Senegal. *Pediatr Infect Dis* J 14: 203–209

233 Maldonado YA, Lawrence EC, DeHovitz R, Hartzell H, Albrecht P (1995) Early loss of passive measles antibody in infants of mothers with vaccine-induced immunity. *Pediatrics* 96: 447–450

234 Markowitz LE, Albrecht P, Rhodes P, Demonteverde R, Swint E, Maes EF, Powell C, Patriarca PA (1996) Changing levels of measles antibody titers in women and children in the United States: impact on response to vaccination. Kaiser Permanente Measles Vaccine Trial Team. *Pediatrics* 97: 53–58

235 Kumar ML, Johnson CE, Chui LW, Whitwell JK, Staehle B, Nalin D (1998) Immune response to measles vaccine in 6-month-old infants of measles seronegative mothers. *Vaccine* 16: 2047–2051

236 Gans HA, Arvin AM, Galinus J, Logan L, DeHovitz R, Maldonado Y (1998) Deficiency of the humoral immune response to measles vaccine in infants immunized at age 6 months. *Jama* 280: 527–532

237 Gans H, Yasukawa L, Rinki M, DeHovitz R, Forghani B, Beeler J, Audet S, Maldonado Y, Arvin AM (2001) Immune responses to measles and mumps vaccination of infants at 6, 9, and 12 months. *J Infect Dis* 184: 817–826

238 Gans HA, Maldonado Y, Yasukawa LL, Beeler J, Audet S, Rinki MM, DeHovitz R, Arvin AM (1999) IL-12, IFN-gamma, and T cell proliferation to measles in immunized infants. *J Immunol* 162: 5569–5575

239 Siegrist CA, Caordova M, Brandt C, Barrios C, Berney M, Tougne C, Kovarik J, Lambert PH (1998) Determinants of infant responses to vaccines in presence of maternal antibodies. *Vaccine* 16: 1409–1414

240 Aaby P, Bukh J, Leerhoy J, Lisse IM, Mordhorst CH, Pedersen IR (1986) Vaccinated children get milder measles infection: a community study from Guinea-Bissau. *J Infect Dis* 154: 858–863

Regulatory issues

The Grand Challenge for the Future
ed. by Stefan H.E. Kaufmann and Paul-Henri Lambert

Regulatory issues in the development of new vaccines with a special emphasis on safety aspects

François Verdier

Sanofi Pasteur, Campus Mérieux, 1541 avenue Marcel Mérieux, 69280 Marcy l'Etoile, France

Introduction

Vaccines represent a major weapon against many infectious diseases. More recently, vaccines have demonstrated promising methods in the prevention or treatment of other types of disorders such as cancer and autoimmune diseases. Their composition has significantly evolved from the whole micro-organism approach (attenuated or inactivated) to the use of crude fractions or purified parts of these organisms (polysaccharides and toxoids) through to protein-polysaccharide conjugates and now to recombinant proteins or polypeptides. Gene transfer products (naked DNA and vector-based vaccines), which are currently in pre-licensing phases, also represent a new approach in vaccinology [1]; they are already successfully used as veterinary vaccines for rabies or distemper. Therefore vaccines are multifaceted products and also act through a highly complex mechanism in which the antigen(s) by itself is not the final acting component of the immune response. Vaccines produce antibodies or activate T cells that are the actual effectors. Obviously, this complexity raises regulatory issues associated with the efficacy and safety assessment of vaccines.

Vaccines fall within the scope of medicinal products (as defined by the amended Council Directive 65/65/EEC [2]) even if they are considered as a separate category as illustrated by the dedicated Office of Vaccines Research and Review within the U.S. Food and Drug Administration – Center for Biologics Evaluation and Research (FDA-CBER) organisation. Therefore they must undergo strict non-clinical and clinical safety evaluation before licensing in line with what is performed with drugs. This classification as a medicinal product associated with the specific status of vaccines implies that documents for pharmaceuticals in general and specific vaccine guidelines provide regulatory guidance for vaccine development. For instance, the WHO publishes appropriate vaccine guidelines covering the nonclinical and clinical development of vaccines only [3, 4].

One of the major differences between vaccines and other pharmaceuticals is the fact that they are given to healthy people, and predominantly to children. As a consequence, safety is a major focus in the assessment of vaccines.

The risk-benefit ratio of vaccination in general is very different between developing countries and developed countries. The recent Rotashield vaccine is a perfect example of this statement. The product has been withdrawn in the US after cases of intussusception in temporal relation to the administration of the vaccine. The withdrawal was a worldwide withdrawal although the benefits of the vaccine in developing countries are still obvious.

The lay public is expecting to receive vaccines which bear a zero risk while the authorities as well as the manufacturers have to deal with an increased number of liabilities. As a consequence, the level of safety requirements has increased tremendously. The time to licensure and the price of the vaccines have increased in parallel.

Vaccine life can be split in three stages: development, licensure and post-licensure. In this document, regulatory aspects will be considered for the development stage with a special emphasis on the nonclinical safety issues as the clinical development will be reviewed in some detail in other sections of this book.

Characterisation of starting materials, production process and final product

Several guidelines present the requirements for the characterisation and control of biological products and/or vaccines prior to licensure. The majority are edited under the International Congress on Harmonization (ICH) process [5–9], by the WHO [4] or by Pharmacopoeia (e.g., European Pharmacopoeia).

Vaccine characterisation starts before the first clinical trial and continues during the clinical development. Based on the test used to characterise the vaccine and also considering previous experience from vaccines from the same category, a range of quality control tests is selected. Vaccine specifications are established from this relevant set of tests. In line with the good manufacturing practice, all these tests must be standardised and validated. Validation may be only partially achievable at the beginning of the vaccine development when innovative techniques are used and the vaccine candidate is not yet in its final formulation.

The particularities of each vaccine imply a product-based strategy for quality control and characterisation and regulatory authorities are able to accept this product-design approach. However, a seed-lot system (for culture of micro-organisms) or a cell-bank system (for culture in cells) is applied as recommended by the European Pharmacopoeia [10] to ensure uniformity and full traceability. The system starts with the Master seed lot (or Master cell bank), continues with the Working seed lot (or Working cell bank) and ends with the final bulk which is filled to obtained the final lot or batch of vaccine. However, when primary cells or embryonated eggs are used, characterisation has to be repeated for every new production run [11].

Quality control includes first the evaluation of the raw or starting materials. This evaluation can start with a supplier audit. Any unwanted endogenous or extraneous agent should be evaluated [12, 13]. For instance, the risk of prion contamination seriously affected the biotechnology industry. The bovine spongiform encephalopathy (BSE) and the related new variant of Creutzfeldt-Jacob Disease (CJD) led to strict rules concerning materials of animal origin. Not only should vaccine manufacturers use BSE-free countries (New Zealand, Australia) whenever feasible for their materials of animal origin, but they should also document the full process from the origin of bacterial or viral seed to their current products. Any undefined step with potential contamination by products of animal origin can require re-derivation of the seed using methods such as RNA transfection.

The absence of other adventitious agents, and particularly viruses, is an essential safety requirement for all biotechnological products. One of the technical difficulties of these tests for live viruses, particularly in early development phases, consists in the requirement for a pre-neutralization of the vaccine virus using specific antibodies. Details about essential phases of viral safety can be found in quality guidelines [8, 12, 13]. Animals are still used for these tests but new *in vitro* methods have been developed recently in addition to animal tests. For instance, the polymerase chain reaction (PCR) amplification can detect fragments of viral contaminants and the product-enhanced reverse transcriptase (PERT) assay is used to identify traces of retroviruses [11].

In addition to viral safety tests, any new cell bank should be studied for their tumorigenicity in chemically or genetically immunosuppressed rodent models (i.e., athymic mice, newborn rodents treated with antithymocyte serum or globulin or thymectomised and irradiated mice that have been reconstituted with bone marrow from healthy mice) with a comparison to a reference tumorigenic cell line. The observation of tumors at the injection site and potential metastases are the endpoints of these tests. *In vitro* methods are also proposed [12]. As a consequence, a limit is required for residual substrate-cell DNA from a tumorigenic cell line (e.g., 10 ng per single human dose based on the European Pharmacopoeia). Bacterial and fungal contaminants are also investigated. Mycoplasmas are carefully screened by culture or indicator cell culture methods [14].

The second quality control phase corresponds to the in-process control. Appropriate in-process controls may eliminate the need for tests on the final product and can allow a reduction of animal use for batch release. A validation of the manufacturing process will concern all aspects of the vaccine manufacturing process including equipment, facilities, and personnel; it allows production of consistent lots. The completion of this validation generally requires at least three released batches.

The quality of the process is also supported by compliance with Good Manufacturing Practice (GMP) and clinical batches should be issued by GMP facilities. Julie Milstien [15] perfectly illustrated the parallel between the "Cutter incident" which occurred in 1955 and then the implementation of GMP rules including those for the development of clinical batches of vaccine. Unfortunately, 260 cases of paralytic polio and 11 deaths were caused by an inactivated polio vaccine in the 50s. Not only did this case result in stricter controls and regulation but also validation, facility inspection, quality assurance implication in protocols and reports required by the GMP safeguarded against such incidents.

Finally quality controls are performed on the final bulk and/or final batch; these include sterility and physico-chemical analysis. Several vaccines still use attenuated or inactivated micro-organisms. Specific toxicity tests are performed as part of the range of quality control tests to verify the attenuation or the inactivation of the micro-organism. As for other tests, *in vivo* methods were the reference technique and are being progressively replaced by *in vitro* techniques [16]. For instance, the rabies vaccine inactivation was tested by the intracerebral route in mice and can be tested on cell culture for non-adjuvanted formulations nowadays. Oral polio vaccine is still tested by an intraspinal route in monkeys for neurovirulence, although alternative methods (molecular-based assay (MAPREC) and transgenic mice expressing the human polio virus receptor) are currently being evaluated and used [16–18]. Neurovirulence tests are also considered for non-neurotropic vaccines but not as a batch-release test. Specific toxicity tests are also used to control the inactivation of bacterial toxins (e.g., diphtheria and tetanus toxins tested by the intraperitoneal route in the guinea-pig or by *in vitro* methods using Vero cells and *Bordetella pertussis* toxin tested by the same route in mice). As a complement to this specific toxicity, abnormal toxicity (also called general safety) tests are also performed at various steps of the vaccine production process (final product, and, in some cases, bulk and primary seed) by intraperitoneal injection of the product in mice and guinea-pigs. Mortality and body-weight decrease are recorded during these tests. These abnormal toxicity tests in animals are intended to detect any toxic substances accidentally introduced in the final vaccine formulation. However, they can be challenged from an ethical perspective and could be irrelevant if the vaccine components are susceptible to triggering false positive reactions due to their reactogenicity by this intraperitoneal route of administration. Therefore, abnormal toxicity tests are removed from several vaccine monographs [19].

To complete this section on safety evaluation, as part of the quality assessment of vaccines, pyrogenicity tests should be carried out particularly for polysaccharide vaccines. The use of the rabbit pyrogenicity test decreases in favor of the *Limulus amoebocyte* lysate test (LAL).

In addition, stability studies are performed not only on the final batch but also on process intermediates using several of the tests mentioned above and, more particularly, safeguarding of potency should be verified.

It would be inappropriate to define a universal list of quality tests due to the diversity of vaccine approaches, each of them being associated with a specific development strategy. Therefore the tests selected for the specifications of a viral vector-based vaccine are presented in Table 1 as an example of the application of the above-mentioned principles. Tests are done on the cells used to produce the virus (i.e., avian cells) and on different steps of the viral suspension preparation from the bulk viral suspension to the finished product.

Results from these release tests (i.e., compliance with specifications), combined with the release of the raw materials and a careful review of the production process and associated data (e.g., data from the environment) allow the release of a vaccine batch for clinical trials. By performing these tests, the manufacturer should verify vaccine safety aspects such as product sterility, but also demonstrate that the manufacturing process is consistent.

Non-clinical safety evaluation

The most exhaustive description of the non-clinical safety requirement is probably included in the recent WHO guideline [4]. This document is the result of concerted work by the WHO, drug agency and industry representatives and represents a global consensus of the diverse regulatory bodies. The description of the main non-clinical safety studies included in this section will comply with this document. However, guidelines applicable to all pharmaceuticals including biotechnology-derived products provide helpful support, such as the ICH S6 guideline entitled "Preclinical safety evaluation of biotechnology-derived pharmaceuticals" [20]. It clearly explains the flexible strategy recommended for biotechnology-derived pharmaceuticals, including vaccines. The scope of this document includes recombinant protein vaccines but does not cover conventional bacterial and viral vaccines or DNA vaccines.

With regard to the specific guidelines, the European document by the European Agency for the Evaluation of Medicinal Product (EMEA), Committee for Proprietary Medicinal Product (CPMP), December 1997, entitled "Note for guidance on preclinical pharmacological and toxicological testing of vaccines" [21] is the only finalised guide solely dedicated to the pre-clinical safety evaluation of vaccines published by the European agency. There is no such guideline in the US and the "Guidance for industry for the evaluation of combination vaccines for preventable diseases: production, testing and clinical studies" [22] only includes a short section dealing with non-clinical studies.

Interestingly, the FDA has recently released a draft guidance document on reproductive toxicology for vaccines intended for women of child-bear-

Table 1. List of the quality control tests selected according to the different manufacturing steps for the specifications of a viral vector-based vaccine produced on avian cells.

	Control cells	
• Observation	• Control cells: Supernatants Bacterial and fungal sterility test	• Test for extraneous agents using cells: - Chick embryo fibroblast cells - Continuous simian kidney cells - Human diploid cells
• Test for haemadsorbing viruses	• Test for mycoplasmas using microbiological culture method • Test for mycoplasmas using indicator cell culture method	• Test for avian leucosis viruses • CoRT test (research of exogenous avian retroviruses on CEF cells)
	Viral suspension	
• Detection of reverse transcriptase by semi-nested PCR (PERT assay)	• Transmissibility assay on human cells	• Identification
• Bacterial and fungal sterility test	• Test for extraneous agents using animals: - Mice - Suckling-mice - Guinea-pigs - Rabbits	• Test for extraneous agents using cells: - Continuous simian kidney cells - Human diploid cells - Chicken embryo cells
• Test for mycoplasmas using microbiological culture method	• Test for extraneous agents using embryonated eggs: - Allantoïc cavity - Yolk sac	
• Test for mycoplasmas using indicator cell culture method		
	Clarified harvest	
• Bacterial and fungal sterility	• Virus concentration	
	Final bulk product	
• Bacterial and fungal sterility	• Assay of residual antibiotic (neomycin)	• Test for removal of intact cells
	Filled product, finished product	
• Appearance • Dissolution time • Appearance after dissolution • Residual moisture content	• PH measurement • Osmolality measurement • Bovine serum albumin content • Bacterial and fungal sterility	• Endotoxin content • Abnormal toxicity test • Identification • Virus concentration

ing age and those which may be used to immunise pregnant women [23]. The recommendations have been adapted from document ICH S5a in order to include the specific properties of vaccines.

For vaccines considered to be in the gene therapy or gene transfer medicinal product category (e.g., pox vector and naked DNA), the following specific guidelines are of use:

- FDA, CBER December 1996: "Points to consider on plasmid DNA vaccines for preventive infectious disease indications" [24]
- FDA, CBER March 1998: "Guidance for human somatic cell therapy and gene therapy" [25]
- EMEA, CPMP April 2001: "Note for guidance on the quality, preclinical and clinical aspects of gene transfer medicinal products" [26].

In addition, the EMEA has recently released a document for consultation called "Guidelines on adjuvant in vaccines" [27].

Guidelines and position papers are regularly published or amended by drug agencies, particularly for new therapeutic approaches or very specific situations such as the development of a smallpox vaccine within the framework of government efforts to combat bio-terrorism or the development of pandemic flu vaccines [28, 29]. The list of documents given is subject to modification and it is recommended that the latest version be checked on the drug agency's web site.

Outline of the proposed studies

With regard to the toxicological studies, animal models remain the best option for mimicking the human situation. Despite many efforts to develop *in silico* and *in vitro* models, such replacement models remain of limited use as they are not able to reproduce the complexity of the human immune system.

Thus, a critical challenge is the identification of the "relevant" animal model. The criteria used include the following (in order of importance): development of an immune response similar to the expected human response after vaccination, demonstration of a similar binding profile for the induced antibodies [30, 31], susceptibility to the targeted pathogen and, perhaps the most difficult to fulfil, the ability to develop exacerbation reactions [32].

These criteria imply the need to be able to generate and interpret immunogenicity data in the species used for toxicological studies. Rats and monkeys remain the most frequently used species. Recently, the use of newborn or aged rodents has been considered for the evaluation of vaccines intended for neonates or elderly people, as the immune responses of these populations present some peculiarities [33, 34].

The evaluation of the potential intrinsic (direct) toxicity of the test article is generally the main outcome of single-dose toxicity studies; therefore the relevance of species selection is less critical than for the subsequent animal studies and rodents are used. The need for this type of study can be challenged. The remarks written about general safety tests and the efforts made to reduce this type of animal study are also applicable to this type of study. Repeated-dose toxicology studies are regularly the pivotal non-clinical safety study before the first human administration.

However, if the single-dose study is the pivotal study supporting a clinical trial, the design should be modified to include more parameters (i.e., clinical pathology and microscopic examination of a limited list of tissues).

The repeated-dose study or studies are considered to be pivotal and should be performed in full compliance with Good Laboratory Practice. Several criteria have to be met in the design of this type of study. The fundamental selection of the animal model was mentioned above. The route of administration and the dosing regimen should mimic the proposed human schedule, although the time between injections can be reduced for practical reasons (e.g., 3 weeks). This is probably the easiest way to fulfil the "be relevant" principle. Dose levels are also widely discussed. Indeed, vaccines and their potential adverse effects do not always follow a linear relationship. The most common approach is to test one full human dose per animal when it is technically feasible. When two dose levels are tested, the lower should correspond to the "pharmacological" dose (the dose known to induce a significant immune response in the selected species) and the higher should be equal to one human dose. Parameters monitored include clinical signs, ophthalmology, clinical pathology (haematology and serum clinical chemistry) and at necropsy, organ weights, gross and histopathological examination. In the interests of reducing animal use and study costs, the assessment of local tolerance during either a single- or a repeated-dose toxicity study can be made when the route of administration used is the same as for humans. In order to take the prolonged action of vaccines through the immune response into account, animals can be split into two sub-groups, the first sub-group sacrificed immediately after the last administration and the second fifteen days later as close as possible to the immune response peak.

During the in-life phase of repeated-dose studies, additional parameters of safety pharmacology, such as body temperature, electrocardiogram and blood pressure, could also be considered. Their inclusion is recommended for cost and ethical reasons as long as they do not interfere with the other parameters. The traditional range of safety pharmacology tests does not seem relevant for vaccines. It was requested as an exception in order to investigate mechanisms potentially involved in human adverse reactions (e.g., convulsion animal models). Efforts to develop vaccine-relevant safety pharmacology parameters, such as interference with existing immune disease, are encouraged.

Indeed, in all pivotal studies, a basic screening of the immune system should be performed (e.g., histopathology of the lymphoid tissues and blood cell counts). Additional immunological indicators (e.g., cytokine production) can be requested on a case-by-case basis, but interpretation of the results remains difficult.

Vaccination of women of child-bearing age (e.g., rabies and meningitis vaccines) and even pregnant women (e.g., influenza vaccine) is common [35,36] and requires an assessment of the embryo/foetal and perinatal toxicity before licensing. Not only is successful gestation dependant on the status of the immune system [37] but antibodies from pregnant animals can also cross the placenta [38] and could have supposedly harmful effects on the foetus.

The classical division of reproductive toxicology studies into 3 segments as used for new chemical entities is not wholly applicable. Treatment design including immunisation(s) before mating is recommended for vaccine embryo-foetal toxicity studies in order to provide antibody exposure during the entire embryo-foetal period. Post-parturition immunisation is suggested for a sub-group of females not submitted to caesarean delivery for foetus examination whose pups will be necropsied at the end of the lactation period in order to study the effects of antibodies in the newborn. A preliminary study to define and justify the laboratory animal species chosen should demonstrate appropriate antibody transfer with exposure of the embryo to vaccine-induced IgG. This is recommended because immunoglobulin transfer during gestation can render the animal model more susceptible to developmental effects following pre-natal exposure to the vaccine immunoglobulin. As part of the study in the main species, foetal examination, developmental monitoring of the litters and pup necropsy should be included.

The above-mentioned studies constitute the core package of the non-clinical safety investigations and even if their design remains flexible, their completion or the accessibility to equivalent data are generally mandatory.

In addition, more product-specific non-clinical safety studies can be judged necessary according to the vaccine category or published safety concern. For instance, hypersensitivity and auto-immune reactions are the most commonly perceived adverse effects associated with vaccination [39, 40]. The ability of animal models to predict these adverse reactions is a real challenge as they are likely to be rare. Systemic anaphylactic models and biological products, including vaccines, have always been a subject of controversy. However, validation data were obtained mainly from chemicals and not from pharmaceuticals. One can regret the lack of research work in this field which would put us in a better position to decide whether to study hypersensibility reactions on new vaccine components.

To focus on auto-immunity, there are two aspects to be considered: the induction *de novo* of auto-immune disease, and the exacerbation of existing auto-immune disorders [41]. In the first category, auto-immune reactions induced by molecular mimicry occur when the host and the microbial/vaccine determinants are largely similar and present in such a way that there is a break in immune tolerance. This molecular mimicry was also suspected with some new vaccines, such as the recently commercialised Lyme vaccine, where the selected antigen, namely the outer-surface protein Osp A from

Borrelia burgdorferi, presents sequence homology with human LFA-1, and it is suspected that it triggers treatment-resistant Lyme arthritis [42]. Risk of molecular mimicry was also considered for a polysaccharidic vaccine against meningitis. The Group B meningococcal capsular polysaccharide used for this vaccine is a polymer of sialic acid which mimics the polysialylated form of neural cell adhesion molecules present particularly on mammalian embryo cells [30]. Recent advances in computer software (e.g., LifeSeq from Incyte) and the availability of the human genome sequence allow rapid comparison between the protein sequence alignment of a vaccine antigen and a host protein. However, results using these tools present some limitations as predictive methods. For instance, for B-cell epitopes, sequence comparison will look for primary structure mimicry but similar antigenic surfaces (conformational mimicry) is technically very difficult or even impossible to detect. However, T-cell epitope mimicry requires not only an appropriate presentation of the identified common peptide by antigen-presenting cells but also the presence of auto-reactive T cells, which can recognise the mimicking peptide-HLA complexes.

From these hypotheses, a recommended strategy would be to avoid any vaccine antigen presenting a mimicry with a host antigen involved in an auto-immune disease. In any case, surrogate markers can be included in the protocol of toxicology and clinical studies to detect any sign of pathogenic auto-immune response.

The second identified category of auto-immune adverse effects is the exacerbation of a pre-existing pathological condition as reported for influenza infection and multiple sclerosis [43]. Animal models for auto-immune diseases (e.g., MRL/Mpj-lpr, NZB/NZW, SJL, NOD mice and BB rats) have been proposed [44] but we do not yet have sufficient validated data. Moreover, observations of biological markers for auto-immune or hypersensitivity reactions are not necessarily linked to pathogenic consequences. For instance, and this is an important point, the presence of auto-antibodies does not necessarily indicate the induction of auto-immune disease.

In order to cover all safety issues related to vaccines, the evaluation of new adjuvants or any other components of the vaccine formulation should also be considered and dedicated studies are usually required. Novel adjuvants are classified as active compounds and they are evaluated as new chemical or biological entities independently from the vaccine formulation. Recommended studies are listed in the recent EMEA guideline [27]. These studies include genotoxicity assays and repeated- and single-dose studies. Specific attention is given to pharmacokinetic studies as illustrated by the work done for *E. coli* and cholera toxins administered by the intranasal route [45]. Specific studies are added, taking into consideration the mechanism of action of the selected adjuvant. For instance, an adjuvant derived from LPS should have been modified to avoid LPS toxic activity. Pre-clinical tests such as endotoxin shock in the mouse should confirm the inactivation of intrinsic properties.

The hard task of removing mercury-containing preservatives because of their potential neurotoxicity emphasises the need to guarantee the safety of extraneous components added to a vaccine formulation. Experimental data should be collected if the scientific literature does not cover all safety aspects.

Conclusion

The development of vaccines has reached a high level of complexity where the safety concerns need to be addressed correctly. Regulatory guidelines and recommendations provide a framework to the manufacturer to develop his products. The final goal is the release and license of high-quality vaccines.

However, for several reasons (desire of zero risk from the lay public, liability issues for the authorities and manufacturers), the weight given to the collected data is not always put into the right perspective concerning the risk-benefit ratio.

Acknowledgement

The author wishes to express his thanks to Bernadette Hendrickx, Laurent Mallet and Alain Sabouraud for their review of the manuscript.

References

1 Bonnet S, Tartaglia J, Verdier F, Kourilsky P, Lindberg A, Klein M, Moingeon P (2000) Recombinant viruses as a tool for therapeutic vaccination against human cancer. *Immunol Lett* 74: 11–25

2 Council Directive 65/65/EEC of 26 January 1965 on the approximation of provisions laid down by law, regulation or administrative action relating to medicinal products (OJ L No 22 of 9.2.1965, p. 369) (As amended by Directives 66/454/EEC, 75/319/EEC, 83/570/EEC, 87/21/EEC, 89/341/EEC 89/342/EEC 89/343/EEC, 92/27/EEC, 92/73/EEC et 93/39/EEC)

3 World Health Organization (2001) WHO guidelines for clinical evaluation of vaccines: regulatory expectations. Technical Report Series 924

4 World Health Organization (2003) WHO guidelines on nonclinical evaluation of vaccines. Technical Report Series. http://who.int/biologicals/Nonclinical_evaluation_vaccines_Nov_2003.pdf

5 ICH (1995) Topic Q5B, Step 4 Note for Guidance on Quality of Biotechnological Products: Analysis of the Expression Construct in Cell Lines used for Production of r-DNA derived Protein Products (CPMP/ICH/139/95 – adopted Dec. 95)

6 ICH (1995) Topic Q5C, Step 4 Note for Guidance on Quality of Biotechnological Products: Stability Testing of Biotechnological/Biological Products (CPMP/ICH/138/95 – adopted Dec. 95)

7 ICH (1997) Topic Q5D, Step 4 Note for Guidance on Quality of Biotechnological Products: Derivation and Characterisation of Cell Substrates used for Production of Biotechnological/Biological Products (CPMP/ICH/294/95 – adopted Sept. 97)

8 ICH (1997) Topic Q5A, Step 4 note for Guidance on Quality of Biotechnological Products: Viral safety Evaluation of Biotechnology Products derived from Cell Lines of Human or Animal Origin (CPMP/ICH/295/95 – adopted April 97)

9 ICH (1999) Topic Q6B, Step 4 Note For Guidance on Specifications: Test Procedures and Acceptance Criteria for Biotechnological/Biological Products (CPMP/ICH/365/96 – adopted March 99)

10 European Pharmacopoeia (2005) 5.2. General texts on vaccines/5.2. 1. terminology used in monographs on vaccines/ 01-2005: 50201

11 Dellepiane N, Griffiths E, Milstein JB (2000) New challenges in assuring vaccine quality. *Bull WHO* 78: 155–162

12 European Pharmacopoeia (2005) 5.2. General texts on vaccines/ 5.2.3. cell substrates for the production of vaccines for human use /01-2005: 50203

13 European Pharmacopoeia (2005) 5.0/02 methods of analysis/2.6. biological tests/2.6.16. tests for extraneous agents in viral vaccines for human use /01-2005: 20616

14 European Pharmacopoeia (2005) 5.0/02 methods of analysis/2.6. biological tests/2.6.7. Mycoplasmas /01-2005: 20607

15 Milstein JB (2004) Regulation of vaccines: strengthening the science base. *J Public Health Policy* 25: 173–189

16 Metz B, Hendriksen CFM, Jiskoot W, Kersten GFA (2002) Reduction of animal use in human vaccine quality control: opportunities and problems. *Vaccine* 20: 2411–2430

17 Dörsam V, Weimer T, Schmeel A, Hein B, Enssle K, Chumakov KM, Fibi MR (2000) Increased safety level of serotype 3 sabin oral poliomyelitis vaccine lots by improved seed virus, and tissue culture and virus infection conditions. *Vaccine* 18: 2435–2443

18 Levenbook I, Dragunsky E, Perkikovc Y (2000) Development of a transgenic mouse neurovirulence test for oral poliovirus vaccine: international collaborative study 1993–1999. *Vaccine* 19: 163–166

19 Schwanig M, Nagel M, Duchow K, Krämer B (1997) Elimination of abnormal toxicity test for sera and certain vaccines in the European Pharmacopoeia. *Vaccine* 15: 1047–1048

20 ICH (1997) Preclinical safety evaluation of biotechnology-derived pharmaceuticals. Step 4 on 16 July 1997. CPMP/ICH/302/95

21 EMEA (1997) Note for guidance on preclinical pharmacological and toxicological testing of vaccines. CPMP/SWP/465/95

22 FDA, CBER (1997) Guidance for Industry. For the evaluation of combination

vaccines for preventable diseases: production, testing and clinical studies. N°97N-0029
23 FDA, CBER (2000) Guidance for industry. Considerations for reproductive toxicity studies for preventive vaccines for infectious disease indications
24 FDA, CBER (1996) Points to Consider on Plasmed DNA Vaccines for Preventive Infectious Disease Indications
25 FDA, CBER (1998) Guidance for human somatic cell therapy and gene therapy
26 EMEA (2001) Note for guidance on the quality, preclinical and clinical aspects of gene transfer medicinal products. CPMP/BWP/3088/99
27 EMEA (2004) Guideline on adjuvants in vaccines. EMEA/CHMP/VEG/134716/2004
28 EMEA (2002) Note for guidance on the development of vaccinia virus based vaccines against smallpox. CPMP/1100/02
29 EMEA (2004) Guideline on dossier structure and content for pandemic influenza vaccine marketing authorization application. CPMP/VEG/4717/03
30 Finne J, Bitter-Suermann D, Goridis C, Finne U (1987) An IgG monoclonal antibody to group B meningococci cross-reacts with developmentally regulated polysialic acid units of glycoproteins in neural and extraneural tissues. *J Immunol* 138: 4402–4407
31 Kantor J, Irvine K, Abrams S, Snoy P, Olsen R, Greiner J, Kaufman H, Eggensperger E, Schlom J (1992) Immunogenicity and safety of a recombinant vaccinia virus vaccine expressing the carcinoembryonic antigen gene in a nonhuman primate. *Cancer Res* 52: 6917–6925
32 Kakuk TJ, Soike K, Brideau RJ, Zaya RM, Cole SL, Zhang JY, Roberts ED, Wells PA, Wathen MW (1993) A human respiratory syncytial virus (RSV) primate model of enhanced pulmonary pathology induced with a formalin-inactivated RSV vaccine but not a recombinant FG subunit vaccine. *J Infect Dis* 167: 553–561
33 Siegrist CA (2001) Neonatal and early life vaccinology. *Vaccine* 19: 3331–3346.
34 Steere AC, Gross D, Meyer AL, Huber BT (2001) Autoimmune mechanisms in antibiotic treatment –resistant lyme arthritis. J Autoimmunity 16: 263–268
35 Munoz FM, Englund JA (2000) A step ahead: Infant protection through maternal immunization. *Pediatric Clinics of North America* 47: 449–463
36 Paradiso PR (2002) Maternal immunization: the influence of liability issues on vaccine development. *Vaccine* 20: S73–S74
37 Raghupathy R (1997) Th1-type immunity is compatible with successful pregnancy. *Immunol Today* 18: 478–482
38 Ghetie V, Ward ES (1997) FcRn: the MHC class I-related receptor that is more than an IgG transporter. *Immunol Today* 18: 592–598
39 Shoenfeld Y, Aron-Maor A (2000) Vaccination and autoimmunity – “vaccinosis”: a dangerous liaison? *J Autoimmunity* 14: 1–10
40 Kumagai T, Ozaki T, Kamada M, Igarashi C, Yuri K, Furukawa H, Wagatuma K, Chiba S, Sato M, Kojima H et al (2000). Gelatin-containing diphtheria-

tetanus-pertussis (DTP) vaccine causes sensitization to gelatin in the recipients. *Vaccine* 18: 1555–1561
41 Wraith DC, Goldman M, Lambert PH (2003) Vaccination and autoimmune disease: what is the evidence? *Lancet* 362: 1659–1666
42 Hemmer B, Gran B, Zhao Y, Marques A, Pascal J, Tzou A, Kondo T, Cortese I, Bielekova B, Straus SE et al (1999) Identification of candidate T-cell epitopes and molecular mimics in chronic Lyme disease. *Nature Med* 5: 1375–1382
43 De Keyser J, Zwanikken C, Boon M (1998) Effects of influenza vaccination and influenza illness on exacerbations in multiple sclerosis. *J Neurol Sci* 159: 51–53
44 Taneja V, David CS (2001) Lessons from animal models for human autoimmune diseases. *Nature Immunol* 2: 781–784
45 Van Ginkel FW, Jackson RJ, Yuki Y, McGhee JR (2000) Cutting edge: the mucosal adjuvant cholera toxin redirects vaccine proteins into olfactory tissues. *J Immunol* 165: 4778–4782

Clinical trials

The Grand Challenge for the Future
ed. by Stefan H.E. Kaufmann and Paul-Henri Lambert

Clinical trials in developing countries: ethical issues

Veronica L.Tallo[1] and Hanna M. Nohynek[2]

[1]Research Institute for Tropical Medicine, Department of Health, Filinvest Corporate City, Alabang, Muntinlupa 1781, The Philippines; [2]National Public Health Instiuute, Department of Vaccines, Clinical Unit, Mannerheimitie 166, 00300 Helsinki, Finland

Introduction

The ethical issues one needs to consider when doing clinical trials in developing countries are so manifold that one could write an entire book on them. In this chapter, we concentrate on the main issues which we have had to consider beforehand (capacities of ethical review committees, truly involving community in research, information process) and during a clinical vaccine trial when things do not go according to plans, when ethical issues arise which need immediate solving. The main ethical principles and guidelines developed are accessible in the already published literature and websites listed in the references. How to apply these guidelines in practice is the golden skill one only learns in the field, by doing, by putting in practice those principles in dialogue with the different stakeholders, and especially the population where trials are being conducted.

Trial design and ethics

Where resources are limited, the decision to do a trial has to be carefully thought through. The choice of trial design, sample size and level of power has ethical implications. It is said that bad ethics makes bad science, and *vice-versa*. Therefore, the trial design has to be fitted to the primary question posed by the research. The primary objective of the trial and the limits of confidence acceptable to its statistical significance dictate the sample size needed for the trial. It is unethical to purposely underpower a study by too small a sample size. Also, an underpowered study implies that an opportunity is lost to do another, possibly better designed, scientifically more robust trial in the community. The gold standard of new vaccine research is the individually-randomized, controlled, double-blinded study. Ideally, the control antigen is a placebo so that absolute rather than relative immunogenicity and efficacy comparisons can be made. The use of a true saline placebo in poverty-stricken conditions has been strongly criticized; the argument has been that at least some protection should be given to the control group as well. Yet if it is very likely that the expected price of the new product will prohibit the introduction of the intervention in these conditions unless the new product is highly efficacious, it is counterargued that it is unethical not to find out the absolute efficacy, thus aiding local decision-makers with relevant data arising from their own circumstances. An often-used compromise is to provide some form of additional benefit to the individuals participating in the trial after the trial is over (see discussion in point "Ethical issues relative to informed consent"). Another way of looking at the benefits given to the trial participant is to consider the care given during the trial, i.e., other additional vaccines, diagnostic tests and medical care during outpatient or hospital visits that the participant is entitled to during the trial. An example is provided by a pediatric pneumococcal conjugate vaccine trial in Asia, the investigators of which were advised by the reviewing supranational ethical committee to provide a comparison between the currently licensed 7-valent vaccine, rather than a saline placebo, and the new 11-valent one. The rationale given was that it would have been unethical not to provide a treatment, i.e., 7-valent vaccine, which already was licensed in some western countries. The investigators argued that even if the 7-valent vaccine was available in some countries, it was not available in the country where the study was to be conducted, and even if it was, it would not be available to the vast majority of children. Also, the researchers argued that given their provision of all other EPI vaccines as well as diagnostic and medical treatment when a trial subject sought medical care for the trial clinical endpoint conditions (i.e., acute respiratory infection, pneumonia, meningitis, sepsis), they provided considerable benefits to all participants. Thus, in the absence of any other non-confounding alternative study vaccines, the saline placebo was accepted as the control vaccine to the study which held X-ray-positive pneumonia as its main endpoint.

The definition of an adequate and/or a standard level of care given to trial participants during the study has been the centerpiece of argumentation in several HIV trials carried out in developing countries (i.e., is the measure for "standard" taken from rich or poverty-stricken settings?). While trials have the general tendency of improving health care in the area where they are conducted, it is also usually not acceptable that trials fundamentally change the care-giving practices for those participating in the trial and thus further create obvious inequality in the trial area. On the other hand, it is clear that any adverse health problem caused by the trial product has to be properly taken care of and compensated for during the course of the trial. It is the role of the Independent Data Safety Monitoring Board (DSMB), among their other duties, to safeguard the trial participants in this respect and provide neutral technical advice to the investigators, even if the ultimate responsibility for the trial participants lies with the investigators and the sponsors.

Capability-building for ethics review committees

In the past decade, there has been an increasing trend of outsourcing clinical trials to developing countries. Admittedly, there are several good reasons for such decisions. For one, sick patients, who are usually the targets of research, are so many in the developing countries, that it significantly shortens trial recruitment and enrolment time. Other trial-related costs, including incentives, treatment and hospitalization, as well as payments for research investigators, are considerably lower in developing countries. Increasingly, however, this trend has given rise to what is perceived as the moral controversy of conducting clinical trials in countries where ethical review committees (ERCs) may not make an effective evaluation of research proposals or at worst are not available at all [1–4].

Requirements of an effective ethical review

We consider the following to be necessary for effective ethical review of research proposals:

1. need for trained and competent ERCs;
2. presence of national regulations and ERC-specific operational guidelines;
3. community representation in ERCs; and
4. independence of ERCs.

Trained and competent ERCs

The number of studies conducted in developing countries has multiplied considerably over the last decade. No parallel development and organization of ERCs, however, has taken place in these countries. There are still some countries which do not have ERCs either at the national or institutional levels, causing reviews to be done either by appointed officials of the health ministry or by *ad hoc* committees. In a survey of health researchers in developing countries, nearly half of the respondents reported that their studies did not undergo any form of review – technical, scientific or ethical – by the health ministry of the country [5]. Very recently, an uproar was raised in India over the conduct of a clinical trial which evaluated the ability of a drug to induce ovulation, indicated for the treatment of breast cancer in post-menopausal women, without ethical approval [6]. And yet, India just recently came up with national ERC guidelines.

In countries with functional ERCs, the concern is about the quality and effectiveness of the ethical reviews made. Observations document that developing-country ethical reviews are done perfunctorily, for formality or rubber-stamping purposes, with minimal or practically no ethical questions raised. A review of the status of health ethics of Asian countries revealed that the existence of national ethics bodies did not equate at the institutional levels with effective evaluation capability [2]. More provocative is the commentary that developed-country ERCs have a "low regard" for the quality or "cosmetic" reviews made by developing-country committees [1]. These observations, whether accurate or not, connote that there may be a number of "unethical" studies being carried out in the third-world countries, because of deficiencies in ethical reviews. This anxiety is further fueled by the increasing complexity and sophistication of new research topics, in the areas of genetic epidemiology and molecular biology for instance, which these ERCs may be too technologically naïve and inexperienced to review effectively.

The different international guidelines for human research are very specific about the need for ethical review as an overt translation of the application of ethical principles. These documents include proposals for the composition, roles and responsibilities of ERCs. There is an urgent need for developing countries to heed this requirement as an initial step towards guiding and regulating the research they will host and participate in and to preclude any possible exploitation of their populations due to inequities in socio-economic conditions and access to health services.

The establishment of ERCs is not sufficient by itself. ERCs should be dynamic, i.e., conversant with the guidelines and their provisions. Its members should be trained in review processes and the mechanisms they can employ to guarantee that only ethically acceptable research is done [2, 7]. ERCs must have a clear appreciation of the relationship between scientifically sound and ethically acceptable research. Like any other ERCs, developing-country ERCs also need training in basic research ethics and should take part in continuing education to keep abreast with ongoing ethics and scientific discourses. There are several online ethical review courses hosted for regulatory authorities, medical schools and the like. Often these are, however, designed to satisfy institutional requirements and rapid accreditation of investigators rather than to encourage critical appraisal of the elements of research proposals. Training programs wherein guidelines are interpreted and applied in case analysis and discussions are needed. These exercises provide insights into what the actual ethical review process is about, how issues should be addressed and conflict resolutions should be made and the difficulties the application and interpretation of the ethics guidelines create in real-life situations.

Presence of national regulations and ERC-specific operational guidelines

The international guidelines for the ethical conduct of research are intended to ensure the protection of the research participants from exploitation and harm. Some of the provisions of the recently revised Declaration of Helsinki (DoH) [8] are still heatedly debated because of varying interpretations, their impact on future research, particularly those with public health implications, and because they do not take into account the unique conditions of developing countries [2, 9]. Also, research is increasingly becoming more complicated and complex. This scenario requires that countries take explicit and unambiguous positions in relation to some provisions in the international guidelines, such as the use of placebos in clinical trials, or whether the "best currently available treatment" is synonymous with the "locally available treatment." This situation may also spell the need for less-developed countries to create a separate set of guidelines as aptly demonstrated by India's development of its own Ethical Guidelines for Social Science Research in Health.

Despite the fact that international guidelines are based on commonly agreed ethical principles, these are open to varying interpretations by the bodies and committees who apply them. This is brought about by varying cultural and value orientations, educational background and access to information. Thus, developing-country ERCs may interpret and apply these intuitively in the review and evaluation of research proposals, as ERCs are very recent and an evolving phenomenon in the developing countries.

One way around this is apparently the establishment of national guidance which will incorporate and reflect a country's local norms and value systems, and procedurally involve wider community participation and consultations. If at all feasible, the practical and operational aspects of its application, such as the selection of ERC chair and members, how administrative and financial support may be provided to ERCs, or how issues may be resolved, should be elucidated. In addition, ERCs at both the national and institutional levels should be urged to develop their own manual of operations or procedures. This could further enhance their appreciation and application of both the international and national guidelines. Its availability provides not only a definite and explicit framework, but also, and more importantly, a set of standards within which ERCs could function and operate. These approaches may pave the way towards a more effective, efficient, as well as a more homogeneous and harmonized ethical review, which is transparent to all parties involved. These reduce the possibility of divergent opinions and different opinions between ERCs, particularly with the escalating multi-center studies, and thus multi-ERC reviews.

Community representation in the ERCs

The potential composition of ERCs is indicated in several documents but most prominently in the guidelines developed by the World Health Organization (WHO) [10]. The purpose of a multidisciplinary and wide diversity in the composition of the committee is that the competency and experience that each member brings into the protocol reviews somehow is a guarantee that all possible ethical and moral issues arising from the scientific and logistics plans described in the research protocols are identified, addressed and appropriately decided on. Ideally the review process should take place in two steps: the scientific soundness should be reviewed by an independent, scientifically qualified review committee, and only if the science is found sound, should the multidisciplinary ethics review follow.

In practice, however, ERCs may be composed primarily of institutionally-affiliated scientists with limited or restricted community representation. In many cases as well, the so-called community representative does not truly exemplify the modal community members, e.g., journalists, and thus may not truly represent their best interests and well-being [11].

More reflection on the selection of community representatives to the ERCs should occur. If a permanent representative is difficult to obtain, then provisions should be made that *ad hoc* representatives of the community where the research will be conducted may be invited during the protocol deliberations. For instance, gay activists or gay HIV-affected individuals could serve as community representatives for an HIV clinical trial intending to recruit participants from the gay community. In this manner, the ERCs are assured that representatives will have a primordial interest in truly protecting the community to which they belong. For instance, they should be able to state whether proposed inducements or benefits are appropriate or whether safeguards for data and personal information are adequate. Community representatives will naturally need orientation and training to be able to participate meaningfully in ethical reviews.

Independence of ERCs

Among the challenges confronting developing-country ERCs is their ability to operate independently of the institutions to which they are affiliated. Independence here is defined as the ability of ERCs to conduct intelligent and effective reviews free of administrative and financial pressures and free from conflicts of interests among its members. This is addressed by the lay membership in the committee, by establishing transparent provisions of lines of accountability and conflicts of interests and providing ERCs with their own logistical support.

The Nuffield report [3] documents that the estimated direct and indirect cost for operating ethics committees in the United Kingdom may amount to £36,000 per annum, while that in the US would reach as much as US$ 500,000 per annum. These are staggering amounts which ERCs in developing countries can ill afford. NBAC [4] learned from its commissioned studies that ERCs in developing countries did not have budgets or access to resources to support the functions of the committee, such as salaries of members, meetings, secretarial assistance, training and networking with other ERCs, and the like. In effect, the institution itself absorbs the operating costs of its ERCs, which although small, may be considerable in relation to their limited resources.

Convincing scholars, lawyers and members of the religious groups or community to sit in the ERCs on a voluntary basis or with minimal incentive, is quite difficult to do. Thus, several developing-country ERCs include researchers and scientists as its members. They perform ethical reviews on top of their research and teaching duties, without any additional compensation for their time and effort. Evidently, questions of conflicts of interest may be raised when these same ERC members present their own proposals or are involved in whatever capacity in the research proposals being evaluated. However, this issue can be addressed by establishing transparent provisions on how the ERCs will handle ethical reviews of its members. Nevertheless, non-compensation of ERC members may cause delays in ethical reviews because of the members' voluntary position or their other competing priorities. On the other hand, ERCs may also be under administrative "pressure" to take favorable decisions on proposals which may result in additional research funds, resources or other benefits for the institution. It is in situations such as these that the independence and integrity of the ERCs may be under suspicion or questioned. These problems, however, are not unique to developing countries; several US institutional review boards have been reported to have similar problems [12].

The functioning of any ERC involves costs. Training of the ERC members is an essential direct cost whose outcome would result in a more relevant and effective review. Equally important is the ERC members' continuing education and networking with other ERCs so that they are kept abreast of the more recent issues or controversies that may affect on their own skills and competencies to conduct ethical reviews.

Capacity-building for ERCs

There is a tremendous gap between the ethical review capabilities and competencies of ERCs of sponsors and that of developing countries. Currently, efforts are being carried out to reduce this gap. The WHO has facilitated the establishment of regional fora of ethical review committees for information exchange, development of national guidelines, standard operating procedures and educational activities for ERC members. There are currently four different fora – the Forum for Ethical Review Committees for Asia and the Pacific (FERCAP), Foro Latino Americano de Comités de Ética en Investigación en Salud [Latin American Forum of Ethics Committees in Health Research] (FLACEIS), Pan African Bioethics Initiative (PABIN) and Forum for Ethics Committees in the Confederation of Independent States (FECCIS). The Strategic Initiative for Developing Capacity in Ethical Review (SIDCER) is an international cooperative endeavor designed to facilitate the development of ethical review of medical research and is currently providing technical and financial support for these four fora. The Fogarty International Centre of the National Institute for Health has also sponsored bioethics training for faculties from developing countries.

Research and medical ethics training should be included as one of the capacity-building activities in all collaborative research as demonstrated by UNAIDS in relation to HIV vaccine research. These efforts can be among the most significant and permanent benefits that a study can provide its developing-country collaborators and could strengthen their relationships. Definitely, increased capacity of a developing country to conduct ethical reviews could lend to more effective collaborative research.

Ethical issues relative to informed consent

As increasingly more clinical trials are conducted in the developing countries, compliance with guidelines governing the conduct of these studies becomes more challenging. The issue of informed consent also gains additional focus as it is progressively applied in countries with culturally diverse settings and which are in a clearly disadvantaged position compared with its research sponsors.

Community research decisions

Several criteria are considered in the selection of a clinical research site, particularly for Phase II or III clinical studies. Obviously, research cannot be conducted in communities which will not accept and support it. Thus, one of these requirements should be the community's acceptance of and consent to research being conducted among its members. Agreement by local scientific collaborators to conduct the investigation is not enough. The acceptance, cooperation and support of local political leaders and health officials should be obtained at all levels – regional, provincial or state as well as at the district and village levels.

All international guidelines [3, 4, 8, 13] agree that the role of community consent is essential. But nowhere are these guidelines on community research decisions more explicitly detailed as in national or country guidance documents. For instance, studies which will be done among Aboriginals and Torres Strait Island communities require that a 'written documentation of consent from the communities' be obtained and to document the reasons where this was not possible [14]. Consultation is prescribed as an essential process in the research relationship and continuing research partnerships between researchers and the Maoris who will be involved in them [15]. The guidelines for the conduct of research in India advocate the general principle of community agreement to all of its research, and specify that the principles of voluntariness and informed consent apply not only to individuals but also to communities [16]. The significance of community approval of research is so critical, that Weijer proposes "respect for communities" as the "fourth" ethical principle relevant to the ethics of research as stated in the Belmont Report [17].

But despite these provisions, there are no suggestions as to how community consent should be obtained. Literature reminds investigators that cultural sensitivity is essential in this process. Just what does this mean for researchers? Apparently, the first step is for researchers to have preliminary discussions with their local collaborators, who are assumed to be knowledgeable about and conversant with the local political hierarchy and structures, its decision-making dynamics, as well as the local culture and mores. They should be able to identify people's organizations or community leaders, possible collaborators, stakeholders or partners in the activity. The procedures and processes to obtain permission to conduct research may be dictated largely by the political protocol, community norms, traditions and practices. It may involve informal one-on-one face-to-face meetings, rites and ceremonies, group or village orientation sessions, an open forum, or structured discussion groups. The tones of these sessions may vary from that of information-giving, to consultation, especially if the research contains contentious issues, and even negotiations, to reach a consensus. It may necessitate only one visit or several return calls and discussions. It is a process which may not be hurried or shortened to meet the researchers' deadlines. The process of obtaining community consent should not be perceived as delaying or complicating the research process. The benefits which can be derived from such community consultation may make the difference between a smooth-sailing clinical research project against one which may be plagued with several conflicts and problems. The significance of the consultation process can be aptly illustrated in the following case study (Box 1).

Individual research decisions

Informed consent embodies the principle of respect for persons and their capacity to make choices. For consent to be valid and genuine, the following elements must be present: (1) complete and relevant information must be provided, (2) the prospective participant must have been given enough time to study her options and choices, (3) the information must be understood and (4) consent was voluntarily given. "Information sheet" will be the term used here to refer to the document used to obtain consent and "informed consent" is defined as a communication process between the researcher and the research participant that, according to CIOMS [13], "begins when the initial contact is made with the prospective subject and continues throughout the course of the study".

Box 1. Consultation as mechanism to ascertain study continuation

In the middle of a 5-year pediatric vaccine trial in Asia, the investigators were informed by the pharmaceutical company that the company had decided to cease clinical development of the vaccine under evaluation [36]. At that particular point, the trial was running smoothly with a monthly enrolment of 93% of the eligible population. The ethical question was: is it ethical to continue the trial knowing that the study vaccine did not have at that point any foreseeable commercial future?

As required, the investigators reported the situation to the appropriate national health authorities, who were for the continuation of the study. The institutional ethics committee, on the other hand, was for the discontinuation of the study, but nevertheless advised the research group to undertake the necessary community consultations.

Assured that safety was not the concern in stopping the clinical development of the trial product, the local stakeholders, i.e., the provincial and town-level health authorities, who considered themselves the "guardians of people's health", considered the risks and benefits provided by the trial to the community, and in appreciation of the evident benefits, voted for the continuation of the study. They took the responsibility of informing the political leadership of their recommendation and the reasons behind them. Upon their recommendations, the researchers also called for a consultation meeting with the midwives, to obtain their opinion and consensus on the issue. Apprehensions and concerns were expressed; explanation and further elucidation were offered by both the researchers and senior health officers. The consultation process concluded with the recommendation for the study to be continued despite the new information released by the vaccine company. The whole consultation process involved several meetings over a period of three months.

Equipped with the support of all the health staff of the trial site, the researchers and representatives of the provincial and town-level health authorities presented themselves to the ethics committee and formally requested the continuation of the pediatric trial.

Provision of complete and relevant information

For consent to be valid the participant should receive "complete, relevant and adequate" information [3]. International guidelines have been clear on, although not totally in agreement with,the information which should be included in these information sheets. Principle 22 of the DoH 2000 [8] states that:

> (I)n any research on human beings, each potential subject must be adequately informed of the aims, methods, sources of funding, any possible conflicts of interest, institutional affiliations of the researcher, the anticipated benefits and potential risks of the study and the discomfort it may entail. The subject should be informed of the right to abstain from participation in the study or withdraw consent to participate at any time without reprisal. After ensuring that the subject has understood the information, the physician should then obtain the subject's freely given informed consent, preferably in writing. If the consent cannot be obtained in writing, the non-written consent must be formally documented and witnessed ([8], as amended in 2000).

Based on the above-mentioned principle, the DoH requires at least 8 essential elements on the information sheet. CIOMS, on the other hand, maintains that in addition to those stated above, 18 more pieces of information are necessary if an educated decision is to be made (Box 2). The International Conference of Harmonization-Good Clinical Practice (ICH-GCP) [18] guidelines agree with the elements proposed by DoH [8] and CIOMS [13], but listed a few more critical information elements which should be included in the information sheet.

With the volume of information required, the development of the information sheet to be used poses several challenges. When all the critical informed-consent elements are present, the information sheet may be as short as one page but could be as long as 15 pages. While it is easier to check the document's compliance with the provisions of the guidelines, its readability is a bit difficult to ascertain. The content of the information sheet is definitely novel, often complex and technical and could be intimidating to the educated, but more so to those who have less education and are unfamiliar with the concept of individual consent. The concepts of randomization, placebo or blinding may not have accurate equivalents in most languages and could thus be difficult to present in a manner ensuring its accurate translation. When Hochhauser [19] reviewed some 12 randomly selected information sheets used in clinical trials, he found out that they were difficult to read, contained several technical words, had a high word density per sentence and were not designed to encourage participants to read them.

As a way towards a more readable information sheet, some ERCs in the United States set an arbitrary grade-level requirement at which information sheets are supposed to be written [20]. Towards this end, some researchers use the Flesch-Kinkaid formula in Microsoft Word to determine whether the information sheet they are writing meets the readability criteria. However, there are arguments on the reliability of such measures [20, 21], making it imperative for researchers to explore other vehicles to ascertain readability.

Information sheets should be translated into the language or the dialect of the area where they are to be applied and used. The prescribed translation and back translation into English (the usual language of research protocols) may not be adequate. The translation may need to be subjected to the more rigorous exercise of pretesting or pilot-testing to ensure its comprehensibility [22]. This pre- and pilot-testing may complement other attempts to guarantee the tool's clarity and simplicity. For instance, the information sheet used in a pediatric Phase III vaccine trial in the Asia was pretested among health workers, mothers and grandmothers. The activity resulted in the validation of words/phrases used in the translation and the re-translation or rephrasing of other parts into the community's every-day language to be better understood. After the pretesting, the tool was further pilot-tested on mothers and caretakers. The exercise provided researchers with insights on how the information sheet was received – the reactions it

Box 2. Essential elements of informed consent according to the different guidelines

Declaration of Helsinki, 2000	CIOMS, 2002
1 Aims and methods of the study	1 Purpose of the study and procedures to be carried out by investigators
2 Sources of funding	2 Similar
3 Possible conflict of interest	3 Similar
4 Anticipated benefit	4 Direct benefit to participant; expected benefit to the community or to the society at large or contributions to scientific knowledge
5 Potential risks	5 Same including risks to partner or spouse
6 Discomforts	6 Similar
7 Right not to participate	7 Similar
8 Right to withdraw	8 Similar
	9 That individual is invited to participate in a research. reasons why the individual is suitable for research
	10 How research is different from routine medical care
	11 The expected duration of the individual's participation and the possibility of early termination of the trial or of the individual's participation in it;
	12 Compensation for participation
	13 That participants will be informed of findings related to their health status and the results of their study in general
	14 That the participants have the right to access their data on demand
	15 Any currently available alternative interventions or courses of treatment;
	16 Institutional affiliation of researchers
	17 Availability to the subjects of any products or interventions proven by the research to be safe and effective after they have completed their participation
	18 Provisions to ensure respect for the privacy of subjects and for the confidentiality of records in which subjects are identified;
	19 The limits, legal or other, to the investigators' ability to safeguard confidentiality, and the possible consequences of breaches of confidentiality;
	20 Whether the investigator is also the participant's physician
	21 The extent of the investigator's responsibility to provide medical services to the participant;
	22 Availability of free treatment, duration, organization providing treatment of specified research-related injuries and uncertainty of funds available for these
	23 How subjects or the subject's family or dependants will be compensated for disability or death resulting from such research-related injury
	24 Whether or not the right to compensation is legally guaranteed;
	25 That the protocol was approved or cleared by an ethical review committee

elicited, the questions it generated and the apprehensions and anxiety it created. The activity further resulted in the identification of procedures by which the information sheet could be applied.

Another concern in information sheet development is its layout and design. Since the document is usually long, it should be "attractive" in form and structure to encourage potential research participants to read and, if necessary, re-read it. There are no studies looking into the significance of layout or design as a stimulus to reading and comprehensibility of information sheets. However, one must recognize that the readability of any document is not only in its contents, but may also be affected by readers' literacy level and vision. Thus, researchers should make the effort to present these increasingly detailed and complex information sheets in a more attention-grabbing style. Consideration should be given to the size and type of printing font, whether the document should be presented in columns, the separation of the long document into Questions and Answers or sections or topics segregated by topic headings and the use of illustrations or boxes to highlight critical information.

Provision of enough time to study options and choices

The potential research participant needs to process an overwhelming amount of information to decide on his/her participation. It is essential that the procedures developed allow potential participants to have open access to the research promotional materials, facilitate continuous discussion and consultations if necessary and offer ample opportunity to thoroughly study and evaluate the information received. The international guidelines are very specific about this. CIOMS states that potential participants should be given the opportunity to ask questions; similarly, NBAC instructs researchers to devote time and effort to devising creative measures to facilitate comprehension of research information. These mechanisms should also be able to address previously identified problems, e.g., variability in the presentation of information and hesitancy of potential participants to ask questions [23].

Are there prescribed steps in obtaining consent? Is there a "preferable" way such that consent obtained is truly informed and voluntary? Cultural feasibility studies [24] or consultations with the community and the target population may be necessary in the development of informed consent. For instance, focus group discussions may result in the setting of systems to capture and identify target participants. These can inform investigators where and when discussions of the information sheets may be efficient, and what recruitment materials may be culturally acceptable. These advice-seeking sessions could also yield information on household decision-making dynamics – who makes decisions, who influences decisions – as a necessary input in targeting who should be invited into these recruitment processes.

Consultations could also result in the easy and well-supported solutions to problems which may deter implementation of trial activities.

The initial dissemination of information about the research activity could be presented to the general population and community through a massive information drive and campaign using both print and mass media and face-to-face interactive discussion groups - village meetings, open fora and the like [4, 25]. Giving lectures during community assemblies, meetings of professional or people's organizations, like medical societies and mothers' classes, may be efficient vehicles for a rapid diffusion of correct information and rapid feedback on people's perceptions of the activity. These introductory mechanisms are expected to generate some awareness about the activity and, it is hoped, create a demand for research-specific information among the target groups.

The information sheet is the commonly accepted mode of communicating research information. These sheets are provided to prospective research participants who are expected to read and understand them, prior to consenting to participate in a research activity. But simply reading the information sheet is not sufficient and satisfactory. Kuczewski and Marshall [26] believe that it should be a dynamic, interactive process, where the potential participant actively demands explanation and clarification, while the researcher provides facts, details and particulars about the trial. It must be conducted in a quiet, unhurried setting, where the participants feel free to read either by themselves or along with the investigator, review the information sheet and ask questions, clarifications or express anxieties and concerns. The potential participant must also be given the freedom to share the information sheet with the significant others in her/his social network or to seek their advice and opinions.

The assimilation of concepts presented in a multiple-paged information sheet may not be easy nor possible in one setting, particularly among less-educated participants. Thus, CIOMS proposes the adoption of a process where prospective subjects are informed orally about the research through repetition and explanation. This implies repeated discussions and consultations, and suggests that it does not take place only once, but rather over a period of time. If time permits, the researcher should allow the future participant to bring the information sheet home, to allow him the opportunity to engage in consultations with or seek the advice of the significant others in his social network. Some of the above-mentioned strategies were employed in clinical trials conducted in the Gambia [25], in rural Africa [27] and in other clinical research projects [28, 29]. The delivery of trial information in a pediatric vaccine trial in the Philippines was timed to coincide with the pregnant woman's/mother's clinic visits, i.e., from her prenatal visits until the newborn's first clinic visit for vaccination (Box 3) [30].

Brady [23] is wary about the ability of this text-based traditional consent procedure to capture the essence of informed consent for several rea-

Box 3. Informed consent in a pediatric vaccine trial in a South East Asian country

Firstly, trial brochures were placed at the health centers and hospitals, primarily for distribution to pregnant women who came for the prenatal check-ups; they were also distributed freely during mothers classes. This material introduced the vaccine trial to the target groups for recruitment. It triggered discussions between the pregnant women and mothers' whose children were already enrolled in the trial. It was the focus of deliberations between the pregnant woman and the health worker, whose advice and opinion about trial participation was also sought. Moreover, it was also used as a vehicle to introduce the EPI program to "new" mothers and reinforced or corrected the information held by the previous users of the service.

Dummy copies of the information sheet were provided to the newly delivered mothers either at the hospitals, during home *postpartum* visits or when the mothers or members of the family brought the newborn to the health center for their BCG vaccination. Upon their receipt of the document, the women were encouraged to read, share and if necessary discuss them with other household members.

A week or two prior to the child's expected clinic visit for the first DPT vaccination, trial staff visited the mothers at home to discuss the information sheet. The decision to make the home visit was gleaned from focus group discussions where child caretakers stated that: (1) they could not go nor stay long enough at the health centers for any reading or discussion of the information sheet because of other competing priorities in the home, i.e., other children, (2) they were shy and uncomfortable to ask questions in presence of other members of the community and (3) they want other household members, specifically the fathers, to participate in the discussion. The women added that although childhood vaccination was a decision mothers may make alone, the prospect of having a new, untested vaccine offered to the infants, is something that fathers should know about.

Depending on the outcome of the first home visit, mothers requested repeat visits at home or clarifications just before the child's vaccination.

sons. The extent and nature of the information presented may be culturally determined and thus obtaining a valid informed consent may be difficult. For instance, it is considered culturally inappropriate to disclose all the potential risks of research participation in Nigeria [4]. Japanese and Russian subjects demonstrate the attitude of "I put myself in your hands, doctors" [24], and thus may participate in clinical research without necessarily getting into the details of their participation. But these examples should not deter researchers from adhering to what are considered essential requirements to obtain valid consent. Therefore, the development of culturally responsive and creative techniques is essential. It is believed that research information could also be presented in culturally accepted media such as prose, stories, dramatization, street theater or ballad singers [3], which may be more suitable when research is conducted among less-literate populations [29, 31]. In more technologically advanced settings the use of network technologies, and employing such "edutainment" tools as illustrations, animation, etc., will greatly enhance informed-consent procedures.

Evaluating comprehension of information sheets

Another basic element for informed consent to be genuine and valid is that the research information should be understood. This implies that some sort of evaluation of the research participant's comprehension of the information sheet is made. The guidelines are not clear-cut about how this should be done and researchers have devised their own evaluation schemes. Fitzgerald et al. [32] required participants to pass some sort of examination using either true or false; Hochhauser [21] documented the use of multiple choice questions for such an evaluation, while others were asked to explain in their own words what they have understood from the information sheets [3]. Hochhauser [21] contends that there are problems inherent in the use of multiple-choice questions in evaluating comprehension and emphasizes that these are not sufficiently sensitive to detect true understanding and thus present limitations and complications in satisfying their element of valid consent [33].

Definitely, more experience and research are necessary to address several and varied issues relative to evaluating comprehension. Among others, these may include:

1. What information in the information sheet should be evaluated for comprehension?
2. When should this comprehension evaluation be done – soon after a discussion of the information sheet is done? Or should there be a gap from when the material was read or discussed by the researcher and the evaluation to be done?
3. How should evaluation of comprehension be done? Should prospective participants be given a pencil and paper test (despite its limitations)? Or should they be asked the questions verbally?
4. Should researchers set a "minimum level of understanding" scores? Who should set these? If the prospective participant fails to reach the minimum level of understanding, should s/he then be not included in the study? Who will make these decisions?
5. How will these evaluation scores be interpreted? Are these scores a function of the readability of the information sheet, the adequacy or deficiency of the informed consent process, a reflection of the reading ability of the research applicant, good or faulty recall of the prospective participant, or true comprehension?

While these issues may appear daunting, it does not justify not taking steps towards the need to find out what potential research participants really understand from the information sheets.

Access to products of research at the completion of the study

Among the controversial provisions in both the DoH and CIOMS guidelines is the access to the benefits of research by the participants, communities or countries. This issue touches the core of the conduct of research in developing countries since the non-availability of the proven intervention to the community from which the participants were drawn is regarded as exploitation. The NBAC report and the Nuffield document have presented exhaustive coverage and discussion of this issue based on expert reviews and discussions. Thus, it would be redundant if the same concerns are reiterated here. This section, however, will attempt to discuss the issue of what happens after the research is over in the case of a vaccine trial.

Vaccines are commodities which have wide public health applications. It takes a mean 15 years before a tried and tested candidate vaccine may be produced; it may take another 3–5 years before the vaccine may be licensed for large-scale use. Moreover, the whole clinical process may take several millions of dollars to undertake. When the proposed vaccine trial protocol is deliberated upon by an ERC for review, the questions in relation to the application of the relevant provisions in the DoH or CIOMs may include the following:

1. Is it the responsibility of the ERCs to be concerned about the future access to the vaccines at the completion of the trial?
2. Is the non-availability of a guarantee of access to the candidate vaccine after trial completion a reason for disapproving a vaccine trial protocol?

We propose that while ERCs are primarily concerned with the immediate risk-benefit ratios for the trial participants, they should look beyond and evaluate plans for providing the benefits of research, particularly those with wide public health impact, specifically when reviewing Phase III vaccine trial protocols. It is assumed here that the decision for bringing a vaccine to a Phase III clinical trial is based on favorable and significant immunogenicity information; in effect the prospects of the vaccine are good. This being the case, the ERCS may be justified in exercising their authority and evoking relevant provisions in the international guidelines when conducting the review. But this is not an easy task for the ERCs to do. They need to obtain answers from the research investigators to several questions prior to any deliberations and decisions they will need to take. Among the questions which should be addressed satisfactorily are:

1. What benefits should be provided to participants in a vaccine trial at its completion? If the vaccine trial had participants who received the placebo, what benefits should they receive at the completion of the vaccine trial? What will happen if the vaccine is not efficacious enough to warrant further production?
2. Is there anybody else who should receive the benefits of a vaccine trial at its completion? Who are these? What benefits should they receive?
3. What should be provided to vaccine trial participants, communities, etc., and should this be affected by the possible outcome of the vaccine trial?
4. What mechanisms should be employed to make these arrangements?

5. Since vaccines are public health commodities, who should make the above decisions?

These are just a few of several questions which investigators need to respond to in front of the ERCs. Moreover, the ERC should be able to appreciate what their responsibilities are in the implementation of the decisions as stated.

The nature of the above questions suggests that the issue of access to the products of vaccine trials needs careful planning, requires multi-level and wide consultations not only with the department of health officials, but also with other stakeholders and, more importantly, the community where the vaccine trial is proposed to be done (see Box 1).

In view of the above scenario, should the non-availability of arrangements for making available the products of a vaccine trial be a reason for disapproving a Phase III vaccine trial protocol? This is not an easy question to answer. In the case of vaccines, its long-term effects may not be readily evident during and immediately after the trial itself, and thus its provision without a long-term surveillance plan may have deleterious effects rather than the benefits expected [34, 35]. On the other hand, Bhutta [2] asserts that the benefits of research should not be viewed narrowly as simply the products of the research activity; these can be in the form of improvements in the health care system, training or technology transfer. This issue needs considerable reflection and deliberation – being very strict and stringent in complying with these provisions would definitely stop significant vaccine trials which may provide the necessary inputs for public health policies.

References

1 Gilman RH, Garcia HH (2004) Ethics review procedures for research in developing countries: a basic presumption of guilt. *Can Med Ass J* 171: 248–249

2 Bhutta ZA (2002) Ethics in international health research: a perspective from the developing world. *Bull WHO* 80: 114–120

3 Nuffield Council on Bioethics (2002) The ethics of research related to health care in developing countries. Nuffield Council on Bioethics, London, p. 76

4 National Bioethics Advisory Commission (2001) Ethical and policy issues in research involving human participants. Vol 1. *Reports and Recommendations of the National Bioethics Advisory Commission*, NBAC, Bethesda, Maryland

5 Hyder AA, Wali SA, Khan AN, Teoh, NB, Kass, NE, Dawson L (2004) Ethical review of health research: a perspective from developing country researchers. *J Med Ethics* 30: 68–72

6 Anonymous. Clinical trials without ethical review under the spotlight. In Focus: 26 March 2004. Accessed from: www.who.int/bulletin/volumes/82/4/feature0404/en. Accessed on October 15, 2004

7 Emmanuel EJ, Wendler D, Grady C (2000) What makes clinical research ethical. *J Am Med Ass* 283: 2701–2711

8 World Medical Association (2000) Declaration of Helsinki. Edinburg

9 Vastag B (2000) Helsinki discord? A controversial declaration. *JAMA* 284: 2983–2985

10 World Health Organization (2000) Operational guidelines for ethics committees that review biomedical research. Geneva

11 Strauss RP, Sengupta, S, Quinn SC, Goepingger J, Spaulding C, Kegeles SM, Millett G (2001) The role of community advisory boards: involving communities in the informed consent process. *Am J Publ Health* 91: 1938–1943

12 Shalala D (2000) Protecting research subjects: what must be done. *New Engl J Med* 343: 808–810

13 Council for International Organizations of Medical Sciences (2002) International ethical guidelines for biomedical research involving human subjects. Geneva

14 National Health and Medical Research Council (1991) Guidelines on ethical matters in aboriginal and Torres Strait islander health research. Wellington

15 Health Research Council of New Zealand (1998) Guidelines for researchers on health research involving Maori. Wellington

16 Indian Council of Medical Research (2000) Ethical guidelines for biomedical research on human beings. New Delhi

17 Weijer C (1999) Protecting communities in research: philosophical and pragmatic challenges. *Cambridge Quart Healthcare Ethics* 8: 501–513

18 Anonymous (1995) Note for guidance on good clinical practice (CPMP/ICH/135/1995). ICH harmonized tripartite guideline. ICH Secretariat/CPMP/World Medical Association

19 Hochhauser M (2000) The informed consent form: document development and evaluation. *Drug Inform J* 34: 1309–1317

20 Paasche-Orlow MK, Taylor HA, Brancat FL (2003) Readability standards for informed-consent forms as compared with actual readability. *N Engl J Med* 348: 721–726

21 Hochhauser M (2004) Informed consent: reading and understanding are not the same. *Appl Clin Trials* 13: April. www.actmagazine.com/appliedclinicaltrials/article/articleDetail.jsp?id=90594

22 Stiffler H (2003) Guidelines for obtaining informed consent for clinical research. *Appl Clin Trials* 12: Nov 2. www.actmagazine.com/appliedclinicaltrials/article/articleDetail.jsp?id=77704

23 Brady JS (2003) Multimedia delivery can enhance the consent process. *Appl Clin Trials* 12: Jan 1 www.actmagazine.com/appliedclinicaltrials/article/article Detail.jsp?id=80369

24 Coreil J, Losikoff P, Pincu R, Mayard G, Ruff AJ, Hausler HP, Desormeau J, Davis H, Boulos R, Halsey NA (1998) Cultural feasibility studies in preparation for clinical trials to reduce maternal-infant HIV transmission in Haiti. *AIDS Educ Prev* 10: 46–62

25 Leach A, Hilton S, Greenwood BM, Manneh E, Dibba B, Wilikns A,

Mulholland EK (1999) An evaluation of the informed consent procedure used during a trial of a *Haemophilus influenzae* type b conjugate vaccine undertaken in the Gambia, West Africa. *Soc Sci Med* 48: 139–148

26 Kuczewski MG, Marshall P (2002) The decision dynamics of clinical research: the context and process of informed consent. *Med Care* 40: 45–54

27 Preziozi MP, Yam A, Ndiaye M, Simaga A, Simondon F, Wassilak SGF (1997) Practical experiences in obtaining informed consent for a vaccine trial in rural Africa. *N Engl J Med* 336: 370–373

28 Stapleton H, Kirkham M, Thomas G (2002) Qualitative study of evidence based leaflets in maternity care. *Br Med J* 323: 1464–1466

29 Benitez O, Devauz D, Dausset J (2002) Audio-visual documentation of oral consent: a new method of informed consent for illiterate populations. *Lancet* 359: 1407–1407

30 Tallo V (2003) Evaluating comprehension of informed consent: how should it be done? Oral Presentation at the 3rd African Conference on Ethical Aspects of Clinical Research in Developing Countries. Kampala, Uganda, March 19–21, 2003.

31 Stober M (2003) Multinational clinical trials: breaking language and cultural barriers. *Appl Clin Trials* 12 Sept 1. www.actmagazine.com/appliedclinicaltrials/article/articleDetail.jsp?id=79882

32 Fitzgerald DW, Marotte C, Verdier RI, Johnson WD, Pape JW (2002) Comprehension during informed consent in a less developed country. *Lancet* 360: 1301–1302

33 Slack C, Lindegger G, Vardas E, Richter L, Strode A, Wassernaar D (2000) Ethical issues in HIV vaccine trials in South Africa. *S Afr J Sci* 96: 291–295

34 Weijer, C (2000) The future of research into rotavirus vaccine. *Br Med J* 321: 525–526

35 Knudsen KM, Aaby P, Whittle H, Rowe M, Samb B, Simondon F, Fine P (1996) Child mortality following standard, medium or high titre measles immunization in West Africa. *Int J Epidemiol* 25: 665–673

36 Anonymous (2002) A dwindling set of manufacturers. GAVI Immunization Focus March 2002, page 4

Vaccine safety and adverse events: lessons learnt

Philippe Duclos, Adwoa D. Bentsi-Enchill and Dina Pfeifer

Vaccine Assessment and Monitoring, Department of Immunization, Vaccines and Biologicals, World Health Organization, 20 Avenue Appia, 1211 Geneva 27, Switzerland

Introduction

The challenge for those who work in the field of vaccination is to collectively gather and present sound scientific evidence of the benefits and risks of vaccination, to recognise, understand and minimize the risks, and to define current vaccination policies as well as the future direction of vaccination. Convincing evidence needs to be presented to health professions, regulatory agencies, governments, and to parents who must decide whether their children should be vaccinated or not, despite uncertainties.

There have been several examples of recently identified serious adverse events being linked to vaccination, some of which were identified after licensure of the product, such as the occurrence of Bell's Palsy following vaccination with a new inactivated intranasal influenza vaccine [1, 2] and that of intussusception with rotavirus vaccination [3]. Some other purported claims of vaccine safety issues, such as that of a causal relationship between measles, mumps and rubella (MMR) vaccination and autism or inflammatory bowel disease or concerns about an "overload" effect of multiple childhood vaccinations on the immune system, have not been supported by scientific evidence but have had a major impact on vaccine acceptance and invited non-compliance [4–7]. These unsubstantiated threats to immunization programmes have had greatest impact in industrialized countries, due in part to a higher media coverage of claims of vaccination risks (whether or not such claims are correct), to the fact that many such claims involve medical conditions more prevalent or better recognized in industrialized countries (such as multiple sclerosis and autism), and to a lesser acceptance of small risks. As concerns in industrialized countries spread in the media or in the scientific literature, it is anticipated that they will have increasing impact in non-industrialized countries as well, potentially undermining vaccination coverage. Often an impact already exists in non-industrialized countries, albeit poorly quantified.

Although much progress has been made with respect to ensuring vaccine safety, with the further development of many additional vaccines and particularly those intended for poverty-related diseases, many safety issues will emerge, particularly in light of the technological needs of these newer vaccines and in light of the fact that some of these vaccines will mostly or even almost exclusively be used in non-industrialized countries. It is therefore of particular importance to acknowledge some of these issues and challenges and to consider the elements critical to overcome them so that safety issues do not later prevent the use and/or development of future vaccines.

In this article we: (1) briefly review the various elements of immunization safety, define the term "adverse events", and describe the steps taken to ensure and monitor vaccine safety; (2) highlight issues and challenges with respect to clinical trials and post-marketing surveillance in general terms and then more specifically with respect to new vaccines and vaccines intended for developing countries; and (3) propose some solutions or steps needed to improve the process, all of which are being promoted by WHO.

Immunization safety, adverse events, and steps taken to ensure and monitor vaccine safety

Scope of immunization safety

Immunization safety can be defined as the process to ensure and monitor the safety of all aspects of immunization, including vaccine quality, vaccine storage and handling, vaccine administration, disposal of sharps and management of waste [8]. In the past there have been dramatic examples of safety issues resulting from faulty production, such as the occurrence of tuberculosis following BCG vaccination in Lubeck in 1929–1930 [9], the episode of jaundice in military recruits following yellow fever vaccination [10] and the occurrence of polio following use of the inactivated Cutter polio vaccine in 1955 [11]. However, the risk of such incidents (most of which have been ascribed to a lack of scientific knowledge, gross negligence and lack of supervision and control in manufacturing procedures) [12], although not inexistent, has become more distant. Countries with properly functional national regulatory authorities have established independent laboratories to test vaccines and have obliged manufacturers to conform to strict standards of efficacy and safety. Detailed control procedures are now essential requirements of good vaccine manufacturing practice. In addition to ever improved and more sophisticated tests, vaccine regulations entail a number of other procedures to ensure safety, including the characterization of starting materials by supplier audits, cell banking, seed lot systems, compliance with the principles of good manufacturing practices, independent release of vaccines on a lot-by-lot basis by national regulatory authorities, and enhanced pre- and post-marketing surveillance [13]. As a result, most of the risk with currently licensed vaccines, particularly in non-industrialized countries with limited health infrastructure, does not come from the vaccine itself but rather from a faulty usage, i.e., unsafe injections given with contaminated equipment resulting in a risk of transmission of blood-borne pathogens (HIV, Hepatitis B and Hepatitis C) following syringe reuse [14] or toxic shock following contamination of reconstituted multidose vaccine vials kept over the recommended period of time [15] or intoxication as a result of reconstitution of lyophilized vaccine with improper diluent or inadvertent inoculation of other drugs. Such incidents have included administration of pancuronium bromide, selenium, and insulin among other substances and have unfortunately resulted in deaths [16].

Innovations in safe vaccine administration such as auto-disable syringes that prevent reuse and other pre-filled devices with similar advantages have now been widely introduced into immunization programs in developing countries and contributed to tremendously reducing the previous risks of unsafe injections [8, 17, 18]. Further efforts are ongoing to prevent infection of health workers through accidental needle stick injuries and to avoid risk to communities through proper sharp waste disposal [8]. Vaccines are now mostly "bundled" with auto-disable syringes and disposal boxes, thus ensuring adequate supplies of equipment to maintain safe injection practices. Developments in needle-free technology are also taking place, particularly focusing on jet injectors using disposable standard single-dose cartridges; multidose jet injectors previously being considered for use in immunization programs are currently faced with virtually insurmountable challenges with respect to demonstrating safety [personal communication Martin Friede, WHO]. Greater attention than ever before is being paid in non-industrialized countries to safe vaccine administration and monitoring and management of adverse events.

Adverse events following immunization

For monitoring purposes, an adverse event following immunization (AEFI) can be defined as an untoward medical event temporally associated with immunization that causes concern and is believed to be caused by immunization but might not be actually caused by the vaccine or the immunization process. This includes true adverse reactions caused by the vaccine's inherent properties, possible programmatic errors caused by faulty vaccine preparation, handling or administration (e.g., use of non-sterile equipment, use of improper diluent for reconstitution as mentioned above) and coincidental events (i.e., an event that happens after but is not caused by immunization). Due to the large number of doses administered, there are indeed many coincidental temporal associations between medical events and vaccine administration. In addition, the fear of injection may result in anxiety reactions, including fainting or other psychogenic illness that are related to the injection itself rather than to the vaccine.

In each individual case, and with few exceptions, particularly for live attenuated vaccines for which the vaccine strain can be sequenced (e.g., yellow fever vaccine-related multi-organ failure [19], mumps vaccine-derived meningitis [20]), there is no pathognomonic syndrome and no clear markers of etiology and it is often difficult to demonstrate or rule out a definite relationship between a vaccine and a particular medical condition.

True vaccine reactions are generally mild. More serious complications are rare. Severe reactions resulting in death or permanent damage are extremely rare. By far not every complication that follows the administration of a vaccine is linked to its antigenic components. Problems can also be attributed to a carrier or excipient rather than to a primary constituent. Vaccines, especially whole bacterial vaccines, often contain pyrogens that cause fever by release of chemicals from macrophages [21]. Adjuvants enhance the antibody response to vaccines but aluminium hydroxide and phosphate may induce local reactions such as induration and swelling. For many years hypersensitivity reactions to measles-containing vaccines were thought to be due to egg protein as the vaccine was produced in chick embryo tissue culture. Yet studies using sensitive techniques have not detected residual egg protein and children who had hypersensitivity reactions after receipt of measles-containing vaccines have been demonstrated to react to the gelatine stabilizer rather than to egg proteins [21–24]. As a matter of fact any vaccine component could arguably be subjected to close scrutiny for its potential capacity to produce serious reactions.

Avoidable adverse events are associated with faulty production (e.g., bacterial or viral contamination or insufficient inactivation, presence of foreign toxin) or programme mistakes mentioned above . A useful and more complete description of adverse events and their causation is provided by Halsey et al. [21]. More information on the occurrence of specific reactions can also be found in WHO reference documents that are periodically updated [25, 26].

Vaccines are said to be victims of their own success. As immunization programs reduce target diseases, adverse events inevitably gain in importance. Negative publicity also tends to put the risk of immunization out of perspective and one loses the sense that most vaccine-preventable diseases still occur and some could re-emerge. The media are prone to propagate vaccine safety issues, and the public to go along with them, at the expense of the recognition of the vaccines' benefits. Anything that occurs after vaccination is likely to be called an adverse event. The saga of the purported risk of autism following MMR vaccination in the UK is an unfortunate example of this [4–6]. Vaccine safety concerns also arise in non-industrialized countries and may be a product of special characteristics of the health service. Fears in India about a potential contraceptive effect of the oral poliovirus vaccine (OPV), possibly related to participation of health workers from routine family planning services in mass OPV campaigns, is such an example [27]. More recent allegations of a contamination of OPV with hormones in northern Nigeria which gravely threatened the global polio eradication effort appeared to have more political motives [28]. False assumptions regarding causality are likely to occur for illnesses without a clearly defined etiology or pathogenesis, allowing for speculation about the role of vaccines or their constituents. In several instances, individual investigators have made observations and speculated way beyond their data to imply causal relationships between vaccines and specific medical conditions.

Steps taken to ensure and monitor vaccine safety

Pre-licensure testing of vaccines includes pre-clinical testing in appropriate animal models as well as three phases of studies in human subjects. Phase I safety and immunogenicity testing involves a small number of low-risk individuals (usually healthy immuno-competent adults) who receive the vaccine to determine tolerability. Phase II dose-ranging studies may involve hundreds of individuals to determine a safe and immunogenic dose. The design of phase II studies may vary and include controls [29]. Phase III studies are the more classic, randomised, double-blind, controlled trials involving thousands to ten thousands of more heterogeneous individuals. These studies are designed to address clinical efficacy in disease prevention, provide further safety information, and serve as the final gate-keepers prior to vaccine introduction to the public market [30]. There are limitations, however, to what we can learn from phase III trials. The nature of pre-licensure trials limits the number of subjects studied and thus limits statistical power. Pre-licensure studies can identify events with a magnitude from 1 in 1,000 to 1 in 10,000. Bigger studies to detect more rare conditions would be conducted at prohibitive cost. According to a mathematical approximation, the rule of three indicates that to detect a given risk you must enrol 3 times more exposed subjects, e.g., 3,000 subjects to detect a risk of 1/1,000 doses. Phase III trials are therefore designed for the detection of common and acute reactions and not generally designed to detect uncommon reactions or reactions with vague or delayed onset. In addition, phase III studies have limitations in their ability to detect interactions and to examine outcomes in special populations and in the general population. As well, difficulties with manufacturing biological products may potentially lead to the inadvertent release of vaccine lots that are not fully protective or that may be more reactogenic and hence are beyond the possibility of detection at the pre-licensure stage.

All of the above points emphasize the importance of post-marketing surveillance for AEFI (including true vaccine reactions). For newer vaccines it is becoming common practice for the National Regulatory Authority (NRA) to require manufacturers to perform post-marketing surveillance or post-market studies to further assess the safety and effectiveness profile of a vaccine. Although it is sometimes appropriate to evaluate new vaccines with randomized control trials after licensure, it is not always ethically acceptable, logistically feasible or even scientifically appropriate to use randomized control trials. For these reasons observational study designs are most commonly used to evaluate the safety and efficacy of a vaccine in the post-licensure stage. Such studies are observational *versus* experimental in nature as the investigator does not allocate subjects to receive alternative vaccines (or interventions) according to any deliberate plan.

The purpose of post-marketing surveillance is (1) to detect, correct and prevent program errors, (2) identify problems with vaccine lots or brands, (3) estimate rates of occurrence of AEFI in the local population, (4) identify signals for unexpected adverse events and generate hypotheses that must be confirmed by controlled studies or laboratory work, and (5) help formulate and adjust contraindications, the risk-benefit equation, and information provided to the patient. Effective post-marketing surveillance in turn will help prevent false blame attributed to coincidental events and maintain confidence in the program.

In the vast majority of countries where it exists, post-marketing surveillance is performed by spontaneous reporting or so-called passive surveillance using various reporting schemes whereby reporting of cases thought to be due to or that could be due to vaccination is expected. The reporting is either linked to or separated from that of adverse drug reactions monitoring. At times reporting is mandatory; however, with a few country exceptions, mandatory reporting seems to provide a weak (if any) incentive to report. Extensive information on this topic and guidelines for reporting of AEFI are available on the WHO website (www.who.int/immunization_safety_en/) [31, 32]. Very few countries enjoy some specific sentinel active surveillance system or specifically targeted active surveillance such as those set up through paediatric hospitals or those set up for mass vaccination campaigns [33, 34].

Issues and challenges

Limits of clinical trials

Because of their relatively large size, phase III trials offer a unique opportunity to evaluate vaccine safety. In past years, however, the approach taken in phase III trials was often to focus on documenting common reactions of mild severity such as fever and pain or erythema at the injection site. Often these trials measured adverse events only in a (at times quite small) subsample of the trial population. Some trials even failed to conduct surveillance for adverse events [30]. In addition, the duration of follow-up is at times too limited to capture some potentially serious AEFIs.

Fortunately, several changes have occurred in the way safety is documented. First, it is recognized that not all adverse events can be easily predicted. For example, intussusception following oral receipt of live rhesus reassortant rotavirus vaccine was not an expected side-effect of the vaccine [3]. Therefore it is inappropriate to limit the focus in phase III trials to those events that can be readily predicted. As well, it is no longer acceptable to target surveillance only to common adverse events or to place only a subsample of participants under surveillance for adverse events. Newer-generation live oral rotavirus vaccines have been or are being tested in phase III trials that are large enough to detect an attributable incidence of intussusception of approximately 1 case in 10,000 vaccine recipients [35].

Ionnanidis and Lau [36] have highlighted that the quality and quantity of safety reporting in randomized trials were often inadequate. The WHO vaccine trial registry, mostly concerned with trials implemented in developing countries, was used to assess whether and how investigators are monitoring AEFIs in vaccine trials [37]. As of August 1999, when analyzed by Val Mayans et al., the vaccine trial registry included 68 trials completed or in progress concerning a wide spectrum of infectious agents and diseases. This review highlighted that AEFIs were mentioned in only 69% of phase III and 42% of phase IV trials; few of the trials provided details on the types of AEFI monitored. The good news was the positive trend toward an improvement over time; 54% of 26 trials started in 1987–1993 mentioned AEFIs, compared with 81% of 42 trials started in 1994–99.

Investigators need to place emphasis on AEFI monitoring methods and include results in any publication along with vaccine efficacy methods and results and it is important that causality assessments be carried out for serious adverse events in clinical trials.

Furthermore, editors and reviewers need to be aware that AEFI data, even when negative and reassuring, are essential information in publications of vaccine trials. Yet there have been many situations where safety information, although it exists and would be critical in the interpretation of other data, is not available to those investigating a particular safety problem.

Limits of post-marketing surveillance

Well-known limitations of post-marketing surveillance include: incomplete data, lack of verification of reported diagnosis, faulty numerator and denominator data, lack of standardization and reporting bias. Post-marketing surveillance data cannot be used for calculating true relative risks or true incidence rates. Causal associations between a vaccine and an adverse event can rarely be determined by specific tests such as identifying a vaccine agent in the affected tissue of patients. In the absence of such data and with the limitations of surveillance data mentioned above, epidemiological studies have to be used to determine if the risk of the condition is increased in vaccinated *versus* unvaccinated individuals. Yet common mistakes include assuming a causal relationship based on a temporal association only or on a series of affected patients. Because vaccines are administered to large segments of the population it is not surprising that a substantial proportion of cases of a particular disease would occur within a given window of time after vaccination, yet surveillance only focuses on those vaccinated individuals expressing a given condition. Determination of the actual risk and causality in epidemiological terms would need consideration of the entire picture and calculation of relative risks, i.e., risk in vaccinated populations/risk in unvaccinated populations.

Fortunately, post-marketing surveillance capability is improving; more countries now have AEFI monitoring systems and more importance is attached to the reporting of suspected links between vaccination and adverse events (termed "signals") and their further investigation. Despite much improvement in the global capacity to monitor adverse events, much progress remains to be made, particularly in developing countries, including addressing a common weakness of limitations in the ability to properly analyze and interpret the data.

Careful studies have demonstrated that many hypothesized (on the basis of surveillance data) causal associations between vaccines and adverse events were not substantiated. Surveillance and signal generation, particularly fishing expeditions in large databases, have the potential to identify spurious associations and generate false hypotheses. Thus one should exert caution before raising a signal and highlighting issues to the general public. It is also fundamental for researchers to differentiate between hypothesis generation and hypothesis testing. Although most of the purported associations have been properly investigated and health risks ruled out, this has created a huge amount of work, public attention and avoidance of vaccination. Because of the many assertions made about vaccine safety and their potential to unduly threaten public confidence in vaccines, there is a need for quick hypothesis testing and for adequate tools for hypothesis testing to be available proactively. It has proven essential that suitably controlled studies be undertaken and completed rapidly when such assertions arise.

Investigating hypotheses

Study designs to investigate signals include case-control studies and cohort studies. The latter are better suited for outcomes that occur shortly after vaccination and where the outcome under study occurs frequently. When an outcome is rare or occurs with a long interval after vaccination, it is usually more feasible to evaluate the vaccine by using case-control designs where cases and controls who did not develop the disease outcome are compared for earlier receipt of vaccination. A more recently proposed design particularly suitable to situations in which coverage is high is referred to as self-controlled case-series analysis in which the incidence of adverse events of interest is compared within two windows of time for the same subject, i.e., a window of vulnerability (the post-dosing interval in which the adverse event is postulated to occur) and a window of invulnerability (another post-dosing interval in which the adverse event is postulated not to occur) [38]. This design was used in particular in the evaluation of intussusception following receipt of the live rotavirus-reassortant vaccine [3] as well as in an evaluation of the potential occurrence of intussusception following receipt of OPV during the same period [39, 40].

Special large linked computerized databases such as the one established by the US Centers for Disease Control and Prevention's Vaccine Safety Datalink [41] or the General Practice Research Database in the UK have a great potential to facilitate the investigation of safety issues [42]. These databases link histories of receipt and non-receipt of vaccines in a defined population with comprehensive records of treatments and hospitalizations. Demographic and socio-economic data are also collected. These databases enable rapid controlled analysis and are getting more and more commonly used in industrialized countries but are still virtually absent from developing countries with the rare exception such as Viet Nam [43]

Only a few countries have the capacity and tools to complete hypothesis testing and international collaboration is therefore vital. The process adopted for the investigation of a potential link between oral polio vaccination and intussuception is a model [39, 40]. International collaboration in hypothesis testing and independent scientific reviews of studies enabled the hypothesis of a causal relationship to be rejected, thereby avoiding the potential damage to vaccine acceptance and the polio eradication objectives.

Specific issues of new vaccines and vaccines for poverty-related diseases

While exciting, the impending flood of new and potential products and technologies must be accompanied by a political commitment to secure the necessary resources to keep up the evaluation of vaccines [44]. Although a number of additional issues and challenges are not exclusively related to vaccines for poverty-related diseases, some need particular emphasis because of the nature of the vaccines under development or the characteristics of the countries where these vaccines would be primarily used. A number of these issues are discussed below.

The first issue concerns adjuvants. During the past decade, a large number of novel adjuvants have been developed and evaluated clinically, several of which are already contained in licensed vaccines. Others are likely to be available in coming years, including oil-based emulsions such as MF59 and Montanide ISA 720, immunostimulators such as monophosphoryl lipid A, CpG oligonucleotides, saponins such as QS21, and mucosal adjuvants based on bacterial exotoxins that have been developed for nasal and oral delivery. A number of these adjuvants will have a bearing on the scientific development, efficacy, safety and quality of new vaccines developed for HIV/AIDS, tuberculosis, malaria, leishmaniasis and other conditions. Safety considerations require a thorough understanding of the effects of adjuvants on the immune response and related mechanisms. Yet there is little understanding of the important field of adjuvant safety [45]. Since adjuvants have their own pharmacological properties, which might affect both the immunogenicity and the safety of vaccines, assessment of adjuvant safety in itself is essential. Adverse events attributable to adjuvants need to be documented and reviewed, and the information made available. Animal models have limitations in predicting adjuvant safety. Validated animal models for adjuvant safety testing do not exist, yet they are required for future vaccine research and development. Short-term and long-term safety evaluation and prediction are important, as is the evaluation of the pharmacokinetics of the adjuvant alone. Safety testing of new adjuvants, once combined with a vaccine, necessitates improved and consistent standards for safety monitoring boards, post-licensure signal generation and evaluation, and surveillance of adverse immunological events. This includes unexpected safety issues. Phase IV studies should accommodate adverse reactions that cannot be anticipated from the biological actions of the vaccine and its adjuvant, including the rare and unusual adverse reactions that are not detected in animal work or in small pre-licensure human studies. All this requires a new clinical, scientific and regulatory approach, with attention to the short- and long-term safety of adjuvants [45]. Since many of the new adjuvants are likely to be used in vaccines for conditions endemic in developing countries, scientists from those countries should be aware of these issues and involved in related discussions.

Another issue is that a surveillance focus and capacity must then be available in countries where vaccines are newly introduced and conversely the choice of where to introduce new vaccines first may have to take into consideration the vaccine-preventable disease and AEFI monitoring capacity of the countries. The case of dengue vaccine development illustrates the point. Dengue virus is a flavivirus with four serotypes and type-specific protective immunity. At least eight vaccines against dengue virus infection are under development. Sensitization to severe dengue illness through pre-existing immunity is a serious safety concern for vaccination. Such sensitization has been observed in the course of sequential dengue epidemics by different virus strains in Cuba [46]. From these and other data, the relative risk of severe disease following secondary heterotypic infection has been estimated to be 15 to 80. While host genetic as well as viral virulence factors might contribute to severe dengue hemorrhagic fever, viral load (infectious pressure) and concentration of antibody also appear to play a role. One of the implications of sensitization to dengue is that dengue vaccines need to elicit a balanced immunity to all four dengue serotypes. The 4–5-year follow-up of a tetravalent vaccine currently under clinical evaluation has not revealed a risk of severe disease among vaccine recipients, but the accrued data are still relatively small. It will be important to study the early immune response, its kinetics, and the relationship of these to vaccine-induced memory. Long-term AEFI follow-up is required. The sero-epidemiology of dengue fever should be determined in order to evaluate dengue vaccine safety before and after general introduction of the vaccine, with special attention to the impact of herd immunity [45, 47, 48].

In the past, vaccines that were developed in the industrialized world were used in the country of manufacture and then gradually reached the developing world, and regulatory authorities in the developing world based their decisions on those taken in the industrialized world. The current situation is that there are vaccines produced in Europe which are only required in developing countries. In view of this situation, the European Medicine Agency (EMEA) has changed its regulations with regard to marketing authorizations for vaccines not marketed in the European Union within 3 years of registration; the license will cease to be valid, as opposed to renewal of the license every 5 years, regardless of the market where the product was placed. Discussions between EMEA and WHO resulted in EMEA article 58. This article states that "the Agency may give a *scientific opinion*, in the context of cooperation with WHO, for evaluation of certain medicinal products for human use intended exclusively for markets outside the Community..." [49]. The process will entail the same thorough assessment as is undertaken for a license, but will end in an opinion on the quality, safety and efficacy of a product, as opposed to a marketing authorization. There are, however, a number of issues which are raised by this new procedure. A key issue is the acceptability of the new procedure in countries that will be recipients of this opinion. This is the subject of ongoing consultation.

Another issue to be considered is that of population risk *versus* individual risk which is particularly critical in developing countries where financial constraints may prevent achievement of a high vaccine coverage. An example of this is in the context of the congenital rubella syndrome. When children are immunized on a large scale against rubella but without reaching coverage levels high enough to interrupt transmission, individuals are less likely to encounter the disease at an early age and gain natural protection before reaching reproductive age. If no consideration is given to immunization of females prior to reproductive age, one runs the risk of an increase in infection during pregnancy and hence of a potential temporary increase in congenital rubella syndrome cases. This risk was unfortunately proven to be real in Greece [50].

Although novel vaccine production methods and delivery technologies could theoretically result in safer, more efficacious, more convenient and potentially cheaper-to-produce vaccines with the added benefit of avoiding injections and therefore improving safety, new vaccines and vaccine delivery technologies are not necessarily safer. This is well illustrated by the recent examples of two non-parenteral vaccines, an oral vaccine against rotavirus and an intranasal influenza vaccine with heat-labile *Escherichia coli* enterotoxin as adjuvant, both of which were withdrawn soon after marketing as a result of adverse reactions: Bell's palsy in the case of the influenza vaccine and intussusception in the case of the rotavirus vaccine already mentioned [2, 3].

Although in the pre-licensure trial of the influenza vaccine no case of Bell's palsy had been reported, during the seven-month period after introduction on the Swiss market (i.e., October 2000 through April 2001) 46 cases of Bell's palsy were reported. A subsequent case-control study estimated that the risk of Bell's palsy in vaccinated as compared with unvaccinated persons was 84 (adjusted odds ratio; 95% CI 20-352) with a relative risk of 19 and an excess risk of 13 per 10,000 vaccinees under the most conservative assumptions. Of the identified 91 intranasally vaccinated patients with Bell's palsy, only 21% had an onset interval of 1 to 30 days after vaccination, i.e., within the duration of follow-up in the context of the pre-licensure trials [2].

Five cases of intussusception were seen among 10,054 infants who received the rotavirus vaccine compared with 1 case among the 4,633 infants in the placebo group [3]. In a case-control study, the incidence rate ratio was estimated at 29 (95% CI 16-54) within two weeks of the first dose. The second dose increased the risk more modestly. Overall there was one case of intussusception attributable to the vaccine for every 4,670 to 9,474 infants vaccinated.

A number of lessons can be learnt from these vaccine withdrawals, some of which have been highlighted by Li Wan Po [51]: first, all vaccines carry some risk of an adverse effect that needs to be balanced against their potential benefits and, second, for diseases for which there are current safe alternatives available, post-marketing surveillance should be intense given the limited pre-marketing testing of some vaccines. In addition, it is important to have the right balance between delaying the benefits and safety concerns. Although the assessment should be country-specific, it is clearly based on the rotavirus experience that the risk/benefit ratio or perception of risk in industrialized countries may unduly influence the decision-making process in developing countries where the ratio may actually be very different.

The growing number of vaccines and limited opportunities for contact with the health care system imposes considerable pressure to combine schedules and antigens within a vaccine to minimize vaccine-related visits as well as the number of injections required. Although on the one hand multivalent vaccines have great advantages such as reduced administration costs and increased coverage, the increased complexity of the antigen mixture makes the determination of adverse event causality very difficult and complicates the assessments of efficacy and safety. As well, the wide-reaching nature of immunization programs in developing countries and limited ability to deliver other preventive and curative health interventions make it tempting and efficient to explore the potential to deliver other health interventions concomitantly with vaccination. Some of these interventions, such as the delivery of intermittent treatment against malaria or antihelmintics, have the potential to interfere both negatively and positively with the immune response and this potential interaction should be assessed.

A major challenge of vaccines against poverty-related diseases is the high prevalence of malnourished children and immunocompromised populations in those countries where the vaccines would be introduced. This may have major implications in terms of safety and should be addressed as early as possible in the life cycle of the vaccine. For example, there is still a paucity of population-based data on the effectiveness of the current live BCG vaccine in preventing severe tuberculosis in HIV-positive infants and on its safety. It has been recommended that population-based studies should be undertaken to determine the efficacy and safety of BCG and other vaccines in both HIV-negative and HIV-positive children where there is a high endemic rate of tuberculosis [52].

For those involved with vaccines aimed at poverty reduction and at prevention of diseases specific to developing countries, it is important to be aware of the prequalification process for vaccines to be provided through the UN system, a needed reality particularly for those countries too poor to afford the vaccines through other purchasing mechanisms. WHO provides a service to UNICEF and other UN agencies that purchase vaccines, to determine the acceptability in principle of vaccines from different sources for supply to these agencies (www.who.int/immunization_safety/en/). This is done through an established procedure for the initial evaluation of candidate vaccines. Reassessment at regular intervals ensures the continued quality of vaccines currently being supplied. The goal is to ensure that vaccines used in immunization programmes are safe and effective and that they meet the specific needs of the program, reflected by the tender specifications: i.e., potency, thermostability, presentation, labelling, shipping conditions, etc. The process relies on the NRA of the producing country, understanding of production process and quality control method, production consistency ensured through compliance with good manufacturing practices, random testing for compliance with specifications, and monitoring of complaints from the field [53]. As a result of this evaluation process, WHO issues a regularly-updated list of vaccines which have successfully fulfilled all the established conditions and can thus be taken into consideration for purchase by UN agencies. This list is public and available on the web and can also be used by countries procuring vaccines directly. The fact that a given vaccine is not included in the WHO list of prequalified vaccine products does not necessarily mean that the vaccine would not meet WHO requirements. It may only mean that it has not undergone the prequalifying process.

One challenge facing the prequalification process is that of vaccines produced in developing countries which, even though they are submitted to the same scrutiny as those produced in the western world and manufactured in top world class facilities, tend to be faced with distrust and the erroneous belief that they are of suboptimal quality. Yet these vaccines, including existing vaccines such as DPT, measles-containing vaccines or hepatitis B vaccines, are of critical importance globally and specifically for developing countries since the global supply, and particularly that procured through the UN system, heavily relies on them.

Solutions

WHO has a critical role to play in ensuring vaccine safety at the global level. First, it has an advocacy and normative role and, second, a role in determining and facilitating sharing of information on the safety profile of vaccines based on the best scientific evidence. Most of all, WHO is providing technical support to help strengthen the capacity of member states, particularly in the non-industrialized countries, to monitor and manage vaccine safety issues. The following provides a description of four major activities/tools that WHO has been involved with in support of the above roles.

Capacity building for the NRA and ability to implement the post-marketing surveillance function

Assessment of NRAs began several years ago with the objective of gaining a clearer idea of how well NRAs were performing and ultimately strengthening them. Initially, the NRA assessment was a capacity-building exercise; it is now linked to prequalification of vaccines. In order for a vaccine to be accepted for prequalification, the NRA of the producing country must have been assessed, with positive results in terms of performance of defined core functions. In view of the link with the prequalification process, there is a need to become more stringent with the criteria that NRAs have to meet and indicators of performance in the various NRA functions have been periodically updated [54, 55]. The review also results in a developmental plan to address weaknesses with support from the Global Training Network (GTN). In June 1996, the GTN was established by WHO to provide educational resources to staff involved in vaccine regulations, programs and production throughout the world. The network consists of 12 training centres which offer instruction in priority areas using approved syllabi and standardized materials [56]. The network provides NRAs, National Control Laboratories, vaccine producers meeting specific requirements and national immunization program staff with training in the following courses: Good Manufacturing Practice; Laboratory Quality Systems; Quality Control Testing; DTP Vaccine Production (for regulatory staff); Regulation of Vaccines; Laboratory Animal Science and Husbandry; Surveillance for Adverse Events Following Immunization; and Lot Release and Laboratory Access [56]. Additional activities to strengthen country capacity include the provision of guidelines and various resource materials, all of which can be found on the WHO safety website at www.who.int/immunization_safety/en/.

Guidelines on clinical evaluation of vaccines: regulatory expectations

Guidelines have been developed and published by WHO to assist regulatory authorities and vaccine manufacturers with the clinical evaluation of vaccines; the document can also be useful for clinical researchers and investigators [57]. These guidelines emphasize that randomized studies must have sufficient power to provide reliable rates of common (>1/100 and <1/10) adverse events, and to detect less common but not necessarily very rare (<10,000) adverse events and provide specific recommendations on post-marketing surveillance and phase IV studies.

Guidelines for preclinical evaluation with a focus on safety have also been developed [58].

Standard definitions

The diversity of case definitions and the variability of assessment methods and cut-off points used in vaccine trials and reports from post-marketing surveillance are huge and concern all types of adverse events or reactions. This was illustrated by Bonhoeffer et al. who reviewed published results from 10 large prospective trials [59]. Such differences in AEFI definitions and categorization limit meaningful comparison or meta-analyses and result in a considerable loss of scientific information. A key element in making different study results comparable is a mutual understanding of the adverse event under study. The Brighton Collaboration was launched in the Fall of 2000 as a global collaboration to facilitate the development, evaluation, and dissemination of high-quality information about the safety of human vaccines through the development of standardized case definitions and monitoring guidelines for AEFI. Voluntary working groups comprised of participants from public health, academia, regulatory organizations and industry develop standardized case definitions and guidelines for data collection, analysis, and presentation through literature reviews and consensus formation [59]. A larger reference group comprising over 500 experts from over 60 countries is offered to review draft documents prior to finalization.

The first six Brighton case definitions and corresponding guidelines to be finalized were for fever, generalized convulsive seizure, hypotonic-hyporesponsive episode, intussusception, nodule at injection site, and persistent crying [60–65]. Sixteen additional definitions are at various stages of development, i.e., abscess and cellulitis at injection site, anaphylaxis, encephalitis, fatiguing illness including chronic fatigue syndrome, local reactions including swelling and induration at injection site, aseptic meningitis, rash, and sudden unexpected death syndrome including sudden infant death syndrome. Altogether the aim is to develop up to 50–100 definitions. More information can be accessed at the Brighton Collaboration web site brightoncollaboration.org. It is important that these definitions are suitable for all settings and that more and more scientists (regulatory authorities, academicians and so on) from developing countries participate in the Brighton Collaboration process.

Global Advisory Committee on Vaccine Safety (GACVS)

As highlighted above, rumours of vaccine risks should be dealt with and investigated urgently and decisively if the potential negative impact on vaccine acceptance is to be prevented or necessary modification of programs to be implemented. Appropriate systems for response are required in every country and international collaboration is needed to deal with safety issues of international or regional concern. National advisory committees or review panels exist in a number of countries to specifically review safety issues. These committees, however, have essentially a national mandate and perspective and may differ in opinion based on a number of factors. Considering its role to serve all countries, the WHO established a Global Advisory Committee on Vaccine Safety in 1999 to provide independent scientific assessments of serious vaccine safety issues of potential global importance [66, 67]. The committee also assesses the implications of vaccine safety issues for practice worldwide and for WHO policies. In doing so, the GACVS often draws on the advice, experience and analysis of outside experts. The committee is particularly useful in helping WHO get the best recommendation and assessment of risks in situations of doubt or uncertainty. One of the first activities of the GACVS was to determine a set of criteria according to which the causality of adverse events following immunization could be judged [68]. The committee has reviewed many safety issues to date, including: macrophagic myofasciitis and aluminium-containing vaccines; health effects of thiomersal-containing vaccines; autoimmune diseases and vaccines; child mortality following routine infant immunization; safety of yellow fever vaccine; risks following immunization in HIV-infected children; safety of BCG vaccine in immunocompromised persons; MMR and autism; multiple sclerosis and hepatitis B vaccination; purported non-specific adverse effects attributed to DTP vaccines in infants; acute lymphatic leukaemia and hepatitis B vaccination; oculo-respiratory syndrome following influenza vaccination; Bell's palsy following vaccination with an inactivated intranasal flu vaccine; and influenza vaccination of women during pregnancy. The outcome of the deliberations of the committee on these and other issues is reported routinely in the Weekly Epidemiological Record [45, 52, 69, 70] and is to be found at http://www.who.int/vaccine_safety/en/.

References

1 Anonymous (2002) Global Advisory Committee on Vaccine Safety, 20–21 June 2002. *Wkly Epidemiol Rec* 77: 389–394

2 Mutsch M, Zhou W, Rhodes P, Bopp M, Chen RT, Linder T, Spyr C, Steffen R (2004) Use of the inactivated intranasal influenza vaccine and the risk of Bell's palsy in Switzerland. *N Engl J Med* 350: 896–903

3 Murphy TV, Gargiullo PM, Massoudi MS, Nelson DB, Jumaan AO, Okoro CA, Zanardi LR, Setia S, Fair E, LeBaron CW et al (Rotavirus Intussusception Investigation Team) (2001) Intussusception among infants given an oral rotavirus vaccine. *N Engl J Med* 344:564–572

4 Miller E (2003) Measles-mumps-rubella vaccine and the development of autism. *Semin Pediatr Infect Dis* 14: 199–206

5 Evans M, Stoddart H, Condon L, Freeman E, Grizzell M, Mullen R (2001). Parents' perspectives on the MMR immunisation: a focus group study. *Br J Gen Pract* 51:904–910

6 Fleck F (2003) UK and Italy have low MMR uptake. *BMJ* 327:1124

7 Offit PA, Quarles J, Gerber MA, Hackett CJ, Marcuse EK, Kollman TR, Gellin BG, Landry S. (2002) Addressing parents' concerns: do multiple vaccines overwhelm or weaken the infant's immune system? *Pediatrics* 109:124–129

8 Duclos P, Delo A, Aguado T, Bilous J, Birmingham M, Kieny MP, Milstien J, Wood D, Tarantola D (2003) Immunization safety priority project at the World Health Organization. *Semin Pediatr Infect* Dis 14: 233–239

9 Anonymous (1931) Lübeck catastrophe general review. *BMJ* 1: 986–988

10 Sawyer WA, Meyer KF, Eaton MD, Bauer JH, Putnam P, Schwentker FF (1944) Jaundice in army personnel in the western region of the United States and its relation to vaccination against yellow fever. *Am J Hyg* 40: 35–107

11 Nathanson N, Langmuir AD (1963) The Cutter incident. Poliomyelitis following formaldehyde-inactivated poliovirus vaccination in the United States during the spring of 1955. II. Relationships of poliomyelitis to Cutter vaccine. *Am J Hyg* 78: 29–60

12 Wilson RJ (1967) The development of new vaccines. 1. General considerations. *Can J Public Health* 58: 145–149

13 Dellepiane N, Griffiths E, Milstien JB (2000) New challenges in assuring vaccine quality. *Bull World Health Organ* 78: 155–162

14 Hauri AM, Armstrong GL, Hutin YJ (2004) The global burden of disease

attributable to contaminated injections given in health care settings. *Int J STD AIDS* 15: 7–16

15 Sood DK, Kumar S, Singh S, Sokhey J (1995) Adverse reactions after measles vaccination in India. *Natl Med J India* 8: 208–210

16 World Health Organization. Information for health-care workers – Managing adverse events: Real-life case histories from the field. Available at: http://www.who.int/immunization_safety/aefi/managing_AEFIs/en/index4.html. Accessed 28 September 2004

17 Anonymous (1999) Safety of injections. WHO-UNICEF-UNFPA joint statement on the use of auto-disable syringes in immunization services. World Health Organization, Geneva, WHO/V&B/99.25

18 World Health Organization (2002) States of the world's vaccines and immunization. World Health Organization, Morges (ISBN 92-4-154578-X).

19 Vasconcelos PFC, Luna EJ, Galler R, Silva LJ, Coimbra TL, Barros VLRS, Monath TP, Rodigues SG, Laval C, Costa ZG et al (2001) Serious adverse events associated with yellow fever 17DD vaccine in Brazil: a report of two cases. *Lancet* 358: 91–97

20 Plotkin SA (2004) Mumps vaccine. In: SA Plotkin, WA Orenstein, PA Offit (eds): *Vaccines*. Elsevier Inc, Philadelphia 441–469

21 Halsey NA (2002) The science of evaluation of adverse events associated with vaccination. *Semin Pediatr Infect Dis* 13: 205–214

22 Duclos P, Ward BJ (1998) Measles vaccines: a review of adverse events. *Drug Safety* 19: 435–454

23 Sakagushi M, Nakayama T, Inouye S (1996) Food allergy to gelatin in children with systemic immediate-type reactions, including anaphylaxis, to vaccines. *J Allergy Clin Immunol* 98:1058–1061

24 Kelso JM, Jones RT, Yunginger JW (1993) Anaphylaxis to measles, mumps, and rubella vaccine mediated by IgE to gelatin. *Allergy Clin Immunol* 91: 867–872

25 World Health Organization (2000) Supplementary information on vaccine safety. Part 2: Background rates of adverse events following immunization. Department of Vaccines and Biologicals, World Health Organization, Geneva, WHO/V&B/00.36

26 World Health Organization (2003) Yellow fever vaccine. WHO position paper. *Wkly Epidemiol Rec* 78: 349–359

27 Kumar S (2002) Polio epidemics hit Uttar Pradesh. *BMJ* 325: 617

28 Heymann DL, Aylward RB (2004) Eradicating polio. *N Engl J Med* 351: 1275–1277

29 Tacket CO, Kotloff KL, Rennels MB (2004) Initial clinical evaluation of new vaccine candidates: investigators' perspective of Phase I and Phase II clinical trials of safety, immunogenicity, and preliminary efficacy. In: Levine MM, Kaper JB, Rappuoli R, Liu M, Good MF (eds): *New generation vaccines*. Third edition, revised and expanded. Marcel Dekker Inc., New York, 19–28

30 Clemens JD, Naficy A, Rao MR, Koo H (2004) Long-term evaluation of vaccine protection: methodological issues for Phase III and Phase IV studies. In: Levine MM, Kaper JB, Rappuoli R, Liu M, Good MF (eds): *New generation*

vaccines. Third edition, revised and expanded. Marcel Dekker Inc., New York, 29–48

31 World Health Organization (1997) Surveillance of adverse events following immunization. Field Guide for managers of immunization programmes. World Health Organization, Geneva. WHO/EPI/TRAM/93.02 Rev 1

32 World Health Organization (1999) Immunization Safety Surveillance. Guidelines for managers of immunization programmes on reporting and investigating adverse events following immunization. Immunization Focus, World Health Organization, Regional Office for the Western Pacific, Manila, WPRO/EPI/99.01

33 Scheifele DW, Halperin SA and members of the CPS/Health Canada, Immunization Monitoring Program, Active (IMPACT) (2003) Semin Pediatr Infect Dis 14: 213–219

34 Pless RP, Bentsi-Enchill AD, Duclos P (2003) Monitoring vaccine safety during measles mass immunization campaigns: clinical and programmatic issues. *J Infect Dis* 187 (Suppl 1): S291–298

35 Roberts L (2004) Vaccines. Rotavirus vaccines' second chance. *Science* 305: 1890–1893

36 Ioannidis JP, Lau J (2001) Completeness of safety reporting in randomized trials: an evaluation of 7 medical areas. *JAMA* 285: 437–443

37 Vall Mayans M, Robertson SE, Duclos P. (2000) Adverse events monitoring as a routine component of vaccine clinical trials: evidence from the WHO vaccine Trial Registry. *Bull World Health Organ* 78(9): 1166–1167

38 Farrington CP (2004) Control without separate controls: evaluation of vaccine safety using case-only methods. *Vaccine* 22: 2064–2070.

39 Sardinas MA, Cardenas AZ, Marie GC, Pena MS, Santiago MA, Sanchez MV, Farrington CP (2001) Lack of association between intussusception and oral polio vaccine in Cuban children. *Eur J Epidemiol* 17: 783–787

40 Anonymous (2000) Oral poliovirus vaccine(OPV) and intussusception. *Wkly Epidemiol Rec* 75: 345–347

41 Chen RT, DeStafano F, Davis, RL, Jackson LA, Thompson RS, Mullooly JP, Black SB, Shinefield HR, Vadheim CM, Ward JI et al (2000) The vaccine safety datalink: immunization research in health maintenance organizations in the USA. *Bull World Health Organ* 78: 186–94

42 Andrews N, Miller E, Grant A, Stowe J, Osborne V, Taylor B (2004) Thimerosal exposure in infants and developmental disorders: a retrospective cohort study in the United Kingdom does not support a causal association. *Pediatrics* 114: 584–591

43 Ali M, Canh do G, Clemens JD, Park JK, von Seidlein L, Thiem VD, Tho le H, Trach DD (2003) The vaccine data link in Nha Trang, Vietnam: a progress report on the implementation of a database to detect adverse events related to vaccinations. *Vaccine* 21: 1681–1686

44 Ward BJ (2000) Vaccine adverse events in the new millennium: is there reason for concern? *Bull World Health Organ* 78: 205–215

45 Anonymous (2004) Global Advisory Committee on Vaccine Safety, 10–11 June 2004. *Wkly Epidemiol Rec* 79: 269–272

46 Guzmán MG, Kourí G, Valdés L, Bravo J, Vázquez S, Halstead SB (2002) Enhanced severity of secondary dengue-2 infections: death rates in 1981 and 1997 Cuban outbreaks. *Pan Am J Public Health* 11: 223–227

47 Sabchareon A, Lang J, Chanthavanich P, Yoksan S, Forrat R, Attanath P, Sirivichayakul C, Pengsaa K, Pojjaroen-Anat C, Chambonneau L et al (2004) Safety and immunogenicity of a three dose regimen of two tetravalent live-attenuated dengue vaccines in five- to twelve-year-old Thai children. *Pediatr Infect Dis J* 23: 99–109

48 Rothman AL (2004) Dengue: defining protective *versus* pathologic immunity. *J Clin Invest* 113: 946–951

49 Anonymous (2004) Regulation (EC) No 726/2004 of the European Parliament and of the Council of 31 March 2004 laying down Community procedures for the authorization and supervision of medical products for human and veterinary use and establishing a European Medicines Agency, Official Journal of the European Union. 136: 1–33

50 Panagiotopoulos T, Antoniadou I, Valassi-Adam E (1999) Increase in congenital rubella occurrence after immunisation in Greece: retrospective survey and systematic review. *BMJ* 319: 1462–1467

51 Li Wan Po A (2004) Non-parenteral vaccines have not lived up to their promise. *BMJ* 329: 62–63

52 Anonymous (2004) Global Advisory Committee on Vaccine Safety, 3–4 December 2003. *Wkly Epidemiol Rec* 79: 16–20

53 World Health Organization (2002) Procedure for assessing the acceptability, in principle, of vaccines for purchase by United Nations agencies. World Health Organization, Geneva, WHO/V&B/02.08

54 World Health Organization (2004) Joint medical products assessment tools of national regulatory system vaccines assessment. http://www.who.int/vaccines-access/quality/nras/NRA_%20jointassessmenttools_vaccines_english_revision_Y2004_R03.pdf Accessed on 28 September 2004

55 World Health Organization (2003) Aide-Mémoire. Strengthening national regulatory authorities. http://www.who.int/vaccines-access/quality/nras/nra_aidememoire_2003.pdf Accessed on 28 September 2004

56 World Health Organization. Global training network on vaccine quality (GTN): Course on adverse events following immunization (AEFI). Available at: http://www.who.int/vaccines-access/quality/gtn/aefi.htm. Accessed 28 September 2004

57 World Health Organization (2004) Guidelines on clinical evaluation of vaccines: regulatory expectations. WHO Technical Report Series, 924, Annex 1

58 World Health Organization Guidelines on non-clinical evaluation aof vaccines. WHO Technical Report Series, *in press*

59 Bonhoeffer J, Kohl K, Chen R, Duclos P, Heijbel H, Heininger U, Jefferson T, Loupi E (2002) The Brighton Collaboration: addressing the need for stan-

dardized case definitions of adverse events following immunization (AEFI). Vaccine 21: 298–302

60 Marcy SM, Kohl KS, Dagan R, Nalin D, Blum M, Connell Jones M, Hansen J, Labadie J, Lee L, Martin BL et al (The Brighton Collaboration Fever Working Group) (2004) Fever as an adverse event following immunization: case definition and guidelines of data collection, analysis, and presentation. *Vaccine* 22: 551–556

61 Bonhoeffer J, Menkes J, Gold MS, de Souza-Brito G, Fisher MC, Halsey N, Vermeer P and The Brighton Collaboration Seizure Working Group (2004) Generalized convulsive seizure as an adverse event following immunization: case definition and guidelines for data collection, analysis, and presentation. *Vaccine* 22: 557–562

62 Bonhoeffer J, Gold MS, Heijbel H, Vermeer P, Blumberg D, Braun M, de Souza-Brito G, Davis RL, Halperin S, Heininger U et al (The Brighton Collaboration HHE Working Group) (2004) Hypotonic-hyporesponsive episode (HHE) as an adverse event following immunization: case definition and guidelines for data collection, analysis, and presentation. *Vaccine* 22: 563–568

63 Bines JE, Kohl KS, Forster J, Zanardi LR, Davis RL, Hansen J, Murphy TM, Music S, Niu M, Varricchio F et al (The Brighton Collaboration Intussusception Working Group) (2004) Acute intussusception in infants and children as an adverse event following immunization: case definition and guidelines of data collection, analysis, and presentation. *Vaccine* 22: 569–574

64 Rothstein E, Kohl KS, Ball L, Halperin SA, Halsey N, Hammer SJ, Heath PT, Hennig R, Kleppinger C, Labadie J et al (The Brighton Collaboration Local Reaction Working Group) (2004) Nodule at injection site as an adverse event following immunization: case definition and guidelines for data collection, analysis, and presentation .*Vaccine* 22: 575–585

65 Bonhoeffer J, Vermeer P, Halperin S, Kempe A, Music S, Shindman J, Walop W and The Brighton Collaboration Persistent Crying Working Group (2004) Persistent crying in infants and children as an adverse event following immunization: case definition and guidelines for data collection, analysis, and presentation. *Vaccine* 22: 587–592

66 Anonymous (1999) Vaccine safety. Vaccine Safety Advisory Committee. *Wkly Epidemiol Rec* 74: 337–340

67 Folb PI, Bernatowska E, Chen R, Clemens J, Dodoo ANO, Ellenberg S, Farrington P, John J, Lambert PH, MacDonald NE et al (2004) A global perspective on vaccine safety and public health: the Global Advisory Committee on Vaccine Safety. *Am J Pub Health* 94: 1926–1931

68 Anonymous (2001) Causality assessment of adverse events following immunization. *Wkly Epidemiol Rec* 76: 85–89

69 Anonymous (2003) Global Advisory Committee on Vaccine Safety, 16–17 December 2002. *Wkly Epidemiol Rec* 78: 17–20

70 Anonymous (2003) Global Advisory Committee on Vaccine Safety, 11–12 June 2003. *Wkly Epidemiol Rec* 78: 282–284

The Grand Challenge for the Future
ed. by Stefan H.E. Kaufmann and Paul-Henri Lambert

Sequential stages of clinical trials and overview of issues to be considered

John D. Clemens and R. Leon Ochiai

International Vaccine Institute, Kwanak P.O. Box 14, Seoul, Korea, 151-600

Introduction

We live in an exciting era in which the fruits of molecular biology and biotechnology are yielding a profusion of new and improved candidate vaccines, delivery systems, and adjuvants that have the potential to control many of the infectious disease scourges of the developing world. Indeed, it has been estimated recently that there are over 350 vaccine candidates currently under development against nearly 100 infectious diseases [1].

Discovery of a new vaccine candidate and demonstration of its safety, immunogenicity, and protectivity in animal models are, however, only the first steps toward licensure and introduction of the vaccine into public health practice. The longest phase of development for most vaccines before licensure, and arguably the most uncertain, laborious, and expensive phase, comprises clinical testing of the vaccine in humans [2]. At a minimum, this clinical testing must demonstrate the vaccine to be acceptably safe and suitably protective in the population that will ultimately be targeted for the vaccine in public health practice [3].

Over the years, regulatory agencies have adopted a standard paradigm for the manner in which new vaccines are tested in humans. A key feature of this paradigm is the phased fashion in which the testing occurs. This chapter describes the phases of vaccine evaluations in humans, including several considerations for the phased testing of vaccines in developing countries.

Rationale for phased testing of vaccines in humans

Vaccines have had a remarkable track record of safety. Nevertheless, even when manufactured flawlessly, some vaccines have caused serious side-effects [4]. The mechanisms for these side-effects are diverse and are sometimes related to such problems as vaccine-induced immunopathology, as occurred with early-generation measles and respiratory syncytial virus vaccines [5, 6]. At times the mechanism may be obscure, as was the case for intussusception induced by quadrivalent rhesus reassortant vaccine against rotavirus diarrhea [7, 8]. Whatever the mechanism, the point to be noted is that such severe side-effects are not always predictable. To minimize potential injuries to subjects caused by vaccine side-effects during re-licensure trials, vaccines are tested in a phased manner. In this phasing, early evaluations are conducted in small numbers of subjects, so that if reactions are observed, they will affect a minimum number of volunteers. And early evaluations are typically conducted in the least vulnerable subjects, often healthy adults, so that if the reactions occur, their severity will be minimized. Successive evaluations of a particular vaccine are then conducted in progressively larger numbers of volunteers, and, as confidence in the safety-profile of the vaccine increases, in subjects in the ultimate target group, including persons who are more vulnerable (e.g., infants). With these successive studies, the complete ensemble of information about the vaccine's safety, immunogenicity, protectivity, and sometimes additional characteristics (e.g., transmissibility) is accrued. Moreover, the large number of subjects ultimately studied ensures estimation of these features in a statistically precise fashion, and, for side-effects, in a way that enables detection of relatively rare events.

Clinical trials for licensing a new vaccine candidate are generally planned in three phases. In the Code of Federal Regulations (USA), the phases of clinical trials are described by using Arabic numerals (Phase 1, Phase 2, Phase 3), while in World Health Organization publications, Roman numerals are generally used (Phase I, Phase II, Phase III). In this paper, we use Roman numerals to describe the phases of clinical trials.

Phase I trials

Phase I trials of experimental vaccines are the first human studies to be conducted after preclinical studies have demonstrated suitable safety, potency, immunogenicity, and, when possible, protectivity. The primary purpose of a Phase I trial is to rule out the possibility of frequent vaccine side-effects. Additional goals include preliminary assessment of vaccine immunogenicity, determination of an appropriate dose and regimen, and, for live vaccines, measurement of vaccine shedding. Phase I trials are typically small, often on the order of 10–50 subjects, usually enroll healthy adults, and may be done with preliminary formulations of the vaccine. Depending on whether there are concerns about potential severe side-effects and the need for biological containment of excreted vaccines, such studies may be done on an inpatient or an outpatient basis. For example, a genetically attenuated, live oral vaccine candidate might well be tested initially on an inpatient basis with containment if there is concern about transmission of fecally excreted vaccine organisms, or about the genetic stability of the candidate during the course of fecal shedding [9]. Often, Phase I studies are designed in an uncontrolled fashion.

Phase II trials

For vaccine candidates that are found to yield promising findings in Phase I trials, Phase II trials may be undertaken. The primary goals of Phase II trials are to evaluate vaccine safety and immunogenicity in larger numbers of subjects, and ultimately in the target population for whom the vaccine is intended. For live vaccines, Phase II trials may also be designed to evaluate vaccine shedding and transmissibility. Phase II trials may also further evaluate different vaccine doses and regimens.

A frequently used strategy for Phase II trials of vaccine candidates intended for infants is to initiate the studies in an older age group, often adults, and to conduct successive studies in progressively younger age groups, with the transition to each younger age group contingent on satisfactory results from the study of the previous age group. In contrast to Phase I trials, which are often done with preliminary formulations, Phase II trials typically evaluate the final formulation of the vaccine, since data from studies of preliminary formulations are not usually eligible for consideration by regulatory authorities in their deliberations about vaccine licensure. Phase II trials are typically larger than Phase I trials, sometimes enrolling 200 or more subjects. By the time that a vaccine candidate has reached Phase II, concerns that would mandate testing it on an inpatient basis have typically been resolved, and outpatient studies are the norm. In contrast to Phase I trials, Phase II trials are conventionally designed as randomized, controlled trials, and control groups typically receive a placebo or an active agent to permit blinding.

For live vaccine candidates, there may be a concern about unintended transmission of the vaccine strain from vaccinees to non-vaccinees with whom they are in contact. Special Phase II trials are sometimes conducted to assess the transmissibility of such vaccine candidates. For example, a Phase II study of the live oral cholera vaccine, CVD03-HgR, in Jakarta, Indonesia, randomly allocated pairs of sibling children within households to either vaccine or placebo, and judged transmissibility of the vaccine candidate by the rate of fecal excretion of the vaccine strain and seroconversion to the vaccine in placebo recipients [10].

Phase II trials may also be done to address environmental concerns about genetically engineered, live vaccine candidates. For CVD03-HgR, for example, open sewers outside the Jakarta homes of children who had received the vaccine were sampled to evaluate whether there was any detectable persistence of the vaccine strain during the 36–40 hours after vaccination [10].

A recent trend in vaccine evaluation is to use Phase II trials to obtain initial data on the level of vaccine protection against targeted, naturally occurring infections. What distinguishes these Phase II trials from conventional Phase III trials (*vide infra*) is that they are smaller in size (although usually larger than Phase II trials geared only to the assessment of safety and immunogenicity) and less able to evaluate vaccine protection with suitable statistical precision than well-designed Phase III trials. Also in contrast with Phase III trials, such Phase II trials may be used to evaluate vaccine prototypes that will be later modified or augmented into final vaccines for licensure (e.g., a vaccine against a single serotype, when a multi-serotype vaccine will be required for the final vaccine), and may attempt to obtain estimates of vaccine protection based on prevention of a surrogate endpoint (e.g., the use of HIV viral load as a surrogate for the rapidity of HIV disease progression).

For certain vaccines, studies are done in volunteers to evaluate the clinical protection against an intentional challenge with the target pathogen. Such studies are sometimes termed Phase IIb trials. In these studies volunteers are typically allocated at random to receive the vaccine or a comparison agent, usually a placebo, and are then challenged at a defined interval after vaccination with an inoculum of the pathogen predicted to cause the target disease in nearly 100% of the control group. The comparative attack rate of the target disease in vaccinees *versus* controls provides an estimate of the conventional measure of vaccine protective efficacy (PE) = (1 minus the relative risk of the disease in vaccinees *versus* controls) × 100%. Estimates of vaccine protection in Phase IIb studies, which are typically small, often conducted in ca. 20–30 subjects, may be helpful in triaging vaccines that are deserving of study in larger and more expensive Phase III trials [11, 12].

In addition to providing estimates of vaccine protection, Phase IIb trials can serve to provide data on vaccine safety, vaccine immunogenicity, vaccine shedding and transmissibility (for live vaccines), and preliminary assessments of immunological responses that correlate with protection. Because such studies entail intentional challenge with pathogens, subjects for the studies should always be healthy adults. The intentional challenge also limits Phase IIb trials to infections for which there is no risk of severe acute complications, significant sequelae, or chronic infection if appropriate therapy is administered promptly upon recognition that the challenge has resulted in infection. Examples of pathogens for which Phase IIb studies have been successfully carried out include cholera, diarrheagenic *Escherichia coli*, *Shigella*, Rocky Mountain spotted fever, malaria, and influenza [13]. It is imperative that such studies be carried out by staff who are highly skilled in the diagnosis and treatment of the infections under study, and it is usually desirable to conduct the challenge phase of these studies under inpatient conditions.

Phase III trials

For vaccine candidates found to be suitably safe and immunogenic in Phase II trials, Phase III trials may be done to provide rigorous evidence about

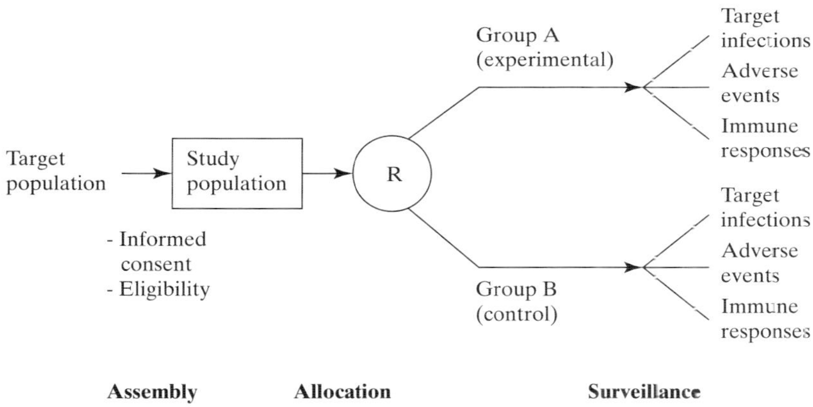

Figure 1. A simplified schematic of a Phase III vaccine trial designed as a two-group, randomized, controlled trial. In such a trial, the study population is assembled from a target population and is then randomized to receive an experimental vaccine or a control agent. The experimental and control groups are followed longitudinally and concurrently to detect the comparative occurrence of target infections, adverse events, and immune responses in the two groups to assess vaccine protection, vaccine safety, and vaccine immunogenicity, respectively.

vaccine protection against naturally occurring infections, and to provide additional data on vaccine safety in larger numbers of vaccinees. Phase III studies are designed as randomized, controlled trials with clear hypotheses, and are conducted in the target group for whom vaccine licensure is desired and in a population that normally experiences the target infection. These studies thus constitute pivotal evaluations that provide the basis for decisions about whether to license a vaccine for use in public health practice [14].

Figure 1 diagrammatically depicts the design of a Phase III trial comparing two groups. In such a trial participants are recruited from a target population and are enrolled for the study after acquisition of informed consent and ascertainment of eligibility. Prior to the trial, a formal randomization scheme is developed to allocate subjects to an experimental vaccine group or a control group, and this randomization scheme is used to allocate the compared agents to consenting subjects who are eligible for participation. To ensure blinding of investigators and subjects to the identities of the compared agents, controls may receive an inert placebo or an active vaccine. If the latter is chosen, it is typically an agent that is identical in appearance to and given with the same regimen as the experimental vaccine, but does not elicit immune responses that are known to protect against the pathogen targeted by the experimental vaccine. After randomization, subjects in the compared groups are followed concurrently with uniform surveillance procedures to detect target infections and adverse events, and the comparative rates of these events in the two groups form the basis for the assessment of vaccine PE and safety. Similarly, participants, or a subsample of participants, are assessed immunologically at baseline and at a defined interval after dosing.

Because Phase III trials must provide statistically meaningful estimates of vaccine PE (calculated in the same way as described above for Phase IIb trials) and because the target disease outcomes to be prevented by vaccination in the trials are typically rare in occurrence, Phase III trials are often quite large, sometimes enrolling tens of thousands of subjects. In addition, because it may be necessary to measure vaccine PE over several years following vaccination in order to provide information necessary to convince regulatory and public health authorities, Phase III trials may entail maintenance and follow-up of study populations for long durations. The large size, lengthy duration, prospective conduct, and extensive quality control and quality assurance procedures needed for Phase III trials make them extremely expensive, often costing millions of dollars.

Measurement of immune responses in Phase III trials is done for two purposes. First, it is necessary to document that the vaccine tested in a Phase III trial elicited the level of immune response expected on the basis of earlier studies. Comparison of immune responses in the vaccine and control groups permits estimation of the proportion of immune responders among the experimental vaccine group that can be attributed to receipt of the vaccine. If vaccine PE proves unexpectedly low in the trial, this assessment will be crucial in helping to explain these results. Assessments to assess whether immune responses were as robust as expected usually require evaluation only of a small subsample of subjects participating in the trial. Second, it is often desirable that a trial define an immunological correlate of vaccine protection – a level of short-term immune response to vaccination that demarcates vaccinees who are protected against the target infection. Immunological correlates of protection are best defined by comparing immune responses to the vaccine in vaccinees who develop the target infection (breakthroughs) *versus* vaccinees who do not.

Definition of immunological correlates of vaccine protection is very important because such correlates permit assessments of the protection of the tested vaccine and ones suitably similar to it in small, short-term studies with immunological endpoints, without resort to full-scale, Phase III efficacy trials with clinical infection endpoints. Phase III trials usually provide the only opportunity before licensure for determining an immunological correlate of protection. Unfortunately, determination of immunological correlates within Phase III trials can be logistically demanding and costly. These problems result from four considerations: 1) it is necessary to contrast short-term immune responses in vaccinees who develop the target infection *versus* those who do not in order to determine an immunological correlate of protection; 2) at the time of vaccination and collection of specimens for immunological assessments it is unpredictable which vaccinees will acquire the target infection ("breakthrough events"); 3) most Phase III trials have very few breakthrough events; and 4) blinding of Phase III trials prevents knowledge of who received the vaccine and who received the control agent. The implication of these considerations is that it may be necessary to obtain suitable specimens from virtually every participant in the trial to ensure that immunological assessments will be available for a large enough number of vaccine breakthroughs to enable statistically meaningful assessments. Moreover, even when arrangements are made to collect the necessary specimens from the required number of subjects, measurement of immune responses in these specimens may not necessarily yield an immunological correlate of the vaccine protection observed in the trial, sometimes for obscure reasons [15].

Other considerations for phased testing of vaccines for developing countries

When in the phased sequence a vaccine should be tested in developing countries

Experience has demonstrated that the performance of a vaccine in affluent populations in industrialized countries cannot be assumed to generalize to persons living in developing-country settings. Examples of vaccines that performed less well in developing-country than in industrialized-country populations have included oral polio vaccine, certain live oral rotavirus and cholera vaccines, and parenteral, polysaccharide-diphtheria protein conjugate *Haemophilus influenzae* type b (Hib) vaccine [16–19]. It is therefore important that new vaccines be tested in developing countries prior to their licensure in these settings.

This raises the question, for vaccine candidates developed in the industrialized world, of when in the phased sequence the candidate should be tested in the developing world. Traditionally, it has been argued, partly over concerns about using poor populations in the developing world as "human guinea pigs", that trials in the developing world should commence only when a vaccine has been fully evaluated and licensed in the industrialized world. Recent changes in thinking have challenged this view. It is now recognized that deferring trials in developing countries to this extent carries the unwanted consequence of significantly delaying the availability of vaccines to populations in developing countries. For example, polysaccharide-protein vaccines against Hib, which have been licensed for over a decade in the United States and other industrialized countries and have nearly eliminated invasive Hib disease in children in many of these settings, are used only to a limited extent today in the developing world [20]. This inequity in use of new-generation vaccines has elicited calls for parallel testing, rather than sequential testing, of new vaccines in industrialized- and developing-world populations. Parallel-testing of new vaccines in the industrialized and developing worlds is now being pursued for both experimental HIV and rotavirus vaccines [21, 22].

Another important trend affecting the testing of vaccines in developing-country populations is the emergence of highly qualified vaccine producers in the developing world, some capable of developing innovative new vaccines. Clearly, it is appropriate that the initial groups for testing of an experimental vaccine developed by such producers be selected from the population of the country in which the vaccine is developed.

Progression of phased studies

Conventional descriptions of phased trials often portray a seamless progression of trials from Phase I to Phase II, and from Phase II to Phase III. In reality, the vast majority of vaccine candidates that are tested in Phase I studies do not progress all the way through Phase III testing, because of disappointing findings or because of a lack of sufficient resources to support the increasingly expensive studies in successive phases [2]. While unwelcome findings at any stage may lead to termination of the clinical development of a vaccine, this need not always be the case. For example, the live-attenuated, oral cholera vaccine, CVD103-HgR, was shown to be safe and highly immunogenic when given as a single dose of 5×10^8 organisms in an extensive series of studies in North American volunteers. However, when the vaccine was subsequently tested in Thai adult volunteers, it proved erratically immunogenic [23]. To address this problem, the vaccine developer raised the dose by one log, to 5×10^9 organisms, and found the vaccine to be suitably immunogenic but still safe in a variety of settings in developing countries [9]. The CVD103-HgR experience illustrates that successful vaccine development may require detours in the phased sequence of clinical trials in order to accommodate necessary adjustments in vaccine dose, schedule, or even formulation in response to findings that emerge during the course of clinical studies. However, because vaccines that appear promising in developed countries not infrequently fail to perform as well in developing countries, and because such detours can greatly increase the expense of clinical development, completion of clinical testing of vaccines for developing countries may be exceptionally challenging.

Alternative endpoints for vaccine licensure

The conventional sequence of phases usually culminates in one or more Phase III trials that are designed to provide pivotal evidence on the clinical protection conferred by the vaccine against the targeted, naturally occurring, infectious disease. Sometimes, however, proof of clinical efficacy in a Phase III trial may not be necessary for licensure of a vaccine. For example, CVD103-HgR vaccine against cholera was licensed in Europe for use in travelers on the basis of Phase I-II studies, together with Phase IIb trials showing a high level of protection against experimental cholera in North American volunteers [24]. However, it is unlikely that Phase IIb evidence from industrialized countries will be taken as a basis for licensure of vaccines in developing countries, in part because of the discrepancies between vaccine performance in developed *versus* less-developed settings and in part because of the uncertainties about whether protection in Phase IIb studies predicts the performance of a vaccine in populations experiencing endemic disease.

In addition, if there is an accepted correlation between a certain immune response (e.g., a serological antibody titer) to vaccination and clinical protection, this immune response may sometimes be used as *prima facie* evidence for judging whether the vaccine is likely to be sufficiently protective to warrant licensure. For example, PRP-CRM$_{197}$ diptheria toxin and PRP-*Neisseria meningitidis* outer membrane protein (OMP) conjugate vaccines against Hib were licensed for infants on the basis of Phase III evidence of clinical protection against invasive Hib disease. Subsequently, PRP-tetanus toxoid conjugate vaccine was licensed for infants in the United States largely on the basis of proven safety and the attainment of protective serum antibody titers to PRP, without corresponding evidence of clinical protection from a Phase III trial [25, 26]. Serological endpoints are also commonly used as a basis for licensure of combination vaccines for which the component vaccines have already been licensed and seroresponse criteria for these components have been established [27].

Some vaccines of public health importance are directed to diseases that cannot be reliably predicted in populations at risk and that cannot be ethically studied in Phase IIb trials. Examples include vaccines against some bioterrorism agents such as anthrax and plague, and vaccines against certain epidemic diseases such as SARS and Ebola. In these situations, decisions about licensure will have to depend on pre-clinical data, demonstration of safety in humans, and assessments of immune responses in humans (even if such immune responses are not known with certainty to be correlated with clinical protection of humans against the target disease).

Good clinical practice

In recent years, considerable attention has been devoted to the ethics, scientific quality, conduct, documentation, and reporting of clinical trials. Several organizations have produced guidelines for these activities, which are subsumed under the rubric of "Good Clinical Practice (GCP)". Guidelines for GCP have been published by the World Health

Organization, the United States Food and Drug Administration, and the International Conference on Harmonization (ICH), among others [13]. Table 1 presents the essential elements of GCP in guidelines issued by the International Conference on Harmonization [28].

The promulgation of GCP has had several implications for vaccine trials in developing countries. Increasingly, the world of vaccines is becoming globalized. Vaccines targeted for a global market may be tested in developing countries to provide initial licensure. For example, a live oral human rotavirus vaccine developed by a major multinational vaccine producer has recently received its initial licensure in Mexico. Moreover, vaccines produced by manufacturers in developing countries are now being used throughout the world. Indeed, the majority of all doses of measles vaccines now administered to children in the world are produced in India.

With the trend toward globalization of vaccines, increasing emphasis has been placed on conducting clinical trials in developing countries in a manner that conforms to international GCP standards. While the benefits of GCP trials are unquestionable, rigid adherence to GCP standards can be a double-edged sword. The expense of clinical trials has risen rapidly in recent years [29]. A portion of this increased expense arises from the extensive documentation and auditing requirements demanded by regulatory agencies as a component of GCP, together with the expense of proprietary products developed to ensure compliance with regulatory requirements, such as proprietary computer software for data management and electronic reporting of trials. While this increased expense can be borne by producers anticipating major markets for their vaccines in affluent markets, it constitutes a disincentive to the clinical testing of vaccines against "orphan diseases" affecting developing countries, for which lucrative markets are not foreseen.

The ethical guidelines for clinical trials in developing countries have been the subject of recent controversy. The ethical principles of respect for persons, beneficence, and justice, which underlie modern clinical trials, are well accepted [30]. Nevertheless, several issues continue to be debated, of which three are touched on here [31–33]. One issue concerns the threshold for the risk/benefit ratio for a vaccine to be tested in developing countries. For example, a live oral, quadrivalent rhesus rotavirus-reassortant vaccine was licensed and then withdrawn from the United States market by its manufacturer because of an association between vaccination and the rare occurrence of intussusception [7, 8]. Understandably, this action had a chilling effect on the testing of this vaccine in developing countries. A meeting of experts organized by the World Health Organization acknowledged the rationale for the company's withdrawal of this vaccine in the United States, where rotavirus diarrhea is a cause of morbidity but not of significant mortality. Nevertheless, there was agreement among participants in the meeting that the burden of mortality of rotavirus in developing countries provided an ethical justification for continued evaluation of this vaccine in these settings [34].

Table 1. Principles of Good Clinical Practice (GCP). From [28]

1. Clinical trials should be conducted in accordance with the ethical principles that have their origin in the Declaration of Helsinki and that are consistent with GCP and the applicable regulatory requirement(s).
2. Before a trial is initiated, foreseeable risks and inconveniences should be weighed against the anticipated benefit for the individual trial subject and society. A trial should be initiated and continued only if the anticipated benefits justify the risks.
3. The rights, safety, and well-being of the trial subjects are the most important considerations and should prevail over interests of science and society.
4. The available nonclinical and clinical information on an investigational product should be adequate to support the proposed clinical trial.
5. Clinical trials should be scientifically sound and described in a clear, detailed protocol.
6. A trial should be conducted in compliance with the protocol that has received prior Institutional Review Board (IRB)-Independent Ethics Committee (IEC) approval-favorable opinion.
7. The medical care given to and medical decisions made on behalf of subjects should always be the responsibility of a qualified physician or when appropriate, a qualified dentist.
8. Each individual involved in conducting a trial should be qualified by education, training, and experience to perform his or her respective task(s).
9. Freely given informed consent should be obtained from every subject prior to clinical trial participation.
10. All clinical trial information should be recorded, handled, and stored in a way that allows its accurate reporting, interpretation, and verification.
11. The confidentiality of records that could identify subjects should be protected, respecting privacy and confidentiality rules in accordance with the applicable regulatory requirement(s).
12. Investigational products should be manufactured, handled, and stored in accordance with applicable good manufacturing practice (GMP). They should be used in accordance with the approved protocol.
13. Systems with procedures that assure the quality of every aspect of the trial should be implemented.

A second controversy over the ethics of trials in developing countries has focused on the use of placebos. As stated in the Declaration of Helsinki, "The benefits, risk, burdens, and effectiveness of a new method should be tested against the best current prophylactic, diagnostic, and therapeutic methods" [35]. There is agreement that a placebo would be inappropriate as a control agent for a trial if a locally licensed standard alternative vaccine exists; there is also general agreement that if such an alternative does not exist, it would be preferable to use for the control group an active vaccine against a different target infection, provided the active control does not cross-protect against the target pathogen and that use of the active vaccine maintains blinding in the trial [36]. However, it remains controversial whether a placebo can be ethically administered to the control groups in trials for which there is no suitable alternative active control vaccine and in which a licensed alternative vaccine against the target infection exists, but the alternative is not licensed in the country for the trial [37].

Yet a third controversy concerns what is owed to the participants at the conclusion of a vaccine trial. The Declaration of Helskinki states that: "At the conclusion of a study, every patient entered into the study should be assured of access to the best proven prophylactic, diagnostic, and therapeutic methods identified by the study" [35]. Few would disagree that if the vaccine tested in a trial is found to be beneficial, it should be provided to all participants in the trial. However, controversy surrounds the boundaries for the group of persons entitled to receive the investigational vaccine at the conclusion of the study – only participants in the trial, all persons living in the same region, or all persons living in the same country? And for how long are these beneficiaries entitled to receive the vaccine?

Increasing expectations for demonstration of vaccine safety before licensure

Because vaccines are administered in public health practice to healthy individuals, most commonly children, there is a higher expectation of safety for vaccines than for many therapeutic agents. In the past, pre-licensure Phase III trials were often designed merely to evaluate the safety profile of a vaccine observed in previous studies. Accordingly, the focus of such trials was on evaluating events that were expected on the basis of earlier studies, that occurred during an interval immediately following vaccination, and that were seen with appreciable frequency. Indeed, a common tactic in older Phase III vaccine trials was to evaluate adverse events only in a small subsample of the total trial population, obviating the possibility of detecting rare but potentially significant side-effects. Modern regulatory agencies now usually require that surveillance for adverse events be undertaken for the total study population rather than for a subsample, at least for events that can be detected passively (e.g., among persons presenting to health care centers for treatment), and that this surveillance be maintained for the duration of the trial.

Increasing concern about vaccine safety has also led to other changes in the design of Phase III trials. Formerly, calculation of sample sizes for such trials was usually geared to enable detection of a certain level of vaccine protection against the target illness, with an acceptable level of statistical power. Detection of rare side-effects was not a typical goal of such calculations. The recent experience with the live oral, quadrivalent rhesus rotavirus reassortant vaccine, which was withdrawn from the United States market because of an association with a small but statistically significant risk of intussusception [7, 8], has led to more stringent regulatory requirements for pre-licensure trials of newer-generation, live oral rotavirus vaccines. The United States Food and Drug Administration, for example, has required that these newer- generation vaccines be tested in numbers of infants sufficiently large to be able to detect whether intussusception is a vaccine side-effect. Current trials of these newer vaccines have therefore enrolled samples of infants many times the number enrolled in pre-licensure trials of the live oral, quadrivalent rhesus rotavirus reassortant vaccine, resulting in greatly increased clinical development costs. Whether the experience with rotavirus vaccines portends regulatory requirements for substantially larger Phase III trials for other new-generation vaccines remains to be seen.

The experience in the United States with the live oral, quadrivalent rhesus rotavirus reassortant vaccine illustrates yet another issue confronting pre-licensure trials. Data from pre-licensure trials of this vaccine showed a suggestive but non-significant elevation of the risk of intussusception [38]. The United States Food and Drug Administration licensed the vaccine with the proviso that the occurrence of this potential side-effect be scrupulously monitored post-licensure. This was possible because of the well-developed systems for post-licensure surveillance for vaccine side-effects established in the United States [39, 40]. Unfortunately, post-licensure surveillance systems capable of detecting and evaluating rare but serious vaccine adverse reactions are absent in most developing countries.

The weaknesses of post-licensure surveillance systems in developing countries place an even greater onus upon pre-licensure trials in these settings to provide reassurance that a vaccine will not cause rare but serious side-effects. However, the large size and great expense of trials capable of detecting rare side-effects present a major dilemma, especially for vaccines against diseases that are primarily limited to the developing world, for which resources for clinical trials are scarce. Clearly, there is an urgent need to develop improved systems of post-licensure surveillance capable of detecting rare but significant vaccine adverse reactions in developing countries.

Recently work has begun to evaluate the methodological challenges and practical feasibility of establishing large population-based, dynamic computerized databases for evaluating potential vaccine side-effects in developing-country settings. Such databases link vaccination histories to severe disease outcomes in defined cohorts, and have been used successfully in industrialized countries for rapid and credible evaluations of putative vaccine adverse reactions [40]. One such database has been successfully established on a pilot scale in Vietnam [41]. Overcoming the challenges of establishing such databases in the diverse settings of the developing world remains a significant but important research agenda.

Concluding remarks

The basic phases of testing of vaccine candidates are relatively straightforward and widely accepted. The successive phases of clinical evaluation of vaccine candidates allow for acquisition of critical information about vaccine safety, immunogenicity, excretion, transmission, and protection in an incremental fashion, while minimizing the risks to subjects who volunteer to participate in these studies.

In recent years we have seen a burgeoning of vaccine candidates against diseases of developing countries, creating breathtaking possibilities for disease prevention in these settings. At the same time, this profusion of vaccine candidates for the developing world has added a layer of complexity to the seemingly straightforward phased sequence of trials.

The factors underlying this complexity are multiple, and include considerations about when in the phased testing sequence a vaccine developed in an industrialized country should begin testing in developing countries; about whether and how to pursue the clinical development of a vaccine when disappointing clinical results are observed in developing countries; about how to meet the scientific, financial, logistical, and ethical challenges of conducting clinical trials in developing countries that conform to contemporary international standards of Good Clinical Practice; and about how to ensure that a vaccine is acceptably safe before and after licensure. The manner in which these issues are addressed in the future will have a great bearing on the success of efforts to accelerate the introduction of new-generation vaccines into programs for the poor in developing countries.

References

1 National Institute of Allergy and Infectious Diseases, National Institutes of Health (2002) *The Jordan report: Accelerated development of vaccines*. The Institute, Bethesda

2 Batson A, Glass S, Whitehead P (2004) Vaccine economics: from candidates to commercialized products in the developing world. In: MM Levine, J Kaper, R Rappouli, M Liu, M Good (eds): *New generation vaccines*. Marcel Dekker, Inc., New York, 57–74

3 Clemens J, Naficy A, Rao M, Koo H (2004) Long-term evaluation of vaccine protection:methodological issues for phase III and IV studies. In: MM Levine, J Kaper, R Rappouli, M Liu, M Good (eds): *New generation vaccines*. Marcel Dekker, Inc., New York, 29–48

4 Wilson GS (1967) *The hazards of immunization*. Athlone Press, London

5 Kapikian A, Mitchell RH, Chanock RM, Shevdoff RA, Stewart CE (1969) An epidemiological study of altered clinical reactivity to respiratory syncytial (RS) virus infection of children previously vaccinated with an RS virus vaccine. *Am J Epidemiol* 89: 422–434

6 Rauh LW, Schmitdt R (1965) Measles immunization with killed virus vaccine, serum antibody titers and experience with exposure to measles epidemic. *Am J Dis Child* 109: 232–237

7 Murphy TV, Gargiullo PM, Massoudi MS, Nelson DB, Jumaan AO, Okoro CA, Zanardi LR, Setia S, Fair E, Le Baron CW et al (2001) Intussusception among infants given an oral rotavirus vaccine. *N Engl J Med* 344: 564–572

8 Kramarz P, France EK, Destefano F, Black SB, Shinefield H, Ward JI, Chang

EJ, Chen RT, Shatin D, Hill J et al (2001) Population-based study of rotavirus vaccination and intussusception. *Pediatr Infect Dis* 20: 410–416

9 Levine MM, Kaper JB, Herrington D, Ketley J, Losonsky G, Tacket C, Tall B, Cryz S (1988) Safety, immunogenicity, and efficacy of recombinant live oral cholera vaccines, CVD 103 and CVD 103-HgR. *Lancet* 332: 467–470

10 Simanjuntak C, O'Hanley P, Punjabi N, Noriega F, Pazzaglia G, Dykstra P, Kay B, Suharyono, Budiarsno A, Rifai A et al (1993) The safety, immunogenicity, and transmissibility of single-dose live oral cholera vaccine CVD 103-HgR in 25-59 month old Indonesian children. *J Infect Dis* 168: 1169–1176

11 Miller FG, Grady C (2001) The ethical challenge of infection-inducing challenge experiments. *Clin Infect Dis* 33: 1028–1033

12 Rosenbaurm J, Sepkowitz K (2002) Infectious disease experimentation involving human volunteers. *Clin Infect Dis* 34: 963–971

13 Tacket, Kotloff K, Rennels M (2004) Initial clinical evaluation of new vaccine candidates: investigators' perspective of phase I and phase II clinical trials of safety, immunogenicity, and preliminary efficacy. In: MM Levine, J Kaper, R Rappouli, M Liu, M Good (eds): *New generation vaccines*. New York: Marcel Dekker, Inc., New York, 19–28

14 Clemens J, Brenner R, Rao M, Tafari N, Lowe C (1996) Evaluating new vaccines for developing countries: efficacy or effectiveness? *J Am Med Assoc* 275: 390–397

15 Kallings L, Olin P, Storsaeter J (1988) Protective effect of two acellular pertussis vaccines in a double-blind, placebo-controlled trial. *Lakartidningen* 85: 1994–1996

16 Patriarca P, Wright PF, John TJ (1991) Factors affecting the immunogenicity of oral polio vaccine in developing countries: a review. *Rev Infect Dis* 13: 926–939

17 Hanlon P (1987) Trial of an attenuated bovine rotavirus vaccine (RIT4237) in Gambian infants. *Lancet* 1: 1342–1345

18 Ward J, Brenneman G, Letson G, Heyward W (1990) Limited efficacy of a Haemophilus influenzae type b conjugate vaccine in Alaskan Native infants. The Alaska *H. influenzae* Vaccine Study Group. *N Engl J Med* 323: 1393–1401

19 Richie EE, Punjabi NH, Sidharta YY, Peetosutan KK, Sukandar MM, Wasserman SS, Lesmana MM, Wangsasaputra FF, Pandam SS, Levine MM et al (2000) Efficacy of a single dose of live oral cholera vaccine CVD 103-HgR in North Jakarta, Indonesia, a cholera-endemicarea. *Vaccine* 18: 2399–2410

20 Watt J, Levine O, Santosham M (2003) Global reduction of Hib disease: what are the next steps? *J Pediatr* 143 (6 Suppl): S163–S187

21 Abram IS (1995) Designing HIV vaccines for developing countries. Harv AIDS Rev Fall: 17–19

22 Glass R, Bresee J, Parashar U, Jiang B, Gentsch J (2004) The future of rotavirus vaccines: a major setback leads to new opportunities. *Lancet* 363: 1547–1550

23 Su-Arehawaratana P, Singharaj P, Taylor D, Hoge C, Trofa A, Kuvanont K, Migasena S, Pitisuttitham P, Lim YL, Losonsky G et al (1992) Safety and immunogenicity of different immunization regimens of CVD 103-HgR live oral choleravaccine in soldiers and civilians in Thailand. *J Infect Dis* 165: 1042–1048

24 Tacket CO, Cohen MB, Wasserman SS, Losonsky G, Livio S, Kotloff K, Edelman R, Kaper JB, Cryz SJ, Giannella RA et al (1999) Randomized, double-blind, placebo-controlled, multicentered trial of the efficacy of a single dose of live oral cholera vaccine CVD 103-Hg-R in preventing cholera following challenge with Vibrio cholerae 01 El Tor Inaba three months after vaccination. *Infect Immun* 67: 6341–6345

25 Santosham M, Wolff M, Reid R, Hohenboken M, Bateman M, Goepp J, Cortese M, Sack D, Hill J, Newcomer W et al (1991) The efficacy in Navajo infants of a conjugate vaccine consisting of *Haemophilus influenzae* type b polysaccharide and *Neisseriae meningitidis* outer-membrane protein complex. *N Engl J Med* 324: 1767–1772

26 Black S, Shinefield H, Fireman B, Hiatt R, Polen M, Vittinghoff (1991) Efficacy in infancy of oligosaccharide conjugate Haemophilus influenzae type b (HibOC) vaccine in a United States population of 61,080 children. The Northern California Kaiser Permanente Vaccine Study Center Pediatrics Group. *Pediatr Infect Dis J* 10: 97–104

27 Goldenthal K, Falk LA, Ball L, Geber A (2001) Prelicensure evaluation of combination vaccines. *Clin Infect Dis* 33 (Suppl 4): S267–S273

28 International Conference on Harmonisation Expert Working Group (1996) International Conference on Harmonisation Guideline for Good Clinical Practice. E6. The Conference, Geneva

29 Greco M (2001) The future of vaccines: an industrial perspective. *Vaccine* 20 (Suppl 1): S101–S103

30 The National Commission for the Protection of Human Subjects of Biomedical and Behavioral Research (1979) *The Belmont report: ethical principles and guidelines for the protection of human subjects of research*. The Commission, Bethesda, 1–8

31 Angel M (1997) The ethics of clinical research in the Third World. *N Engl J Med* 337: 847–849

32 Shapiro HT, Meslin EM (2001) Ethical issues in the design and conduct of clinical trials in developing countries. *N Engl J Med* 345: 139–142

33 Varmus H, Satcher D (1997) Ethical complexities of conducting research in developing countries. *N Engl J Med* 337: 1003–1005

34 Weijer C (2000) The future of research into rotavirus vaccine. *Br Med J* 321: 525–526

35 World Medical Association (2002) Declaration of Helsinki: Ethical Principles for Medical Research Involving Human Subjects. The Association. Available from: URL: http://www.wma.net/e/policy/b3.htm

36 Joint United Nations Programme on HIV/AIDS (2000) Ethical considerations in HIV preventive vaccine research. UNAIDS, Geneva

37 World Medical Association (2001) When are placebo-controlled trials ethically acceptable? (Press Release: November 28, 2001) Available from: URL: http://www.wma.net/e/press/2001_1.htm

38 Clemens J, Keckich N, Naficy A, Rao M (1999) Public health considerations for

the introduction of new vaccines against rotavirus: a case study of the rhesus rotavirus-reassortant vaccine. *Epi Rev* 21: 24–42

39 Chen RT, Rastogi SC, Mullen JR, Hayes SW, Cochi SL, Donlon JA, Wassilak SG (1994) The Vaccine Adverse Event Reporting System (VAERS). *Vaccine* 12: 542–550

40 Chen RT, Glasser JW, Rhodes PH, Davis RL, Barlow WE, Thompson RS, Mullooly JP, Black SB, Shinefield HR, Vadheim CM et al (1997) Vaccine Safety Datalink project: a new tool for improving vaccine safety monitoring in the United States. *Pediatrics* 99: 765–773

41 Ali M, Canh DG, Clemens J, Park J-K, von Seidlein L, Thiem VD, Tho LH, Trach DD (2003) The vaccine data link in Nha Trang, Vietnam: a progress report on the implementation of a database to detect adverse events related to vaccinations. *Vaccine* 21: 1681–1686

The Grand Challenge for the Future
ed. by Stefan H.E. Kaufmann and Paul-Henri Lambert

Practical aspects of phase 3 vaccine trials in developing countries

Brian Greenwood

Department of Infectious and Tropical Diseases, London School of Hygiene and Tropical Medicine, Keppel St., London WC1E 7HT, UK

Introduction

Setting up and successfully conducting a large vaccine trial is a major undertaking in any circumstances. Additional problems arise when a trial is done in a poor country with limited resources, for it is no longer acceptable for clinical trials to be conducted in developing countries in any less rigorous a way than in more affluent societies. In this chapter, some of the practical issues that face those wishing to undertake a large vaccine trial in a developing country that meets the highest standards of Good Clinical Practice (GCP) are discussed. Some of these trials will be true phase 3 studies, that is to say a trial of a definitive product used in the target population for which it has been developed and which will contribute to licensure. However, many of the same issues apply to vaccine trials that are not strictly phase 3 studies as they involve a product that is already licensed or one for which licensure is not being sought.

Background studies

Before any phase 3 vaccine trial is contemplated, it is essential that the background epidemiology of the infection against which the vaccine is directed is documented carefully in the proposed study area. This is especially important in the case of infections such as malaria and schistosomiasis whose prevalence and epidemiological pattern can vary widely over short distances, even from village to village [1].

It is also essential that immunogenicity and safety data are obtained in the area where the phase 3 trial is to be undertaken, or in an epidemiologically similar one, and not just in the country where the vaccine has been developed, as substantial differences in vaccine responses may occur between communities [2]. Prior exposure to the organism in question or to related organisms, for example atypical mycobacteria in the case of a tuberculosis vaccine [3], may influence the vaccine's immunogenicity and safety.

Acquiring the background epidemiological and immunogenicity data necessary to undertake a phase 3 trial can take several years. An example of this is the programme of research on *Haemophilus influenzae* type b (Hib) infection in The Gambia (Fig. 1) which led to a successful phase 3 vaccine trial and to the introduction of this vaccine into routine use [4]. However, this process can be accelerated by the development of trial sites where a series of trials of related vaccines can be undertaken. Although epidemiological patterns can change over time, and this needs to be watched, evaluation of a second or third vaccine may progress much more rapidly than the first if the background epidemiology of the disease in question has been well documented and surveillance systems have been set in place.

Selection of the trial site

Selection of the site for a large phase 3 trial is often a complex process involving political, social and logistical as well as scientific considerations.

Scientific considerations

Although many factors play a role in deciding the site of a trial, an essential requirement is that the incidence of infection in the target age group is high enough for a trial of manageable size to be able to achieve its endpoint with sufficient statistical power. It is also important that the incidence of the infection is stable from year to year or known to vary in a predictable manner. Planning a trial in an area where the pattern of infection is highly unpredictable and subject to fluctuations from year to year is a risky strategy; a number of trials have come to grief when the incidence of infection fell below that predicted from studies carried out in previous years because of a drought or other climatic change.

Establishing the surveillance system needed to measure the impact of a vaccine in a developing country frequently requires provision of support to the routine curative and preventative health services. This may have an impact on the overall incidence of the infection that is the subject of the trial. For example, increasing the availability of an effective cure for malaria in the study area may result in a reduction in malaria transmission and a lower incidence of infection in the control group than had been predicted from initial epidemiological studies [5]. This possibility must be borne in mind when sample size calculations are being done. Although this indirect effect of a trial has the drawback that it may necessitate a larger sample size than had originally been envisaged, it has the major advantage of providing some benefit from participating in the trial to those in the control group.

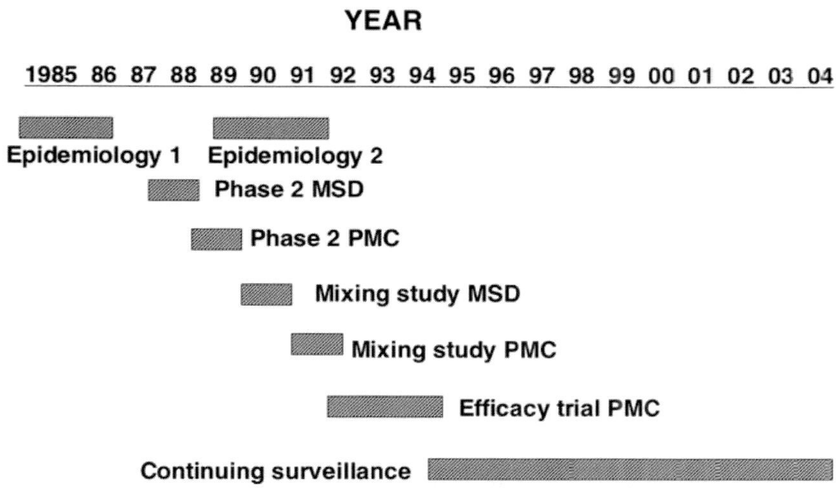

Figure 1. Time scale for a programme of Hib vaccine research in the Gambia (MSD = Merck, Sharpe & Dohme; PMC = Pasteur Merieux Connaught, now Sanofi Pasteur).

Political considerations

Large phase 3 trials are extremely demanding and difficult to accomplish in poorly-resourced countries in the best of circumstances. Thus, it is unwise to embark on a large trial in a politically unstable area, unless the objective of the trial is to investigate the impact of a particular intervention, for example measles or meningococcal vaccination, in a refugee or chronic emergency situation. Even when a politically stable site is chosen, some degree of risk remains because of the unpredictability of the political environment in many developing countries and this needs to be recognised by the sponsors. A risk-management strategy should be developed and kept up to date throughout the course of the trial.

Strong pressures may be applied by the Ministry of Health or regional health authorities to conduct a trial in a particular area for political reasons. For example, a particular health official may push for the trial to be conducted in his/her home area because of the improvements to the health services in that area that are likely to accrue and because of the job opportunities that the trial will create for those resident in his/her constituency. Provided that the area meets the scientific criteria needed to conduct the trial successfully, there are advantages in meeting requests of this kind as this is likely to guarantee a high level of political support once the trial is underway. However, problems can arise when there is a conflict between the scientific suitability of a particular site and the political imperative to conduct the trial there or when there is a change in political leadership during the course of the trial.

Political and administrative issues may influence the choice of a trial site at the local as well as at the national or regional level. Some communities operate cohesively, perhaps because of the presence of an especially able village head, whilst neighbouring ones do not. This is generally recognised although not openly discussed. Enquiries among local community workers, for example agricultural extension workers or local NGOs, may quickly identify communities that are unsuitable for inclusion in a complex trial because of poor leadership and internal dissension within the community. Failure to recognise this possibility may result in the vaccine trial becoming the basis for a struggle between different sections of the community, seriously compromising its chance of success.

Sociological considerations

Knowledge of the causes of a particular disease and the ways in which it can be prevented can vary widely from community to community over a small area because of ethnic group or religious differences. The attitudes of a community to intervention studies may be influenced markedly by the views of an individual traditional or religious leader. Collection of blood samples can be a particularly contentious issue, especially the collection of venous blood samples from small children. In some communities, the need for the collection of blood samples is well understood and accepted, whilst in others local beliefs about the consequences of blood collection, for example the view that blood is used to make medicines or sold overseas, may already be widespread or be fomented by an individual in the community who is antagonistic to the trial. Deeply entrenched views of this kind are difficult to change. It is often recognised locally that some communities are 'difficult' to work in, perhaps as a result of problems encountered in a previous research study. Such communities are best excluded from a complex trial.

Logistical considerations

Logistical factors that may influence the choice of trial site are summarised in Box 1.

Obtaining approval for the trial

A complex set of approvals is likely to be required before a large phase 3 vaccine trial can be started. This process can take many months so it is essential that it is started as soon as the trial site and study protocol have been defined. In the case of a large and complex trial, obtaining regulatory

Box 1. Practical issues that may influence the choice of trial site

1. *Access to the research centre.* Transport can account for a substantial part of the budget of a large field trial and vehicle maintenance is often a problem. Thus, whenever possible, the trial should be conducted in communities which are easily accessible by road to the centre where laboratory tests and data entry will be done.
2. *Access to an international airport.* If it is known that samples will require shipment out of the country on a regular basis, easy access to an international air-port is a bonus. This will also be appreciated by the many overseas visitors, such as trial monitors, that a large trial is likely to attract.
3. *Communications.* Mobile phones are becoming an increasingly important component of field work but areas of effective coverage are distributed patchily in many developing countries. An ability to communicate regularly with field staff and peripheral sites using mobile phones may add to the attraction of a particular site.
4. *Health care.* Participants in a trial must be provided with health care that achieves the highest standards prevailing in the country where the trial is being conducted. This may be difficult to achieve if the trial is conducted in a remote area with few health facilities. Access to health care, for example to a functional district or mission hospital, may influence the choice of study site.

and other approvals may warrant the employment of a project manager. Several types of approval are likely to be required.

1. *Approval by the regulatory authorities.* Regulatory issues are discussed in detail in the chapter by F. Verdier. If the trial is being conducted with an unlicensed product manufactured in an industrialised country, then the trial will require approval by the regulatory authorities of the country of manufacture. This will usually be accepted by the authorities of developing countries that do not have their own regulatory authority but formal approval by the Ministry of Health will usually be required. In countries that do have a regulatory body, local approval as well as approval in the country of manufacture will be needed.
2. *Ethical approval.* Ethical issues related to trials in developing countries are considered in the chapter by V.L. Tallo and H.M. Nohynek. Before a phase 3 trial can start in a developing country, approval of the relevant local ethical committee or committees is essential. In addition, if investigators from outside the country are involved, approval by their host institutions is likely to be required. Finally, if an international organisation such as WHO is participating in the trial, approval by an additional committee may be necessary. Investigators need to decide whether to submit the proposal to several committees simultaneously or to submit in sequence. The former can save time but difficulties may arise when different committees pick on different issues that each require changes to the protocol, necessitating a further round of distribution to all committees. It is generally sound practice to seek approval locally before progressing to committees outside the country where the trial will be undertaken.

3. *Research approval.* In some developing countries, all research sponsored from outside the country, whether involving interventions or not, requires approval from a central authority. This may require payment of a registration fee.

In addition to obtaining the scientific and ethical approvals required for the trial, it can be very helpful to develop formal memoranda of understanding between the partners involved in the trial, including the investigators, sponsors and local and national authorities. These should define the responsibilities of each partner in areas related directly to the conduct of the trial, but it may be helpful to include also topics such as the provision of routine clinical care for the study community during the course of the trial, training and the use of the assets acquired for the trial on its completion. Written agreements are essential as, during the course of a long trial, there may be replacement of the staff who made the initial agreements by others with different expectations.

Communication

Activities that ensure that all sections of the community understand why a trial is being undertaken, what participation will entail and the consequences of a successful outcome are always investments well made. People who need to be informed about a large phase 3 vaccine trial include central, regional and district health authorities, political and religious leaders and local health staff, community leaders, school-teachers and opinion leaders. Most importantly, efforts must be made to educate the whole community of the area covered by the trial about its objectives and not just those who will participate directly, as discussions within the community are likely to influence the willingness of families chosen to join the trial to participate. Obtaining community consent is a much more complex process than administration of information sheets to those who will be involved directly in the trial. Some of the approaches that have been used to gain community support are summarised in Box 2. Which of these activities will be most relevant for a particular trial will depend upon factors such as its size and profile but some activities, such as meetings with key opinion leaders, village meetings and the distribution of information sheets, are essential for all studies if good community participation is to be ensured.

It is generally wise to approach the dissemination process in a hierarchical manner beginning with the most senior health and political authorities before moving to village level activities.

Community meetings (Fig. 2) can be particularly helpful in ensuring that the reasons for a trial and its potential risks and benefits are properly understood, especially if the discussion can be guided by a skilled facilitator so as to provoke a debate among those attending the meeting. A trial

Box 2. Methods used to inform a community about a new vaccine trial

- Individual meetings with key political officials, religious leaders and educational and health officials in the district or region where the trial will be undertaken.
- Radio or television programmes and newspaper articles describing the background to the trial.
- Posters placed in health centres, schools and other key sites.
- Travelling singers or actors using songs or plays to describe the background to the study.
- Individual meetings with community and religious leaders at the study site.
- Presentations at schools in the study area.
- Village meetings in the study area.
- Distribution of information sheets in a comprehensible language to all households in the area where the trial will be done.

that involves a major pharmaceutical manufacturer may require, for legal reasons, lengthy information and consent forms which provide a detailed account of the procedure of the trial and its risks and benefits, but which may not be fully comprehended by the audience for which they are intended. Thus, many investigators conducting trials in developing countries now place as much emphasis on the activities listed in box 2 as a means of obtaining informed consent as on administration of the information and consent forms.

Development of the trial site

Once a trial site has been chosen, a number of activities needs to be undertaken before the trial can start. The amount of background work required will depend to some extent upon whether the site has been used previously for similar studies but it is likely to require a period of several months. Pre-trial activities that may be needed include the following:

1. *Undertaking an initial assessment of the relevant components of the local health services.* A joint assessment by members of the research team and local health services of the improvements in infrastructure, staff numbers and training that will be needed to implement the trial successfully should be carried out and agreement reached as to how the changes needed will be addressed and who will be responsible for bringing them about.
2. *Strengthening the EPI programme.* This is especially important if the trial vaccine is to be delivered through the routine EPI system. Areas likely to require support include the cold chain, transport to outreach vaccination centres and record-keeping. Although provision of extra staff for vaccination clinics and salary supplements for existing staff who undertake additional duties will improve the conduct of the trial, care is

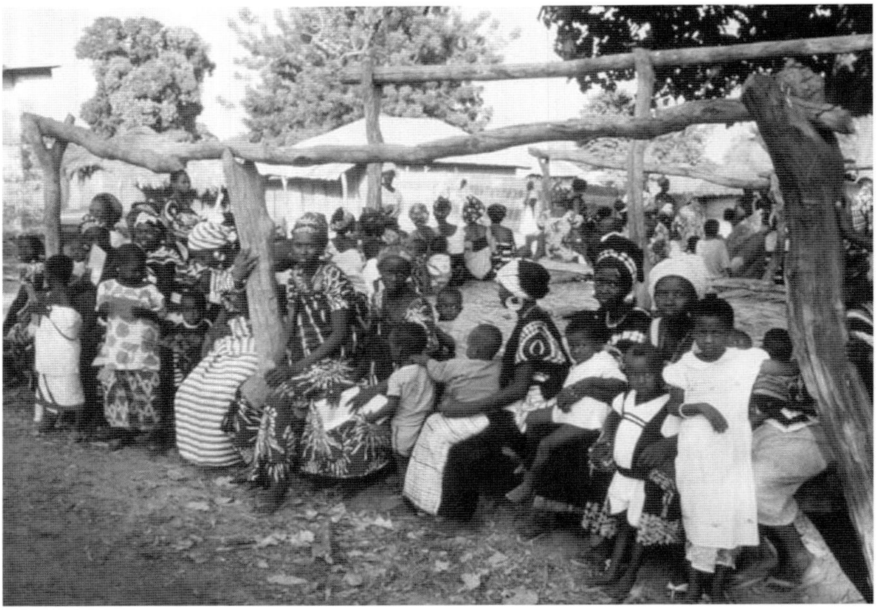

Figure 2. Communication through a village meeting.

needed not to establish a system that cannot be sustained after the trial is over (see below).

3. *Strengthening the routine health services.* This may be required for ethical as well as logistical reasons, as discussed in the chapter by V.L. Tallo and H.M. Nohynek. If hospital admission with a particular condition comprises a major trial end-point, then in-patient services may need to be up-graded and quality control procedures introduced. In the case of trials in which out-patient diagnosis at peripheral centres is an important study end-point, some infrastructure and staff support to peripheral health centres may be needed. Strengthening of both in-patient and out-patient services may be required to ensure that any adverse events resulting from vaccination are detected and documented properly. Laboratory assays that will be used in the trial must be validated and comply with the standards of Good Laboratory Practice (GLP).
4. *Conducting or updating a census.* If the trial is to be conducted in an area which already has a demographic surveillance system in place, the quality of the data being collected should be reviewed and any deficiencies addressed. However, if no census data are available, the investigators need to consider carefully whether it is necessary to conduct a full or partial census of the study area, perhaps concentrating on the target group of special interest. Sustaining a demographic surveillance system is expensive, about $1 per person per year, and demanding of staff, so

clear evidence that this will benefit the trial is needed before this investment is made.

5. *Establishing or improving an established data management system.* Careful consideration is required before the trial starts of the type of data processing system that will be used to support the study. Expert advice may be needed to ensure that an appropriate system is set in place or that an existing system is modified to meet the needs of the trial. Factors likely to influence these decisions are: previous experience of data management at the trial site, the infrastructure available for data management, ease of communication including linkage to the internet, the availability of staff with data management experience and, if needed, the ability to recruit senior staff to work on site. Some regulatory authorities have rules about the types of database that they will accept, so they may need to be consulted. Decisions that will need to be made include:
   - Whether to employ a Contract Research Organisation (CRO) to undertake all data management or to do this "in-house" using staff employed directly by the project. However, whichever route is taken, it is important that the opportunity provided by a large trial to contribute to local capacity development should be taken.
   - Where data entry will take place. There are advantages in undertaking data entry close to the trial site so that queries can be detected soon after data collection and remedial action taken. However, improvements in communication, which allow rapid transfer of large data sets, are making this less essential than was previously the case.
   - Whether to use a paper or an electronic system for the collection of data or a combination of the two with key entry on scanned documents. Electronic systems are likely to play an increasingly important role in large trials in the future although they are still not widely accepted by regulatory bodies.

   Whatever system is put in place, it is essential that all relevant members of the trial team are involved in establishing the system, understand how to use it and appreciate the need to collect high-quality data throughout the length of the trial. Standard operating procedures (SOPs) need to define clearly who has responsibility for following up queries and who has authority to make changes on paper forms or to the data base.
6. *Monitoring.* The investigators, acting in conjunction with the trial's sponsors, need to establish systems for monitoring the trial. A quality management plan is a useful tool for the principal investigator and should be developed early. The trial's sponsors will require monitoring of data collection and management procedures so as to comply with GCP. If the trial is sponsored by a pharmaceutical company, this may be done by staff from the company. Alternatively, staff from a CRO may be hired for this purpose. In addition, a number of independent investigators have been trained in GCP by WHO and other organisations and may be available to undertake the monitor's role.

It is likely that the sponsors and the investigators will wish the trial to be guided by an independent Data and Safety Monitoring Board (DSMB). The terms of reference for this group need to be established carefully before the trial starts; they are likely to include monitoring adverse events, conducting an interim analysis of the trial results when this is appropriate and making recommendations on the extension of the trial or its premature termination. When the majority of the members of a DSMB are based outside the country where the trial is being conducted and communications are difficult, it can be helpful to have a local safety monitor based at the trial site who can act on behalf of the DSMB and who can provide immediate advice to the investigators.

Training

Training is such an important pre-trial activity that it warrants separate discussion. The extent of training required for a particular trial will be influenced by whether the trial site has been used for a major intervention study before and whether a team of trained staff can be inherited for the new study. However, even if the latter is the case, a substantial degree of training may be required.

Who needs to be trained?

Training may be required for a wide range of staff including some or all of the following:
- Senior clinical staff involved in making measurements in study individuals,
- Health services staff who will be responsible for the routine medical care of subjects in the trial when they are ill,
- EPI staff involved in vaccine administration and documentation,
- Laboratory staff,
- Field staff involved in the follow-up of study subjects,
- Data entry clerks.

There may be substantial changes in staff during the course of a long trial so repetition of courses held before the trial starts may be needed as it progresses.

Training methods

The key to a successful training programme for a large vaccine trial is the development of a detailed set of SOPs that sets out clearly who is responsible for each component of the trial and exactly what they are required to do. SOPs are needed for activities such as the use of specialised equipment and transport as well as for the conduct of clinical and follow-up procedures. SOPs can be bound into an overall document that becomes the foundation for the trial and the basis for training sessions. This must be a flexible document that allows changes to established SOPs to be made and new SOPs to be developed as the trial progresses.

It is very important that staff at all levels are given an opportunity to contribute to the development of SOPs and questionnaires. This can usually be done best at workshops held before the trial starts. Workshops provide an opportunity for pilot testing of questionnaires, translation into relevant local languages and back translation. This is needed to ensure that comparable information is collected across the trial community which may include several linguistic groups. For example, finding the correct way to elicit a history of convulsions that is uniform across several language groups requires skill and may involve several iterations of the questionnaire.

Uniformity in the description of clinical findings

A trial may require detection of a clinical sign that contributes to an important trial end-point such as respiratory indrawing or pallor. When clinical observations are made by several investigators, it is important that they are consistent. Thus, an important pre-trial training activity can be clinical sessions aimed at reducing inter-observer variability in the detection of clinical signs and the interpretation of radiographs. An important recent development that has facilitated the conduct of trials that employ radiological signs of pneumonia as a trial end-point has been the generation of a consensus between experts on how to do this and production of a set of training films that are available on a CD [6]. Refresher courses may be needed to ensure that comparability in clinical observations between observers is sustained throughout the trial.

Good clinical practice and ethics

All phase 3 vaccine trials conducted in developing countries should follow the requirements of GCP as set out in the International Conference on Harmonisation (ICH) and similar guidelines (http://www.who.int/medicines/library/par/ggcp/GCPGuidePharmatrials.pdf). This may require specific training for various groups within the study team on issues such as record keeping, data management and good laboratory practice. Training in ethics may be required for senior staff and this is now available through various residential and on-line courses.

Safety

Safety of the staff conducting a trial is now seen to be as important as the safety of those participating in the study. This may require some specific training on issues such as the collection of blood and other biological samples and the safe use of project transport such as the need to use a crash helmet or seat belt.

Conduct of the trial

The first few months of a large trial are likely to make heavy demands on the study team which lessen as staff begin to work effectively together and become familiar with the SOPs for which they are responsible. However, in the case of a trial that lasts for several years, a new set of problems emerges as the trial progresses. Maintenance of the high standards set at the beginning of the study can be a particular problem. Some of the issues that may arise during the course of the trial are discussed in this section of the chapter.

Management

Management of a large vaccine trial is a complex process covering a wide range of activities including:

- Staff management. A large trial may employ several hundred people who need support on personal issues.
- Financial management. A large trial may have several donors so that managing its finances and financial reporting systems can be complicated.
- Management of a transport fleet. This may be large and demanding of resources.
- Maintenance of equipment.
- Dealing with emergency situations resulting from natural or man-made causes.

Although the host institution may have administrative staff who work in each of these areas, the demands of a large trial may be too large for them to cope effectively with the trial in addition to their other responsibilities, and the trial may need its own administrative team. Senior scientific staff should not be required to undertake all these functions.

Logistics

As the trial progresses, vehicles are likely to have accidents, vaccine refrigerators to break down and essential laboratory and x-ray equipment to expire under the strains of operating in an inhospitable environment. Maintaining the logistical support for a large phase 3 vaccine trial can make heavy demands on the study team. It is essential that when the initial budget for the trial is developed, provision is made for the replacement of vehicles and essential items of equipment during the course of the trial if this will take several years to complete – the life-time of a motorcycle used every day on bush roads is only two to three years. Inclusion in the initial budget of a contingency fund for unexpected equipment failures is wise if the donors will allow this.

Staff

Maintaining staff enthusiasm and morale during a long trial can be difficult for staff who may be required to collect the same kind of clinical or laboratory data over a prolonged period without any apparent outcome. This can tempt staff into taking short-cuts or even into inventing data. A number of approaches can be used to sustain staff morale in addition to those of good, general staff management. These include:

1. *Regular staff meetings*. Regular staff meetings for all categories of staff, at which problems arising during the conduct of the trial can be discussed, are essential.
2. *Refresher training courses*. Lessons learnt during workshops held at the beginning of the trial need to be re-inforced by follow-up workshops and discussion groups on topics relevant to the conduct of the trial.
3. *Staff awards*. Introduction of a competitive element in which staff are given awards based on performance during the past month can help to maintain enthusiasm among those required to collect or enter repetitive data.
4. *Changing staff roles*. It may be possible to alternate staff between different roles, for example between collection of questionnaires and data entry.
5. *Ancillary studies*. It may be possible to establish studies related to the main trial which provide an opportunity for team members to take a leading role.

However, regardless of how well staff have been looked after during the course of a long trial, as the end of the study approaches staff will seek new employment and the most able staff are likely to be the first to obtain a new position. This can make the last few months of a large trial difficult to manage. This problem is difficult to avoid unless the trial is conducted at an established site which has a core complement of trained staff on long-term contracts and where a series of trials can be planned to take place in a sequential manner.

Maintaining standards

The most important way of ensuring that standards are maintained throughout a trial is to ensure that its staff are well trained and well supported. However, regular evaluation of the performance of individual members of staff is essential to ensure the maintenance of standards. Some under-performers may benefit from additional training whilst, inevitably, some will need disciplining. Disciplinary procedures must be transparent and understood by everyone who joins the trial team.

In addition, some form of external control over standards may also be required. In the case of a study that is being undertaken to support licensure of a new product, it is likely that the pharmaceutical company that has developed the product will establish a detailed system of monitoring that involves regular visits to the site by a team of monitors. This should ensure that the quality of the record keeping and data entry is maintained throughout the trial and that it meets full GCP standards. However, some additional measures may be needed to ensure the accuracy of laboratory data. A quality assurance system should be established to ensure that the quality of laboratory observations is maintained and it may be possible to introduce other quality control procedures. For example, 10% of the x-rays collected during the course of the Gambian pneumococcal conjugate vaccine trial have been read by an independent panel and the results communicated to the two primary readers.

After the trial is over

On completion of a large and complex clinical trial, local staff are likely to move on to new studies and senior staff to take up new positions, perhaps in a different country. However, their responsibilities and those of the trial's sponsors do not end with the completion of the study. Some of the post-trial issues that must be addressed are considered in the final section of this chapter.

Communication of the results of the trial

A prime responsibility of the investigators is to ensure that the results of the trial are communicated to the community where the trial has been done, even when the results are disappointing. It is essential that the results of the study are presented first to the health authorities in the area where the trial has been done and to the trial participants, perhaps through a series of community meetings, before the results are disseminated internationally. Health officials are understandably annoyed if the first information that they receive on the outcome of an important trial conducted in their country comes from a report on the BBC's overseas service or from a poster at an international meeting.

Maintaining improvements established during the course of the trial

As discussed earlier in the chapter, it may be necessary to improve the routine health care delivery system in order to undertake a large vaccine trial in a country with limited resources. The investigators and their sponsors have an ethical responsibility to ensure that as many of these improvements as possible are sustained on completion of the study. This may not be easy to accomplish: for example, additional staff may have been employed to support clinical or immunisation services and their sudden withdrawal can be very disruptive. However, it may be possible to persuade the Ministry of Health to maintain support for some additional staff when it has been shown that their employment greatly increases the quality of care provided, for example provision of a laboratory assistant to read malaria blood films in an out-patient clinic. When withdrawal of additional staff cannot be avoided, this should be done in a phased and orderly manner that has been agreed previously with the health authorities. New and more efficient practices, such as the way in which children are managed in a vaccination clinic, may have been introduced during the course of the trial that can be sustained subsequently without added costs. Finally, vehicles and equipment may be bequeathed to the government health services on completion of the trial but these may be of little value unless funds can be found to support their maintenance and running costs. It is important that at the beginning of a trial, a plan for hand-over and maintenance of equipment purchased for the trial is developed and agreed.

Introduction of the new intervention

The most contentious issue likely to result from a successful trial in a developing country is the question of the introduction of the intervention if it has been found to be highly effective [7]. In a wealthy country, the national health authorities will usually take up fairly rapidly a new intervention that has been shown to be highly effective and cost-effective. However, this may not be the case in a developing country where there are many conflicting priorities for a limited health budget, even when it has been shown that the new intervention is cost-effective.

It is generally accepted that the investigators and the sponsors have a responsibility to those involved directly in the trial. For example, if a new vaccine is shown to be highly efficacious, a strong case can be made for offering it to those in the control group if they are still at risk. This has the disadvantage of making it impossible to determine the duration of the protective effect conferred by the vaccine but this approach will usually be required on ethical grounds. The information sheet and consent form provided to the trial participants at the beginning of the trial should set out clearly what is planned in this respect.

A more contentious issue is whether the investigators or their sponsors have any responsibility to provide the intervention to a wider group, for example the whole community where the study was done or even the whole region or country. Pressure on the company is likely to be particularly strong if the results of the trial have helped in the registration of a product that will be used widely outside the country where the trial was done and which is highly profitable to the manufacturer. However, if the company agrees to make a donation, how big should this be and for how long should vaccine be supplied? There are no easy answers to these questions and views on what is appropriate are evolving. However, it has become clear that the time to begin to address these issues is not after the trial is over but before it has begun.

Conclusion

The international community is at last paying appropriate attention to some of the major health problems of the developing word such as HIV, tuberculosis and malaria and funds for the control of these infections are becoming available on an unprecedented scale through organisations such as the Global Fund on AIDS, Tuberculosis and Malaria and the Global Alliance for Vaccines and Immunization (GAVI). Much can be done by implementing existing interventions but new tools, including vaccines, are needed if these infections are to be finally brought under control. Thus, there is likely to be a major expansion in the number of clinical trials conducted in developing countries in the next few years. Lessons learnt about the conduct of large vaccine trials in developing countries during the past few years, some of which have been discussed in this chapter, should help to ensure that these trials are conducted ethically and efficiently.

Acknowledgments

I thank Felicity Cutts, Amanda Leach, James Beard and Geoffrey Targett for their many helpful comments and suggestions.

References

1 Greenwood BM (1989) The microepidemiology of malaria and its importance to malaria control. *Trans R Soc Trop Med Hyg* 83 (Suppl): 595–598

2 Puumalainen T, Dagan R, Wuorimaa T, Zeta-Capeding R, Lucero M, Ollgren J, Käyhty H, Nohynek H (2003) Greater antibody responses to an eleven valent mixed carrier diphtheria- or tetanus- conjugated pneumococcal vaccine in Filipino than in Finnish or Israeli infants. *Pediatr Infect Dis J* 22:141–149

3 Fine P (1995) Variation in protection by BCG: implications of and for heterologous immunity. *Lancet* 346: 1339–1345

4 Mulholland K, Hilton S, Adegbola R, Usen S, Oparaugo A, Omosigho C, Weber M, Palmer A, Schneider G, Jobe K et al (1997) Randomised trial of *Haemophilus influenzae* type-b tetanus protein conjugate for prevention of pneumonia and meningitis in Gambian infants. *Lancet* 349: 1191–1197

5 D'Alessandro U, Leach A, Drakeley CJ, Bennett S, Olaleye BO, Fegan GW, Jawara M, Langerock P, George MO, Targett GA et al (1995) Efficacy trial of malaria vaccine SPf66 in Gambian infants. *Lancet* 346: 462–467

6 World Health Organization Pneumonia Vaccine Trial Investigators' Group (2001) Standardization of interpretation of chest radiographs for the diagnosis of pneumonia in children. World Health Organization, Geneva

7 Nuffield Council on Bioethics (2002) The ethics of research related to healthcare in developing countries. Nuffield Council on Bioethics, London

Vaccination programmes

The Grand Challenge for the Future
ed. by Stefan H.E. Kaufmann and Paul-Henri Lambert

Issues to be considered for the introduction of new vaccines into national vaccination programmes

Bjarne Bjorvatn

Centre for International Health, University of Bergen, Armauer Hansen Building, Haukeland University Hospital, N-5021 Bergen, Norway

Introduction

In 1974, the World Health Organization (WHO) recommended six vaccines for worldwide routine use within the Expanded Programme on Immunization (EPI), namely vaccines against tuberculosis (BCG), poliomyelitis (OPV), diphtheria-tetanus-pertussis (DTP) and measles[1]. In 1988, WHO recommended yellow fever (YF) vaccination of all infants in countries endemic for this disease and in 1992 hepatitis B (HepB) vaccine was added to the EPI list. In 1997, the scientific advisory group of the WHO global immunization programme endorsed use of the conjugated vaccine against *Haemophilus influenzae* type b (Hib), according to national capacities and priorities, in countries where Hib disease is recognized as a public health problem. Since 1998, the WHO policy concerning the use of novel vaccines has been published in the Weekly Epidemiological Record (http://www.who.int/wer).

Whereas the initial six vaccines cover approximately 80% of the annual global birth cohort, introduction of the vaccines against YF and HepB into the national immunization programmes (NIPs) has been relatively slow. As of August 2004, 33 of the 44 at-risk countries in Africa and Latin America have included the YF vaccine in their national programmes, but in many high-risk areas less than 50% of the young children were covered by this vaccination. Of the 214 countries and territories reporting to the WHO, about 160 had adopted infant vaccination against HepB. By 2003, the Hib vaccine had been introduced into the programmes of 88 of the 192 WHO member states, most of which belong to the industrialised world. Several other vaccines, such as the rubella, typhoid, and pneumococcal vaccines, are of documented public health value, but are clearly underused so far. It is therefore important to identify common hurdles to the introduction of new vaccines and to search for mechanisms that may facilitate world-wide acceptance of essential childhood immunization.

This chapter reviews some of the issues to be considered before appropriately licensed, new vaccines may be introduced into the NIPs. Some examples are added to illustrate issues that are characteristic of particular vaccines. Emphasis is on introducing new vaccines into NIPs of developing countries. It is realised, however, that also in developing countries considerable vaccination activities may occur outside the national programmes. In some major cities of the developing world as much as 25–45% of all vaccinations are carried out in the private sector [2]. Immunization in the private sector may therefore have considerable impact on the local epidemiology of the target diseases.

The decision-making process

Decisions to adopt new vaccines into a NIP are commonly based on assessments of disease burden, vaccine characteristics such as protective efficacy, safety and price, cost-effectiveness analyses, professional as well as public acceptance of the vaccine, as well as on programmatic and socio-economic considerations. Around the world, there are a number of organizational models for this decision process [3]. In most countries the Ministry of Health (MOH) appoints one or more advisory committee(s) whose mandate includes evaluation of new vaccines for the national programme. To avoid possible conflicts of interest, the professional and economic integrity of members of the advisory committees should be ensured and the decision process kept transparent. Suggestions for new vaccines may originate from experts within the MOH, the medical community (usually paediatricians), pressure groups such as concerned parents, international agencies such as the WHO and UNICEF, non-governmental organizations, or from the vaccine manufacturing industry. Occasionally, major outbreaks of vaccine-preventable diseases may prompt large-scale vaccination as a consequence of broad public demand. In most cases coinciding input from several different sources are at play.

Even when recommended by the advisory committee, the introduction of new vaccines may sometimes be delayed by opposition from the ministry of finance, the anti-vaccine lobby, and occasionally by the vaccine programme managers who may be already overwhelmed with the existing programme. Although inclusion of new vaccines into the NIP is ultimately a question of political will, at least in democratic settings, politicians are strongly influenced by public perception of the magnitude and urgency of the problem.

Disease burden

National records of disease incidences before and after introduction of large-scale immunization provide pertinent information on programme performance and effectiveness of the vaccine. Unfortunately, most developing countries lack the infrastructure required for comprehensive infectious disease surveillance. On the other hand, it may not be necessary that every country undertake full-scale epidemiological surveys before introducing a new vaccine. Where the actual disease is recognized as a major public health problem, surveillance from comparable epidemiological settings, possibly combined with limited national prevalence studies, may suffice to justify the introduction of documented safe and effective vaccines. In some situations, targeted serological surveys can provide the necessary information on the burden of the target disease. For example, screening of hepatitis B surface antigen (HBsAg) in representative segments of the population permits acceptable estimates of the burden of chronic hepatitis and hepatocellular cancer in the population at large. Similarly, serological surveys of rubella susceptibility in adolescents will allow qualified predictions of the number of children likely to be born with congenital rubella syndrome in the population concerned. In other situations, laboratory or clinical parameters suitable for disease-burden assessments may be very difficult to achieve. For example, in most cases of bacterial pneumonia the exact aetiology remains unknown. In the case of Hib, indirect aetiological evidence was obtained from trials comparing the total incidence of pneumonia among Hib vaccinated groups *versus* the control groups [4]. Similar indirect approaches are likely to work with other vaccine-preventable infectious agents. WHO has prepared rapid assessment tools for surveillance of several vaccine-preventable diseases [5].

Although scientific assessments of disease burden are mandatory for rational planning, the figures obtained are not necessarily representative of the disease burden as perceived by the population at large. For example, in the 1970–90s Norway experienced a protracted outbreak of meningococcal disease due to *Neisseria meningitides* type B. In 1983 the incidence peaked at 10 (in the northernmost region almost 20) per 100000 inhabitants. Children below 5 years of age and adolescents were most commonly affected and fulminant meningococcal septicaemia with high case-fatality rates occurred frequently. In this situation, the burden of meningococcal disease as perceived by the general public greatly exceeded the perceived burden of cancer in the same age groups, although their respective incidence rates were similar (statistics from the Norwegian Institute of Public Health and the Cancer Registry of Norway).

The vaccine

According to the WHO [6], new vaccines for large-scale public health use should

1) meet WHO's quality requirements;
2) be safe and have a significant impact on the actual disease in all target populations;

3) if intended for infants or young children, be easily adapted to schedules and timing of the national childhood immunization programmes;
4) not interfere significantly with the immune response to other vaccines given simultaneously;
5) be formulated to meet common technical limitations, e.g., in terms of refrigeration and storage capacity;
6) be appropriately priced for different markets.

Modern vaccines that are licensed internationally have been manufactured according to strict quality requirements and have proven to be safe. In most countries, a national regulatory authority (NRA) provides the local "license" for all locally manufactured or imported medical products, including vaccines. Vaccines that have been procured through UNICEF have all been pre-qualified according to standardized WHO procedures [7]. In addition to the efficacy and effectiveness profiles, the expected duration of protection is an essential parameter in the planning process. Also, the formulation, route and number of administrations and adaptability of the new vaccine to existing programmes are important factors to be considered as they affect public acceptance of the vaccine, the workload of the programme managers, and vaccine wastage [8]. Combination vaccines have the great advantage of providing several antigens in a single dose. This aspect becomes increasingly important with the growing number of vaccines that are offered in the NIPs. In addition to decreasing discomfort for children and parents and reducing the workload for programme officers, a reduced number of injections results in less needles and syringes and thereby reduced risk of transmitting blood-borne pathogens [9].

Vaccine efficacy and effectiveness

Vaccine efficacy is a measure of the protection obtained under the relatively ideal conditions of a clinical trial, whereas effectiveness measures the level of protection achieved in the real setting of a large-scale immunization programme. Effectiveness is negatively influenced by factors such as suboptimal transportation and storage, inadequate administration of the vaccine and by possible vaccine-induced replacement of preventable serotypes of the actual pathogen. In some cases, such as with the Hib vaccine, effectiveness may be positively influenced by herd immunity. The measured effectiveness is normally lower than the corresponding efficacy, but in well-functioning immunization programmes this difference may be relatively small. When optimally applied on their respective target groups, the best vaccines will reach protection rates of at least 90%.

No vaccines will be adopted into a national programme without evidence of high disease-preventing efficacy in the target population. Ideally, this type of information is obtained nationally through well-conducted clinical trials and in many countries a favourable outcome of national vaccine trials may be a prerequisite for adoption of new vaccines. However, where resources are limited or in emergency situations the decision to adopt a new vaccine may be based on experiences gained in comparable settings, for example in neighbouring countries. Naturally, trial results should always be interpreted cautiously, particularly when no comparable studies are available to confirm the findings. Different trials may arrive at dissimilar figures for protective efficacy simply because the period of observation or the outcome criteria are defined differently. Furthermore, differences in the definition of clinical disease or disease-specific mortality or in the inclusion and exclusion criteria may strongly influence the outcome of clinical studies. The problems of misclassification may be avoided using all-cause mortality rather than pathogen-specific mortality as the endpoint [10]. In trials applying serological correlates of protection, the diagnostic method and choice of cut-off values between positive and negative results are critical.

Despite comparable study design, there are many examples of vaccines that have worked well in one epidemiological setting, but less well in others. This may reflect ethnic differences in the study populations or differences in terms of average age, nutritional status or co-infections. Also local differences between prevailing microbial strains may play a role in some situations. For example, the 7-valent pneumococcal conjugate vaccine is based on the serotypes that most commonly cause invasive pneumococcal disease in western countries. This vaccine may provide no or limited protection against some important serotypes (e.g., types 1, 3, 5, 7) found in Asia and other parts of the world. In western countries the most feared manifestation of Hib is meningitis in young children, whereas in most developing countries its aetiological role in childhood pneumonia may be far more important. Obviously, the excellent results of Hib vaccination against meningitis in western countries do not necessarily imply similar success rates against pulmonary manifestations of the pathogen in other parts of the world.

Vaccine safety

Although safety issues are given top priority throughout the vaccine development process, no vaccine is absolutely free from adverse effects. To disclose possible rare complications, proper follow-up through post-licensure studies is mandatory. Where a dangerous, vaccine-preventable disease is prevalent, most people consider active immunization as an important life insurance. However, when the disease is under control, childhood immunization may appear less important and remote risks associated with vaccination rather than frequent complications of natural infection are emphasised. For example, in recent years fear of measles and oral polio vaccines rather than of measles and poliomyelitis has been reported by western media, although the risk of developing encephalitis or paralysis following immunization is about 1000-fold less than the corresponding risks accompanying the target diseases [11]. Also, in the 1970s unsubstantiated fear of serious adverse events caused by whole-cell pertussis vaccine (wP) contributed to falling vaccination coverage and resurgence of the disease in countries such as Sweden, England and Wales, and Japan [12]. Unfortunately, there are several examples of reduced compliance with immunization following scientifically poorly documented allegations of causal links between vaccination and serious adverse effects. Such examples include vaccination against measles, mumps and rubella (MMR) allegedly causing autism and inflammatory bowel disease and vaccination against hepatitis B allegedly causing multiple sclerosis. Also the inclusion of thiomersal and aluminium in some vaccines prompted major public concern, and resulted in reduced coverage of important vaccines in some countries. Although none of these allegations were supported by independent and thorough scientific analyses [13–15] public trust in immunization has suffered significantly, and it may take a long time to rebuild confidence.

In order to be pro-active, all countries should have access to a standing committee of independent, highly qualified experts who could look into cases of possible vaccine-related adverse events as soon as such concerns are brought up. Intra-regional collaboration in this area should be encouraged. It must be realised, however, that severe events due to programme failures are much more common than severe events caused by inherent properties of the vaccine, in particular where the programme infrastructure is poor [16]. Where a causal link to the vaccine is proven or likely and where no personal or programmatic failure is identified, mechanisms should be at hand to compensate the victims from public sources.

Vaccine price

When supplied by UNICEF, the 2004 price of the traditional EPI vaccines required for fully vaccinating an infant is approximately US$ 0.8. Adding HepB vaccine increases vaccine costs to US$ 1.6, and when also Hib vaccine is added the vaccine price increases to approximately US$ 10 per infant [5]. In NIPs personnel costs, supervision and management have traditionally accounted for the largest expenses and the vaccine itself for only about 5% of all costs [17]. Where the more expensive HepB and Hib vaccines are added to the programmes, the price of vaccines increases to 40% of the total costs of immunization and becomes the single most expensive component [18]. Although current regulatory requirements guarantee safe and efficacious products, the required manufacturing process has become very expensive. The current price per dose of the sophisticated 7-valent pneumococcal conjugate vaccine is 40–50 US dollars. Such vaccines are obviously not affordable for governments of most developing countries. The limited use of HepB vaccine in many endemic countries shows that it is economics, not the epidemiology, which dictates introduction of vaccines into national programmes [19].

Developing countries pay more than 80% of the total costs of their NIPs. Purchase of the EPI vaccines is commonly negotiated through UNICEF or other international organizations and mostly acquired from WHO-authorized manufacturers in developing countries. Also, WHO and UNICEF in collaboration with the pharmaceutical industry have launched a tiered pricing system whereby essential vaccines may be purchased at prices that are dependent on the gross national product (GNP). Countries with the lowest income *per capita* may receive up to 75–90% of the purchase costs through international funding. In recent years, several organizations, including the Global Alliance for Vaccines and Immunization (GAVI), sponsor the provision of vaccines for developing countries [20]. The support is for a limited period of time and may be gradually reduced. A well-functioning national programme is a prerequisite for international funding. It has been suggested that the minimum national contribution towards vaccine procurement should be 0.01% of the GNP. Where this percentage is insufficient to purchase the essential EPI vaccines, global funds should meet the shortfall [21]. It is essential that novel mechanisms of pricing and purchasing are fully utilized in order to speed up the introduction of new vaccines in the developing world.

Cost-effectiveness

Several methods are used to estimate whether investing in vaccines is worthwhile. Regardless of method, all estimates show that in developing as well as in developed countries, all EPI vaccines are highly cost-effective (cost per year of life gained is below national *per capita* GNP), and mostly cost-saving (ratio of benefits divided by costs >1.0). Also the recently introduced and technically more sophisticated vaccines are cost-effective in spite of their high prices [18]. Calculations of the cost-effectiveness of new vaccines are increasingly used as a tool to measure their value in economic terms and to establish priorities between vaccines [22]. Cost analyses should have both a short-term and long-term perspective, and include direct as well as indirect costs. Direct costs include the price of the vaccine, personnel costs, transportation and storage as well as the costs of possible adverse events following vaccination, whereas indirect costs may include loss of working hours when extra visits to vaccination centres are required [23]. A prediction of the *additional* costs associated with the inclusion of a new vaccine into a NIP may be obtained through consensus cost-estimates of each component of the existing vaccination programme, and extrapolation of the extra resources needed for the new vaccine component [24].

Similarly, both direct and indirect costs must be considered when calculating the economic impact of the target disease, such as hospital costs, costs caused by possible sequelae of the natural infection and, when applicable, wardens' absence from work during the disease. The savings achieved through vaccination include not only reduced societal costs due tò control or even elimination of the disease, but also reduced private spending on, for example, treatment. When possible, the cost-effectiveness of vaccination should be compared with the cost-effectiveness of other medical interventions, such as medication. This may help overcome the perception that vaccines must be cheap in order to be highly cost-effective, in particular as vaccines protect not only individuals and groups, but society at large [9].

Standardised tools of assessment facilitate comparison between different vaccines and allow a rational choice between different programme strategies. Mathematical modelling is increasingly used to compare the effects of different vaccination policies. The WHO has developed methodology and software to estimate programme costs [5]. Cost-effectiveness of immunization is often expressed in terms of DALYs, i.e., the cost of a disability-adjusted life-year gained through the intervention. For example, the cost per DALY gained by immunization in low-income countries was 12-17 US dollars. This cost should be compared to 200-350 US dollars per DALY saved through limited therapeutic care [25].

In spite of their usefulness, it should be remembered that cost-effectiveness analyses represent approximations only, the quality of which depends upon the correctness of the underlying data. Even with increasing quality of such data, fear, grief and physical suffering remain aspects of the disease burden that are hard to compare and to translate into economic terms.

Professional and popular acceptance

It is important that paediatricians, infectious disease specialists, vaccine programme managers and other concerned experts are well informed about an extension of the NIP before a large-scale information campaign is launched for the general public. In many countries official recommendations given by medical associations on the use of vaccines carry considerable weight and have become crucial elements of vaccine advocacy. The political impact of such expert recommendations increases considerably when adopted by non-professional pressure groups, such as non-governmental organizations or groups representing victims of vaccine-preventable diseases.

Social mobilization and positive publicity through mass media are key elements of successful introduction of new vaccines into the NIP also in developing countries. Considerable efforts should be made in advance to provide concise and balanced information to the general public. Adapting this information to local conditions and perceptions is decisive for national acceptance. In addition to presenting the facts concerning the target disease and data on vaccine efficacy and adverse events, one should emphasise the right of all children to be protected against vaccine-preventable diseases. Also, the importance of achieving high immunization coverage should be underlined. It is unwise to omit mentioning possible allegations concerning adverse effects, but independent scientific reasons for rejecting such claims must also be presented and explained carefully.

When science is played against emotion, science is likely to lose. The "anti-vaccine movement" is hardly an organization in the strict sense of the word, but rather a number of groups that for a variety of reasons argue against immunization, particularly when executed in early childhood. Some of these groups perceive immunization as "un-natural" as opposed to immunity following "natural" infection. Others advocate individual rights over the welfare of the community. Physicians recommending vaccination are sometimes perceived as promoting mainly the interests of the vaccine-manufacturing industry. Adverse effects of vaccines, alleged or real, may be used as arguments against the vaccination recommended by the medical establishment. Interestingly, the small risk of adverse events associated with vaccines appears less acceptable to the general public than the considerably higher risk associated with use of most therapeutic drugs. It is rather peculiar that the anti-vaccine movement seems to recruit most followers in countries where large-scale immunization programmes have been most successful. Unfortunately, anti-immunization attitudes are sometimes conveyed to worried parents by poorly informed members of the medical profession.

Psychologically, the concept of the single, courageous dissident fighting the medical establishment, or the desperate victim of adverse effects standing up against the powerful pharmaceutical industry has a natural public appeal. Therefore, both dissident and victim are likely to be presented very favourably by those mass media that have no ambition to provide documented facts. The immensely beneficial impact of immunization is easily lost from the headlines.

Programmatic issues

In spite of the overall success of the EPI programme, coverage is still low (40–50%) in many developing countries and in some areas vaccination coverage seems to be falling. Strong vaccination programmes with highly motivated and appropriately supported staff is a prerequisite for successful extension of the immunization services [26]. Before adding new vaccines to the NIP, there is a need to improve immunization services in communities where coverage of existing vaccines is low [27]. As a rough rule of thumb, no new vaccine should be included before coverage for the basic EPI vaccines has reached a sustainable level of at least 80%. Weak programmes are more likely to collapse than to gain strength when adding new vaccines, however important they may be. Besides, immunization against some diseases, for example rubella, may cause more harm than benefit when coverage is too low (see below).

The addition of a new vaccine to an existing NIP represents an extra burden on the programme managers, distribution lines and storage capacity. Hence, as part of the planning process the programme managers' current workload, motivation and training, as well as the financial sustainability and technical capacity of the programme, should be carefully assessed. In populations where the private sector is responsible for a considerable proportion of the total vaccination coverage, as may be the case in major cities also in the developing world, the epidemiological impact of private immunization activities should be analysed.

Age-specific background data on the disease burden will disclose at which age the concerned vaccine should be offered to maximise its preventive potential. On the other hand, new vaccines should be incorporated into existing schedules in such a way that extra visits to the vaccination centre are avoided. Most new vaccines can be easily administered simultaneously with the traditional EPI vaccines. Combined vaccines result in less injections and are in principle preferable where funds are available. Regional harmonization of immunization programmes and vaccination schedules will ultimately benefit both customers and service providers. Such harmonization could also stimulate improved coverage and thereby reduce dissemination of vaccine-preventable agents from areas with low vaccination coverage.

The recent "Vaccine Introduction Guidelines" from the WHO summarize pertinent programmatic issues related to the introduction of new vaccines [5].

Socio-economic and political issues

A number of political and socio-economic factors influence the rate at which developing countries incorporate new vaccines. The most important of these factors may be the appreciation of national governments and international agencies of the value of these vaccines [28]. However, unless political as well as economic commitment is ensured for continuous long-term immunization, the addition of a new vaccine into the national programme should not normally be considered [9]. Funding for NIPs will have to compete with other important public needs. Although vaccines are the most cost-efficient tool in the field of public health, it is often easier to raise money for curative than for prophylactic purposes.

In areas where a particular disease never existed as a public health problem, for example HepB in the Nordic countries, the cost-effectiveness of HepB immunization will be low. Hence, these countries have not yet followed the WHO recommendation to immunize all infants against HepB. Similarly, in many industrialised countries it may be hard to get public acceptance for continued vaccination against diseases that disappeared from the area many years ago, such as diphtheria, poliomyelitis and measles. It should be emphasised, however, that a high level of social acceptance of vaccines in rich countries is not only desirable in itself, but influences both the availability of vaccines in low-income countries and the industrial choices of new vaccines to be developed [29].

Vaccine-specific issues to be considered

Universal infant immunization against HepB and vaccination against YF in endemic countries are both part of existing WHO recommendations for NIPs. Several other vaccines may be of considerable public health value in countries where the respective diseases are prevalent. Examples of typical issues to be discussed when considering the inclusion of such vaccines in national programmes are summarized below.

Hepatitis B vaccine

Specific issues include: reaching the newborn within 24 hours also when delivered at home. Motivating long-term investments in health.

Infant vaccination against HepB will drastically reduce the incidence of chronic hepatitis, thereby preventing subsequent development of liver cirrhosis and hepatocellular cancer. Where perinatal transmission of HepB virus is common, for example in South-East Asia, the first of the three HepB vaccine doses should be given as soon as possible after birth, preferably within 24 hours, using monovalent vaccine. Vaccination at birth may be difficult to organize especially in areas where most deliveries take place at home. Furthermore, as the positive impact of immunization becomes apparent only decades later, it may be difficult for parents as well as health workers to fully realise the importance of this vaccine in infants [30].

Yellow fever

Specific issues include: improving YF surveillance and strengthening the infrastructure of NIPs in remote high-risk areas. Organization of immunization campaigns to avoid major outbreaks.

In African and South American countries where YF is prevalent, inclusion of the 17D vaccine into NIPs is strongly recommended. The vaccine is cost-effective, very safe and seems to induce life-long protection. Unfortunately, several high-endemic countries have not yet, or only incompletely, implemented routine childhood vaccination against YF, partly because cases tend to occur in remote areas where the infrastructure is weak. Improved surveillance is mandatory to identify all populations at risk of infection. In high-risk areas, infant immunization against YF should aim at ≥80% coverage and in addition, mass vaccination campaigns should be organized to prevent devastating outbreaks in non-immunized segments of the population [31].

Measles vaccine

Specific issues include: achieving at least 80 % coverage in every district and subpopulation. Coping with anti-vaccine activists and allegations concerning vaccine safety.

Live, attenuated measles vaccines are very safe and effective and relatively inexpensive. Combinations of measles vaccine with rubella (MR), or rubella and mumps vaccines (MMR) are equally immunogenic, but more expensive than measles vaccine alone. The cornerstones of the WHO/UNICEF strategic plan for measles mortality reduction are improved surveillance and – to account for the extremely contagious nature of measles – global vaccination coverage of at least 80% even in remote districts. A challenge for the NIPs is to convey the scientific evidence of the safety of measles vaccine in view of the widely published allegations of vaccine-associated autism and inflammatory bowel disease [32].

Rubella vaccine

Specific issues include: achieving at least 70-80 % vaccination coverage in order to avoid an increase rather than a decrease in the burden of congenital rubella syndrome (CRS). Reaching the majority of adolescent girls and young women with rubella vaccine. Co-ordination of public and private sector immunization.

Rubella infection in early pregnancy may result in foetal lesions termed the CRS. Prevention of CRS is the rationale for large-scale vaccination against this otherwise relatively mild childhood disease. Where rubella is highly endemic, most females contract the infection before childbearing age and vaccination may not be indicated. On the other hand, rubella vaccination is recommended in countries of low or medium endemicity where a proportion of females of childbearing age remain susceptible to the infection. To ensure sufficiently high vaccination coverage and reduce the number of injections, large-scale immunization against rubella should be offered only as a combined MR (or MMR) vaccination, and only where coverage is likely to reach at least 80%. Paradoxically, partial vaccination coverage (<70%) may increase rather than decrease the CRS burden. This situation could occur in, for example, large cities with extensive private sector rubella vaccination, but no rubella vaccination as part of the NIP. It is therefore essential that where childhood rubella vaccination is initiated, coverage should be high and sustainable. To avoid a temporal increase in the rate of CRS following initiation of childhood immunization, all adolescent girls and women of childbearing age should be offered rubella vaccination for the 12–15 years it takes to close the "susceptibility gap" [33].

Pneumococcal vaccine

Specific issues include: establishing the burden of pneumococcal disease and sub-type profiles in developing countries. Encouraging large-scale manufacturing of conjugate vaccines with optimal sub-type profiles for children in the developing world. Stimulating political will and long-term funding commitment to pneumococcal vaccination in developing countries.

Invasive pneumococcal disease in infants and young children belongs to the most important public health problems in developing countries. However, in many areas the exact burden of the disease as well as the most important pneumococcal serotypes involved are poorly defined. The traditional 23-valent polysaccharide vaccine is unreliable in children less than 2 years of age, whereas the new conjugate vaccines induce protection also in infants. The currently available 7-valent conjugate vaccine is mainly designed for western markets, whereas the 9–11-valent vaccines that are now under evaluation include more serotypes that are relevant also in developing countries. Unfortunately, the vaccine price increases with increasing number of serotypes. In developing countries pneumococcal conjugate vaccine will be available only where there is strong political will to invest in health and where the vaccine price can be brought down through long-term, large-scale delivery agreements between manufacturers, the governments concerned and international sponsors [34].

Rotavirus vaccine

Specific issues include: leadership in international public health. Funding of essential vaccines for developing countries. Co-ordinated action from the MOHs of developing countries to secure threatened, essential vaccines for their NIPs.

Rotaviruses are the most common cause of severe diarrhoeal disease in infants and young children worldwide and are an important cause of infant death in developing countries. In 1998, a tetravalent rotavirus vaccine (RRV-TV) was licensed in the United States. The vaccine provided 70% protection against all rotavirus diarrhoea and >90% protection against severe rotavirus disease in young children. Initially, the RRV-TV vaccine appeared to be practically free from serious adverse effects. However, following immunization of about one million US children, vaccine-associated infantile intussusception was reported at a (consensus) frequency of about one per 10000 vaccinees. For this reason, the rotavirus vaccine was withdrawn from the US market. The vaccine has not been further tested since then, and is not licensed in other parts of the world. Unfortunately, the RRV-TV vaccine had undergone limited testing in developing countries prior to its licensure in the United States. A few trials in South America showed that the vaccine worked very well in some settings, less so in others. Although other rotavirus vaccines have been developed in China and recently also in Europe (licenced in Mexico), these vaccines are still unavailable in most development countries.

The underlying problems here are of medical, economic and moral nature. Should very rare, but potentially life-threatening adverse events that make the vaccine unacceptable in the western world prevent an otherwise excellent vaccine from further trials and possible use in developing countries? The answer to this question is likely to be no. Without disregarding the inherent problems, this vaccine should have been adopted by relevant international agencies and submitted to further carefully conducted trials in different parts of the developing world in close collaboration with the manufacturer and interested countries [35, 36].

A successful case: Hib vaccination in Latin America

The most important manifestations of Hib infections, namely meningitis and pneumonia, occur in children under 5 years of age, mainly in infants. The novel conjugate Hib vaccine has been shown to be very safe and in most cases highly efficient even in children below 12 months of age. Besides, through reduction of nasopharyngeal carriage, the vaccine shows considerable herd effect. In spite of limited epidemiological information from large areas of Asia and Africa, WHO considers diseases caused by Hib to be sufficiently important to warrant inclusion of this vaccine in NIPs all over the world. Hib vaccine was adopted by many industrialised countries already in the early 1990s, for example in the United States in 1990 and in Canada in 1991. However, due to mainly financial constraints, this very successful vaccine has not yet been adopted by the majority of developing countries.

The first states in Latin America to include Hib vaccine into their NIPs were Uruguay in 1994 and Chile in 1996. As a consequence, the incidence of diseases due to Hib dropped dramatically in both countries. In 1997 the Pan American Health Organization (PAHO) recommended the inclusion of Hib vaccine in the regular immunization programmes of all member states and to establish surveillance systems to monitor Hib illness and its consequences. It was also decided to use the PAHO Revolving Fund for joint purchases of vaccines. This contributed to considerable price reductions, allowing even low-income countries in the region to adopt the Hib vaccine. By the year 2000 more than 90% of the birth cohort in the Americas had been vaccinated or had Hib included in their vaccination schedule. Furthermore, a number of the Latin American states had introduced the combined Hib-HepB vaccine, thereby adding two essential vaccines to their programmes at the same time.

The Americas were the first to eliminate polio. The governments in this region have once again shown a high level of political and financial commitment to immunization and again they have been very successful [37, 38].

References

1 Henderson RH (1995) Vaccination: Successes and challenges. In FT Cutts, PG Smith (eds): *Vaccination and world health*. John Wiley & Sons, Chichester, 3–16

2 Atkinson S, Cheyne J (1994) Immunization in urban areas: Issues and strategies. *Bull World Health Organ* 72: 83–94

3 Wenger JD, DiFabio J, Landaverde JM, Levine OS, Gaafar T (1999) Introduction of Hib conjugate vaccines in the non-industrialized world: experience in four "newly adopting" countries. *Vaccine* 18: 736–742

4 Mulholland K, Hilton S, Adegbola R, Usen S, Oparaugo A, Omosigho C, Weber M, Palmer A, Schneider G, Jobe K et al (1997) Randomised trial of *Haemophilus influenzae* type b-tetanus protein conjugate for prevention of pneumonia and meningitis in Gambian infants. *Lancet* 349: 1191–1197

5 World health Organization (2004) Vaccine Introduction Guidelines (WHO/V&B/04/00) Geneva, WHO, 2004. Available at http://www.who.int/vaccines-documents/DocsPDF04/www000.pdf

6 World Health Organization. Document WHO/VSQ/GEN/96.02 available from the VAB documentation centre, WHO, 1211 Geneva, Switzerland

7 World Health Organization (2002) Procedure for assessing the acceptability, in principle, of vaccines for purchase by United Nations agencies (WHO/V&B/02.08) Geneva, WHO, 2002. Available at http://www.who.int/vaccines-documents/DocsPDF02/www675.pdf

8 Mulholland EK, Bjorvatn B (2003) Introduction of new vaccines in the health care system. In: BR Bloom, P-H Lambert (eds): *The vaccine book*. Academic Press, San Diego and London, 391–410

9 Di Fabio JL, de Quadros C (2001) Considerations for combination vaccine development and use in the developing world. *Clin Infect Dis* 33 (Suppl 4): S340–S345

10 Jaffar S, Leach A, Smith PG, Cutts F, Greenwood B (2003) Effects of misclassification of causes of death on the power of a trial to assess the efficacy of a pneumococcal conjugate vaccine in The Gambia. *Int J Epid* 32: 430–436

11 Halsey NA (2003) Vaccine safety: real and perceived issues. In: BR Bloom, P-H Lambert (eds): *The vaccine book*. Academic Press, San Diego and London, 371–389

12 Gangarosa EJ, Galazka AM, Wolfe CR, Phillips LM, Gangarosa RE, Miller E,

Chen RT (1998) Impact of anti-vaccine movements on pertussis control: the untold story. *Lancet* 351: 356–361

13 Institute of Medicine (1994) Adverse events associated with childhood vaccines: Evidence bearing on causality. National Academy Press, Washington, DC

14 Confavreux C, Suissa S, Saddier P, Bourdes V, Vukusic S (2001) Vaccinations and the risk of relapse in multiple sclerosis. Vaccines in Multiple Sclerosis Study Group. *N Engl J Med* 344: 319–326

15 Ball LK, Ball R, Pratt RD (2001) An assessment of thimerosal use in childhood vaccines. *Pediatrics* 107: 1147–1154

16 Cutts FT, Olivé J-M (1999) Vaccination programs in developing countries. In: SA Plotkin, WA Orenstein (eds): *Vaccines* (3d ed). Saunders, Harcourt, Philadelphia, 1047–1073

17 Creese A, Sriyabbaya N, Casabal G, Wiseso G (1982) Cost-effectiveness appraisal of immunization programmes. *Bull World Health Organ* 60: 621–632

18 Hinman AR (1999) Economic aspects of vaccines and immunizations. *C R Acad Sci III* 322: 989–994

19 Batson A (1998) Sustainable introduction of affordable vaccines: the targeting strategy. *Vaccine* 16 (Suppl): S93–S98

20 Global Alliance for Vaccines and Immunization. Immunization financing options – A resource for policy makers. Available at http://www.gaviftf.org/docs_activities/briefcase/briefcase_ web.pdf

21 Mahoney RT, Ramachandran S, Xu Z (2000) The introduction of new vaccines into developing countries II. Vaccine financing. *Vaccine* 18: 2625–2635

22 Clemens J, Brennen R, Rao M, Tafari N, Lowe C (1996) Evaluating new vaccines for developing countries. Efficacy or effectiveness? *JAMA* 275: 390–397

23 Trotter CL, Edmunds WJ (2002) Modelling cost effectiveness of meningococcal serogroup C conjugate vaccination campaign in England and Wales. *BMJ* 324: 809–812

24 Edmunds WJ, Dejene A, Mekonnen Y, Haile M, Alemnu W, Nokes DJ (2000) The cost of integrating hepatitis B virus vaccine into national immunization programmes: a case study from Addis Ababa. *Health Policy Planning* 15: 408–416

25 World Bank (1993) World Development Report 1993. *Investing in Health*. Oxford University Press, Oxford, 1–329

26 Streefland PH (2003) Introduction of a HIV vaccine in developing countries. Social and cultural dimensions. *Vaccine* 21: 1304–1309

27 Suresh K, Saxema D (2000) Trends and determinants of immunization coverage in India. *J Ind Med Assoc* 98: 10–14

28 Hausdorff WP (1996) Prospects of the use of new vaccines in developing countries: cost is not the only impediment. *Vaccine* 14: 1179–1186

29 Balinska MA (2003) Vaccination in tomorrow's society. *Lancet Infect Dis* 3: 443–447

30 World Health Organization (2004) Hepatitis B vaccine. WHO position paper. *Weekly Epidemiol Record* 79: 255–263

31 World Health Organization (2003) Yellow fever vaccine. WHO position paper. *Weekly Epidemiol Record* 78: 349–359
32 World Health Organization (2004) Measles vaccine. WHO position paper. *Weekly Epidemiol Record* 79: 130–142
33 World Health Organization (2000) Rubella vaccine. WHO position paper. *Weekly Epidemiol Record* 75: 161–169
34 World Health Organization (2003) Pneumococcal vaccines. WHO position paper. *Weekly Epidemiol Record* 78: 110–119
35 World Health Organization (1999) Rotavirus vaccines. WHO position paper. *Weekly Epidemiol Record* 74: 33–40
36 World Health Organization (2003) Rotavirus vaccines, an update. *Weekly Epidemiol Record* 78: 2–3
37 World Health Organization (1998) *Haemophilus influenzae* type b conjugate vaccine. WHO Position paper. *Weekly Epidemiol Record* 73, 64–71
38 Anonymous (1999) Introduction of Hib vaccines in the Americas: lessons learned. *EPI Newsletter* 21: 4–5

Index

The BAID-Series
Birkhäuser Advances in Infectious Diseases

Homepage: http://www.birkhauser.ch

Infectious diseases remain a substantial drain on human well-being and economies despite the availability of modern drugs. New pathogens emerge and known pathogens change their geographical distribution and their susceptibility to the available drugs. An understanding of the structure and function of infectious disease pathogens is a major scientific challenge with important potential applications.

This new cross-disciplinary monograph series will provide up-to-date information on the latest developments in infectious disease research. The multi-authored volumes will cover basic biology and biochemistry of pathogens as well as applied medical aspects and implications for public health and policy.

The contributions are written by leading infectious disease researchers and pharmaceutical scientists with a wide range of expertise.

The envisaged readership includes academic and industrial researchers in medicine and infectious diseases as well as clinicians and others involved in diagnostics and drug development.

Forthcoming volumes:
Poxviruses, A. Mercer, A. Schmidt, O. Weber (Editors), 2006

Available volumes:
Coronaviruses with Special Emphasis on First Insights Concerning SARS, A. Schmidt, M.H. Wolff, O. Weber (Editors), 2005

Capitalism's latest global crisis and slump have made Geoff Pilling's work newly relevant. His essays on value and crisis, and on Marx vs. Keynes and Marx vs. Sraffa, that are brought together here are especially timely. Keith Gibbard's intellectual biography of the author, which introduces the volume, is lucid and masterful. One of the foremost contributors to the revival of the Marxian critique of political economy a generation ago, Pilling carried forward a tradition that did not divide theory from practice or economics from philosophy. And his precise, accurate scholarship remains a model; he understood well that one must get Marx right before judging whether Marx got it right. As someone who learned a lot from him, I highly recommend this book.

Andrew Kliman, author of *Reclaiming Marx's 'Capital': A Refutation of the Myth of Inconsistency* and Professor of Economics at Pace University, New York, USA

Marxist Political Economy

The free market can no longer be trusted to bring prosperity. The financial market has had to be rescued by socialisation. The problem is the greed of bankers and speculators, and a lack of sufficient regulation. These are the opinions of world leaders and finance ministers. But there have been no analyses of the deep-seated and fundamental problems of the capitalist system.

Geoff Pilling, leading Marxist theoretician makes just such analyses in this collection of essays, which he was preparing for publication before his death in 1997. In an essay remarkably prescient of today's situation, he analyses the crises of post-war capitalism. Other essays in the book explain fundamental concepts of Marx's analysis of capitalism, their irreconcilability with Keynes's theoretical system, and refute the contention that all Marxist theoretical development post-Marx was distorted by Stalinism. Pilling also shows how problems in British capitalism were the forerunners of those in world capitalism. And he defends Engels's contention that the greatest significance of the industrial revolution was the development of a working class that was forced to fight against its conditions of oppression.

Geoff Pilling's work shows that Marxist theory is relevant to those struggling to understand the problems of capitalist society today, and that the work not only of Marx and Engels but also that of later Marxist theorists, including Lenin is worth studying. It also shows that to understand the problems of today's society needs more than narrow specialist economic analysis, but a deep awareness of current developments in society.

Geoff Pilling was a prominent political economist who devoted his life to the achievement of socialism and a 'truly human society'. Geoff taught Economics at Sheffield and Bradford Universities and at Middlesex Polytechnic (later University), where he developed an MA in Political Economy and was awarded a readership. In addition to a distinguished academic career, in which he published several books, he was a prolific writer in the left-wing press, including *Labour Review*, *Fourth International*, *Workers' Press* and the *Dockers Charter*. He sadly died in 1997.

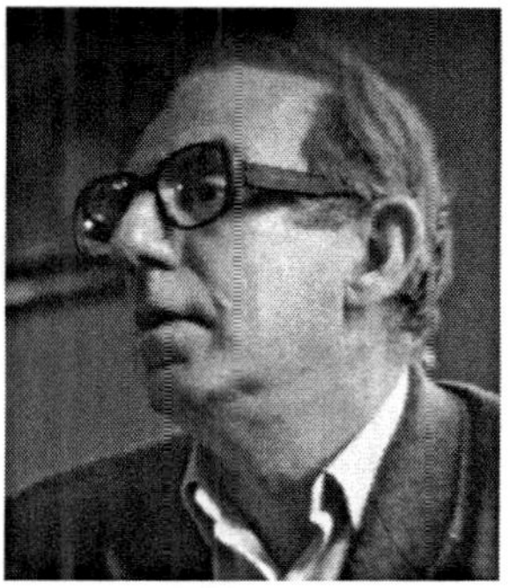
Geoff Pilling

Doria Pilling was Geoff's wife and is an Honorary Senior Fellow at the School of Health Sciences at City University London, UK.

Routledge studies in the history of economics

1 **Economics as Literature**
Willie Henderson

2 **Socialism and Marginalism in Economics 1870–1930**
Edited by Ian Steedman

3 **Hayek's Political Economy**
The socio-economics of order
Steve Fleetwood

4 **On the Origins of Classical Economics**
Distribution and value from William Petty to Adam Smith
Tony Aspromourgos

5 **The Economics of Joan Robinson**
Edited by Maria Cristina Marcuzzo, Luigi Pasinetti and Alesandro Roncaglia

6 **The Evolutionist Economics of Léon Walras**
Albert Jolink

7 **Keynes and the 'Classics'**
A study in language, epistemology and mistaken identities
Michel Verdon

8 **The History of Game Theory, Vol. 1**
From the beginnings to 1945
Robert W. Dimand and Mary Ann Dimand

9 **The Economics of W.S. Jevons**
Sandra Peart

10 **Gandhi's Economic Thought**
Ajit K. Dasgupta

11 **Equilibrium and Economic Theory**
Edited by Giovanni Caravale

12 **Austrian Economics in Debate**
Edited by Willem Keizer, Bert Tieben and Rudy van Zijp

13 **Ancient Economic Thought**
Edited by B.B. Price

14 **The Political Economy of Social Credit and Guild Socialism**
Frances Hutchinson and Brian Burkitt

15 **Economic Careers**
Economics and economists in Britain 1930–1970
Keith Tribe

16 **Understanding 'Classical' Economics**
Studies in the long-period theory
Heinz Kurz and Neri Salvadori

17 **History of Environmental Economic Thought**
E. Kula

18 **Economic Thought in Communist and Post-Communist Europe**
Edited by Hans-Jürgen Wagener

19 **Studies in the History of French Political Economy**
From Bodin to Walras
Edited by Gilbert Faccarello

20 **The Economics of John Rae**
Edited by O.F. Hamouda, C. Lee and D. Mair

21 **Keynes and the Neoclassical Synthesis**
Einsteinian versus Newtonian macroeconomics
Teodoro Dario Togati

22 **Historical Perspectives on Macroeconomics**
Sixty years after the 'General Theory'
Edited by Philippe Fontaine and Albert Jolink

23 **The Founding of Institutional Economics**
The leisure class and sovereignty
Edited by Warren J. Samuels

24 **Evolution of Austrian Economics**
From Menger to Lachmann
Sandye Gloria

25 **Marx's Concept of Money**
The God of Commodities
Anitra Nelson

26 **The Economics of James Steuart**
Edited by Ramón Tortajada

27 **The Development of Economics in Europe since 1945**
Edited by A.W. Bob Coats

28 **The Canon in the History of Economics**
Critical essays
Edited by Michalis Psalidopoulos

29 **Money and Growth**
Selected papers of Allyn Abbott Young
Edited by Perry G. Mehrling and Roger J. Sandilands

30 **The Social Economics of Jean-Baptiste Say**
Markets and virtue
Evelyn L. Forget

31 **The Foundations of Laissez-Faire**
The economics of Pierre de Boisguilbert
Gilbert Faccarello

32 **John Ruskin's Political Economy**
Willie Henderson

33 **Contributions to the History of Economic Thought**
Essays in honour of R.D.C. Black
Edited by Antoin E. Murphy and Renee Prendergast

34 **Towards an Unknown Marx**
A commentary on the manuscripts of 1861–63
Enrique Dussel

35 **Economics and Interdisciplinary Exchange**
Edited by Guido Erreygers

36 **Economics as the Art of Thought**
Essays in memory of G.L.S. Shackle
Edited by Stephen F. Frowen and Peter Earl

37 **The Decline of Ricardian Economics**
Politics and economics in post-Ricardian theory
Susan Pashkoff

38 **Piero Sraffa**
His life, thought and cultural heritage
Alessandro Roncaglia

39 **Equilibrium and Disequilibrium in Economic Theory**
The Marshall–Walras divide
Michel de Vroey

40 **The German Historical School**
The historical and ethical approach to economics
Edited by Yuichi Shionoya

41 **Reflections on the Classical Canon in Economics**
Essays in honour of Samuel Hollander
Edited by Sandra Peart and Evelyn Forget

42 **Piero Sraffa's Political Economy**
A centenary estimate
Edited by Terenzio Cozzi and Roberto Marchionatti

43 **The Contribution of Joseph Schumpeter to Economics**
Economic development and institutional change
Richard Arena and Cecile Dangel

44 **On the Development of Long-run Neo-Classical Theory**
Tom Kompas

45 **F.A. Hayek as a Political Economist**
Economic analysis and values
Edited by Jack Birner, Pierre Garrouste and Thierry Aimar

46 **Pareto, Economics and Society**
The mechanical analogy
Michael McLure

47 **The Cambridge Controversies in Capital Theory**
A study in the logic of theory development
Jack Birner

48 **Economics Broadly Considered**
Essays in honour of Warren J. Samuels
Edited by Steven G. Medema, Jeff Biddle and John B. Davis

49 **Physicians and Political Economy**
Six studies of the work of doctor-economists
Edited by Peter Groenewegen

50 **The Spread of Political Economy and the Professionalisation of Economists**
Economic societies in Europe, America and Japan in the nineteenth century
Massimo Augello and Marco Guidi

51 **Historians of Economics and Economic Thought**
The construction of disciplinary memory
Steven G. Medema and Warren J. Samuels

52 **Competing Economic Theories**
Essays in memory of Giovanni Caravale
Sergio Nisticò and Domenico Tosato

53 **Economic Thought and Policy in Less Developed Europe**
The nineteenth century
Edited by Michalis Psalidopoulos and Maria-Eugenia Almedia Mata

54 **Family Fictions and Family Facts**
Harriet Martineau, Adolphe Quetelet and the population question in England 1798–1859
Brian Cooper

55 **Eighteenth-century Economics**
Peter Groenewegen

56 **The Rise of Political Economy in the Scottish Enlightenment**
Edited by Tatsuya Sakamoto and Hideo Tanaka

57 **Classics and Moderns in Economics, Volume I**
Essays on nineteenth and twentieth century economic thought
Peter Groenewegen

58 **Classics and Moderns in Economics, Volume II**
Essays on nineteenth and twentieth century economic thought
Peter Groenewegen

59 **Marshall's Evolutionary Economics**
Tiziano Raffaelli

60 **Money, Time and Rationality in Max Weber**
Austrian connections
Stephen D. Parsons

61 **Classical Macroeconomics**
Some modern variations and distortions
James C.W. Ahiakpor

62 **The Historical School of Economics in England and Japan**
Tamotsu Nishizawa

63 **Classical Economics and Modern Theory**
Studies in long-period analysis
Heinz D. Kurz and Neri Salvadori

64 **A Bibliography of Female Economic Thought to 1940**
Kirsten K. Madden, Janet A. Sietz and Michele Pujol

65 **Economics, Economists and Expectations**
From microfoundations to macroeconomics
Warren Young, Robert Leeson and William Darity Jnr.

66 **The Political Economy of Public Finance in Britain, 1767–1873**
Takuo Dome

67 **Essays in the History of Economics**
Warren J. Samuels, Willie Henderson, Kirk D. Johnson and Marianne Johnson

68 **History and Political Economy**
Essays in honour of P.D. Groenewegen
Edited by Tony Aspromourgos and John Lodewijks

69 **The Tradition of Free Trade**
Lars Magnusson

70 **Evolution of the Market Process**
Austrian and Swedish economics
Edited by Michel Bellet, Sandye Gloria-Palermo and Abdallah Zouache

71 **Consumption as an Investment**
The fear of goods from Hesiod to Adam Smith
Cosimo Perrotta

72 **Jean-Baptiste Say and the Classical Canon in Economics**
The British connection in French classicism
Samuel Hollander

73 **Knut Wicksell on Poverty**
No place is too exalted
Knut Wicksell

74 **Economists in Cambridge**
A study through their correspondence 1907–1946
Edited by M.C. Marcuzzo and A. Rosselli

75 **The Experiment in the History of Economics**
Edited by Philippe Fontaine and Robert Leonard

76 **At the Origins of Mathematical Economics**
The economics of A.N. Isnard (1748–1803)
Richard van den Berg

77 **Money and Exchange**
Folktales and reality
Sasan Fayazmanesh

78 **Economic Development and Social Change**
Historical roots and modern perspectives
George Stathakis and Gianni Vaggi

79 **Ethical Codes and Income Distribution**
A study of John Bates Clark and Thorstein Veblen
Guglielmo Forges Davanzati

80 **Evaluating Adam Smith**
Creating the wealth of nations
Willie Henderson

81 **Civil Happiness**
Economics and human flourishing in historical perspective
Luigino Bruni

82 **New Voices on Adam Smith**
Edited by Leonidas Montes and Eric Schliesser

83 **Making Chicago Price Theory**
Milton Friedman–George Stigler correspondence, 1945–1957
Edited by J. Daniel Hammond and Claire H. Hammond

84 **William Stanley Jevons and the Cutting Edge of Economics**
Bert Mosselmans

85 **A History of Econometrics in France**
From nature to models
Philippe Le Gall

86 **Money and Markets**
A doctrinal approach
Edited by Alberto Giacomin and Maria Cristina Marcuzzo

87 **Considerations on the Fundamental Principles of Pure Political Economy**
Vilfredo Pareto (Edited by Roberto Marchionatti and Fiorenzo Mornati)

88 **The Years of High Econometrics**
A short history of the generation that reinvented economics
Francisco Louçã

89 **David Hume's Political Economy**
Edited by Carl Wennerlind and Margaret Schabas

90 **Interpreting Classical Economics**
Studies in long-period analysis
Heinz D. Kurz and Neri Salvadori

91 **Keynes's Vision**
Why the great depression did not return
John Philip Jones

92 **Monetary Theory in Retrospect**
The selected essays of Filippo Cesarano
Filippo Cesarano

93 **Keynes's Theoretical Development**
From the tract to the general theory
Toshiaki Hirai

94 **Leading Contemporary Economists**
Economics at the cutting edge
Edited by Steven Pressman

95 **The Science of Wealth**
Adam Smith and the framing of political economy
Tony Aspromourgos

96 **Capital, Time and Transitional Dynamics**
Edited by Harald Hagemann and Roberto Scazzieri

97 **New Essays on Pareto's Economic Theory**
Edited by Luigino Bruni and Aldo Montesano

98 **Frank Knight and the Chicago School in American Economics**
Ross B. Emmett

99 **A History of Economic Theory**
Essays in honour of Takashi Negishi
Edited by Aiko Ikeo and Heinz D. Kurz

100 **Open Economics**
Economics in relation to other disciplines
Edited by Richard Arena, Sheila Dow and Matthias Klaes

101 **Rosa Luxemburg and the Critique of Political Economy**
Edited by Riccardo Bellofiore

102 **Problems and Methods of Econometrics**
The Poincaré lectures of Ragnar Frisch 1933
Edited by Olav Bjerkholt and Ariane Dupont-Keiffer

103 **Criticisms of Classical Political Economy**
Menger, Austrian economics and the German historical school
Gilles Campagnolo

104 **A History of Entrepreneurship**
Robert F. Hébert and Albert N. link

105 **Keynes on Monetary Policy, Finance and Uncertainty**
Liquidity preference theory and the global financial crisis
Jorg Bibow

106 **Kalecki's Principle of Increasing Risk and Keynesian Economics**
Tracy Mott

107 **Economic Theory and Economic Thought**
Essays in honour of Ian Steedman
John Vint, J. Stanley Metcalfe, Heinz D. Kurz, Neri Salvadori and Paul Samuelson

108 **Political Economy, Public Policy and Monetary Economics**
Ludwig von Mises and the Austrian tradition
Richard M. Ebeling

109 **Keynes and the British Humanist Tradition**
The moral purpose of the market
David R. Andrews

110 **Political Economy and Industrialism**
Banks in Saint-Simonian economic thought
Gilles Jacoud

111 **Studies in Social Economics**
Leon Walras
Translated by Jan van Daal and Donald Walker

112 **The Making of the Classical Theory of Economic Growth**
Anthony Brewer

113 **The Origins of David Hume's Economics**
Willie Henderson

114 **Production, Distribution and Trade**
Edited by Adriano Birolo, Duncan Foley, Heinz D. Kurz, Bertram Schefold and Ian Steedman

115 **The Essential Writings of Thorstein Veblen**
Edited by Charles Camic and Geoffrey Hodgson

116 **Adam Smith and the Economy of the Passions**
Jan Horst Keppler

117 **The Analysis of Linear Economic Systems**
Father Maurice Potron's pioneering works
Translated by Christian Bidard and Guido Erreygers

118 **A Dynamic Approach to Economic Theory: Frisch**
Edited by Olav Bjerkholt and Duo Qin

119 **Henry A. Abbati: Keynes' Forgotten Precursor**
Serena Di Gaspare

120 **Generations of Economists**
David Collard

121 **Hayek, Mill and the Liberal Tradition**
Edited by Andrew Farrant

122 **Marshall, Marshallians and Industrial Economics**
Edited by Tiziano Raffaelli

123 **Austrian and German Economic Thought**
Kiichiro Yagi

124 **The Evolution of Economic Theory**
Edited by Volker Caspari

125 **Thomas Tooke and the Monetary Thought of Classical Economics**
Matthew Smith

126 **Political Economy and Liberalism in France**
The contributions of Frédéric Bastiat
Robert Leroux

127 **Stalin's Economist**
The economic contributions of Jenö Varga
André Mommen

128 **E.E. Slutsky as Economist and Mathematician**
Crossing the limits of knowledge
Vincent Barnett

129 **Keynes, Sraffa, and the Criticism of Neoclassical Theory**
Essays in honour of Heinz Kurz
Neri Salvadori and Christian Gehrke

130 **Crises and Cycles in Economic Dictionaries and Encyclopaedias**
Edited by Daniele Bensomi

131 **General Equilibrium Analysis: A Century after Walras**
Edited by Pascal Bridel

132 **Sraffa and Modern Economics, Volume I**
Edited by Roberto Ciccone, Christian Gehrke and Gary Mongiovi

133 **Sraffa and Modern Economics, Volume II**
Edited by Roberto Ciccone, Christian Gehrke and Gary Mongiovi

134 **The Minor Marshallians and Alfred Marshall: An Evaluation**
Peter Groenewegen

135 **Fighting Market Failure**
Collected essays in the Cambridge tradition of economics
Maria Cristina Marcuzzo

136 **The Economic Reader**
Edited by Massimo M. Augello and Marco E.L. Guido

137 **Classical Political Economy and Modern Theory**
Essays in honour of Heinz Kurz
Neri Salvadori and Christian Gehrke

138 **The Ideas of Ronald H. Coase**
Lawrence W.C. Lai

139 **Anticipating the Wealth of Nations**
Edited by Maren Jonasson and Petri Hyttinen, with an Introduction by Lars Magnusson

140 **Innovation, Knowledge and Growth**
Edited by Heinz D. Kurz

141 **A History of Homo Economicus**
The nature of the moral in economic theory
William Dixon and David Wilson

142 **The Division of Labour in Economics**
A history
Guang-Zhen Sun

143 **Keynes and Modern Economics**
Edited by Ryuzo Kuroki

144 **Macroeconomics and the History of Economic Thought**
Festschrift in honour of Harald Hagemann
Edited by Hagen M. Krämer, Heinz D. Kurz and Hans-Michael Trautwein

145 **French Liberalism in the 19th Century**
An anthology
Edited by Robert Leroux

146 **Subjectivisim and Objectivism in the History of Economic Thought**
Edited by Yukihiro Ikeda and Kiichiro Yagi

147 **Marxist Political Economy**
Essays in retrieval: selected works of Geoff Pilling
Geoff Pilling
Edited by Doria Pilling

Marxist Political Economy

Essays in retrieval: selected works of Geoff Pilling

Geoff Pilling

Edited by Doria Pilling

Routledge
Taylor & Francis Group
LONDON AND NEW YORK

First published 2012
by Routledge
2 Park Square, Milton Park, Abingdon, Oxon OX14 4RN

Simultaneously published in the USA and Canada
by Routledge
711 Third Avenue, New York, NY 10017

Routledge is an imprint of the Taylor & Francis Group, an informa business

British Library Cataloguing in Publication Data
A catalogue record for this book is available from the British Library

Library of Congress Cataloging in Publication Data
Pilling, Geoffrey.
Marxist political economy: essays in retrieval: selected works of Geoff Pilling/by Geoff Pilling; edited by Doria Pilling.
p. cm.
1. Capitalism 2. Marxian economics. I. Title.
HB501.P437 2012
335.4′12–dc23
2012002307

ISBN: 978-0-415-67852-0 (hbk)
ISBN: 978-0-203-10723-2 (ebk)

Typeset in Times New Roman
by Wearset Ltd, Boldon, Tyne and Wear

To Dylan and Travis, Geoff's grandsons, and all their generation, to whose future Geoff devoted his life's work.

Contents

Foreword

What follows is the very slightly edited text of a speech that I delivered at a memorial meeting for Geoff nearly 15 years ago. In contributing a foreword to this select edited collection from his work, I had expected to expand and revise upon the text of the speech. But, having reviewed the collection and, in particular, the other recollections, I consider it unnecessary to do so. What I spoke, and wrote, then still stands today and represents the most important things I have to say about Geoff's work and its influence upon me personally.

But, nonetheless, it is recognisably inadequate for two reasons. The first is my contribution focuses unduly, indeed solely, on Geoff's contribution to value theory. As this collection, and recollections, make abundantly clear, his work of the same level of insight and scholarship ranges over a much broader terrain of political economy. I was aware of this work but it has had lesser influence and prominence than his value theory.

Second, the value theory resides at a more abstract and general level than much of his other work. This inevitably renders the value theory more long lasting, as is the enduring interest upon it. For example, the critical dissection of Keynesianism is of potentially more significance, and prominence, when it has both some prospect of being adopted and historical experience of its successes and failures are closer to hand. Thirty years of neo-liberalism have so much removed Keynesianism from the analytical and policy environment that it is now only re-emerging, where it has managed to survive, in the weakest policy forms of throwing as much money at the banks as is deemed necessary to use them as the source of stimulus to effective demand (and, of course, to sustain their solvency and rewards). Meanwhile, corresponding fiscal deficits arising out of rescuing the banks and recession are deployed as a rationale for attacking the living standards of working people who bear no responsibility for the crisis by any account.

In short, no matter how much neo-liberal policy and scholarship have, or have not, been shaken by the global financial crisis at time of writing, only when some genuine version of Keynesian resurrection accrues as response to our current and continuing travails will its critical inadequacies themselves be once more in need of full exposure. Indeed, it is striking how weak and compromised are the perspectives of mainstream Keynesian dissidents, with their raised exposure more a consequence of crisis than any genuine renewal of reflection over its causes. Their perspective is to make *markets* work, not to expose the ways in which capital exploits and with what consequences.

By different tokens, Geoff's contributions around the classic texts and issues of Marxism, such as imperialism and unequal exchange (and the salience in principle, practice and methodology of world economy as starting point), and the revolutionary potential of the working class, are not so much dated by the passage of a few years in events and ideas, as the raw materials for the renewal of corresponding intellectual endeavours in light of what has occurred and how it should be addressed. For the latter, as is abundantly clear from what follows, Geoff's enduring legacy is a personal and collective commitment to the principles of scientific socialism in theory and practice.

This is evident, for example, in Chapter 2 which, given that the era of relatively rapid capital accumulation and corresponding class compromises are over, focuses on the prospects for the British working class in historical and global perspective. And it inevitably does so by reference to the world economy and politics, the significance of faltering accumulation, the end of the Cold War, and the rise of US hegemony, and (with considerable prescience) recognition of the rise of finance and immiseration across much of the globe. Of course, the exact contours of the current crisis could hardly have been anticipated, but the methods to address it are fully present, not least the emphasis on 'the epoch of *world* economy and *world* politics' without which is spread the illusion and delusion that national policymaking is both obliged to, and capable of, resolving the problems of global capitalism on its own if only working people will tighten their belts in the interim. At least with the crises around the euro, the illusion of national solutions to the problems of global capitalism has been shattered.

Speech at Memorial Meeting, 19 November 1997

It is with an overwhelming sense of sadness that I talk to you today for obvious reasons, but that sadness is also tinged with a considerable honour and pleasure, for reasons which I hope to be able to explain later on. The pleasure that I got from thinking about this talk comes from recalling the value debates in political economy which we had in the late 1960s and 1970s and in which Geoff made a major contribution which I think is very easily overlooked for two separate reasons. The first reason, the obvious one, is that political economy, value theory, particularly of the sort that Geoff contributed has gone out of fashion, and with its going out of fashion many of the qualities that shone like beacons out of Geoff's work have also gone out of fashion. I've noticed the words used by both of the previous speakers about Geoff – the rareness of the qualities he had, in particular the intellectual integrity of his scholarship, and I'm afraid there is also the fading of these qualities in others in academia, especially in an economics that has excised, as it were, political economy, its method, and the history of economic thought.

What are the qualities of the scholarship that marked Geoff out even at the time he was writing – and which are even rarer today? First of all Geoff had a very profound knowledge of the history of his own discipline, of political economy and of economics. And this is very rare in economics. The only person you have to know about is the last person to write an article on the subject that you are interested in. I was shocked in teaching some LSE graduates in economics this year, some of whom didn't even know who Samuelson was. And there's no reason for them to do so – because Samuelson is an early neo-classical economist and he's been superseded by those who have written subsequently. The second feature of Geoff's work is an equally profound knowledge of economic history to provide a background context for the understanding of economics as a discipline. Again economists who know about economic history are becoming increasingly rare. The third quality is the commitment to address the political implications of the economic theory that he puts forward. Unfortunately I would say that this is no longer rare among economists but the fashion in which they undertake their understanding of politics is relatively simplistic. A fourth feature of Geoff's work is the way in which he contributed a very close, informed and scholarly reading of other people's works. And that's very, very important for developing his own views and criticising those of others. Again these are very rare qualities in economists today. A fifth feature is the extraordinary sophistication of the methodology that he brought to bear in his work. Again I'm in the unfortunate position of slagging off my own profession but I would say that the vast majority of economists are the hyenas of the philosophy of methodology. And the last, and by no means least, quality of Geoff's work is a very limited respect for the prestigious figures within his own discipline, unless they deserved it in the light of his own intellectual standards. I have to say there was something almost cold or, more accurately, clinical about the skill with which Geoff dissected the work of others. Yet I think that his work also combined both a passion and a respect for the work that he admired, especially obviously that of Marx, Lenin, Engels and others, whom he considered incorporated the qualities he considered to be, quite rightly, essential to appropriate scholarship. In some respects I think it is very unfortunate for Geoff to be so cold, clinical, and accurate about the writings of others, for he often reserved his sharpest criticisms for those who believed that they were promoting the very sort of political economy that he sought to promote himself. I can obviously mention figures such as Maurice Dobb and Ronald Meek, huge figures in political economy as we began the venture of promoting political economy in the late 1960s and early 1970s. Of course there were many who were very unhappy about these figures being criticised because this was undermining our own supporters. So, in this respect, it was unfortunate for Geoff. I also think that it was very fortunate, in the long run, to use an economists' expression, because this means that the standards of scholarship could move forward in assessing critically, accurately and appropriately the work of those who had gone before.

It was one of Geoff's major contributions to reject what was called the Ricardo–Marx theory of value as an interpretation of Marx that was offered by

Dobb and Meek and very substantially taken up by many other writers subsequently. Now what I would say is that the decline of political economy, and particularly of value theory within political economy as a serious alternative in economics, has meant that these qualities of Geoff's are not liable to be recognised, certainly by the profession as a whole. And even those who are working within Marxist political economy, and who are influenced by Geoff's work, are liable to be influenced in ways that they no longer recognise. They no longer recognise them because they have become part of schools or ways of looking at political economy and value theory without continuing reference to the contribution that Geoff made.

And as I said earlier for this reason I want to try to make clear some of my own debt to Geoff's work, and it is something that informs my thinking most frequently. In particular, there is Geoff's criticism of what's happened to what he would have called the instrumentalist approach to value theory. By value theory we mean the idea that the understanding of the capitalist economy must be based on Marx's theory of value, by which we mean the labour theory of value. In the approaches that Geoff particularly wanted to criticise, the instrumentalist approach, the labour theory of value is constructed as a theory like an instrument and examined for the purposes to which it might be put. Is it a good theory of price, is it a good theory of crisis, is it a good theory of economic level of activity? And in contrast Geoff said the issue is not, is this a good theory of price or not, is this a good theory of this that and the other or not, shall I invent a theory and see if it works for my economic purposes or not, which of course has led many orthodox economists, as well as many political economists to reject Marx's value theory. Geoff really wanted to start with the question: does value exist? And in what societies does value exist? If I can show that value exists then I must explore its relationship to the other economic and social relations within that society. In other words he put forward the method in which it is necessary to look at the world as it is and how capitalist relations and processes can be incorporated theoretically within the concepts that are employed. Now I can't go into detail into the significance of this, but I think a very neat way of demonstrating the validity of this approach is demonstrated by reference to the work of Adam Smith. Adam Smith argued in his own value theory that the labour theory of value would only hold in the 'rude' society. The 'rude' society is that primitive stage of society where you go out and get your deer or your beaver according to your needs. You go out and hunt them, and if it takes twice as long to catch a deer as it does a beaver then one deer will exchange for two beavers. Adam Smith said that the labour theory of value will hold in this society but as soon as you emerge from that society where the only factor of production that is rewarded is labour and, instead, where there are rewards through wages, and also through profits and rent, then the labour theory of value will not hold. It is the perfect example of the instrumental approach to the labour theory of value. Let me invent the labour theory of value and see if it applies in the rude society – yes – does it hold in the commercial society – no. There is one major problem with this approach – you don't need a labour theory of value in the rude society.

People if they want a deer will go out and get a deer and if they want a beaver will go out and get a beaver. There is no need for any exchange at all. This completely illustrates the fallacy of the instrumental approach: that your theoretical concepts should be drawn from the society that you wish to examine. And I think that that is something which I continue to try to employ in my work – that is, the theory that I employ should correspond to the societies that I seek to examine, and I should not simply construct a theory ideally and attack problems with it. And that's a lesson that I learned from reading Geoff's work. And there are many other lessons that I learned as well.

Perhaps I can finish by saying that I have been familiar with much of Geoff's work. And in 1986 I was asked by the editors of *Economy and Society* to edit a book of contributions to that journal on value theory. I was a little bit annoyed by this as the reason they wanted to do this was to make money by re-printing articles from their own journal, so they wouldn't have the cost of re-setting articles from other journals and I was confined in my choice to articles that had appeared in *Economy and Society.* One thing that I was not annoyed about was that I could include Geoff's contribution, as the first contribution to *Economy and Society* and it's the best contribution that could have been made on value theory and would grace any collection on value theory. And the same is true of his book on Marx's *Capital* which does represent as I tried to suggest earlier the highest level of scholarship for reasons of the qualities that I indicated. Now the other speakers and I have also suggested that the qualities that characterised Geoff's work are not sufficiently recognised both by virtue of the developments within the discipline itself as well as by virtue of the rarity and lack of respect for what are the highest levels of scholarship. But I would say so strong are the contributions that Geoff has made – particularly in these two contributions as far as I am concerned – that I believe that they will serve as a fitting memorial to him and his scholarship long after, very long after, the orthodoxies for which today you see the highest honours, have long since been forgotten.

Professor Ben Fine, School of Oriental and African Studies,
University of London

Acknowledgements

Above all I would like to thank Andrew Burgin, without whose encouragement I would not have succeeded in putting this book together. I am very grateful to Professor Ben Fine for writing the Foreword to the book. I am also particularly grateful to Keith Gibbard, who not only wrote the Introduction but has been exceedingly patient in answering many queries, and whose advice has been invaluable. I would like to thank those who so readily agreed to contribute to the Recollections chapter, Professor Kazuto Iida, Dot Gibson and Faruk Ibrahimović. I am also very indebted to Bob Archer, Terry Brotherstone and Andy Blunden, all of whom have taken considerable pains in answering my queries. As editor, of course, I take full responsibility for decisions made and for any errors.

I am very grateful to copyright holders who have given permission for copyrighted material to be used. This is as follows: to Informa UK for G. Pilling (1972) 'The law of value in Ricardo and Marx', *Economy and Society*, 1 (3): 281–307 and G. Pilling (1973) 'Imperialism, trade and "unequal exchange": the work of Arghiri Emmanuel', *Economy and Society*, 2 (2): 164–185 – these articles can be seen on the *Economy and Society* website, online, available at: www.tandfonline.com/toc/reso20/current; to Porcupine Press for G. Pilling (1996) '"Globalisation" and the British working class: an essay in economic analysis and political prognosis' T. Brotherstone and G. Pilling (eds) *History, Economic History and the Future of Marxism: Essays in Memory of Tom Kemp;* to Workers International to Rebuild the Fourth International for G. Pilling 'On disinterring Karl Marx: Cyril Smith, *Marx at the Millennium*, Pluto Press, London, 1996, 182 pp.', *Workers International Press*, 3, June 1997, p. 11 and to John Lea who holds joint copyright with Geoff Pilling to G. Pilling (1996) 'Engels and the industrial revolution' in J. Lea and G. Pilling (eds) *The Condition of Britain: Essays on Frederick Engels*, London: Pluto Press. Without these permissions this book would, of course, have been impossible.

Doria Pilling, December 2011

Note on references

To provide consistency, as far as has been possible, references are given to the following versions of Marx's, Engels's and Lenin's works:

Marx, K. (1961) *Capital* vol. I Moscow and London: Foreign Languages Publishing House and Lawrence & Wishart, online, available at: www.marxists.org/archive/marx/works/1867-c1/ (accessed 16 December 2011).

Marx, K. (1957) *Capital* vol. II Moscow and London: Foreign Languages Publishing House and Lawrence & Wishart, online, available at: www.marxists.org/archive/marx/works/download/pdf/Capital-Volume-II.pdf (accessed 16 December 2011).

Marx, K. (1959) *Capital* vol. III Moscow and London: Foreign Languages Publishing House and Lawrence & Wishart, online, available at: www.marxists.org/archive/marx/works/download/pdf/Capital-Volume-III.pdf (accessed 16 December 2011).

Marx, K. (1969) *Theories of Surplus Value*, Part I, London: Lawrence & Wishart, online, available at: www.marxists.org/archive/marx/works/1863/theories-surplus-value/ch02.htm (accessed 16 December 2011).

Marx, K. (1969) *Theories of Surplus Value*, Part II, London: Lawrence & Wishart.

Marx, K. (1972) *Theories of Surplus Value*, Part III, London: Lawrence & Wishart.

Marx, K. and Engels, F. (1975–2004) *Karl Marx Frederick Engels Collected Works* (50 volumes), Moscow and London: Progress Publishers and Lawrence & Wishart, online, available at: www.marxists.org/archive/marx/works/cw/index.htm (accessed 16 December 2011).

Marx, K. and Engels, F. (1956) *Selected Correspondence*, Moscow and London: Foreign Language Publishing House and Lawrence & Wishart.

Lenin, V.I. (1960–1980) *Collected Works* (47 volumes), Moscow and London: Progress Publishers and Lawrence & Wishart, online, available at: www.marxists.org/archive/marx/works/cw/index.htm (accessed 16 December 2011).

It should be noted that specific references are given at the end of each chapter, and that these may refer to a different version where this was used originally by Geoff Pilling.

Introduction

As a leading figure in the Trotskyist movement, Geoff Pilling was fully involved over many years in every aspect of the life of the international working class. In reviewing his intellectual contribution, it is important to remember at the outset that his was not the life of an armchair theorist. Rather his writing was inseparable from his daily activity as an agitator, teacher, journalist and editor of socialist newspapers and journals. His writing, spanning over 30 years of work on history, philosophy, politics and economics charts the course of the breakup of the period of relative capitalist stability following World War II through to present times.

In his first articles, written as a young man in his twenties, published in periodicals such as *Labour Review* and the *Fourth International* in the early 1960s, he set about the task of providing an analysis of the state of post-war capitalism. With remarkable foresight, and much earlier than most, Pilling argued in 1964 on the basis of a detailed empirical study, that the period of global expanded reproduction was coming to an end.[1] In a talk given at the University of Sheffield in 1965, fully six years before the final collapse of the Bretton Woods international monetary system, he explained the contradictions within world economy and the impossibility of sustaining the gold–dollar link in the face of the growing pool of dollar reserves held outside the United States.[2] Going behind the monetary appearance of the crisis he showed its significance in terms of the uneven development of world imperialism and the fact that the inflationary nature of the period was a sign of capitalism's weakness in the face of the international working class – in particular with respect to the financing of the Vietnam War. That early work was instrumental in orienting whole new layers of students and young people coming into the socialist movement towards an understanding of capitalism's laws of motion and the need for a serious re-examination of Marx's *Capital*, at a time when left social democracy still held out the panacea of capitalist stability through a benign Keynesian policy. In addition, as those early contributions show, it was at this time that Pilling began to develop his views on two issues which were to grow into major areas of research for the future: first Marx's philosophy and second the economics of John Maynard Keynes.[3]

Pilling's work on Marx's method came to the attention of a much wider readership with the publication in 1972, in the newly-established journal *Economy and Society*, of his 'The law of value in Ricardo and Marx'. It is necessary to recall the scarcity of well-established writers on the subject of Marxist 'economics' at that time. Dobb and Meek in Britain, Paul Sweezy in the United States along with Belgian Trotskyist Ernest Mandel held sway in a very limited field. It was these authorities who were the subject of Pilling's critical attention. In uncompromising style he set himself the task 'to show that many of Marx's aims and methods have been seriously misrepresented by the majority of commentators who would wish to be designated "Marxist economists" '.[4] In particular, he attacked their attempts to conflate Marx's ideas with those of classical political economy, on the basis of a 'Classical-Marxist tradition' and a common 'labour theory of value'. In place of Ricardo's fruitless search for an invariable measure of value, Pilling correctly argued that:

> The task of Marx's critique of political economy was *not* one which involved him finding a 'constant' in terms of which everything could be quantified but of establishing the laws of mediation through which the essence of phenomena manifested itself as appearance.[5]

The article drew a rather injured response from Ronald Meek to the effect that the differences of approach were matters of emphasis rather than substance. Pilling's implacable reply served not only to reconfirm the gulf with those who he considered were distorting Marx's work, but also located its historical roots:

> it seems clear that the major source for the degeneration of Marxism was undoubtedly the emergence of Stalinism inside the Soviet Union and the parties of the Third International. From the mid 1920s onwards an entire layer of writers and intellectuals became 'hired prizefighters' on behalf of Stalin's pronouncements as certainly as the political economists had become 'hired prizefighters' for the bourgeoisie in the years following 1830. Nowhere was this more true than in the field of political economy.[6]

The positions taken in that article, with its intention of reclaiming a Marxism based on dialectics, contradiction, historical specificity and the distinction between form and content, were given a much fuller treatment with the appearance in 1980 of Pilling's first book, *Marx's Capital: Philosophy and Political Economy.*[7] The validity and significance of his approach had in the interim been confirmed by the re-publication in English of I.I. Rubin's *Essays on Value*, followed by Marx's *Grundrisse* and the subsequent appearance shortly afterwards of Rosdolsky's book on Marx's *Capital*.[8] In addition to these writings, Pilling's understanding of the centrality of Marx's method had developed, in particular through his study of the writings of the Soviet philosopher, Evald Ilyenkov, whose books had begun to appear in English in the late 1970s.[9] Together these works were instrumental in providing the methodological basis for a refutation of the Ricardian interpretation of Marx's value theory which was dominant among followers of Piero Sraffa.[10]

Whilst developing his earlier themes, Pilling extended the scope of his critique to include the, then influential, work of the French structuralist school of Louis Althusser and his followers. The book argues convincingly that Marx's method cannot be metaphysically separated from the whole history of western philosophy. It pays particular attention to the advance made by Hegel over the system of thought developed by Kant, with his insistence on the a priori categories of reason. According to Pilling, the acceptance of Kant's outlook was the fundamental flaw in Althusser's work, encapsulated in Althusser's claim that 'history features in *Capital* as an object of theory, not as a real object'.[11] In other words, for Althusser, the extensive historical evidence in Marx's chief work was selectively refracted through a pre-existing conceptual framework based upon Marx's reading of classical political economy. Pilling gave a detailed refutation of this sceptical outlook, through a spirited defence of the dialectic, re-examining the fundamental concepts of *Capital* itself, while in addition – possibly influenced by his study of Rosdolsky and Rubin – emphasising the importance to our understanding of Marx, of grasping the overall structure of *Capital* as a whole work. The book concludes with a detailed examination of the nature of commodity fetishism, the process exclusive to capitalism whereby the natural human relation of man to man is transformed into a relation between 'things'. In a very real sense this issue suffused Pilling's Marxism, a leitmotiv running throughout his work, based upon a clear understanding that the socialist goal was the achievement of a 'truly human society'.

In his second major work, *The Crisis of Keynesian Economics: A Marxist View*,[12] Pilling produced a fascinating all-round study of Keynes's ideas and their influence. It was published in 1986 at the height of the Thatcherite onslaught in Britain, in a period when Keynesianism was thought to be officially buried. The attempted revival of Keynes's ideas in some circles in the 1990s gives Pilling's critique a fresh relevance. In particular the book takes issue with those sections of the left, who, from the 1930s onwards, saw in Keynes's vision either a viable alternative to Marxism or the possibility of a reconciliation between them. J.K. Galbraith, for example, was not alone in believing that the advent of the Keynesian revolution had 'brought Marxism in the advanced (*sic*) countries to a total halt'.[13] Alternatively, Joan Robinson, left-leaning member of Keynes's circle at Cambridge, declared that 'the systems of Keynes and Marx stand together'.[14]

Pilling showed that Keynes's claim to have made the decisive theoretical break with a pre-existing free-market orthodoxy was somewhat wide of the mark. With the advent of monopoly capitalism in the late nineteenth century, and the rapid increase in the size of the urban working class, the English policy of laissez-faire had been gradually abandoned. The state, crucial to capitalist development since its inception, in Britain at least since the Tudor Period, had come to play an increasingly central role in economic life. The ideas of academic economists for a generation before Keynes's work had reflected that shift. Nor was Keynes's attack on the rentier and on financial speculators particularly new. Similar views were being expressed by late nineteenth-century Fabian authors decades before, partly in response to the growing separation between the ownership and management of capital. Pilling's critique of Keynes's theoretical system focused principally on two major themes. First, drawing on his earlier work on Marx's method, Pilling discussed the abstract, ahistorical nature of the categories on which Keynes's economics is founded – investment, consumption, etc. – revealing their inadequacy, based as they are on a crude empiricism, as a means to comprehend the dynamics of capitalism. Second, he assessed Keynes's contribution to the long history of underconsumptionist theorists, noting his influence on a group of post-war writers in the Marxist tradition, from Baran and Sweezy to advocates of the 'permanent arms economy' thesis. Above all, Pilling's work on Keynes still provides a theoretical sheet-anchor in the battle against all those 'third-way' remnants of reformism in the labour movement, based as they are upon the (largely nostalgic) notion of the ability of the national state to insulate the majority of its citizens from the shrill winds of 'turbo-capitalism' at the millennium. His analysis confirmed him in the view that the period when it was possible for capitalism to grant concessions to the working class via the actions of the national state was over. As he wrote in the conclusion to the book: 'British capital is at the mercy of world forces over which she now has little or no control.'[15]

In his books, Pilling acknowledged a number of comrades and co-thinkers from within the Trotskyist movement who had helped to shape his own ideas. If one stands out it must be Tom Kemp, formerly Reader in Economic History at the University of Hull. It was Kemp who first interested Pilling in Marx's *Capital.* Following Kemp's death in 1993, Pilling turned his attention to the broader questions of the historical development of capitalism, a subject in which Kemp was an established scholar. To mark the centenary of Engels's death in 1885, Pilling co-edited with John Lea *The Condition of Britain*, a collection of essays which reflected upon 'the condition of the English working class' 100 years after Engels's classic study.[16] His own contribution to the book was a comparative historiography of the industrial revolution and Engels's place in it. He surveyed and then criticised three positions taken in that century-long debate. First, that Engels uncritically accepted Carlyle's romantic vision, based upon a critique of social inequality and the possibility of a new religion founded upon the 'cult of labour'. Second, that, measured in terms of rates of economic growth (to the nearest percentage point), the long period of capitalist development in England was marked not by revolution, but by gradualness. Finally, that the industrial revolution should be conceived principally in terms of the development of technique, as a period of rapid scientific and technical progress. Paradoxically, as Pilling shows in that essay, those who have interpreted the industrial revolution largely in terms of technique, at the expense of any consideration of the broader questions of social and political context, constitute an eclectic intellectual grouping. They ranged from early economic historians intent upon repudiating Marx, who identified the industrial revolution with changes in technology, through to Stalin's own crude distortion of historical materialism with its rigid distinction between the 'forces' and 'relations' of production. Pilling shows the baleful influence of such ideas even upon some of Stalin's erstwhile critics. Thus, for example, for Mandel: 'The first industrial revolution had been based on the steam engine, the second on the electric motor and the combustion engine. The third industrial revolution is based on the release of nuclear energy and the use of electronic machinery.'[17] Against such interpretations, Pilling argued persuasively, in defence of Engels, that at the heart of the industrial revolution was a profound transformation in social relations whose roots lay in the creation, for the first time in human history, of an industrial working class, developing in Manchester's textile districts.

Pilling was also a moving force behind the publication in 1996 of a memorial volume for Tom Kemp, jointly edited with Terry Brotherstone: *History, Economic History and the Future of Marxism.* In a chapter devoted to the impact of economic globalisation, Pilling responded to the free market triumphalism of the new world order that followed the fall of the Berlin wall. Using United Nations data he examined the growth in poverty, hunger and indebtedness on a world scale showing that for millions the question of 'socialism or barbarism' was not one to be resolved in some future period for barbarism was already a 'terrible ever-present reality'.[18] As he demonstrates, the essential features of the international economy in the 1990s – the dominance of the multinationals, the rapid growth in financial speculation and predatory merger activity leading to ever greater monopoly – had been mapped out long ago in Lenin's study of *Imperialism*. In the main body of the essay, Pilling returned to issues which had concerned him throughout his career, the history of the post-1945 period, the break-up of the Bretton Woods monetary system and the collapse of Keynesianism, drawing out the implications for the current Labour government in Britain.

As the essays in this volume testify, Pilling never succumbed to the pressure in academic life to become a narrow specialist doggedly pursuing a single theme. This was the result of more than mere intellectual curiosity, something that he had in great measure. Rather, I believe, it sprang from a recognition that to grasp the concrete, living reality required the 'concentration of many determinations' to use Marx's phrase. He paid careful attention to the latest developments in all aspects of society, testing the 'facts of experience' against his current conceptions, both within the areas of his own expertise and beyond, whether in the fields of philosophy, politics or economics. As global capitalism lurches from one crisis to the next, Pilling's work stands as an invaluable contribution to our understanding in the battles to come.

Keith Gibbard

Notes

1 Pilling, G. (1964) 'The crisis of post-war capitalism', *Fourth International*, 1 (2): 56–63.

2 Pilling, G. (1966) 'Imperialism and the liquidity crisis', *Fourth International*, 3 (1): 3–9. The argument was possibly influenced by Robert Triffin's (1961) *Gold and the Dollar Crisis*, New Haven: Yale University Press.

3 Pilling, G. (1966) 'An evaluation of John Maynard Keynes', *Fourth International*, 3 (4): 163–176.

4 Pilling, G. (1972) 'The law of value in Ricardo and Marx', *Economy and Society*, 1(3): 285.
5 Pilling, G. (1972) 'The law of value in Ricardo and Marx', *Economy and Society*, 1(3): 284.
6 Pilling, G. (1973) 'A reply to Professor Meek', *Economy and Society*, 2 (4): 505.
7 Pilling, G. (1980) *Marx's Capital: Philosophy and Political Economy*, London: Routledge & Kegan Paul.
8 Rubin, I.I. (1972) *Essays on Marx's Theory of Value*, Detroit: Black and Red; Marx, K. (1973) *Grundrisse*, Harmondsworth: Penguin; Rosdolsky, R. (1977) *The Making of Marx's Capital*, London: Pluto.
9 Ilyenkov, E. (1977) *Dialectical Logic*, Moscow: Progress Publishers.
10 As a contribution to that refutation, Pilling's 1972 article was subsequently republished in Fine, B. (1986) *The Value Dimension: Marx versus Ricardo and Sraffa*, London: Routledge & Kegan Paul.
11 Cited in Pilling, G. (1980) *Marx's Capital: Philosophy and Political Economy*, London: Routledge & Kegan Paul, p. 78.
12 Pilling, G. (1986) *The Crisis of Keynesian Economics: A Marxist View*, London: Croom Helm.
13 Pilling, G. (1986) *The Crisis of Keynesian Economics: A Marxist View*, London: Croom Helm, p. 3.
14 Pilling, G. (1986) *The Crisis of Keynesian Economics: A Marxist View*, London: Croom Helm, p. 17.
15 Pilling, G. (1986) *The Crisis of Keynesian Economics: A Marxist View*, London: Croom Helm, p. 160.
16 Lea, J. and Pilling, G. (eds) (1996) *The Condition of Britain: Essays on Frederick Engels*, London: Pluto Press.
17 Lea, J. and Pilling, G. (eds) (1996) *The Condition of Britain: Essays on Frederick Engels*, London: Pluto Press, p. 72.
18 Brotherstone, T. and Pilling, G. (eds) (1996) *History, Economic History and the Future of Marxism: Essays in Memory of Tom Kemp*, London: Porcupine Press, p. 15.

1 Recollections

Doria Pilling writes:

Geoff was planning a publication of a collection of his academic work before his untimely death in August 1997. The title of the present volume, the major part of its content, and the order of the chapters are as he planned. Chapter 5, 'A "third industrial revolution"? Marxism and the productive forces' is published here for the first time. Chapter 8, 'A very peculiar capitalism' appeared originally in *Thames Papers in Political Economy*, but the version included here was considerably re-worked by Geoff. Chapter 7, 'On disinterring Karl Marx' was also extensively re-written by Geoff since it appeared as a book review in *Workers International Press* in 1997. The other chapters consist of previously published articles and chapters from his books.

Geoff was born in 1940 in Ashton-under-Lyne in Greater Manchester, formerly a thriving cotton mill town, famous for its market. His parents were working-class, his father being a self-employed window cleaner for many years, and then working in the market. His mother worked as a secretary for a firm of carpet-fitters. Both parents encouraged him educationally and he went to Audenshaw Grammar School and then Leeds University to study economics. He obtained his BA in 1961 narrowly missing getting a first-class degree. He held posts as a lecturer in economics at Sheffield and Bradford universities, and joined Middlesex Polytechnic (later Middlesex University) in 1969, where he eventually obtained a readership. In 1983 he obtained a PhD from Kingston Polytechnic entitled *The Nature and Significance of Marx's Critique of Classical Political Economy.*

The originality and impact of Geoff's academic work are detailed in the speech that Ben Fine made at his Memorial Meeting at Middlesex University in November 1997, which is included in the Foreword to this book, and in Keith Gibbard's Introduction to the book. His ideas reached across the world, as is made clear in the specially written contribution by the Japanese economist, Kazuto Iida, translator into Japanese of Geoff's *The Crisis of Keynesian Economics: A Marxist View.*[1]

Geoff's penetrating and painstaking critiques of orthodox British Marxist political economists and of Keynesianism were never made in the pursuit of academic recognition. As Cliff Slaughter, lecturer at Leeds and Bradford Universities and Marxist scholar, wrote to me, after Geoff died:

> Everybody knows that he had great talent, but most important of all, about Geoff, was that he never had a single thought of directing that talent to any other purpose than the cause of the working class from which he came. He had no thought of personal 'success' or self advancement, but proceeded always with great intellectual courage to defend the cause of working class emancipation and the theory necessary to achieve that emancipation, against every enemy of the working class and socialism, and against all those who falsified those theories and ideals.... He gave his whole life to what he passionately believed in, and no more can be said of any man.

That he could have had such recognition was obvious in the comments of his academic referees when he was eventually persuaded to apply for a readership at Middlesex University because it would give him more time for writing and research. They could not understand why he had not applied for a readership, or a professorship, years earlier.

Geoff was an inspiring teacher. His colleague, John Lea, said at the funeral

> his attitude, his meticulous thoroughness, the depth of his knowledge of the classics in his field and his healthy scepticism toward the temporary fads and fashions which come and go in the social sciences.... This, combined with his engagement with what was happening in the world today and with the need to understand it and his unfaltering optimism that things could be different, made him one of the best teachers that it has been our privilege to work with.

Geoff set up and ran an MA in Political Economy, and also taught some modules on it. One of the students on the course, Andy Denis, now Director of Undergraduate Studies in the Department of Economics at City University London wrote to me

> It was a great course, and was absolutely critical for my own development. In opposition to the formalist technocracy of the neoclassical mainstream, the course located controversy in economics in its historical and philosophical context. Again, instead of presenting economics as a monolith, space was made for dissenting points of view such as Austrianism, Marxism and all the various shades of Keynesianism.

Geoff was deeply worried for his young grandsons, Dylan and Travis, and all future generations about what would happen if capitalist society were not replaced by socialism. He would be even more convinced of this need today. He would be alarmed at the ever-present threat of terrorism and the prospect of a prolonged European – and even a global – recession. He would be saddened by continuing conflicts in Africa, the Middle East and elsewhere and appalled that a world with abundant food resources could still produce so much hunger and malnutrition. In the United States, he would see signs of rising class tension and even talk of American secular decline as evidence of an existential crisis at the heart of western capitalism. If his lifetime views are anything to go by, he would doubtless be watching such momentous developments with a mixture of anxiety and optimism. The socialist society Geoff envisaged bore no relationship to the so-called communism of the Soviet bloc. Indeed, he saw the collapse of that bloc, and of Communist parties, as providing a tremendous opportunity to build a new political party which would be a step towards creating a socialist society.

When a student at Leeds University, Geoff was introduced by Cliff Slaughter to the ideas of Leon Trotsky, and became convinced that Trotsky's analysis of the degeneration of the 1917 October revolution in Russia as due to Stalin's theory of 'Socialism in One Country' was correct. Geoff subsequently joined the Socialist Labour League (SLL) (which later became the Workers' Revolutionary Party (WRP)), to which Cliff Slaughter had been attracted when he left the Communist party because of Khrushchev's revelations about Stalinism and the Soviet Union's crushing of the 1956 Hungarian revolution. Another of these ex-Communist Party scholars, Tom Kemp, lecturer in economic history at Hull University, also had a profound influence on Geoff, introducing him to Marx's *Capital.*

Having joined the SLL, Geoff immediately became involved in lecturing at a summer camp. He became a frequent contributor on economic and historical questions to the party's daily newspaper, *Workers' Press* after its launch in 1969. He took numerous classes on Marxism, and lectured regularly at the Derbyshire College of Marxist Education after its establishment. He never wavered in his conviction of the correctness of Trotsky's analysis or the need to overthrow capitalism but he made several attempts to leave the party, having grave misgivings about the way theoretical differences within the party were treated. Lack of an alternative movement to which he could commit himself always drew him back. Whatever difficulties he was having within the party, though, he never allowed these to divert him from his intensive study of Marx's *Capital*, of political economy and of philosophy.

A revolt in 1985 led to the end of the old leadership of Gerry Healey in the WRP and gave Geoff new political energy. He was at the forefront in activities which brought the party closer to working class struggles. He edited for a time the now weekly *Workers' Press*, opening it to wider theoretical debate. He took part in the discussions and demonstrations of migrant workers and refugees. He was an enthusiastic initiator and organiser of 'Workers' Aid for Bosnia', our small study becoming deluged with faxes from Zagreb, as the first convoy taking food struggled to find a way of reaching its destination, the besieged multi-ethnic city of Tuzla. Faruk Ibrahimović, unable to return home to Tuzla because of the war and working at the Tuzla Logistic Society in Zagreb, which was trying to organise supplies to the city, became a leading member of Workers' Aid. He writes about Geoff's role in this Recollections chapter. In the summer of 1995 a 24-hour Whitehall picket was organised, demanding a lifting of the one-sided arms embargo, and an end to genocide in Bosnia, and Geoff regularly got a very early tube train into London to take part. He also forged a close relationship with the leaders of the Liverpool dockers, fighting for reinstatement of 500 dockers dismissed for 'being in breach of their contract of employment', for refusing to cross a picket line. In the paper published by the Liverpool Dock Shop Stewards Committee, the *Dockers' Charter*, Geoff wrote about how the dockers' demand for 'The People's Charter for Social Justice' was in the tradition of the People's Charter 160 years earlier, Chartism being a movement which he had studied closely and for which he had great sympathy.

Geoff had a biting wit, and could hold an audience spellbound, in the local pub as much as in the lecture theatre or on a political platform. His interests were wide. He loved classical music, and could provide a detailed commentary on Beethoven's symphonies or Haydn's. He was particularly fond of opera, Verdi's Rigoletto, Mozart's Magic Flute and Bizet's Carmen being among his favourites. But he'd also often listen to Tony Bennett, Neil Diamond or Elkie Brooks. He loved Shakespeare, read French rather than English nineteenth-century novels, liked crime novels and humorous books, including those of P.G. Wodehouse and Tom Sharp. He loved comedy, from Chaplin and the Marx Brothers to 'Sergeant Bilko', 'Hancock's Half Hour' and 'Yes Minister'. 'Inspector Morse' was a favoured means of relaxation. He was an excellent cook, inventing rather than following recipes, and enjoyed showing off his skills to guests. He was fascinated by technology, and we possessed an infuriating (as it was always breaking down) word processor he'd asked a friend to make before the Amstrad came on the scene. Coming from Ashton-under-Lyne in Greater Manchester, Geoff was a devoted Manchester United supporter, but after moving to London he also became a strong supporter of our local football club, Brentford, and when he had time we'd spend Saturday afternoons there. He was proud of his son's table tennis talent, and was as well known at our local club as at the university. Geoff had an interest in, and could make almost everything, interesting.

This interest included that in the cancer that indirectly killed him. He bore this distressing illness with immense fortitude. He seemed to be on the road to a good recovery, and was planning much future work, so it was a tremendous shock when he died unexpectedly from a thrombosis which was probably an effect of the surgery he had undergone.

Geoff's death was devastating not only to me and our son David, and his parents, but to many of his friends, colleagues and political comrades. Now, almost 15 years later, friends often ask me what Geoff would have thought about the current political situation, or some particular issue. It is hoped that the present book will inspire others to carry out meticulous analyses of capitalist society, as he did, in the pursuit of changing it for a better society.

In writing this introductory section I have drawn heavily on the obituary written for the Guardian *by Terry Brotherstone and on that written by Bob Archer in the* Workers International Press, *11, 97.*

Kazuto Iida, Professor of Political Economy, Meiji University, Tokyo, writes:

It was in 1988 that I met Dr. Pilling for the first time. Of course, I had known of him and read some of his works before then. They were 'The law of value in

Ricardo and Marx', 1972,[2] *Marx's Capital: Philosophy and Political Economy*, 1980,[3] and *The Crisis of Keynesian Economics: A Marxist View*, 1986.[4]

His treatise of 1972 is well-known amongst Marxist economists in Japan. It was translated into Japanese and included in the book, *New Development of Western Marxist Economics* (in Japanese) published in 1979, which gathered the works of famous authors, including for example, Maurice Dobb 'The Sraffa system and critique of the neo-classical theory of distribution', 1979; Ronald L. Meek 'Marginalism and Marxism', 1972 and Bob Rowthorn 'Neo-classicism, neo-Ricardianism and Marxism', 1974. This was the first work of Dr. Pilling's that I read.

When I read his book published in 1980, I wanted to meet him and ask him about his views on Marx's economics directly. In this book he emphasised the significance of the notion of fetishism as the critical idea for understanding Marx's critique of political economy. Studying Marx's *Capital* from such a viewpoint would be uncommon among western Marxist economists. However, this kind of study has been very popular in Japanese academic circles. He has been highly estimated in Japan as a unique economist amongst western Marxists. In this book he examined the opening chapters of *Capital* in detail, to define Marx's method of philosophy and political economy. Through this examination, he demonstrated that the opening chapters of *Capital* have a decisive significance for the work as a whole and that fetishism is a key concept for Marx's system. I agree with his understanding on the Marx's method.

Moreover, he applied the same method as in Marx's critique of political economy in his second book, *The Crisis of Keynesian Economics: A Marxist View*, published in 1986. After reading this book I decided to translate it into Japanese, because it would be very useful for Japanese Marxist economists to know about his theoretical standpoint in criticising Keynesian economics.

Fortunately I was given sabbatical leave by the university in 1988. So I planned to visit London for this period and to translate his book after discussing it with him. It was in April of 1988 that I was able to go to London and meet him.

Dr. Pilling wrote this book conscious of J. Hicks' work, *The Crisis in Keynesian Economics*.[5] We can easily see this from the title of his book, *The Crisis of Keynesian Economics: A Marxist View*. However, the purpose of Hicks' work was to realise the reconciliation of Keynesian economics with neo-classical economics, that is, the neo-classical synthesis. In contrast Dr. Pilling's book was so critical of the Keynesian economics in itself that the validity of the 'Keynesian revolution' in the received popular view of the history of economics was denied.

He strongly advocated in this book that it was necessary for the Marxist economist to go back to the origin of Marx's method, the critique of political economy. He demonstrated that a superior framework for the analysis of modern capitalism could only be posed in this way, as he showed in his book. He believed, I think, that Marxist economics should be developed in this direction. He advocated this to the Marxist economist in the English-speaking area, and it also applies to the Marxist economist in Japan.

My sabbatical year in London was successful. I could talk over, while translating his book into Japanese, the various matters of modern economics with him. We used to drink and discuss with each other in a pub in the university. It is my precious memory in London.

The Japanese version of his book was published in March of 1991. It was one and half years after I came back to Japan. Through this publication, he became more widely known among Japanese Marxist economists. They discovered again that Dr. Pilling was a unique theorist, as his treatise of 1972 had shown.

After that, he told me in a letter about his plan for his next publication. The theme was, as far as I remember, a study of the history of currency controversy since the nineteenth century. Thereby he would aim to open up a new field in the study of money. He would apply the same method in this book too, that is the critique of political economy.

Now I am very sorry that he was not able to realise it. If this book had been published, the name of Geoffrey Pilling would be unassailable as an excellent economist. Then, of course, I would have been the first candidate for the translator of the Japanese version of the book.

Presentation at the Memorial Meeting for Geoff organised by the Workers International to Rebuild the Fourth International on 25 April 1998 by WIRFI Secretary Dot Gibson:

It is difficult at a meeting like this to know where to begin and what to leave out. Over the 12 years, since we expelled Gerry Healy and his supporters from the Workers Revolutionary Party in 1985 until Geoff Pilling's death on 20 August last year, he and I worked together closely on all aspects of party activity and got to know each other's thoughts and reasoning very well.

Our political paths were different. Geoff had a university education and made a constant study of Marxism. I had no such education and had spent 20 years before 1985 in party administration of the most oppressive kind. As usual and in common with other comrades in the leadership of the party our development in those 12 years took place through contradiction and conflict. Between us there was often political antagonism, but not personal animosity.

I will treasure always the memory of Geoff's total unselfishness with his knowledge and abilities – his patience, his constant striving for a truly communist party in all aspects of his life. He was painstaking in his efforts to explain and understand; he was never tired of assisting us to write in *Workers Press*, to suggest reading material and to think about and come back to our doubts and questions as his own concerns. This did not mean that he gave any quarter in the cut and thrust of political and theoretical battle as many here know. But there was nothing aloof about Geoff.

What I am pleased about is that in the last two years of Geoff's life we witnessed and participated in what we recognised to be an important development and break in the working class movement, particularly reflected in the leadership of the Liverpool dockers' struggle, and this came together with our understanding in the Workers Revolutionary Party that the working class needed its own new socialist party.

The development of the Liverpool dockers' struggle made more acute the question that was uppermost in Geoff's mind – what he considered to be Marxism's greatest single discovery – the revolutionary nature of the working class and its struggle.

In 1995 jointly with John Lea he had edited the book *The Condition of Britain*, to mark the 100th anniversary of the death of Frederick Engels and the 150th anniversary of Engel's book *The Condition of the Working Class in England.* In his chapter in that commemorative book 'Engels and the industrial revolution' Geoff rejected the opponents of Engels's view and demonstrated that the industrial revolution was not simply the development of machinery and factories, it produced the modern working class that was forced to fight its oppression and 'help itself'. As Geoff was fond of quoting, Engels said it 'was not simply a hopeless, trampled-down class, but one that was forced to fight against the conditions into which it had been plunged'.

Geoff explained that taking up the question of the nature and consequences of the industrial revolution was part of a wider project. To use his words, 'the rescuing of Engels and Marx from the fate that befell them after their deaths'.

'Their creative work,' he said 'become distorted beyond belief, in part in the lifetime of the Second International, but above all in the period when the Stalinist bureaucracy ruled the Soviet Union and controlled a significant sector of the world's labour movement'.

Geoff was absorbed by a deep desire to get underneath the skin, so to speak, of Engels's thinking and method, when Engels said that 'The condition of the working class is the *real basis and point of departure* of all social movements of the present because it is the *highest and most unconcealed* pinnacle of the social misery existing in our day.' Geoff said that this 'allowed Engels to speak of the "world historical significance" of the transformation he studied.'

As part of the preparation for the chapter in *The Condition of Britain* Geoff gave four lectures on Chartism and Socialism. They were not just on history as something in and of itself, he said. They were conducted, organised and written from the standpoint of Britain today, which is now at a decisive historical turning point in the history of the working-class movement.

At the first of these lectures Geoff recalled that he had been working on a lead for *Workers Press*, and was toying with the idea of a headline 'Death of the welfare state', but thought that maybe this was too dramatic. However he bought the *Guardian* and saw that it too had reported on the speech by Labour's front bench spokesman on welfare matters saying that it heralded the end of the welfare state. He realised that this was a warning to us not to underestimate the depth of this historical crisis and the enormous shock for millions of workers.

The Chartist movement was born out of deep shock among millions of workers and poor people. They had supported and taken part in the campaign for the reform of parliament against the landed aristocracy, only to find that the reformed parliament in the hands of the new arising capitalist class enforced the Poor Law against them, sending millions of unemployed and poor people into virtual imprisonment in Workhouses.

A Labour government returned on 1 May 1997 with millions of workers looking for some respite to 18 years of Toryism. But this party, which has been the political expression of millions of workers for nearly 100 years must now more than ever before come out in its true colours and attack workers on behalf of the capitalist state it represents. We are experiencing just that kind of historical turning point which brings great shocks and must bring great convulsive events.

Geoff was convinced that a renewed study of Chartism was vital for today, and he was deeply interested when the Merseyside Port Shop Stewards Committee published their draft Charter and held the March for Social Justice in April last year. This had followed the call by stewards for a political/industrial committee and 'representative democracy' for the working class. Geoff recognised the significance of an industrial dispute turning its attention to all layers in the workers' movement, calling for a united struggle.

He wanted to study further Lenin's estimation of Chartism as the 'first truly mass and political organised proletarian revolutionary movement'. Lenin did not mean that it was the first in Britain, said Geoff. It was the first in the world. And he referred to Trotsky's statement that 'every fundamental problem of the working class movement was posed by Chartism'.

Explaining the empire as the very solid historical foundation for reformism in the British working-class movement, nevertheless Geoff argued that this should not be absolutised. There has always been a revolutionary element in the working-class movement that represented the real historical aspirations of the working class, and it was from this point of view that he wanted to tackle further study for today's situation.

Engels had said it was evident that the workers' movement was divided into two sections. The Chartists and the Socialists (meaning mainly Robert Owen). 'The Chartists are theoretically the more backward, the less developed, but they are genuine proletarians all over – the true representatives of their class,' said Engels. 'The Socialists are more far seeing. They propose practical remedies against distress, but proceeding originally from the bourgeoisie are for this reason unable to amalgamate completely with the working class'.

'I suggest this is our problem,' said Engels. 'The union of socialism with Chartism will be the next step and has already begun. Then only – when this has been achieved – will the working class be the true intellectual leader of England. Meanwhile political and social development will proceed and will foster this new party, this new departure for Chartism.'

Geoff considered that this is the task we now face as Marxists. The Trotskyist movement had been bedevilled by discussions about the correctness of this, the correctness of that, the correctness of the other, he said. But often, through no fault of its own, it was quite remote from the living real problems of the millions of ordinary people.

He was proud that it was our movement which had predicted from the 1970s that capitalism had entered a new period of real structural fundamental world crisis, had opposed those who said that the Keynesian settlement was final, that the Soviet Union was building socialism, that the days of crisis and catastrophe were over and we were in the era of peaceful co-existence. In fact he wrote the decisive document on the world crisis in the 1970s, and it was on the basis of his theoretical work on the crisis that our perspectives were based. But he was concerned that it wasn't simply 'being right' that created the possibilities for the new socialist party that the working class needs.

He was proud to write for the *Dockers Charter* the article on the 149th anniversary of the Chartists' march from Kennington Common, and an answer to the Thatcherite economist Professor Patrick Minford when he attacked the dockers. But more than anything else, he was most happy when he could meet the dockers and listen to them. To hear what they thought about the political movement, about the problems of their struggle, about their experiences, about their methods of organising internationally. They have so much to teach us; we have so much to learn, he said. If we don't understand that we will never be able to participate in the building of the new party.

Our party, with others had initiated the Movement for Socialism. Geoff was concerned that it should not be directed towards the overtly political people but that it should be integrated into workers' struggles. He saw this as part of the reconstruction of the Fourth International and did not back down from making his views on this known out of fear that workers would be put off. In any case this reconstruction could not be separated from the need for Marxists to be joined to the workers' movement, and Engels had pointed the way when he talked of 'the new departure for Chartism'.

Geoff had had no problem whatsoever in discussing this with the dockers, even those who had grown up in the Communist Party. He saw no reason to somehow hide the fact that we are Trotskyists. He was looking forward to inviting them to our own Workers International congress to report on their experiences and listen to what we saw as our problems and tasks.

Mainly he was confident that the way forward was to work in theory and practice on the revolutionary nature of the working class and its struggle. He would continue to collaborate with others to develop an understanding of the world crisis of capitalism and to participate to the full in the workers' struggles coming into being.

He was looking forward to resuming these tasks. There is no doubt that he would have been at the heart of fighting for the second March for Social Justice on 30 May and for the development of the *Dockers Charter*.

Faruk Ibrahimović, a leading member of Workers' Aid for Bosnia, writes:
I am a Bosnian and you may wonder what relationship I had with Geoff Pilling. The story is long but I'll try to make it short.

The war in Bosnia was raging and I was stuck in Zagreb (Croatia) on my way back to Tuzla from Holland. There I heard about the Workers' Aid for Bosnia convoy. We, at the Tuzla Logistic Centre in Zagreb, were very happy that somebody from a European country was supporting Tuzla and its multi-ethnicity.

It was the summer of 1993. The people that arrived on the convoy were untidy and unshaved. But, they were brave and sincere friends of Bosnia and

Tuzla people. They had organised demonstrations in the United Kingdom in support of Bosnia and Tuzla and against their own government, which considered the aggression on Bosnia as an 'ethnic war'. That convoy did not manage to get through to Tuzla, but the desire to organise another one, bigger, with more aid and people was evident. The first convoy that reached Tuzla came in the spring of 1994.

While the convoy members were collecting necessary documents to leave Croatia two people in the United Kingdom were the brains of all the activities. They made links with Croatian Trade Unions animating them to support Bosnians in their fight against the nationalism and division of the country. Later in October 1993 I met them both in the United Kingdom.

One of them was Geoff Pilling. He had the power of attracting people and making people listen to him. He and most of the people around him were Trotskyists. From what I had learned in school Leon Trotsky was an outlaw. Now I had a chance to meet his followers. At that moment I did not think that we would become friends.

His and his wife's house in Acton Town became my starting point, my logistic base, for numerous trips in the United Kingdom. Both of them were very hospitable. They took me as a family member. They answered telephone calls, took messages, directed me on how to reach a certain place, and supported me. Geoff seized every opportunity to advise me on what to say, and sometimes helped me to write my speeches. Once I wanted to write a letter to the editor of the *Guardian*. Geoff told me that my text should not exceed 300 words. When I finished, the text was more than 700 words. He did a lot of work to make it under 300 words. Then he faxed it and the following day the text appeared in the paper.

Geoff inspired, organised and participated in many demonstrations in support of oppressed peoples. He told me about the first demonstration in support of Bosnia. They had gathered together at Hyde Park Corner and marched to Trafalgar Square. It was so windy and freezing cold that only six people arrived at Trafalgar Square to deliver their speeches.

After the fall of Srebrenica we organised big demonstrations, involving many other organisations. At that time the Workers Press had a very small office in the basement of a bookstore. Geoff telephoned his friends – colleagues – asking them for donations. We needed the money to pay for an advertisement on the cover page of the *Guardian.* Geoff looked very tired. After a while he took a cushion from an armchair, folded it, lay down on the floor and put his head on it. He slept only for a short while as the office was very busy.

It was around Christmas. I was preparing to leave for Tuzla on a mid-day flight. Geoff wanted to buy me a present for Christmas, although I am a Muslim. He knew that I am interested in computers and he decided to buy me a motherboard – the motherboard of all motherboards, as he said – with a high speed processor. So we left Acton early in the morning and arrived in Tottenham Court Road just before the shop opened. Paying for the goods he said that we had plenty of time and that we could have a Belgian beer and he took me to a pub near Leicester Square. Later on I realised that his mother had given him some money for Christmas, and that he wanted to share it with his friends. He left nothing or very little for himself.

The war in Bosnia was over, I got a job in Tuzla and my visits became less frequent. Then I was told that Geoff had some health problems and would have to undergo an operation. The operation went well.

Some time later I got a sad message from a friend in Manchester that Geoff had passed away. I did not know what to do since it was the first time in my life that my friend, who lived in a foreign country, had died. Tradition and culture are different. But I knew for sure that I had to call Doria and express my sympathy. I promised her I would come for the funeral. At the funeral his friends spoke about his work, both at the university and in his party. I was proud of the friend I had, although unfortunately it was not for so long. I was coming and spending days and nights in his house but he did not have the opportunity to come to Bosnia, the country he was striving for so fiercely.

Notes

1 Pilling, G. (1986) *The Crisis of Keynesian Economics: A Marxist View*, London: Croom Helm.
2 Pilling, G. (1972) 'The law of value in Ricardo and Marx', *Economy and Society*, 1 (3): 281–307.
3 Pilling, G. (1980) *Marx's Capital: Philosophy and Political Economy*, London: Routledge & Kegan Paul.
4 Pilling, G. (1986) *The Crisis of Keynesian Economics: A Marxist View*, London: Croom Helm.
5 Hicks, J. (1974) *The Crisis in Keynesian Economics*, Oxford: Basil Blackwell.

2 'Globalisation' and the British working class

An essay in economic analysis and political prognosis[1]

Introduction

This chapter is concerned with the developing contradictions of post-war capitalism and with some of their political implications in Britain. One basic consideration must be emphasised – that in the twentieth century we live in the epoch of *world* economy and *world* politics. The chapter begins by looking at the catastrophe overtaking millions upon millions of people, especially in Africa, Latin America, and Asia. It is argued that this is by no means a manifestation of the problems of those areas: it can be explained only from the standpoint of the nature of the world capitalist system in the epoch of its decline and decay. Likewise, when we turn to the particular features of British capitalism, its crisis and related developments in the class struggle: these cannot be artificially abstracted from their world context.

Capitalism on the eve of the twenty-first century

The collapse of the states of Eastern Europe and of the Soviet Union between 1989 and 1991 brought a predictable response from apologists for the bourgeois social order: 'Socialism is dead'. In the year the Berlin Wall fell, Francis Fukuyama (1992) notoriously declared that the 'end of history' had arrived. The idea that the Stalinist regimes were ever socialist is, in my view, absurd, but that question must be left aside. But where does *capitalism* actually stand in the mid-1990s? What has the much-celebrated 'market economy', as its apologists currently prefer to call it, achieved on the eve of the twenty-first century? If we start with the colonial and semi-colonial countries, we find that the United Nations (UN) – which Marxists, developing Lenin's analysis of its forerunner, the League of Nations, have seen as one of the chief instruments of the contemporary capitalist order – itself gives a grim answer to this question. Towards the end of 1994, the UN issued a series of figures produced as part of the preparation for a World Summit for Social Development held in March 1995. They reveal that of the world's 5.6 billion people, one in five live in poverty – defined by the UN as those in receipt of an income below \$275 a year. Over 1.5 billion lack access to clean drinking water or basic sanitation. After 50 years of 'development plans' and the like launched by the World Bank and cognate bodies the situation gets worse, not better. At the time of writing (late 1995), half a billion people go to sleep hungry each night and on the basis of present trends, a further 200 million people in the colonial countries alone will be plunged into grinding poverty by the end of the century. Of the planet's nearly three billion labour force there are 120 million people actively looking for work – but in the great majority of cases without result or hope. But what is particularly striking about these data is that although, not surprisingly, poverty is concentrated in the colonial and semi-colonial countries, it is growing rapidly in North America and western Europe where one in six currently live below the poverty line. Technical changes in production, dominated as they are by the needs of capital, far from bringing the 'affluent society' nearer, are destroying jobs in the 'rich' and 'poor' countries alike. London, still one of the world's leading financial centres, has 40,000 registered homeless; there are 10,000 with no home in Paris, out of a total of 50,000 homeless in France as a whole. Nearly a quarter of a million New Yorkers have stayed in shelters over the last five years. This is more than 3 per cent of the city's population and includes more than one in 12 of its black children. Over 26 million people in the United States are on food stamps – one in ten of the population.

Women represent 70 per cent of the poverty-stricken people of the world, followed by the elderly and children. Infant mortality rates are about 175 per 1,000 live births in Africa and close to 100 in India. In the big capitalist countries the figure is 15 per 1,000 live births. Imperialism has created conditions where whole continents are rotting away. In Africa half the population is impoverished; the major agencies show that in terms of national food consumption, food production, sources of food, and income levels, 27 African countries can be defined as 'at risk', that is, vulnerable at any time to famine. The 1980s have been a nightmare for the vast majority of the population in sub-Saharan Africa. UN (1993) figures reveal that at the end of the 1980s some 35 per cent of the people in that region (totalling 175 million) were living in a state of 'chronic under-nourishment'. This represented an increase of over 80 million compared with ten years earlier. The number of people in the world as a whole who were chronically under-nourished came to a staggering 786 million at the end of the 1980s. Between 1980 and 1986, per capita GDP in sub-Saharan Africa fell by 20 per cent, the terms of trade by 34 per cent, and the real minimum wage by 20 per cent. Per capita imports dropped by 65 per cent over this period. These trends are, on average, between two and three times worse than for Latin America. In 1988, Africa's debt-service burden accounted for 60 per cent of export earnings and the states of the sub-Sahara paid the International Monetary Fund some $1 billion more than they received in 'grants' and 'aid'. Austerity in the shape of state reductions in health services, limited capacity to import food in times of crisis, growing income inequalities and unemployment, and a compelling pressure to generate export revenue from the rural sector makes these countries less and less resistant to famine and disease (see Watts 1991). Figures of this sort reveal that 'socialism or barbarism' is not simply a theoretical alternative posed for the future. For millions and millions of people barbarism is a terrible, ever-present, reality. The bubonic plague, which many thought had been consigned to history, returns to strike down innocent people in India, and other diseases that were long ago held to have been eradicated are once again in evidence.[2] Yet at the same time the world is increasingly dominated by a handful of giant monopolies and financial institutions, some of which have incomes in excess of many of the largest colonial and semi-colonial countries.[3]

These facts exemplify, not a series of discrete 'area' problems, but the contradictions of post-war capitalism as a whole. The system's overall crisis, in other words, is the real context of what appear as particular local problems. The same consideration applies when we come to look at the particular features of British capitalism and of the impact of its crisis on the working class and the labour movement.

Imperialism and the crisis in Britain

Naturally the development of capitalism, including the (changing) forms taken by its crisis, exhibit definite peculiarities in each country. Thus the particular features of British capitalism in large measure result from the fact that as an industrial power it was 'first in the field'. This pioneering role not only made Britain, albeit for a relatively brief period, the 'workshop of the world' but also helps explain the decline of her industries over a period stretching out over the last century. Likewise, Britain's historical primacy in industrialisation also explains the peculiar role of the City of London in the functioning of British capital. Understanding this is, in its turn, important for an appreciation of the pre-eminence of the banks and other financial institutions over industrial capital – a factor much lamented by the Keynesians and others.

With the arrival of the twentieth century, capitalism entered the stage of its development, more strictly speaking its decline, known to Marxists as imperialism.[4] In the most general sense, imperialism is characterised by the fact that capitalism had, by the start of the present century, reached a stage where humankind's productive forces came into historical conflict with the social relations within which they had previously developed. Lenin placed great emphasis on the point arrived at in the socialisation of production and the stage it had reached with the advent of the present century, and this will be a major theme of this chapter's efforts to analyse some of the key developments in world economy since Lenin wrote his pamphlet on imperialism. Referring to those who drew attention to the increasing 'interlocking' of financial and industrial capital, Lenin noted:

> [B]ut underlying this interlocking, its very base, are the changing social relations of production. When a big enterprise assumes gigantic proportions, and on the basis of an exact computation of mass data, organises according to plan the supply of primary raw materials to the extent of two-thirds, or three-fourths, of all that is necessary for tens of millions of people; when the

> raw materials are transported in a systematic and organised manner to the most suitable places of production, sometimes situated hundreds or thousands of miles from each other; when a single centre directs all the consecutive stages of processing the material right up to the manufacture of numerous varieties of finished articles; when these products are distributed according to a single plan amongst tens of hundreds of millions of consumers ... then it becomes evident that we have socialisation of production, and not mere 'interlocking'.
>
> (Lenin 1964: 302–303)

Quite obviously the processes that Lenin outlined have advanced enormously since 1916, to the point that he could hardly have imagined. The following factors are important in considering the way in which the socialisation of production has proceeded in the intervening eight decades:

1 One expression of this socialisation process in the post-war period was the fact that international *trade* in industrial products grew at two-and-a-half times the rate of the production of such goods. In other words an ever-greater share of the production of each country was sold on the world market. It is instructive to look at these trends in historical perspective. If we break down the period from the start of the eighteenth century to the early 1960s into three roughly equal periods (of some 80 years each) the following pattern emerges. In the first period, from 1720 until 1800, world trade increased somewhat less than fivefold; in the second stage (1800 until circa 1880) it expanded tenfold. In the third period, from 1880 until 1960, slightly less than tenfold. Thus, overall, the rise of capitalism is associated with an accelerating growth of world trade. But it is significant to note that in the last four decades of the nineteenth century the rate of growth suffered a considerable setback. Here already was an anticipation of the increasing restrictions that capitalism was placing on the growth of the productive forces and the international division of labour. This was the period of the rapid industrialisation of countries that were already successfully challenging Britain's position as 'workshop of the world'. Germany and the United States built up their industries behind various protectionist walls, and this found its reflection in the slowdown in the expansion of world trade. Even more significant are the figures relating the share of world trade to world output, a rough indicator of the division of labour in world economy. According to these data, the share of world trade fell back significantly in the last two decades of the nineteenth century, to rise rapidly again in the period immediately prior to World War I. During the period of that war and in the slump of the 1930s it fell rapidly again. Even though the share rose steadily in the period after 1945, in 1960–1962 it still lagged significantly behind the 1876–1880 level. Comparing the world output of manufactured goods with the volume of exports of manufactures, we find the following: in 1929, the latter (exports) was equivalent to 89 per cent of the former

(production); by 1937 the figure had dropped to 64 per cent; in 1948, on the eve of the post-war boom it was 55 per cent and thereafter rose steadily until the end of the long boom when it was 123 per cent.[5]

2 The trend towards the concentration of capital, for Lenin one of imperialism's key features, has continued apace in the post-war period. Thus in the United States, the number of company mergers or take-overs in the manufacturing industries and in mining rose from 3,365 in the period 1955–1959 to 8,213 a decade later. In Britain in the early 1970s 100 firms accounted for half of overall manufacturing production; in France the top 100 firms were responsible for two-thirds of overall manufacturing output. In the United States the top 500 corporations were responsible for over three-quarters of total sales.

3 This socialisation of production is also expressed in the increasing preponderance of the multinational corporations in world economy. Thus United Nations statistics show that in the quarter-century 1951–1975 alone, the 180 biggest US transnational corporations operating in the manufacturing sphere founded or bought out some 14,000 branches or subsidiaries abroad.

4 Even more significant as a reflection of the globalisation of economic activity has been the huge increase in the export of capital over the last two decades especially. By the end of the 1980s, direct investment made by the capitalists of all countries outside their national borders had reached $1.5 trillion. But what is significant is not so much the sum involved as the speed of its growth over the last two decades. For the figure almost tripled in the 1980s alone. Put another way: for the period 1983–1989 the outflows of direct investment to other countries rose by almost 29 per cent each year, whereas world exports rose much more slowly – at about 9 per cent a year – and world domestic product even more slowly. And the investment involved went far beyond manufacturing and the extraction of raw materials. To an ever-greater extent it involved such areas as finance, real estate, insurance, advertising and the media. In the 1950s and early 1960s most foreign investments came from US corporations, although Britain, which was able to reinvest earnings from previous investments, was also important in this respect. But, as part of her relative loss of power, the United States had to face increasing competition from other countries in the field of foreign investment. Thus whereas in 1960 almost half of all direct foreign investment originated from the United States, by the end of the 1980s this had dropped to under 30 per cent. The figure for Japan had risen from under 1 per cent to over 11 per cent during the same period.[6]

5 There has been an astronomical growth of bank lending across national frontiers. In the past such activity was regarded as abnormal. As recently as the mid-1960s the volume of international banking reached only approximately 10 per cent of the combined national incomes of the capitalist countries. By the mid-1980s that figure had doubled. The comparison with world trade is even more striking. A normal function of international banking is to facilitate world trade and some 30 years ago the volume of banking activity

across national borders came to about 10 per cent of world trade. Over the last two decades that volume has swollen out of all proportion with world trade, and by the middle of the last decade it actually exceeded the volume of trade of the capitalist countries. This is how one leading financial institution sums up these trends:

> The [economic and financial instability of the 1970s] engendered government deficits and external imbalances that required financing on a scale unprecedented in peacetime and that exceeded the capacity or willingness of the traditionally fragmented financial markets to cover. These financing needs joined with the advances in technology and communications to spawn a host of innovations ranging from securitisation in place of intermediated bank credit to new derivatives including swaps. Taken together these financial innovations have helped overwhelm traditional and regulatory segmentation of national markets and thereby have contributed much to the effective integration of financial markets globally.
>
> (Morgan Guaranty Trust Company 1991)

Or as another writer puts it:

> [World trade in goods and services] amounts to around $2.5 trillion to $3 trillion a year. But the London Eurodollar market, in which the world's financial institutions borrow and lend to each other, turns over $300 billion each working day, or $75 trillion a year, a volume at least 25 times that of world trade. In addition, there are foreign exchange transactions in the world's money centres, in which one currency is traded against another. These run around $150 billion a day, or about $35 trillion a year – 12 times the world-wide trade in goods and services. Of course, many of these Eurodollars, yen, and Swiss francs are just being moved from one pocket to another and may be counted more than once. A massive discrepancy still exists, and there is only one conclusion: capital movements unconnected to trade – and indeed largely independent of it – greatly exceed trade finance.[7]
>
> (Drucker 1986: 782)

Thus the last two decades have seen an astonishing growth in the funds devoted purely to speculation. This period witnessed the appearance of quite new exotic financial instruments that have the most tenuous connection with the production or even circulation of commodities but which both extended greatly the credit base while at the same time opening wide the gates for speculation. For instance, financial futures markets – where bets are laid on what interest rates will be at a specified date in the future – first emerged in the early 1970s and are now reckoned to total over $1 trillion worldwide, although in truth nobody really knows their magnitude.[8] There has been an even faster growth in interest and currency swaps. These consist of swaps between two parties who possess interest-bearing securities or future-currency contracts, the purpose being to hedge and/or seek additional speculative gains. There are now over $2.5 trillion worth of such contracts outstanding in the financial markets, yet they were almost unknown before 1980.

Thus the tendency towards socialisation does not come to a dead halt with the arrival of the epoch of imperialism. It does however take on more perverted, even crazy, forms. And second, it is a tendency subject to violent and inevitable disruptions which threaten the future of mankind. Thus the present century has been marked by two world wars, the slump of the 1930s, when economic nationalism, protectionism and even autarchy re-asserted themselves with great force. In short, imperialism, in its own way, both unites world economy while at the same time breaking it up.[9]

Two points should be made about this increasing globalisation of capital. In the first place, far from creating the conditions for a smoothly-operating world economy, as some daydreamers hope, the globalisation of capital was itself a response to the intensifying contradictions of the world economy. The great increase in the export of capital seen over the last two decades or so was an expression of the growing rivalries among states and corporations as they sought out more surplus-value to counteract downward pressure on the rate of profit. Similarly, with the arrival of the 1970s the explosion of debt and speculation became an increasingly important prop for the big capitalist powers. Government budgetary deficits, along with the mushrooming of corporate and personal debt, shored up demand and helped sustain the production of goods and services.

Second, deregulation of financial markets, the growth of international telecommunications and the creation of highly sophisticated computer software have not only encouraged aggressive speculation in new weird and wonderful financial instruments, they have also rendered virtually impossible the attempt by any state, even the largest, to carry out an 'independent' economic policy. Indeed it is now perfectly possible for the speculators, should they object to a particular government's policies, to create a run on any currency they choose. They are so powerful that they have:

> effectively created an international market in government policies. Speculators who doubt the ability of a national government to maintain a particular exchange rate can destroy the government's position by betting against the currency, as one individual, George Soros, did to great effect in 1992. The search for market credibility has already imposed a deflationary straight-jacket on European economies, led by high interest rates across Europe in the last 15 years, and the power of individual economies to buck these trends is severely restricted.
>
> (Commission on Social Justice 1994)[10]

In other words, we are witnessing a return – although on a much wider and deeper scale – to the 1930s when the 'bankers' ramp' forced governments out of office, including the British Labour Government in 1931.

The displacement of capitalism's contradictions after 1945

The advent of the epoch was announced by the first imperialist war, to be followed by the slump of the 1930s, a second world war and a series of wars and crises that have engulfed capitalism during the last half century. This chapter sketches out the main lines along which capitalism developed after the end of World War II and seeks briefly to locate the crisis of British capitalism within that framework.

The long boom that lasted for more than a quarter of a century after 1945 led many to conclude that capitalism had found new ways of overcoming the sort of world crisis it had experienced in the 1930s. And there certainly was a boom. Thus from 1948 to 1971 the annual average rate of growth for world industrial production was over 5 per cent; phrases such as the 'silver fifties' and 'golden sixties' reflected the widespread complacency among capitalism's apologists that the system had at last found the key to a permanent, crisis-free future.[11]

But there was another question involved: did the boom indicate that capitalism had overcome its fundamental *historical* contradictions? In fact the very length of the boom was an indication of the depth of the crisis into which capitalism plunged in the 1930s and during the period of World War II. As the war ended there was a need for massive reconstruction of a shattered European capitalism and the necessity of rebuilding foreign trade links. Under the aegis of US capital, and given an unprecedentedly large peacetime military expenditure, a long investment boom ensued, centred on military investment which carried production and trade forward to new heights. But beneath the surface the basic contradictions of capitalism developed and intensified, and capitalism has been unable to overcome them. Thanks to the unresolved crisis of leadership in the working class, capitalism survived the immediate post-war convulsions and in so doing was able, for a period, to displace its fundamental contradictions. But this displacement in no way implied that such contradictions had been *overcome*.[12] On the contrary: the contradictions continued to exist and develop, albeit taking new forms and notwithstanding the fact that they were in part hidden below the immediate surface of economic relations. We have now reached a point where these contradictions threaten to break surface with renewed virulence and under conditions where the ruling class has lost the main props through which it established its order in the post-war period – the Stalinist bureaucracy, which was of course aided and abetted throughout the period by the reformists in the labour and trade union movement of western Europe. It was precisely because the *fundamental* contradictions of capital were not overcome in the post-war period (and this fundamental contradiction is, in the final analysis, one between the need of the productive forces to develop under conditions where they are historically constricted by the social relations of capital) that the boom that followed 1945 bore all the marks of the epoch in which it took place. Because *finance* capital dominates all economic relations, the entire post-war period was marked at first by creeping inflation and then, from the 1970s onwards, by ever-greater currency and financial instability; by chronic imbalance in the state budgets of most of the leading capitalist powers; by an ever-increasing unevenness of development of capitalism on a world scale, with large areas of the globe condemned to stagnation and in many cases absolute regression; by the secular decline of industry in many of the advanced capitalist countries, with a consequential rise in long-term, structural, unemployment; and, despite all the efforts by US imperialism to impose a regime of free trade on the rest of the world, by growing trade rivalries and the emergence of trade blocs based on Europe, Japan and the United States.[13]

At the same time, the collapse of Stalinist regimes in Eastern Europe is history's verdict on the theory that socialism can be established within national boundaries. In the most general sense it was the deepening crisis of capitalism that lay at the base of the collapse of the USSR and the states of Eastern Europe. Simultaneously, this series of collapses creates acute tensions for the world capitalist system. Here is one important source of the considerable strains placed on German economy in particular and European economy generally by the attempts to restore capitalism in the former Eastern Europe. These strains find vivid expression in the crisis in the European monetary system and the growing realisation that an integrated financial system and a common currency in the European Union are, to put it mildly, by no means easily attainable objectives.[14]

A new stage of capitalism?

In short, the renewed period of extended reproduction after the end of World War II was no sign of capitalism's new-found vigour, no indication that it had entered a new, progressive stage of its development, that it had found new ways of overcoming its inherent contradictions. According to the reformists, this is precisely what had happened with the arrival of what they called 'welfare capitalism'. From now on, thanks to Beveridge and Keynes, capitalism had been tamed; given suitable social policies and measures to bring about a redistribution of income, the class struggle could be confined to the past, Marx pronounced a 'dead dog' and 'welfare capitalism' declared victorious. The current position of the social democrats – the principal advocates of such ideas – testifies to the superficiality of such 'theories'. For today social democracy declares that to all intents and purposes it has finished with Keynes and the 'welfare state'. This is an international phenomenon – in Britain, France, Italy, and even that 'dreamland' of social democracy, Sweden.[15]

The Stalinists likewise referred to the 'scientific and technological revolution' as distinguishing marks of 'contemporary capitalism'. These ideas represented a decisive break with the Marxist analysis of imperialism as the highest stage of capitalism. But it was not only Stalinism and reformism that rejected this thesis, although in many cases the rejection was implicit rather than explicit. The late Ernest Mandel was to the fore with similar ideas. Mandel saw the post-war period as marking the advent of a 'third industrial revolution' based on the development of new 'hi-tech' industries and the growing involvement of the state in the economy. He coined the phrase 'neo-capitalism' to describe this new and distinct phase in the development of capitalism. Writing in the late 1960s he had the following to say:

> I do not care very much for the term 'neo-capitalism' which is ambiguous, to say the least.... Nevertheless I am quite convinced that starting either with the great depression of 1929–32 or with the Second World War, capitalism entered into the third stage of its development, which is as different from monopoly capitalism or imperialism described by Lenin, Hilferding and others as monopoly capitalism was different from classical nineteenth century laissez-faire capitalism. We have to give this child a name; all other names proposed seem even less acceptable than neo-capitalism. State monopoly capitalism, the term used in the Soviet Union and the 'official' communist parties, is very misleading because it implies a degree of independence of the state which, to my mind, does not at all correspond to present-day reality. On the contrary, I would say that today the state is a much more direct instrument for guaranteeing monopoly surplus profits to the strongest private monopolies than it ever was in the past. The German term *Spaetkapitalismus* seems interesting, but simply indicates a time sequence and is difficult to translate into several languages.[16]
>
> (Mandel 1974)

The implications of such a passage are obvious, and have nothing to do with semantics. 'Neo-capitalism' is as different from imperialism as imperialism was from classical, nineteenth-century, capitalism, says Mandel. For Marxists, imperialism represented a *qualitative* change within the capitalist system; the features that characterised capitalism throughout much of the last century – free competition, free trade etc. – turned into their opposite with the advent of imperialism.[17] Now if neo-capitalism represents such a qualitative change compared with imperialism, this can only mean that imperialism proved to be not the *highest* stage of capitalism, as Lenin claimed. Likewise with the idea of a 'third industrial revolution': this involves a break with the fundamental conceptions of historical materialism. The industrial revolution that started in Britain in the eighteenth century was based on the emergence of *new social relations*, those of industrial capitalism. The industrial revolution cannot be narrowed down simply to a series of inventions, as with Mandel.[18] It meant not merely a series of inventions – in the textile industries and so on – but new social relations of production (the factory), new relations between town and country and, above all, the appearance of the modern working class. The post-war period has seen no such qualitative transformations, nor are they possible on the basis of capitalist property relations.

US capitalism's dominant position

The ability of capitalism to enter a new phase of extended reproduction after World War II rested not upon some new-found vigour on the part of capitalism but essentially on the counter-revolutionary role of reformism and Stalinism after 1945. Stalinism was able to behead the revolutionary movement of the working class that erupted throughout western Europe – in Italy, France and Greece in particular. In Britain the reformists, elected to government with a huge majority, were able to buy off the working class who, throughout the war itself as well as in the election that brought the Atlee government to office, had shown the most powerful desire for fundamental social change. Without the treacherous activities of these bureaucracies the 'restabilisation' of Europe (naturally, it was a relative restabilisation) would have been impossible.[19]

It was on this basis that US imperialism emerged from the war as the world's dominant power. US imperialism alone possessed the resources to prevent the complete collapse of European capitalism. The war had brought about a decisive shift of economic power to North America and it was this power that enabled the United States to finance the Marshall Plan and carry out the reconstruction of Japanese capitalism. As the leading imperialist power, the United States arranged the basic institutional structures of what was the then 'new world order'. Foremost among them were the monetary arrangements established at the Bretton Woods conference of 1944. It was at this conference that the rest of the world was obliged to acknowledge the United States' dominant role in the post-war period.[20] The decisive aspect of the decisions reached at Bretton Woods was that the leading capitalist states agreed to build the post-war monetary system around the dollar. They undertook to buy and sell their own currencies in order to preserve a fixed exchange rate with the dollar. In return the US government agreed to exchange dollars for gold at a fixed rate: $35 to an ounce of fine gold. This arrangement meant that US firms would always have funds to finance their international activities and in addition it gave US imperialism the power to force economic policies on to other governments. The power of US capital was reflected in the fact that it effectively controlled the various institutions established to regulate the post-war era: the International Monetary Fund (designed to deal with short-run economic and financial disturbances), the International Bank for Reconstruction and Development (set up to deal with long-term economic 'development') and the General Agreement on Tariffs and Trade (established to facilitate the reduction of trade barriers, a move which obviously benefited the United States). Even where the United States was unable to break down barriers to the sale of its exports in world markets, the establishment of production facilities in Europe by the big US multinationals gave US firms access to the markets of her competitors. Between 1950 and 1965 the value of foreign assets held by US firms grew at approximately twice the rate of US gross domestic product. In terms of the importance of this foreign investment to profits, foreign earnings as a share of after-tax profit of US non-financial corporations rose from 10 per cent in 1950 to 22 per cent by 1965.

This period has often been referred to as that of 'Pax Americana' to draw attention to the parallel with 'Pax Britannica' in the mid-nineteenth century when Britain exercised similar dominance over world economics and politics. But there are strict limits to this parallel. For Britain's hegemony was established in a period when capitalism was still able to develop the productive forces, albeit in a contradictory manner, not in the period of its decline. In particular, Britain dominated a world in which rival capitalist powers were still in the process of emerging. The United States established its power when conditions were quite different, even the opposite, of those existing in the last century – in an age when already well-established, albeit weaker, rivals existed ready to challenge that dominance whenever they could. Thus the enormous capital outflows from the United States, while in the short term strengthening the position of the US multinationals, meant the build-up of the economies of Japan and Europe. Firms based in Japan and Europe came to challenge the United States throughout the world, including in the US market itself; thus from the mid-1960s onwards the share of foreign direct investment held by US-based multinationals began to fall as a percentage of the world total, with Japanese and German firms in particular accounting for a rapidly-increasing share. The development of capitalism after 1945 proved the old adage that while US capitalism might be extremely powerful the contradictions of world capitalism were even more powerful.

These contradictions manifested themselves more clearly as US power began to ebb in the 1960s; and as US hegemony came under even more severe pressure in the 1970s following the collapse of Bretton Woods, a sequence of events was set in motion that led to a new role for banking and debt in the international economy. One of the key elements giving US imperialism its power was the very Bretton Woods system, which afforded the dollar a privileged role in the world monetary system. The fact that dollar balances piled up in the reserves of Europe and Japan indicated that the US government, firms, and private individuals were buying more abroad than foreign interests were purchasing from the United States. (It was like an individual being able to write cheques on their bank account in the sure knowledge that many would never be cashed.) Not least of the advantages accruing to the United States from these international monetary arrangements was that they allowed the strongest capitalist power to export its inflation. As non-US governments received ever-greater inflows of dollars they were faced with a dilemma. They could refuse to increase the supply of their own currency to the extent necessary to buy the extra dollars; but this would increase the downward pressure on the dollar and thereby threaten the stability of the international monetary systems. On the other hand, if they inflated their domestic currency to accommodate the inflow of dollars this would increase inflationary pressures in their own economies. In practice they took the second course, one which made their exports less competitive compared with US exports. But the situation could not last indefinitely, and faced with a massive shift out of dollars in 1970, the US administration was forced to end the convertibility of the dollar and with it the cornerstone of Bretton Woods.

Turning to non-monetary factors, the secular boom starting in the 1950s was characterised by a long investment boom that greatly increased the productive capacity of those industries producing means of production – Department I industries – far above their pre-war level. This investment, by creating a high demand for labour power, enabled working-class consumption levels to rise and this in turn created the basis for the new investments in Department II industries, those producing means of consumption. But over time, as the build-up of capacity proceeded in the older capitalist countries, the market for new plant and machinery began to shrink in both departments. By the late 1960s and early 1970s the crisis began to reveal itself in a downward pressure on the rate of profit, further discouraging new investment. Growth rates fell off and unemployment began to appear on a large scale for the first time since the end of World War II. Unlike in previous periods, prices began to rise rather than fall. This combination, which defied the logic of Keynesianism,[21] was dubbed 'stagflation' by bourgeois economists. But here was an expression of the in many ways *artificial* character of the post-war boom. It did not represent a healthy revival of capitalism, which, to emphasise the point again, had been unable to overcome the crisis of the 1930s. The post-war boom bore all the hallmarks of the epoch in which it occurred. For it was marked by powerful inflationary pressures and currency disruptions which by the early 1970s had undermined the post-war monetary arrangements. To maintain the boom required the constant creation of new sources of liquidity which, under the conditions of Bretton Woods, had to be provided by the US Federal Reserve Board. It was the continual flow of dollars into the world financial system that made it possible for the national and thus the commercial banks to issue increasingly large volumes of credit-money which provided the means to finance ever greater government budget deficits and business investment. Here lay the financial basis for the economic 'miracles' of the 1950s and 1960s – but the price had to be paid by capitalism in terms of increasingly strong inflationary pressures which became more and more difficult to control without triggering off a severe depression.

The collapse of Bretton Woods

By 1971 Bretton Woods had collapsed. The United States could no longer finance the export of dollars on a scale sufficient to sustain the old arrangements. Nor were other governments prepared to accept an ever-increasing influx of dollars, the purchasing power of which was increasingly uncertain. Some governments, with the French in the lead, demanded that the United States actually implement its pledge, and large quantities of gold moved across the Atlantic as the governments of Europe cashed in their dollar reserves for that 'yellow devil', gold. The system of fixed exchange rates, with all leading currencies tied to gold via the dollar was replaced with floating rates. It was the ending of Bretton Woods that unleashed considerable inflationary pressures. Whereas in the past no one country could inflate out of line with others without inducing a balance of payments crisis, now inflation simply brought a depreciation of the exchange rate. With the uncertainty that existed after 1971, governments had increasingly to resort to deflationary measures to avoid balance of payments crises, currency breakdown and a succession of bank failures that such breakdowns would have entailed. However, after the ending of dollar convertibility and fixed exchange rates, the need to create new means to finance US foreign requirements and to finance overseas military and other expenditures continued. Without this flow of liquidity there would have been a sharp aggravation of the crisis. In fact the US balance of payments deficit continued its inexorable growth throughout the 1970s and 1980s. Despite the complaints of other countries, especially in western Europe, there was nothing that they could do.[22]

As we have noted, the need to find ever-greater sources of liquidity led to the growth of new forms of 'fictitious capital' – the Eurodollar market becoming an increasingly important source of credit for big corporations, public utilities etc. A characteristic of the Eurocurrency market was the virtual absence of any regulation.[23] Severe competition between the banks and other financial institutions pushed them into ever-riskier loans and towards holding a smaller and smaller proportion of deposits as reserves.[24] Equally important, with the growth of the largely unregulated Eurocurrency market, individual governments had much less control over the supply of their currencies. When, for instance, banks holding dollars abroad loan out these dollars they create new dollars, that is, new claims on goods and services in the United States. Dollars can be lent, and then, when the borrower deposits new funds in the banking system, they can be re-lent: the only limit to the process is the willingness of banks to take on risk. The vast increase of this unregulated money and credit – greatly swollen with the arrival of 'petrodollars' following the rise of revenues accruing to OPEC (Organization of the Petroleum Exporting Countries) member governments – meant that the establishment of a 'national economic policy', along the lines envisaged by Keynes and his followers, became less and less possible, especially for the weaker capitalist powers.

In any case the result was a vast increase in international financial deals. Pushing money around on the part of speculators and 'money managers' became much more profitable than the direct extraction of surplus-value in the process of production.[25] In Britain, for instance, while whole industries have been shut down and industrial communities devastated, the business and profits of the City of London have continued to soar. But, contrary to what the reformists say, this is not the result of policy decisions by the Tories but is a graphic expression of the nature of imperialism as the epoch of capitalist decay, of the ever-more parasitic character of capital in that epoch. At the same time, such activities sharpen enormously the contradictions of capitalism. For financial services do not create surplus-value. They merely create an ever-greater lien on surplus-value generated elsewhere and thus the struggle for surplus-value became ever-more acute, a tendency which necessarily finds its reflection in the class struggle. The acceleration of inflation following the detachment of the dollar from gold in 1971 – the Nixon shock – was followed by a steep increase in commodity prices and the end of the era of cheap fuel, as the oil producers adjusted oil prices in line with general inflation. But the scrapping of Bretton Woods in 1971 and the sharp increase in oil prices in the two shocks of 1974 and 1979 were expressions of the crisis, not its fundamental cause, though in turn these developments undoubtedly exacerbated the crisis.

The collapse of Bretton Woods was due not to 'technical' factors, as the apologists for capitalism claim. Monetary relations are a reflection of economic relations, that is ultimately a reflection of class relations. Thus a powerful factor in creating the monetary crisis of 1971 was the Vietnam war. The United States faced the prospect of financing what was a deeply unpopular war at a time of considerable social tensions in the United States itself; these tensions, especially amongst poor workers in the decaying inner cities, had forced vast increases in health, education, employment and welfare programmes. The combination of welfare and war spending obviously necessitated sharp tax increases but the government was desperately concerned about opposition to the war. So there were no tax increases, the consequence of which was a growing budget deficit combined with considerable increases in the money supply. As domestic industry was turned to the needs of the war, imports rose sharply to maintain consumption levels and the result was a widening balance of payments gap. It was the attempt to finance this deficit by simply pouring out yet more dollars to the rest of the world that was the proximate cause of the monetary breakdown of 1971. In short, the Vietnam war and the resistance to it of the Vietnamese masses, was a potent factor that made impossible the maintenance of the exchange rates agreed at Bretton Woods. These factors contributed to a new phase of the crisis which began around 1973 and one which resulted in the first world-wide depression since the 1930s. From that point onwards we can say that the 'boom' was over, Keynesianism was on its last legs, and that the slowdown of world economy, though uneven, was increasingly generalised, with only short-lived revivals here and there. It is this phase of the post-war crisis which today assumes ever-acuter forms: rising long-term unemployment, growing tensions between and within the three rival trading blocs in world economy, currency instability, mounting budget and external debts, which imply a huge destruction of fictitious capital if 'stability' is to be restored, even in the short-term.

In the intensified competition which marked this new phase in the crisis some countries – notably Japan and the four hungry tigers in the Pacific zone – increased their share of the world market and underwent a further process of expanded reproduction.[26] Unemployment began to rise sharply in the advanced countries, especially long-term unemployment, with industry facing higher costs both of inputs of constant capital (especially fuel) and of variable capital (wages).[27] It was now that the social concessions made previously by the ruling class to the working class in certain countries entered more directly as factors in the crisis. As budget deficits mounted, the capitalist class found it increasingly difficult to finance these concessions. From this point onwards the struggle to take back previous concessions has been joined in all the major countries, although it has proceeded at different rates and taken different forms. A period had arrived when not only was it no longer possible to grant further reforms to the working class, but all previous gains had to be taken back from it.[28]

This in turn meant a decisive change in class relations, especially in the relationship of the working class to its reformist leadership in countries such as Britain, France and Germany. The ability of these reformists to betray the working class rested on their capacity to extract certain concessions for the working class, or at least a minority of its members. Reformism is no longer able to play this role. In Britain, in Germany, in France and even in Sweden the reformist leaders of the working class now spearhead the attack on the social gains won by the working class in the post-war period.[29] This is not to say that the class character of reformism has not altered. Since 1914 the trade union and labour bureaucracy became counter-revolutionary agents of capitalism within the working class movement. But this bureaucracy is now called upon to perform *new* services for imperialism, to become more directly its agent in taking from the working class the fruits of its previous conquests. This has particular significance for a country such as Britain, the home of reformism. It is increasingly clear that no concessions will be possible under a future Labour government, indeed the leaders of the Labour Party say as much. The Labour leaders have made clear that they will continue the attacks of the present government [i.e. the Conservative government of John Major – ed.] against the working class, seeking to dismantle the system of welfare benefits established particularly after 1945; they will continue the attempts to undermine the trade union movement, the movement from which the Labour Party was born at the start of the century.

It was in 1974, just as a new stage of the post-war crisis opened, that the Labour government attempted to avert a growing unemployment crisis by resort to a classical Keynesian reflationary boom. Almost immediately those efforts ran into the sand as the City went on strike, refusing to finance the government's borrowing requirement, and the International Monetary Fund (essentially US imperialism) stepped in and warned the Labour government that further loans would only be forthcoming on the basis of attacks on welfare spending. It was then, on the eve of a sterling devaluation (the second since the end of the war) that Callaghan warned the Labour Party that the days of Keynes were over.[30]

At the point of production the crisis manifested itself principally in a struggle for relative surplus-value – for example new systems of wage payment, cutbacks in the labour force, resistance to trade union demands for wage rises in line with inflation. The giant corporations began systematically to search out ways of increasing absolute surplus-value as well as relative surplus-value[31] by shifting manufacturing facilities from their old centres to areas where there was a plentiful supply of cheap labour.[32] The result was a flood of cheap commodities back into the advanced capitalist countries and the resultant destruction of whole industries in Europe and the United States. In this way the giant corporations were able, within certain limits, to combat the tendency for the rate of profit to fall but only at the expense of further aggravating the crisis. In a highly uneven way, new centres of capitalism grew while others declined – absolutely as well as relatively – in Europe and North America, with some industries remaining profitable even in their old centres.[33] But there were no outlets sufficiently large to counteract completely the downward pressure on the rate of profit. Meanwhile, the dependent capitalist countries also reflected the growing crisis in an uneven way. Some became centres of a new industrialisation drive fostered by the multinationals; others benefited from the high price of their oil, others were plunged into stagnation and poverty or famine; yet others found a temporary lifeline by borrowing on a massive scale.

Funds for international loans for the so-called 'developing countries' came from the recycling of oil money, or were based on bank credit and the continuous creation of fresh money by the Federal Reserve Bank in the United States to finance that country's growing balance of payments and budget deficits. The borrowing countries found themselves entangled in a vicious debt trap, with interest and debt repayment absorbing an ever-greater share of their foreign earnings. By the mid-1980s this meant heavily-indebted countries were unable to go on buying commodities from the advanced capitalist countries without further borrowings. At the same time the commercial banks of Europe and America found themselves with a sheaf of bad debts, with the prospect that unless more credit was shovelled into the debtor countries they would face collapse. At the centre of all these relations stands the United States, as still the hegemonic capitalist country: with a huge balance of payments problem, and a massive and unprecedented budget deficit. While still the leading capitalist power, whole sectors of this economy have been devastated: by the fall in investment, by the impact of technological change, the growth of foreign, especially Japanese, competition and the shifting of manufacturing facilities abroad by the multinationals. The US economy has kept afloat by sucking in great quantities of foreign money to finance the budgetary and balance of payments deficits and by continuing to pay for its needs with newly-created credit money ('fictitious capital').[34]

The recent past has been dominated by the collapse of the USSR and the states of Eastern Europe, with implications that we have noted above. Far from opening up a new period of capitalist prosperity and expansion as many believed, this great change has intensified the contradictions of world capitalism. The Russian economy remains on the edge of disintegration, with all the social and political implications that this implies.[35] US imperialism, even if it were willing to provide the funds for the reconstruction of the Russian economy on capitalist foundations (and in so doing it would only be building a powerful rival for itself) lacks the resources to carry out this task. Whereas in the immediate post-war period US capitalism's position was unchallenged, the period since the war has seen its steady relative decline, a decline measured in its share of world production, of world markets, the position of the dollar in the system of world finance. As one writer puts it:

> No one doubts that the United States remains the leading power among capitalist nations, but the joint ability of US government and business to set the rules of international affairs no longer exists. The US government cannot readily impose economic policies on its allies. US business is no longer unchallenged – quite the contrary. It has had to adjust to challenges from Japan and Europe, from rising economic powers such as Korea and Brazil, and from the OPEC nations.
>
> (MacEwan 1990: 44)

Whereas in 1950 per capita industrial output in the countries of the Common Market was 31 per cent of that in the United States, 20 years later the figure was

58 per cent. Over the same period, per capita GDP in the EEC rose from 38 per cent of the US level to 62 per cent. In the case of Japan the rise was from 16 per cent in 1950 to 53 per cent in 1970. In 1960 the United States was responsible for 44 per cent of the aggregate GDP of the capitalist countries. Some 20 years later this figure had dropped to under 37 per cent. Over the same period the share of Japan had risen from under 7 per cent to almost 14 per cent.

It was US capitalism, through the Marshall Plan that laid the basis for the regeneration of European economy in the late 1940s. But at that time it dominated world industry, it monopolised the supply of mined gold. The situation it now finds itself in bears little resemblance to that position. But if US imperialism is unable to find the resources to rebuild the Russian economy, then certainly no other power is in any position to carry though this task. The nature of the 'capitalism' that is being established in Russia and Eastern Europe is all too plain to see. It is a capitalism dominated by the Mafia which in turn is the instrument through which the imperialists set out to plunder the resources of the USSR by the most primitive means.

The period since the collapse of the USSR is characterised by growing tensions between the capitalist powers. Thus the mounting threats by US imperialism to launch a full-blown trade war against Japan, which, despite countless 'agreements', adamantly refuses to open up its markets to US exports. Roughly half the current US trade gap is accounted for by its deficit with Japan. The electoral victories of the Republican Party in the mid-term Congressional elections and the possibility that the next president will be a Republican strengthen the forces towards protectionism in the United States. From this point of view, the important thing about the last round of GATT [the General Agreement on Tariffs and Trade, superseded in 1994 by the World Trade Organization – ed.] negotiations (the so-called 'Uruguay Round') was not that they were eventually signed but that they took such a long time to conclude.[36] Within the three main trading blocs, tensions mount. These are most clearly manifest within Europe. Virtually every ruling class within the European Union is bitterly divided over the question of European integration. All the signs are that a serious trade war is being prepared in which economic protection and nationalism will reassert themselves as they did in the 1930s, the decade that saw the preparations for a world war for the division and redivision of the world amongst the Great Powers. Under these conditions Rosa Luxemburg's alternative 'socialism or barbarism' takes on a new and sinister meaning.

The crisis in Britain

It is clear that despite the shrill counter-claims, the 'Thatcher experiment' – with its 'monetarism' and 'supply-side economics', its battery of anti-union laws and its attempts to cutback state spending – has singularly failed to arrest the decline of British capitalism. Far from having found their way to an economic nirvana, the Tories have superintended a continuing decline of British capital throughout the 1980s and 1990s, one that in some respects has proceeded at an accelerated rate. Emerging from World War II in a greatly-weakened state, having been forced to liquidate a great slice of its foreign assets to finance the war against Germany, Britain has declined uninterruptedly over the last half century or so.[37] Whole industries – steel, shipbuilding, marine engineering, coal mining and others – have collapsed or are in a parlous state. This involves a sharply increased struggle for surplus-value from the workers in the industries that remain, which in turn is not possible without the greater disciplining of workers, the attacks on their rights. A point has been reached where the relative decline of British capitalism – which can be traced back to the last quarter of the nineteenth century – now threatens to become absolute.

Such stuttering 'revival' as did occur in 1994 in Britain was almost entirely the result of the sharp sterling devaluation following the exit from the European Monetary System in 1992. That humiliating ejection from the European Exchange Rate Mechanism (ERM) was itself an indication of the parlous state of British capital; long ago unable to 'look the dollar in the face', sterling was no longer able to maintain parity with the D-mark or the French franc. Divisions in the British ruling class had made entry into the European exchange rate mechanism impossible in 1985. But from 1987, the British chancellor of the exchequer, Nigel Lawson, began the policy of shadowing the German currency as the best available means of controlling inflation. The policy collapsed when, because of the crisis in the German economy brought about by the attempt to assimilate the eastern German Länder, interest rates began to rise sharply. Britain, having joined the ERM, was forced out and a general crisis in the European currency system rapidly ensued. The lira soon followed sterling and was devalued heavily, to be quickly followed by the Portuguese and Irish currencies. Norway and Sweden were obliged to abandon their policy of pegging their currencies to the D-mark.

But even the respite provided by that sterling devaluation seems likely to be of the shortest duration; already inflationary pressures are starting to build up again, indicating that the problem of 'stagflation' – the combination of heavy unemployment and inflation – remains. In any case the resort by the British ruling class to such a measure again is highly problematic, inviting as it would retaliatory actions from the rest of Europe, and raising the spectre of the sort of 'devaluation cycle' that in the 1930s expressed the desperate struggle amongst the major capitalist powers for a larger slice of a stagnant or shrinking world market following the 1929 Wall Street crash.

Not unexpectedly, the leaders of the Labour Party blame this continued decline and crisis on the 'wrong' policies pursued by the Tories during their long period of office. They complain in particular about the privileged role afforded the City of London, to which they attribute the collapse of large swathes of manufacturing industry. But there is no evidence that the crisis of British capitalism over the post-war period could have been tackled on the basis of different 'policies'. Indeed, one of the features that has emerged with ever-greater clarity during the period since 1945 is the growing inability of the British ruling class to pursue an 'independent' economic policy on the world arena, under conditions of the ever-increasing globalisation of capitalism.[38] The very opposite of the position advanced by the Labour leaders is in fact the case: the sickness of capital in Britain, the first industrial capitalist power in the world, is a reflection of the malaise of capitalism as a whole as it nears the end of the twentieth century. The increasingly parasitic nature of the British ruling class, the fact that it is more and more dominated by speculation and dubious money-dealing, if not straight fraud, is a graphic expression of the character of capitalism as a whole in the epoch of imperialism. It is not, as the reformists pretend, something 'exceptional' to be put right by sagacious policies. Just as it did in the last century, so today British capital holds up a mirror to the rest of the world.[39]

The search for a policy that would allow the British ruling class to pursue its 'own' interests was one of Keynes's chief preoccupations. This was the source of his opposition to the return to the gold standard in the 1920s – he believed it would severely restrict the ability of British capitalism to pursue an economic and financial policy independent of US capital. Likewise, as World War II drew to a close it was Keynes who fought for a set of post-war monetary arrangements which would, he fondly hoped, free a severely debilitated British capitalism from the pressures of the world market. Needless to say in the ensuing struggle with the representatives of US imperialism it was the Keynes Plan that lost out, with the United States imposing its own monetary system on to the rest of the world, just as British imperialism had done in the previous century via the mechanisms of the gold standard.

It was Keynes who provided the ideological basis for reformism in post-war Britain. Throughout the 1960s, that 'Keynes had put paid to Marxism' was commonplace amongst Labour's 'theoreticians', such as C.A.R. Crosland.[40] Thanks to the techniques of Keynesian 'demand management' the scourge of mass unemployment could be eliminated; given sufficient spending on welfare services the chronic poverty suffered by millions in the 1930s would be a thing of the past; with a policy of income redistribution the worst inequalities of income could be eradicated. In short the class struggle could be overcome in this new 'welfare capitalism' to which the Labour and trade union leaders were wedded. These fond ideas can be put into some perspective when we consider that as the century draws to a close, the leaders of the Labour Party are busily severing their last links with Keynesianism. Labour is no longer the party of high taxation and high spending, pleads Tony Blair. These leaders now pledge their support for that strange animal, 'the social market economy'.

The *Financial Times* (28 September 1994) commented approvingly on 'the new model Labour Party':

> It has jettisoned much cumbersome baggage. Gone is the commitment to demand expansion as a remedy for unemployment. Gone is the simplistic commitment to taxing and spending. In their place come recognition of the constraints imposed by the global economy and a willingness to build on the improvements in the macro-economic policy framework of the past two years.

The roots of this somewhat undignified abandonment of Keynesianism are not hard to seek. In the first place, Keynesian-style spending on welfare benefits was possible only to the extent that world capitalism continued to expand at a sufficient rate. Thus while US imperialism was able to regulate an inflationary expansion of world economy after 1945, it was possible, within limits, for the ruling class in countries such as Britain, West Germany, Sweden and France to make certain concessions to the middle class and sections of the working class. Once the United States was unable to sustain this role – the collapse of the Bretton Woods monetary arrangements in the late 1960s and early 1970s indicated when that point was reached – then Keynesianism became untenable.

In the second place, the operation of a traditional Keynesian policy became increasingly untenable given the 'globalisation' of finance which occurred with such rapidity in the 1970s and 1980s. The collapse of Bretton Woods and with it the abandonment of fixed exchange rates after 1971, the appearance of Euromarkets in bank credit and bonds, and the ever-greater operations of multinational banks made it impossible for the Thatcher government to regulate the domestic money supply, as the doctrine of 'monetarism' demanded. Indeed the 'deregulation' of the financial markets, amongst the first of Thatcher's acts, stood in stark contradiction with the other arm of the policy that was supposedly guiding the policy of her government: a strict control over the money supply. Any effort to regulate the supply of money and credit within Britain could be easily overcome by the importation of credit from abroad. And in any case, attempts by the Bank of England to curtail the activities of the banks operating in London would have weakened the competitiveness of the City against foreign centres.[41]

The forces at work revealed themselves in the aftermath of the demise of Bretton Woods. When the Labour government assumed office in 1974 it was faced with rising unemployment:[42] the Wilson government attempted a Keynesian-style reflation of the economy. It came into office with what it claimed was a 'new industrial strategy', with bodies such as the grandiosely-named National Enterprise Board set up to regenerate British industry. Money was poured into industry and grants for 'regional development' increased sharply. While such expenditure did nothing to improve the competitiveness of British firms in the world market, it did contribute to a sharp increase in the public sector borrowing requirement, which went up from the equivalent of 6.5 per cent of the GDP in 1973 to 11.0 per cent of GDP in 1975. Faced with a severe depreciation, the Wilson experiment soon came to a halt as the City of London in effect went on strike, refusing to finance the government's borrowing needs, and the International Monetary Fund made clear to the government that any loans made to Britain were dependent on severe cutbacks in welfare spending. Wilson and Callaghan duly obliged: in July 1976 a package of cuts was made and the government announced that as part of the attempt to curb inflationary pressures, targets for the growth of the money supply would be implemented. Thus did the Labour leaders prepare the way for the Tories after 1979 to begin a systematic dismantling of the 'welfare state'. It was then that the 'counter-revolution' against Keynesianism got underway and the doctrine of monetarism, associated particularly with Milton Friedman (1990), replaced the old, now discredited, orthodoxy.

It is the same forces that now oblige the Labour leaders to explicitly ditch any adherence to Clause IV of the Labour Party constitution – that clause that committed the Labour Party to the nationalisation of the means of production, distribution and exchange. Although this clause had little to do with socialism (it could correctly be called a reflection of state capitalism) in the minds of the majority of workers, this measure *is* associated with socialism. At least in theory, between the two world wars the social democrats still stood for the social ownership of the means of production, that is to say the abolition of the capitalist system. They simply claimed that this could be achieved gradually within the framework of existing institutions. Things have changed dramatically since the war, with the leaders of the Labour Party merely the latest 'reformist' party to abandon in words such a goal.[43]

But this opens up a crisis for the working class, marks a turning point in its development. For the last 90 years or so the majority of workers have seen the Labour Party as the instrument through which they could realise their political aims. By keeping their unions strong and winning concessions from the employers, the working class could periodically elect a Labour government that would legislate in the interests of the workers. This period is over. It is over because a point has been reached in the world crisis of capitalism where no further concessions can be made to the working class in the advanced countries, let alone in the colonial and semi-colonial countries. The purpose of this chapter has been to make an effort to re-examine this crisis, and suggest the political implications that flow from it.

Notes

1 This chapter started life as a series of brief theses drafted by Tom Kemp in 1985. [*History, Economic History and the Future of Marxism: Essays in Memory of Tom Kemp* (Brotherstone and Pilling 1996), in which this chapter first appeared, was a *Fetschrift* to Tom Kemp, originated by the editors, one of whom was Geoff Pilling, when Tom Kemp was diagnosed with cancer in 1993. Born into a London working class family in 1921, Tom Kemp won a scholarship place at a south London grammar school, Emmanuel, and then at the London School of Economics, his university career being disrupted by war-time service in the Royal Navy. After an initial post at University College Southampton, he moved to the economic history department at the University of Hull, where he remained till his retirement in 1986, belatedly being appointed to a readership. He was a prolific academic author, starting with *Theories of Imperialism* in 1967 and including a series of books on industrialisation which became popular with students and lecturers in the United Kingdom and many other countries. He had joined the Young Communist League, aged 16, in 1937, tearing up his Communist Party card after the events of 1956, Khrushchev's 'secret speech' denouncing Stalin, and the Soviet invasion of Hungary. To Kemp this raised questions about the history of the Soviet Union since its inception in 1917, and how such crimes could be committed in a 'socialist' society, leading to his need to study the hitherto forbidden books of Trotsky and make contact with those who had fought against Stalinism – the Trotskyists. After joining the Trotskyist group led by Gerry Healy, which became the Socialist Labour League and then the Workers Revolutionary Party, he became one of its main theoreticians, writing and giving theoretical classes. He was one of the key figures writing for the journal *Labour Review*, which played an important role in the

discussion of Trotskyism. As indicated elsewhere, it was Tom Kemp who introduced Geoff Pilling to Marx's *Capital.* However, by the late 1970s he became uneasy with the direction the party was going, which sometimes seemed guided more by the desire to build the party rather than achieve socialism, and by the early 1980s, he became much less active, though he continued some writing. After Healey's expulsion in 1985 he returned to writing prolifically in the party newspaper, and full party activity – ed.].

2 Cholera and hepatitis, caused by contaminated food and drinking water, is spreading rapidly; malaria resulting from mosquito bites is estimated to have killed one million people in 1993; typhoid, likely where water supplies and sanitation are poor, has flared up recently in Eastern Europe. Tuberculosis claimed 2.7 million victims in 1993. The capitalist class tries to blame 'nature' for these deaths. New, virulent strains of old diseases have emerged which are immune to traditional treatments, it is said. The true causes of the re-emergence of these diseases is primarily the lack of basic decent living conditions for millions of people as well as the lack of research into the causes and treatment of such diseases. As is general, what are exclusively *social* causes are attributed to *nature*.

3 To give some idea of the magnitude of this situation: in 1975 the joint value of the five largest US corporations (Exxon, General Motors, Ford Motor, Texaco and Mobil) came to $197 billion. In 1974 the combined gross domestic product of 55 African states was $147 billion. The GDP of India, with a population at that time of 600 million, was $80 billion.

4 To avoid any misunderstanding: the term imperialism is not used here as a synonym for 'colonialism'. It marks a definite stage in the development of capitalism, which, according to Lenin (1964), has several decisive economic features. Imperialism involves the concentration of production to the point where monopolies become decisive in the system's functioning; bank and industrial capital merge to create a situation where finance capital becomes the dominant form of capital; the export of capital, rather than the mere export of commodities, becomes crucial; international capitalist monopolies emerge which share out the world market among themselves; the territorial division of the world is completed among a handful of Great Powers.

5 For a summary of the main trends see Jozsef Nyilas (1982).

6 See 'Globalisation – to what end?' (*Monthly Review* 1992). There is much useful information in this article.

7 The figures are so big as to be almost incomprehensible and they have certainly shot up since these calculations/guesses were made. The *daily* turnover on the foreign exchange markets is now around $1 trillion. One further striking statistic: at the start of the 1970s, 90 per cent of currency flows across the exchanges were based on trade and only 10 per cent on speculation; today, a quarter of a century later, the proportions have been reversed.

8 It was this sort of activity that in 1995 brought down Barings – Britain's oldest and most prestigious merchant bank. Barings had been forced into high risk-taking activities in the Far East in an effort to compete with its more powerful North American rivals.

9

> By drawing the countries economically closer to one another and levelling out their stages of development, capitalism, however, operates by methods *of its own*, that is to say, by anarchistic methods which constantly undermine its own work, set one country against another, and one branch of industry against another, developing some parts of world economy while hampering and throwing back the development of others. Only the correlation of these two fundamental tendencies – both of which arise from the nature of capitalism – explains to us the living texture of the historical process.
>
> (Trotsky 1974: 16)

10 The fact that this could appear in the Report of the 'Commission on Social Justice', the body set up by the late leader of the British Labour Party, John Smith, is highly ironic.

11 By the end of the 1980s there was a growing mood of doubt about the future of the system, well captured in the following sort of passage:

> The economic crisis of the 1970s has not gone away; rather, in the 1980s it has been brushed under the carpet. Now it shows signs of emerging again but on a larger and much nastier scale. The world economy in the 1980s has consisted of a remarkable juggling act in which the three chief sets of actors on the world economic stage – multinational corporations, banks and the governments of countries – have all striven to gain maximum advantage whilst simultaneously promoting economic recovery. The act has produced a world-economic order which is more and more uncertain and yet which is also more and more inured to that uncertainty. It is a world-economic order which is addicted to the knife edge. It is a world-economic order hooked on speed.
>
> (Thrift 1989: 16)

12 To insist that imperialism constitutes an epoch of crisis is not to say that in some simplistic sense the crisis always and everywhere takes the same form. Despite the fact that imperialism marks a stage in human history where the material conditions for socialism have been achieved, this does not imply that there can or will be an *automatic* transition to socialism. For capitalism there are no impossible situations, or permanent crises. The defeat of the working class at the end of the war meant that the conditions for a certain restabilisation of capitalism were created. Naturally this restabilisation was relative and took place in an epoch which in a fundamental sense is one of crisis. Cf. Lenin:

> [It becomes evident] that private economic and private property relations constitute a shell which no longer fits its contents, *a shell which must inevitably decay if its removal is artificially delayed*, a shell which may remain in a state of decay for a fairly long period ... but which will inevitably be removed
>
> (Lenin 1964: 303, emphasis added)

13 For trends at work in long-term unemployment see OECD, *Economic Outlook* table quoted in Dicken (1992: 426). [Similar figures are available in Ljungqvist, L. and Sargent, T.J. (1997) *The European Unemployment Dilemma*, Table 1. Online, available at: http://swopec.hhs.se/iuiwop/papers/iuiwop0481.pdf (accessed 12 December 2011) – ed.]

14 The September 1994 meeting of the International Monetary Fund (IMF) in Madrid was unable to agree on further loans from the Fund to Russia. This decision came hard on the heels of the warning from the director of the National Bank of Switzerland that the IMF was in danger of following Gresham's Law and pouring good money after bad in Russia; in so doing it was threatening the very stability of the fund itself. The tensions within the European Union (EU) recently found graphic expression with the failure of Britain's representative, Sir Leon Brittan, to be given responsibility for relations between the EU and Eastern Europe. It is clear that Germany intends to take the lead here and establish its own interests in the area.

15 Professor Fritz Scharpf, a leading political economist in Germany, expresses this demise of Keynesianism in the bluntest terms.

> National governments in highly industrialised countries in the 1970s lost the ability to maintain or regain full employment through demand reflation; in the 1980s they have lost (or abdicated) the power to protect their own industries against intensified competition from other first-world countries; and they are now for the first time confronted with the possibility that world markets may be

> captured by high-quality industrial goods (and services) produced at low costs in what used to be third-world or second-world countries.
>
> (Commission for Social Justice 1994: 66)

16 This did not prevent Mandel from calling one of his subsequent publications *Late Capitalism*!

17 An interesting feature of capitalism in its decline is the manner in which it exhibits tendencies that characterised it in its youth. Thus the rise of capital is distinguished by its heavy reliance on the state, by its efforts to suppress competition, by its opposition to the principle of free trade. These features reappear in the twentieth century and find their expression in a variety of forms including, for example, Keynesianism.

18

> With the 1940s appeared the warning signs of a third industrial revolution. The first industrial revolution had been based on the steam engine, the second on the electric motor and the internal combustion engine. The third industrial revolution is based on the release of nuclear energy and the use of electronic machinery.
>
> (Mandel 1968: 605)

Contrary to Mandel, the history of capitalism has been characterised by technical changes that have brought first one industrial sector and then another to a leading position. Thus it was textiles, cotton in particular, that in Britain occupied such a position in the early period of the industrial revolution; at a later stage heavy industry, concentrated on the iron and steel industry, occupied the leading position; it was subsequent developments in the engineering and chemical industries that later made new means of transportation possible, especially the motor car. According to one writer,

> The so-called 'industrial revolution' actually had precious little that was industrial about it in a technological sense: it consisted to a great extent of changes in the organisation and management of work, in new methods of marketing, finance and the control of enterprises.
>
> (Smith 1984)

For a discussion of the Marxist conception of industrial revolution see Geoff Pilling, 'Engels and the industrial revolution', 1996 [Chapter 9 of this book – ed.].

19 For a detailed examination of the role of Stalinism in creating the conditions for the survival of Japanese capitalism after 1945 see Moore 1983.

20 One of the conditions for the loans made by the United States to Britain after the war was that the latter had immediately to ratify the terms of the Bretton Woods Agreement, with its provision for rapid trade liberalisation and the early convertibility of sterling. It is clear that the United States was using her economic power to break up what remained of the British Empire so that it could be opened up to US capitalism as a source of raw materials and an outlet for her exports. There were similarly stringent conditions attached to the granting of Marshall Aid; each recipient had to sign an agreement promising to balance its budget, stabilise its exchange rate and devise a plan for the elimination of the majority of its trade controls.

21 According to Keynesian theory, inflation only becomes a problem near the top of the economic cycle, that is, as full employment is reached. The idea behind this was that as unemployment rises, inflation will be lowered since unemployment will reduce the level of wages; unemployment will then fall as the demand for labour increases as a result of declining real wages. (Keynes never rejected the idea that wages would have to fall in times of heavy unemployment; he believed that this fall was best brought about through a drop in *real* wages brought about by rising prices.) Keynesians argued that in times of heavy unemployment the government would allow a budget deficit sufficiently large to restore full employment, whereas in times when the economy was 'overheating' a budget surplus would be run to curb inflationary pressures. The other major problem that the Keynesians encountered concerned budget deficits. They

argued that any such deficit incurred during a recession would be compensated for in periods of economic upswing. But during the 1980s a pattern emerged where not only did governments incur borrowing requirements that far exceeded anything in the previous quarter century, but such deficits persisted even when the economy started to expand. In other words, a good proportion of the deficits run up by governments in the 1980s and 1990s were the result not simply of problems associated with the economic cycle but were *structural* in character – long-term unemployment, changing demographic factors, etc. This phenomenon has been described by some as the 'fiscal crisis of the state'.

22 During the 1950s and the early 1960s, the total value of US foreign investment in real terms (that is taking into account price changes) increased at the rate of 7 or 8 per cent per annum. During the late 1960s and throughout the 1970s the rate dropped to between 4 and 5 per cent per annum, while in the 1980s the real value of the stock of US foreign direct investment declined somewhat. Equally significant was the changing *structure* of these investments. Thus in 1960 receipts from *direct* investment constituted over 80 per cent of total receipts from overseas assets held by US firms and government agencies. By the late 1980s this had dropped to around 12 per cent. The other side of the coin was the rapidly-growing importance of income from portfolio investments, predominantly *loans* made by US imperialism. By 1987 such receipts represented almost 90 per cent of returns on overseas assets. Here was the growing significance of usury imperialism, itself an expression of the decay of capitalism. For a discussion of this issue see MacEwan (1990).

23 In origin, Eurodollars were dollars held outside the United States banking system, largely by countries like the USSR and China which wanted to avoid US control over their dollars. Once it was understood that such dollars were free of US banking laws, such as those dealing with reserve requirements and the payment of interest, their rapid growth was inevitable. One writer sums up the significance of the Eurodollar market thus:

> [It] was perhaps the most important international financial development of the 1960s, growing, within a decade, from a market worth a few hundred million dollars and handling issues between \$2 million and \$5 million each in the mid-1960s to a market worth several hundred billion dollars a year and handling issues of between \$200 million and \$500 million a time. Now it is worth \$300 billion a year and it is a market whose development can be charted very much in terms of reaction to regulation within the domestic financial systems of the USA, Europe and Japan.
>
> (A. Hamilton, *The Financial Revolution*, 1986: 21, quoted in Dicken 1992: 365)

24 In other words, those operating in the Eurocurrency market were not subject to the sort of controls to which domestic banks are subject, including the requirement to maintain a certain proportion of their assets in liquid form.

25 Paul Sweezy sees in the development of such activities over the last 20 years or so a new feature in world capitalist economy.

> What I am talking about is the development in the last twenty years or so of a relatively independent – relative, that is, to what went before – financial superstructure sitting on top of the world economy and most of its national units. It is made up of banks – central, regional, and local – and a host of dealers in a bewildering variety of financial assets and services, all interconnected by a network of markets, some of which are structured and regulated, others informal and unregulated. Such an entity is multi-dimensional, and there is no conceptual unit that could be used to measure its size.
>
> (Sweezy 1994: 7)

26 Expanded reproduction involves the turnover of capital on an ever-larger scale.

27 Prior to the first oil price shock, the unemployment rate within the European Union stood at below 3 per cent. Thereafter it rose remorselessly, peaking at 11 per cent in 1985; it then fell to a little over 8 per cent by the end of the decade, but has increased again and is now over 10 per cent. Bourgeois economics has no explanation for this phenomenon which remains, in the words of one writer, 'a major puzzle'. See Bean (1994: 573–619). As we have noted, one source of the enigma was that during the mid-1970s increasing unemployment was associated with rising prices, something that defied the logic of Keynesianism. Just as significant was the growth in the number of *long-term unemployed*, defined in the official statistics as those out of work for a year or more. Comparing 1979 with 1988, we find that the percentage of long-term unemployed amongst those unemployed rose from 29.3 per cent to 54.8 per cent in the European Union as a whole. Some 40 per cent of those currently out of work in the European Union have never had a job. In the United States long-term unemployment in the decade after 1979 rose from 4.2 per cent to 7.4 per cent, while in the case of Japan the rise was from 16.5 per cent to 20.6 per cent. It is obvious that these changes have implications for the sort of welfare programmes that were introduced in many advanced countries after 1945. The growth of youth unemployment (that is amongst those under 25) has been particularly sharp in western Europe over the recent past. In Spain it is currently above 40 per cent; in Ireland around 30 per cent, in France approximately 25 per cent, in Italy over a third. See *The Economist*, 1994. Such unemployment is concentrated in inner-city areas and is especially heavy among ethnic minorities. In the city of Manchester for example, in 1991 almost 44 per cent of non-white males were without work, with the figure for females being not much lower. See Symes (1995: 82). It is clear that the old welfare spending programmes cannot cope with large-scale, long-term unemployment. It is one thing to operate a welfare system when the rate of unemployment is 2 or 3 per cent, as it was for the first quarter century after 1945, and when most unemployment is short-term. It is another thing when that rate rises and at the same time people are unemployed not for a few weeks or months but for years, and perhaps even permanently.

28 The importance of the safety net provided by welfare benefits was well understood by the ideologists of capitalism. Thus the United Nations *World Economic Survey* for 1993 notes,

> The difficult situation of workers in the 1980s was not as salient politically as it might otherwise have been because real consumption levels grew more rapidly than compensation [earnings]. To some degree this was made possible by growing official transfers, including social security payments to the elderly and unemployment benefits that have been relatively generous in some countries. It was also the result of a major and irreversible social change, the entry of large numbers of women into the labour force and the increasing number of households with more than one wage-earner. But it was the result as well of increases in household borrowing, collateralised largely by rising house values.

29 These social gains represented an inroad into the surplus-value of the ruling class. Given that the working class, at least in the advanced capitalist countries, was able to maintain a subsistence (living) wage, all the social benefits paid to workers were in fact diminutions from surplus-value. One writer has recently pointed to the great increase in the number of unproductive workers (that is, for example, those involved in the mere circulation of surplus-value, as well as those engaged in speculative and banking activities) and sees this as the principal source of the reassertion of the law of the tendency of the rate of profit to fall over the last two decades. According to one estimate, the number of workers involved in the circulation of surplus-value as well as those engaged in supervisory activities on behalf of capital rose in the United States from 10.5 million in 1947 to 25.5 million in 1977, while over the same period the number of productive workers (that is those producing surplus-value) rose at a far

slower rate – from 29.6 million to 39.6 million. See Moseley (1991). No doubt the growth of an increasing layer of unproductive workers (that is those not producing surplus-value) was one of the sources of the capitalist crisis that increasingly manifested itself from the mid-1970s onwards. But whether this was the *cause* of this crisis is a different matter. The fact is that capitalism was less and less able to sustain a growing number of unproductive workers. The task is therefore to establish why this was so, and the key to the answer lies in the inability of capitalism to raise the productivity of labour at a pace sufficient to offset the tendency of the rate of profit to fall.

30 Speaking at the Labour Party Conference in 1976, James Callaghan made the following statement:

> We used to think that you could spend your way out of a recession, and increase employment by cutting taxes and boosting government expenditure. I tell you in all candour that option no longer exists, and in so far as it ever did exist, it only worked on each occasion since the war by injecting a bigger dose of inflation into the economy. And each time that happened the average level of unemployment has risen. Higher inflation followed by higher unemployment. That is the history of the last 20 years.

Thus was the demise of Keynesianism pronounced. And this was not simply a British question. In 1981 François Mitterrand, in alliance with the Communist Party of France, was elected president of France on the basis of a project that he said 'had nothing in common with the corrupt compromises of a Schmidt or a Callaghan, let alone a Mollet'. Within the first months of office, the new government had raised the minimum wage by 10 per cent, old age pensions by 20 per cent and family allowances by 30 per cent. To deal with rising unemployment, over 60,000 jobs were created in the public sector, with the promise of a further 150,000 to follow shortly. The state acquired 100 per cent of the shares in five major conglomerates and public ownership of the banking sector was further extended. But faced with a severe run on the franc, within less than two years the government had executed a u-turn on economic policy, imposing austerity on the working class and providing incentives for the rich. Removed from office in the 1986 parliamentary elections, the 'socialists' were returned again in 1988 but they showed no inclination to reverse the wholesale privatisations carried out in the intervening period. See David Singer (1988) and Marc Lombard (1995).

31 Relative surplus-value involves the increase in surplus-value *within* a given working day. The increased production of absolute surplus-value involves the prolongation of the working day.

32 The enormous pressure, even in the advanced capitalist countries, to increase surplus-value in its absolute form – that is by attempting to lengthen the working day and/or increase the intensity of labour in a given working day – is symptomatic of the historical stage in which capitalism finds itself. For in the period of its heyday capitalism relied more on the extraction of *relative* surplus-value, that is, surplus-value obtained through increases in the rate of exploitation brought about principally by the mechanisation of production. Capitalism is more and more driven back to the methods of exploitation that characterised its infancy when it was still in struggle against feudalism. This is a general feature of capitalism in its decay: it resorts to methods and forms that are reminiscent of its infancy. Thus it increasingly *plunders* the colonial and semi-colonial countries after the fashion of the conquistadors: this is the only 'plan' that the monopolies and financial institutions have for Eastern Europe and the former USSR. This is reflected in the trend noted above for capitalism to exploit the colonial and semi-colonial countries increasingly by means of loans, rather than through the exploitation of labour through investment of industrial capital.

33 It seems clear that the stark division between the 'backward' countries on the one hand and the 'advanced' countries on the other is in itself inadequate in grasping the profoundly uneven development of the capitalist system. This is certainly true for the

imperialist epoch as a whole, but even more so as we approach the end of the twentieth century. The fact is that this unevenness of development manifests itself just as much within the colonial countries as it does within the metropolitan countries. Thus sectors or areas of the economies of the former countries become the basis for important 'hi-tech' industries which are able to take advantage not simply of cheap labour power but often an appropriate educational and training environment provided by the host state. In countries such as Brazil the contrast between some of the most advanced productive equipment in the world in rapidly-growing cities such as Sao Paulo alongside equally backward social conditions is a reflection of a more universal trend. For a detailed examination of this with the computer industry in mind see Henderson (1989).

34 This is undoubtedly one of the pressures currently forcing the US administration to keep its interest rates high, for it has to be able to attract enough money from abroad to finance its twin budget and external deficits, a problem exacerbated by the very low savings ratio in the United States.

35 The gross domestic product of the economies of the former Soviet Union and the countries of Eastern Europe fell by an incredible 42 per cent in the period 1990 to 1993. See United Nations (1993).

36 'Had the Uruguay Round failed to culminate in agreement, there would have been a real prospect of a descent into 1930s-style trade policies, with the major industrial powers engaging in cycles of retaliation and counter-retaliation' (Watkins 1995: 129). The report goes on to stress the 'highly unbalanced' outcome of the Uruguay Round, with a projected two-thirds of the benefits going to the big industrialised countries. Sub-Saharan Africa stands to lose absolutely from the agreement. The transnational corporations will gain directly from the terms of the Uruguay Round for under them the power of governments to regulate foreign investment has been further curtailed. This will give the transnationals even more scope to exploit national differences in social and environmental standards by locating their investments in the sites of maximum profitability. See Watkins (1995: 10).

37 Britain's overseas liabilities had increased from £542 million in June 1939 to £3,354 million in June 1945, while its reserves of gold and US and Canadian dollars had risen by only £121 million to £624 million between August 1939 and June 1945. The diversion of industry to the needs of war meant that in 1945 exports stood at only 46 per cent of 1938 volume and the enforced sale of overseas assets meant that income from a pre-war level of nearly £170 million fell to £50 million in 1945, during which period prices had approximately doubled (Sayers 1956).

38 In this connection it should be stressed that the expansion of British capitalism after the war had nothing to do with the successful application of Keynesian policies by British governments. It was US imperialism with its 'global Keynesianism' of money and debt expansion that provided the framework for any expansion in Britain. This is now recognised by the more intelligent bourgeois commentators.

39 For a detailed defence of this position see Meiksins Wood (1991).

40 It is interesting to compare the stance of a person such as Crosland in the mid-1960s with the positions of the current Labour leadership. Thus some three decades ago Crosland had the following to say:

> The two remaining aspirations – the concern with social welfare, and the desire for an equal and classless society – still have a perfectly clear relevance. The first implies an acceptance of collective responsibility and an extremely high priority for the relief of social distress or misfortune, in contrast to the much lower priority it would receive in a 'free' economy guided mainly by individualistic philosophy. This is the contemporary version of the traditional welfare and social-service philosophy of the Labour movement, and of the instinct to side automatically with the less fortunate and those in need.
>
> (Crosland 1964: 76)

The Commission on Social Justice Report (1994), with its stress on 'individual responsibility' and its rejection of the old 'collectivism', indicates how far the Labour leaders have shifted to the right, itself an expression of the depth of capitalism's crisis.

41 For a discussion of these matters see Jerry Coakley and Laurence Harris (1992). The authors argue that while Thatcher aimed to strengthen the position of the City at the expense of the further decline of British industry, even this aim was not achieved during her years of office.

42 The rise in unemployment from 2.6 per cent in 1974 to 6.2 per cent in 1977 was far worse than anything experienced since the 1930s; in addition this was combined with unprecedented rates of inflation which reached 26 per cent in 1975. Again these changes were not due principally to domestic factors but to changes in world economy. Thus from 1951 until 1973 Britain benefited from an expanding international economy and stable world prices, whereas after 1973 she was hit by a world recession and inflationary pressures arising from sharply rising commodity prices, especially the price of oil.

43 For a discussion of the meaning to be attached to the term 'reformist' in the light of these sorts of factors see Singer (1994).

References

Bean, C.R. (1994) 'European unemployment: a survey', *Journal of Economic Literature*, 32 (2): 573–619.

Brotherstone, T. and Pilling, G. (eds) (1996) *History, Economic History and the Future of Marxism: Essays in Memory of Tom Kemp*, London: Porcupine Press, pp. 13–50.

Coakley, J. and Harris, L. (1992) 'Financial globalisation and deregulation', in J. Michie, (ed.) *The Economic Legacy 1979–1992*, London: Academic Press.

Commission on Social Justice (1994) (the Borrie Report) *Social Justice: Strategies for National Renewal*, London: Vintage.

Crosland, C.A.R. (1964) *The Future of Socialism*, London: Cape.

Dicken, P. (1992, second edition) *Global Shift: The Internationalization of Economic Activity*, London: Paul Chapman Publishing.

Drucker, P.F. (1986) 'The changed world economy', *Foreign Affairs*, 64 (4): 768–791.

The Economist (1994) 'The slippery slope. Europe and the underclass', 332 (7874): 19–21.

Friedman, M. (1990) *Monetarist Economics*, Oxford: Basil Blackwell.

Fukuyama, F. (1992) *The End of History and the Last Man*, London: Hamish Hamilton.

Henderson, J. (1989) *The Globalisation of High Technology Production*, London: Routledge.

Lenin, V.I. (1964) 'Imperialism, the highest stage of capitalism', in *Collected Works*, vol. 22, Moscow and London: Progress Publishers and Lawrence & Wishart, pp. 185–304.

Lombard, M. (1995) 'A re-examination of the reasons for the failure of Keynesian expansionary policies in France, 1981–1983', *Cambridge Journal of Economics*, 19 (2): 359–372.

MacEwan, A. (1990) *Debt and Disorder: International Economic Instability and US Imperial Decline*, New York: Monthly Review Press.

Mandel, E. (1968) *Marxist Economic Theory*, London: Merlin Press.

Mandel, E. (1974) 'Workers under neo-capitalism', in E. Mandel and G. Novak, *On the Revolutionary Potential of the Working Class*, New York: Pathfinder Press, pp. 13–28.

Meiksins Wood, E. (1991) *The Pristine Culture of Capitalism: A Historical Essay on Old Regimes and Modern States*, London and New York: Verso.

Moore, J. (1983) *Japanese Workers and the Struggle for Power 1945–47*, Madison: University of Wisconsin Press.

Monthly Review (1992) 'Globalization – to what end? Part 1', 43 (9): 1–18.

Morgan Guaranty Trust Company (1991) *World Financial Markets*, April.

Moseley, F. (1991) *The Falling Rate of Profit in the Post-war United States Economy*, London: Macmillan.

Nyilas, J. (1982) *World Economy and its Main Development Tendencies*, The Hague: Nijhoff.

Pilling, G. (1996) 'Engels and the industrial revolution', in J. Lea and G. Pilling, (eds), *The Condition of Britain: Essays on Frederick Engels*, London: Pluto Press, pp. 58–83.

Sayers, R.S. (1956) *Financial Policy 1939–45*, London: HMSO and Longmans, Green.

Singer, D. (1988) *Is Socialism Doomed? The Meaning of Mitterrand*, New York and Oxford: Oxford University Press.

Singer, D. (1994) 'Europe's crises', *Monthly Review*, 46 (3): 86–100.

Smith, K. (1984) *The British Economic Crisis: Its Past and Future*, Harmondsworth: Penguin.

Sweezy, P.M. (1994) 'The triumph of finance capital', *Monthly Review*, 46 (2): 1–11.

Symes, V. (1995) *Unemployment in Europe: Problems and Policies*, London: Routledge.

Thrift, N.J. (1989, second edition) 'The geography of international economic disorder', in R.J. Johnston and P.J. Taylor (eds) *A World in Crisis? Geographical Perspectives*, Oxford: Basil Blackwell, pp. 16–78.

Trotsky, L.D. (1974) *The 3rd International After Lenin*, London: New Park Publications. 1929 *Militant*, New York version. Online available at www.marxists.org/archive/trotsky/1928/3rd/index.htm (accessed 13 December 2011).

United Nations (1993) *World Economic Survey*, New York: UN.

Watkins, K. (1995) *The Oxfam Poverty Report*, Oxford: Oxfam.

Watts, M. (1991) 'Entitlements or empowerment? Famine and starvation in Africa', *Review of African Political Economy*, 19 (51): 9–26.

3 The law of value in Ricardo and Marx

There can be little doubt that for academic economists at least, the main object of their attack against Marxism continues to be the Marxist theory of value. This is as true of Marx's 'friends' (such as Joan Robinson [see, for example, Joan Robinson (1966, second edition) *An Essay on Marxian Economics*, London: Macmillan – ed.] and many of her colleagues in the Cambridge School) as it is of his enemies. We do not propose to answer all these attacks. This would be impossible in the space available here; in any case most of them have failed to advance over those issued by Bohm-Bawerk more than 70 years ago.

Instead we intend to restate as simply as possible the essential features of this law and the place it occupied in Marx's work as a whole. In the light of this statement we wish to suggest that fundamental errors have been committed particularly by English writers, many claiming to write as Marxists, in their treatment of this law. Finally we intend to examine these errors in the light of Marx's relationship to classical political economy, and in particular to David Ricardo (1953).[1]

Perhaps the best statement which Marx made about his law of value – an account which Lenin advised all students of *Capital* to consult carefully – is to be found in his famous letter to Dr. Kugelmann of 11 July 1858. The critical passage reads as follows:

> even if there were no chapter on 'value' in my book, the analysis of the real relationships which I give would contain the proof and demonstration of the real value relation. The nonsense about the necessity of proving the concept of value arises from complete ignorance both of the subject dealt with and of the method of science. Every child knows that a country which ceased to work, I will not say for a year, but for a few weeks would die. Every child knows too, that the mass of products corresponding to the different needs require different and quantitatively determined means of the total labour of society. That this necessity of distributing social labour in definite proportions cannot be done away with by the *particular form* of social production but can only change the *form it assumes*, is self evident. No natural laws can be done away with. What can change, in changing historical circumstances, is the *form* in which these laws operate. And the form in which this

> proportional division of labour operates, in a state of society where the interconnection of social labour is manifested in the *private exchange* of the individual products of labour, is precisely the *exchange-value* of these products. The science consists precisely in working out *how* the law of value operates. So that if one wanted at the very beginning to 'explain' all the phenomena which apparently contradict that law, one would have to give the science *before* the science.
>
> (Marx 1934: 73–74)

In our view this is an extremely important passage and in a sense the rest of this chapter will be a commentary on the ideas we feel are implicit in it. Marx evidently wished to stress one basic idea – the historico-relative character of all the categories of political economy. For him none of the categories met with in political economy – such as 'production', 'division of labour', etc. – can be understood except in their relations to the specific mode of production of which they formed a part.

'The categories of bourgeois economy ... are forms of thought expressing with social validity the conditions and relations of a definite, historically determined mode of production, viz., the production of commodities' (Marx 1961: 76).[2] But this recognition of the relative character of economic categories – recognition that the theory of historical materialism required – did not mean however that there were not features common to many if not all modes of production. This was inevitable in that all societies had this much in common: they involved some mechanism for the allocation of social labour between the various branches of the economy. Socialist society will be no different in experiencing this universal need. However, and this is crucial, the *form* which this mechanism takes differs widely from society to society. The differences depend ultimately upon the structure of the productive relations and it was one of Marx's chief preoccupations to establish – in opposition to the vulgar school – the dependence of 'distribution' on 'production'.

Having made clear the precise nature of his task, Marx shows that the *specifica differentia* of the capitalist mode was the dominant position achieved within it of commodity production, and the transformation of the category 'labour' into the category 'labour power'. Given this, how was the allocation of social labour between the different branches effected? It was effected, answered Marx, only through the exchange of commodities as equivalents, through their exchange-values. And, as we shall see, this category 'exchange-value' was but the phenomenal form of 'value'. In other words, for Marx, the law of value reflected the only possible, indirect, mechanism whereby social labour could be distributed in a commodity-producing society. *The law of value reflects the specific social relations which operate under commodity (and particularly capitalist commodity) production, and under these conditions alone.* Speaking of socialist economic organisation, Engels said 'People will be able to manage everything very simply, without the intervention of the much-vaunted "value"' (Engels 1977: 375).[3]

In his letter to Kugelmann, Marx wished to draw his friend's attention to another point which will particularly concern us in this chapter – namely the fact that capitalism was also unique in another sense in that the value relation (a social relation) appeared as a relation between things. *Capital* is concerned, that is, with both quantitative problems (the exchange ratios prevailing between commodities) and qualitative problems (that behind these quantitative ratios stood social relations). For Marx, the attachment of social relations to things was no 'illusion'. For under capitalism the social relations between the labour of individuals constituting society could only manifest themselves, or *appear as* the relations between objects of material wealth. These appearances were, as Marx puts it, 'necessary appearances'.

> A social relation of production appears as something existing apart from individual human beings, and the distinctive relations into which they enter in the course of production appear as the specific property of a thing – it is this perverted appearance, this prosaically real, *and by no means imaginary mystification* that is characteristic of all social forms positing exchange-value.
>
> (Marx 1971a: 49, emphasis added)

Or again

> the relations connecting the labour of one individual with that of the rest appear, not as direct social relations between individuals at work, *but as what they really are* material relations between persons and social relations between things.
>
> (Marx 1961: 73, emphasis added)

A very important result flowed from this conception of appearances as *necessary* appearances: they could only be destroyed by overthrowing the economic categories which sustained them. Marx did not see his task merely as one stripping away the illusions of capitalism, to reveal things 'as they really were'. This conception is indeed implicit in all those treatments of *Capital* which seek to reduce its method to a variety of sociological 'model building'. Thus one prominent writer, Maurice Dobb (1940: 11) puts the matter this way in discussing his requirements for such a 'model': 'But to permit all the full quantitative statements to be made, such governing dimensions or entities to which the price-variables are connected must be related in a way which enables them to be reduced to a common term.' For him, Marxism is superior in an 'operational' sense in that 'labour' provides such a constant to which all the other entities in the model can be reduced.

For Marx, no such task presented itself. His aim was not to *reduce* all the phenomena of the system (such as the structure of prices) to the determination of value by labour time, but on the contrary one of *explaining* these phenomena by demonstrating how they could be reconciled with the operation of the law of value. Hence his scorn for all those intent on 'proving' the law of value, rather than seeking to find out how it *operated.*

While not anticipating Marx's solution to this problem, this much can be said: the entire method of *Capital* is based upon the conception that the thing in itself (in this case 'value') can only present itself through its contradictory opposite, its appearance (to continue with the illustration, 'exchange-value' is the form of appearance of 'value'). In other words, Marx rejected Kant's separation of the 'thing in itself' from its 'appearance' in favour of Hegel's method. The task of Marx's critique of political economy was not one which involved him in finding a 'constant' in terms of which everything could be quantified but of establishing the laws of mediation through which the 'essence' of phenomena manifested itself as 'appearance'. 'Hence law is not beyond Appearance, but is immediately present in it; the realm of laws is the quiescent counterfeit of the existing or appearing world' (Hegel 1929: 133). While Ricardo grasped the nature of the problem facing political economy, it was his method which prevented him from arriving at a satisfactory solution to it.

Marx, we have suggested, traces the many links between 'essence' and 'appearance', demonstrating the necessary nature of the latter. This is why he is able to write:

> Its discovery [of the determination of the magnitude of value by labour-time – G.P.] while removing all appearance of mere accidentality from the determination of the magnitude of the values of products, yet in no way alters the mode in which that determination takes place.
>
> (1961: 75)

In other words, only a reorganisation of society can abolish fetishism:

> The life process of society, which is based on the process of material production, does not strip off its mystical veil until it is treated as production by freely associated men, and is consciously regulated by them in accordance with a settled plan.
>
> (Marx 1961: 80)

Or as he notes a little earlier, after the discovery by science of the component gases of air, the atmosphere itself remained unaltered (1961: 74).

So far we have elaborated a number of points which are implicit in the letter to Kugelmann. To state matters from a different angle: Marx intended to remind his friend of what he had already said nine years earlier with the publication of the *Critique* – that the 'guiding thread' for his work was the materialist conception of history. This was the theory that started from the proposition that the social relations of production form the 'real foundations' of society on which arose a political, legal, etc. 'superstructure'. Specifically, Marx set himself the task over the three volumes of *Capital* of tracing out the manifold interconnections between the social relations of production (under capitalism, the reflection of which is to be found in the category 'value') and all the other phenomena within the system, including the class struggle. This implied a method entirely opposed to that of Ricardo, as Marx's letter already suggests.

But many of Marx's aims and methods have been seriously misrepresented by the majority of commentators who would wish to be designated 'Marxist economists'. The leader in this field is Maurice Dobb. He opens his major theoretical work in the field of value theory with a chapter entitled 'The requirements of a theory of value' (Dobb 1940, ch. 1). Immediately he presupposes a method alien to that of Marx; we have already argued that the analysis of 'value' cannot be disembodied from a work the aim of which was to 'lay bare the law of motion of modern society'. If Dobb has in mind *Marx's* value theory (as against that of Ricardo, for example) then the concern of the chapter would appear to be misplaced. For our only answer would consist of an exposition of the value analysis as developed in *Capital*. If on the other hand Dobb has in mind a *general concept* of value (as indeed the remainder of the work shows him to have) he is guilty of starting from an abstract concept and not as Marx insisted we must, from an examination of the process of social labour as it appears in 'modern society'. Marx evidently had this type of error in mind when he replied to the charges of A. Wagner; the latter had accused him of 'illogicality' in 'splitting the concept of value into exchange-value and use-value'. Marx said:

> Above all I do not start from 'concepts' thus not 'from the concept of value'. What I start from is the simplest social form in which the product of labour in the present form of society presents itself; and this is 'commodity'.
>
> (Marx 1972: 50)

Marx is here pointing out to Wagner and others that he started as a materialist from 'real active living men' and not as an idealist who starts always from 'concepts'. In this respect Dobb is firmly in the camp of Wagner, against Marx.

Similarly, when Ronald Meek writes a book 'to try and build some sort of bridge between Marxian economists and their non-Marxian colleagues' and sets out to convince Joan Robinson that Marx's value theory 'was good sense' (1956: 7) his task is as ill-conceived as Dobb's starting point – the comparison of the 'adequacy' of 'models' is wrong. Marx's avowed aim – of exposing the ever-sharpening contradictions of a particular mode of production – is one necessarily abandoned by vulgar economy. We need only recall, that for Marx, if not Meek, '1830 sounds the knell of scientific bourgeois economy'. If we do accept this judgement, then we are forced to the inescapable conclusion that 'modern economics' with which Meek is so keen to forge links, cannot have a theory of *value*, 'adequate' or otherwise. It was Marx's point that with the emergence of the working class, increasingly consciously ranged against the capitalist class and its political economy, the latter inevitably degenerated into shallow apologetics for the existing order, ultimately to become a branch of technology. All modern 'price theory' (it still occasionally masquerades as a 'value theory') derives from the category 'utility' or the relationship between 'wealth' (for Marx the aggregate of use-values) and the 'individual consumer'. The point about such theories is that because they are ahistorical they are necessarily asocial. For individuals *always* confront 'nature' whatever the mode of production; because such theories concern only the individual's relationship with nature and not with his fellow man they are devoid of social content. Thus it is impossible that 'economics' can have a category 'value' which, we insist, is not a 'thing' but a social relation. Yet running through the work of many of those who would wish to 'defend' Marx or 'praise' him is the conception that they have a rival value theory to answer. Dobb writes of 'the two major value theories which have contested the economic field' (1940: 12) and proceeds to suggest that both (he means the 'labour' theory of value and marginal utility analysis) meet his formal requirements of 'adequacy': 'Quite a number of theories of value can be derived with no means of choice between them except their formal elegance.' And in a later work he repeats this view in even stronger terms (Dobb 1955, *passim* but particularly pp. 110–111). In the same fashion, Meek accepts Pareto's and Bohm-Bawerk's utility analysis as constituting an alternative value theory to that of Marx which he seeks to defend (1956, ch. 6). Both these writers wrongly see their task as merely exposing the penumbra of approbation with which these theories surround capitalism. Put another way, the mistake they both make is to fail to see the significance of the profound distinction which Marx and political economy – however unclearly in the latter case – drew between 'wealth', the sum of material objects and *value*, a social relation specific to conditions of commodity production and especially to capitalism.

This is not a minor point of difference with these writers. For it is closely connected with a number of equally erroneous conceptions which they hold about value theory. Dobb, for example, has tried to answer the question: Why did Marx choose labour as the basis for his value theory? Why not choose capital or land as the category in terms of which everything else is computed? Here is the answer:

> In the case of land or capital, clearly there were serious practical objections to taking them as a basis: difficulties which would have exceeded any of those which were charged against the labour theory.... Acres are more dissimilar than man-hours of labour. In the case of capital there was the crucial objection that it was itself a value, depending upon other values, in particular upon profit to be earned.
>
> (Dobb 1940: 18)

These, apparently were insurmountable difficulties. Thus labour is chosen! Thus the labour theory of value! In a sense we cannot analyse the nature of the answer which Dobb provides for his own question. *For it is in the very posing of the question that the fundamental error is committed.* With good reason did Lenin (1934: 12) on one occasion speak of 'the so-called "labour" theory of value'. We must repeat – Marx is concerned with the analysis of the social relations of production and his work never strays outside of these limits. Man's social relations under capitalism appear only through the relations between 'things' (commodities). Leaving aside their particular properties as use-values – which Marx says is an area of concern appropriate to commerce – their one common property is that they are products of abstract labour, the quantitative measure of which is *time*. In other words, the category 'value' is one entirely subordinate, in both a logical and a historical sense, to the commodity. As Dobb would have it, Marx 'chose' labour – a subjective act – because it enabled him to solve certain 'practical' problems:

> The statement which the labour theory of value implied was that the exchange-values bore a certain relation to the output and using up of human energies and in so doing provided a term which gave some meaning to the distinction between a gross and net product and to the concept of surplus, and a criterion for differentiating one type of income from another.
>
> (Dobb 1940: 22)

Here a number of issues are raised, all of them of great importance for a correct interpretation of Marx's work. First we see Dobb moving directly in the direction of Ricardo with the emphasis he places upon the question of *distribution*. We need to recall that it was *Ricardo*, not Marx, who defined the task 'To determine the laws which regulate this distribution [of the social product between rent, profit and wages] as the principal one facing political economy' (Ricardo 1953: 55).[4] In following Ricardo, Dobb is playing into the hands of all those, from Bernstein onwards, who have falsely accused Marx of 'using' his value theory to 'prove' the existence of exploitation under capitalism. But was the quantitative problem – that of the distribution of the social wealth between the classes which constituted capitalist society – Marx's main preoccupation? It was not. A surplus over and above the needs of immediate consumption is inevitable and necessary in all but the most primitive societies. Value theory merely reflects the particular form, with capitalism, of this more general relation.

This leads us to another matter, also implied in the same quotation – that Marx's value theory can in some sense be empirically 'verified', unlike the value theory of marginal utility analysis. Ernest Mandel's widely-read textbook states:

> The neo-classical theory [this refers to the theory formulated by Jevons in England and Walras, Menger, Pareto and others on the Continent in the last quarter of the nineteenth century – G.P.] is not only divorced from social reality as a whole. It is also divorced from the practical reality of everyday life. The labour theory can be demonstrated empirically, even if only in the sense that, in the last analysis, all the elements of the cost of production of a commodity tend to be reduced to labour, and to labour alone, if one goes back far enough in the analysis.
>
> (Mandel 1968: 716)

Dobb echoes this point when he writes:

> It seems clear, from the nature of the subject matter and the type of statements which it required to make, that an economic theory must be quantitative in form; the determining relation or relations which figure in the equational system should be capable of expression in terms of quantitative entities in the real world.
>
> (1940: 11)

But what, we must ask of those who share this standpoint, are these 'quantitative entities in the real world'? If the phrase has any meaning it must refer to entities such as 'price', 'rate of profit,' 'rate of interest' etc. It deals, that is, with the realm of *appearances* to which the vulgar school is exclusively confined, the realm where 'equality and Mr. Bentham' reign supreme.

Specifically, we can ask Dobb: how do you propose to 'measure' or quantify 'capital' or 'socially necessary labour time'? For Marx, capital was a social relation, the means of production in a specific social form – confronting the sellers of labour power as an alien, coercive power. In the same way, how can we 'calculate' the amount of socially necessary labour time incorporated into a commodity? As we have said, this latter is but the quantitative equivalent of Marx's abstract labour which as a category cannot appear empirically within the capitalist system. In any case the exchange-value of any commodity does not depend on the productivity of the labour in the branch of capitalist economy in which it has been produced; it reflects the productivity of labour on a social scale. In dealing with 'microscopic' entities we are forced to consider phenomena of a macroscopic dimension. In other words, no one commodity can be abstracted from the totality of commodity production; as we shall see, Ricardo's false method of abstraction forced this erroneous view upon him. Society, not Mr. Mandel, can be the only accountant of socially necessary labour time.

It is clear that the last few matters we have briefly considered are not isolated questions that flow from a series of 'particular' mistakes. For they all involve a distortion of Marxism in the general direction of positivism. Mandel, for example, (1968: 716) makes this clear when he suggests that one aspect of the superiority of the Marxist value analysis lies in the fact that businessmen, albeit unconsciously, price their products according to the labour theory of value. Sweezy also takes this position when he writes:

> Marx's value theory thus has the great merit, unlike some other value theories [he here incidentally accepts that there can be rival value theories to that developed by Marx out of his critique of classical political economy] of close correspondence to the actual accounting system of capitalistic business enterprise.
>
> (1946: 63)

Dobb makes essentially the same point, if from a slightly different angle, when he states: 'An economic law or tendency must state the possibility of some actual course of events occurring' (1940: 29), and earlier: 'The ultimate criterion [for the "adequacy" of a theory] must be the requirement of practice: the type of question which one requires to answer, the purpose of the inquiry in hand' (1940: 8). Here we have a thinly disguised form of instrumentalism, the method which selects its categories, not according to their congruence with historical and social forces but simply by virtue of their ability to sustain predictions 'in the real world'.[5]

It was positivism that falsely decreed that the only 'real' sciences were those dealing with natural phenomena: 'real' in the sense that they alone were exact enough to make predictions. But Marxism involves the view that the future evolution of events can be 'predicted' only to the extent that the material and social world consists of a series of fixed quantities. But the entire method of *Capital* is based on entirely the opposite view – that 'quantity' ('commodity' for example) is constantly in the process of transformation into other quantities and qualities ('money' to continue with the example) and thence into new quantities and qualities ('capital' in this case); this method further insists that far from being automatic, such transformations occur only under definite historical and social circumstances, which must be established by science. Marx also made clear that because the capitalist system is fundamentally an anarchic one – that is, cannot be subjected to a priori conscious regulation – each law of the system asserts itself as a 'blindly working average' – as he makes clear in connection with the law of value.[6] Given that this is so, the predictability of future events cannot be dealt with in the peremptory manner Dobb and others would have us believe.

To cite but one case: In what sense can Marx's law of the falling rate of profit enable us concretely to predict the future course of capitalist development? Its author certainly made no such claims on its behalf. In formulating this law of tendency, he wished to draw attention to the fact that (a) the rate of profit was the regulator of the entire accumulation process and (b) that this process was profoundly contradictory and must lead to periodic crises. But he never pretended that the precise *forms* taken by such crises could be predicted, nor even their exact magnitude or timing. As Marx makes clear in many places in *Capital*, each crisis was in a sense unique, determined by the whole past process of capital accumulation; it was therefore obligatory to examine each crisis in its concreteness and not by means of simple formulae. Precisely *because* capitalist social relations were antagonistic – that is based on the struggle of classes whose historical interests were diametrically opposed, that is qualitatively different – no predictions of a concrete nature about the evolution of economic categories was possible. More precisely, in connection with the movement of the rate of profit, Marx made clear that he was stating a general *law of tendency*, which in all cases, inevitably produced 'counter-acting' forces to its operation which modified its functioning in important respects. These included the strength and determination of the working class, the 'weight' of which could in no sense be known beforehand in that it depended upon both objective and subjective factors, amongst which had to be numbered the role which a knowledge of this law would have within the working class movement.[7] Here Marx, was, in effect, warning against the old mechanical materialism which thought that the world could be understood in a purely *contemplative* manner.

These distortions of Marx's method are doubly important because they also involve, in our view, another danger. This is the tendency to reduce Marxism to the level of 'political economy' particularly in the latter's Ricardian form. We wish therefore briefly to review Marx's attitude to his predecessors in the classical school in order to establish what we consider to be the fundamental break which his work represents with this school. Marx's studies in the history of political economy provide no mere 'appendix' to *Capital*; in every sense *Theories of Surplus Value* must be considered as the final volume of *Capital*, as indeed Marx intended it to be. For contained in the *Theories* is a detailed examination of the evolution of the categories 'value' and 'surplus-value' as reflected in the work of the principal French and English economists. But this work should not be taken as 'history' in the conventional sense; it was intended as Engels at one point notes to provide

> a detailed critical history of the pith and marrow of Political Economy, the theory of surplus-value, and develops parallel with it, in polemics against predecessors, most of the points later investigated separately in their logical connection in the manuscripts for Books II and III.
>
> (Engels, 'Preface' to Marx 1957: 2)

Marx writes this work always 'critically', from the vantage point that is of his own theory (historical materialism), just as the anatomy of the ape must be studied from the standpoint of its higher, further development, in man. He is interested not merely in tracing the origin of his own ideas, in paying his intellectual debts, as it were. Nor is he interested only in exposing the limitations of the classical school – of which he was fully conscious. He aims, throughout the *Theories*, to probe the contradictions in the writings of Smith, Ricardo, etc. because he sees in them only a 'purer', more abstract and therefore heightened expression of the real economic contradictions of the capitalist system which was their real underpinning.

It is from this standpoint that the work of Ricardo is judged, in an all-round fashion. Marx never saw his problem as one merely of correcting the 'distortions' in Ricardo's work, nor of analysing capitalism in a naive manner, from the 'standpoint of the working class'. Indeed, as anyone acquainted with the *Theories* will know, Marx was always insistent upon drawing attention to Ricardo's great 'disinterestedness' (objectivity) as against the special pleading of Malthus – 'this shameless sycophant' 'that bought advocate of the ruling classes' as Marx contemptuously dubs him. But Marx stresses always that Ricardo's sincere insistence that the needs of production should be placed above the sectional claims of any class (herein lay the 'disinterestedness' of this rich financier) coincided with the needs of the rising capitalist class only in that period when the bourgeoisie had every interest in the further development of the productive forces. With the emergence of the modern working class, the most decisive of all the productive forces, this progressive interest was finished and scientific political economy died. That is why the period around 1830 spells for political economy its 'final crisis'; Ricardo's doctrines become the basis, albeit in a confused and unsatisfactory manner, for the political economy of Utopian Socialism.

What were the main periods which Marx discerns in the history of political economy up to its ignoble collapse in the first quarter of the nineteenth century? While Petty can be regarded as the founding father of the science, French Physiocracy represents the first true school in political economy. The writers who formed this school grasped that forms of production were *physiological* forms, arising out of the necessities of production and independent of will and politics. Seeing value in production, the school then proceeds to trace the connections between production and circulation. The weakness of Physiocracy was that 'production' was still seen concretely and not abstractly, for according to Quesnay and his followers, labour on the land was alone productive of value. But this limited view, a reflection of the limited stage reached in the evolution of the eighteenth century French economy, was nonetheless decisive for the future analysis of the capitalist system. For the contradictions at the heart of Physiocracy arose essentially from its attempt to explain feudalism from a more consistently bourgeois point of view.

Adam Smith's *Wealth of Nations* marks a new leap forward in that it sees 'labour in general' as value-creating. It was from this time onwards that political economy could be placed upon a much firmer theoretical basis. But again, Marx sees the material basis for the advance which Smith's work constitutes. The category 'abstract labour' which Smith correctly sees as forming the basis of value was an expression of the economic categories which were being created by the development of the class struggle; for here was reflected a society where the organic bond between an individual and his labour was in the process of violent rupture. Smith's indifference to the particular type of labour when considering value – his real point of criticism against Physiocracy – implied the existence of highly developed varieties of concrete labour, none of which was predominant.

But, as in the case of Physiocracy, so now with Smith: his advance in theoretical understanding was severely limited and necessarily so. He was a 'transitional' figure in every sense. This was particularly so in the fact that his work continues the classificatory and descriptive emphasis of his British predecessors – as seen most clearly in Petty's *Political Arithmetick* [Petty 1690 – ed.] – and the more abstract approach which was to be found in Ricardo's writings some 50 years later. The matter can be put this way: Smith was on the one hand concerned with a search for those abstract laws which would accurately express the innermost workings of capitalism as a system – hence the importance for his work of the concept of the 'hidden hand'. This side of his work – which Marx refers to as its 'esoteric' element is seen in his famous phrase 'It is not from the benevolence of the butcher the brewer or the baker that we expect our dinner but from their regard to their own interest' (Smith 1976, vol. 1, book 1, ch. II: 26–27). On the other hand Smith's work contains also a considerable 'exoteric' element, that is, a concern not for the inner-structure of phenomena, but for their outward manifestations. Many examples of this naive 'duality' of which Smith was unaware could be drawn from the *Wealth of Nations*, and elsewhere. But it is seen most clearly in his conception that the law of value only holds in a 'rude and primitive' state of society, and must be abandoned once 'modern' society is reached. Smith was thus guilty of allowing immediate impressions of competition between the branches of economy to intrude into and ultimately overthrow his basic theoretical starting point.

In this respect, Ricardo's work involved a significant advance. We should in any case remember that he first took up the study of political economy as a result of the feeling of dissatisfaction he experienced with the theoretical and practical answers provided by the *Wealth of Nations.* For Marx, his work represents a decisive attempt to establish political economy as an *abstract science* dealing with the laws which governed the workings of the capitalist system. Ricardo, in effect insists that the science can no longer operate with 'description' on one hand and 'analysis' on the other. It must, starting with its basic principle – the determination of value by labour time – make all the outward appearances of the system 'answerable' to it.

This advance in method, what Marx at one point calls 'Ricardo's great service to the science' can be judged by an examination of the latter's *Principles.* This work consists, in its third edition, of 30 chapters; the essential theoretical matters are however given in the first two – the rest consist of elaborations or applications of principles enunciated at the start of the work. How does Ricardo proceed? He starts with a statement of the determination of value by labour time which is much less ambiguous than that to be found in Smith. In the next sections he takes up a number of questions – the movement of relative wages between different branches of economy, the varying structure of capital between the different sectors, etc. Of each he asks: to what extent do they overthrow or force the modification of the law of value as already stated? We give, as an example of this procedure, the opening paragraph of the section dealing with rent: 'It remains to be considered whether the appropriation of land, and the consequent creation of rent, will occasion any variation in the relative value of commodities, independently of the quantity of labour necessary to production' (1953: 67). He thus tries to 'hold fast' to the law of value, whereas Smith had concluded as we have noted, that it had to be rapidly abandoned in the face of the immediate appearances of the emerging economic system.

Thus it can be said that Ricardo posed correctly the problem facing political economy. Hence for Marx the 'great theoretical satisfaction' afforded by the earlier chapters of the *Principles* as against the 'diffuse and meandering' work of Smith. The whole bourgeois economic system was based firmly upon one law and all phenomena which seemed to conflict with it were examined in its light. Here is the clue to the real meaning of the English adage 'It's the exception that proves the rule'; for Ricardo, after neatly setting forth the law of value 'demonstrates that this law governs even those bourgeois relations of production which apparently contradict it most decisively' (Marx 1971a: 60).

Here, however, Marx's praise for Ricardo's great historical achievement ends. Each advance in political economy can be seen as a 'criticism' of previous writers – Smith of Mercantilism; Ricardo of the *Wealth of Nations*, etc. But Marx's attitude towards Ricardo cannot be seen as in any way analogous. For each of the writers who preceded Marx accepted that the laws of the capitalist system were akin to the laws of nature. As we have seen this was Marx's main objection to their work which he sees as the source of its ultimate break-up.

But it was an objection directly tied in with another: a recognition that empiricism dominated the method of classical economy. In this connection the central role which Marx ascribed to Locke should not be forgotten: 'his philosophy served the basis for all the ideas of the whole of subsequent English political economy' (1969: 367). Again: 'With all later bourgeois economists, as with Adam Smith, lack of theoretical understanding needed to distinguish the different forms of economic relations remains the rule in their coarse grabbing at and interest in the empirically available material' (1969: 92).

All Ricardo's weaknesses reflect this empiricism and resolve themselves into this: that while he starts correctly from the law of value he attempts *immediately* to deal with all the phenomena which conflict with this law. Hence Marx's reference to the 'faulty archetectonics' of his work. What is lacking in the *Principles* is any treatment of the process of *mediation* by which the 'forms of appearance' in bourgeois society are connected to their origin, the law of value.

This makes it imperative to highlight the differences between Ricardo's method and that of Marx, as reflected in the structure of *Capital.* While Ricardo feels obliged to take up all the phenomena which appear to overthrow the law of value in the very opening chapters of his work, Marx only comes to deal with the realm of 'appearance' with the opening of the *third* volume, after an exhaustive study of the fundamental processes of production and circulation. Marx explains his procedure at the very opening of this third volume and we reproduce the key passage from the first chapter:

> In Book I we analysed the phenomena which constitute the *process of capitalist production* as such, as the immediate productive process, with no regard for any of the secondary effects of outside influences. But this immediate process of production does not exhaust the life span of capital. It is supplemented in the actual world by the *process of circulation*, which was the object of the study in Book II. In the latter, namely Part III, which treated the process of circulation as a medium for the process of social reproduction, it developed that the capitalist process of production taken as a whole represents a synthesis of the processes of production and circulation. Considering what this third book treats, it cannot confine itself to a general reflection relative to this synthesis. On the contrary, it must locate and describe the concrete forms which grow out of the *movements of capital as a whole.* In their actual movement, capitals confront each other in such

> concrete shape, for which the form of capital in the immediate process of production, just as its form in the process of circulation, appear only as special instances. The various forms of capital, as evolved in this book, thus approach step by step the form which they assume on the surface of society, in the action of different capitals upon one another, in competition, and in the ordinary consciousness of the agents of production themselves.
>
> (Marx 1959: 25)

Here Marx explains that the process of movement to the realm of appearances cannot be an immediate one. All the manifold links, missing in Ricardo, have to be established between the outward form of things and their inner source. For Marx, this was precisely what he had in mind when he suggested to Kugelmann that the problem was to establish how the law of value operates. So when the realm of appearances was finally reached they were not considered as isolated, disembodied phenomena, as in the vulgar conception, nor were they merely counterposed to their source, the law of value, as in classical economy. They were now grasped as *necessary appearances*, contradictory, opposite, manifestations of definite, historically determined social relations of production. To take one illustration of this method: at one point Marx writes of the transformation of value and price of labour power into the form of wages:

> This phenomenal form, which makes the actual relation invisible, *and, indeed, shows the direct opposite of that*, forms the basis of all the juridical notions of both labourer and capitalist, of all the mystifications of the capitalist mode of production, of all its illusions as to liberty, of all the apologetic shifts of the vulgar economists.
>
> (1961: 540, emphasis added)

We must now indicate the connection between Ricardo's faulty abstractions (Marx calls them 'violent' at one point) and the grave errors which he made on all the questions of political economy which left his work open to ready attack by his opponents. This question cannot be systematically dealt with; we shall merely indicate some important issues. In the first place, Ricardo failed to see that under capitalism, prices could never coincide with values, but were transformed into 'prices of production' around which prices in turn oscillated, according to the fluctuations of supply and demand.[8] Because Ricardo tried *directly* to reduce all prices to values (and this is the method of procedure that writers like Dobb would have us adopt) he ended up, as Marx shows, with a false theory of *rent*, a serious matter in his case as it constituted the cornerstone of his system. Ricardo tried *directly to* uphold the law of value; this forced him to deny the possibility of *absolute* rent (rent on the least fertile land) and he focused his attention exclusively on the movement of *differential rent* (rent earned on land of varying fertility). Marx, in his critique of Ricardo, establishes the possibility of absolute rent, by demonstrating the indirect operation of the law of value, via prices of production.

Ricardo also consistently confused the generic category, surplus-value, with one of its specific forms, profit. This resulted from his faulty conception of capital, which he saw only in its immediately available form as 'stored up labour'. This in turn stemmed from his wrong understanding of the relation between the source of a category (in this case surplus-value) with its various forms of appearance (rent, interest, profit). Marx shows in volume I of *Capital* that surplus-value is created in the sphere of production, in the antagonistic relations between wage labour and capital. It is subsequently divided between the three classes who live on this surplus according to definite and objective laws, but laws which are only analysed at a later stage. Not that this procedure could be reversed, by moving from the realm of appearance back to essence, as Marx makes clear:

> The transformation of surplus-value into profit must be deduced from the transformation of the rate of surplus-value into the rate of profit, not vice versa. And in fact it was rate of profit which was the historical point of departure. Surplus-value and rate of surplus-value are, relatively, the invisible and unknown essence that wants investigating, while rate of profit and therefore the appearance of surplus-value in the form of profit are revealed on the surface of the phenomenon.
>
> (1959: 42–43)

Because Ricardo wrongly identified the category 'profit' with the more general category 'surplus-value' he wrongly concluded that the rate of profit could only change if the value of wage goods changed – in other words, and using Marx's terms, only if the rate of surplus-value altered. Marx rejected this conclusion. By dividing capital into *variable* capital (that portion of capital advanced in the form of wages) and *constant* capital (that portion expended on raw materials, heat, light power, machinery, etc.) Marx was able to arrive at his category the 'organic composition of capital', the ratio of constant to variable capital. This was placed at the centre of his theory of capital accumulation and the potential breakdown associated therewith. Here indeed was a revolutionary development. The only possible barrier to the further development of the productive forces which Ricardo's work had allowed was associated with *agriculture.* Ricardo had assumed that what Marx scornfully termed the 'so-called law of diminishing returns' operated in agriculture; the working of this law would ultimately, said Ricardo, force up the price of corn which would in turn lead to an increase in wages and produce a tendency for the rate of profit to decline – a prospect which sent shivers down the spine of the millionaire banker.[9] Hence the need for a 'heavy class struggle' against the landed interest if this ominous tendency were to be checked. Marx was able to show, however, that there were forces quite *internal* to the accumulation process which provided potential sources of breakdown; he was thus able to reject all 'explanations' of capitalist crisis which rely upon the importation of 'outside' factors – in Ricardo's case from the sphere of agriculture which Marx recognised was rapidly becoming a force increasingly subordinate to industrial capital. Marx went on show that with the 'progress of industry' there was an inexorable tendency for the rate of profit to decline through a tendency for the organic composition of capital to rise. (We should recall, however, what was said above about the possibility of this tendency being modified in its operation.)[10]

But the inadequacies of classical economy were revealed most clearly and fundamentally in its analysis of the commodity. It is this question which we now wish to deal with in that it will enable us to highlight some of the criticisms we have already made of the treatment of the law of value. We have seen that classical economy had noted the distinction between the value of a commodity and its use-value. But it had singularly failed to grasp the implications of this distinction, which for Marx was to provide the key for his entire analysis. Marx commences with an analysis of the commodity both because the commodity is the basic expression of the relations between man and man in capitalist society and second because the development of commodity production was a necessary precondition for the development of capitalist social relations. As we know, Marx went on to show that these two aspects of the commodity were reflected in his distinction between *concrete labour* and *abstract labour* (the source of use-values and exchange-values respectively). This examination of the twofold nature of labour contained in the commodity was, according to the author of *Capital*, 'the pivot on which a clear comprehension of Political Economy turns' (Marx 1961: 41), just as the confusion of Ricardo and others on this question constituted the 'weak point' of the classical conception. Marx explains the importance of the distinction when he writes:

> tailoring if one considers its physical aspect as a distinctive productive activity produces a coat, [a use-value – G.P.] but not the exchange-value of the coat. The exchange-value is produced by it not as tailoring as such but as abstract universal labour, and this belongs to a social framework not devised by the tailor.
>
> (Marx 1971a: 36)

Here Marx wishes to stress that, unlike the classical school, he not only sees labour as the *measure* of value, but as its *substance.*

In the first chapter of *Capital* we find the following observation 'It is one of the chief failings of classical economy that it has never succeeded, by means of its analysis of commodities, and, in particular, of their value, in discovering that form under which value becomes exchange-value' (1961: 80–81). Commenting on Petty in an earlier work he says: 'His case is striking proof that recognition of labour as the source of material wealth by no means precludes misapprehension of the specific social form in which labour constitutes the source of exchange-value' (1971a: 54).

Let us look more closely at the manner in which Marx investigates the nature of the commodity. In his *Marginal Notes on Wagner* mentioned above he tells us

> I analyse this [the commodity] and indeed, first in the form in *which it appears.* Here I find that on the one hand it is in its natural form a *thing of use*, alias a *use-value*, on the other hand *a bearer of exchange-value*, and in this respect itself 'exchange-value'. Further analysis of the latter shows me that exchange-value is only a '*phenomenal form*', an independent mode of representation of the *value* contained in the commodity.
>
> (1972: 50)

Hence, accurately speaking Marx was 'wrong' as he himself recognised:

> When, at the beginning of this chapter, we said, in common parlance, that a commodity is both a use-value and an exchange-value we were, accurately speaking, wrong. A commodity is a use-value or object of utility and a value. It manifests itself as this twofold thing, that it is, as soon as its value assumes an independent form – viz., the form of exchange-value. It never assumes this form when isolated, but only when placed in a value or exchange relation with another commodity of a different kind. When once we know this, such a mode of expression does no harm; it simply serves as an abbreviation.
>
> (1961: 60)

The most generalised value form taken by commodities was of course the *money form* (one coat = £2). *Marx seeks in his analysis of the value form, to trace the genesis of this money form from the internal structure of the commodity and to demonstrate its further development in the form of capital.*

> Here, however, a task is set us, the performance which has never been attempted by *bourgeois* economy, the task of tracing the genesis of this money-form, of developing the expression of value implied in the value-relation of commodities, from its simplest almost imperceptible outline, to the dazzling money-form.
>
> (Marx 1961: 47–48)

In general, Marx was once more showing the origin of all the 'appearances' within the capitalist system and at the same time pointing to the basis for their overthrow. Thus he explains that the contradictions within a single commodity (as a unity of a use-value and a value) are necessarily overcome only through the relations between two commodities in what Marx calls the 'accidental' or 'elementary' form (one coat = 20 yards of linen). 'Hence the elementary form of value of a commodity is the elementary form in which the contrast contained in that commodity, between use-value and value, becomes apparent' (Marx 1961: 61).

Here are two crucial points. First, the category value can only appear as *exchange-value;* the two cannot be torn apart, as some imply they can when they argue that the category 'value' could continue to exist in socialist economy while its form of appearance, exchange-value would disappear.[11] Second, and connected with this point Marx insists that 'exchange-value' arises from the category value, and not vice versa. 'Our analysis has shown that the form or expression of the value of a commodity originates in the nature of value, and not that value and its magnitude originate in the mode of their expression as exchange-value' (Marx 1961: 60). Here we have seen one aspect of the different conception of Marx from the later vulgar economy which taught that exchange could be examined quite independently of the relations of production.

Marx now subjects the 'elementary' form to detailed examination. He discusses the three 'peculiarities' of the form '20 yards of linen (the relative form) = one coat (the equivalent form)', when he examines the role of the equivalent.

> The first peculiarity that strikes us ... is this: use-value becomes the form of manifestation, the phenomenal form of its opposite, value ... the second peculiarity ... is, that concrete labour becomes the form under which its opposite, abstract human labour, manifests itself ... a third peculiarity ... namely, that the labour of private individuals takes the form of its opposite, labour directly social in its form.
>
> (Marx 1961: 56–59)

Next we see how this accidental form leads to the 'expanded' form along with the development of capitalism. This is given by 20 yards of linen = one coat or 10 lbs of tea, or 4 lbs of coffee, etc. This form brings out what was only implicit in the accidental form. 'It becomes plain, that it is not the exchange of commodities which regulates the magnitude of their value; but, on the contrary, that is the magnitude of their value which controls their exchange proportions' (Marx 1961: 63). But this expanded form suffers from grave 'defects' in that it is an incomplete form – the creation of every new commodity lengthens the chain and thereby furnishes the material for a fresh expression of value. Hence out of these contradictions arises the 'general' value form (one coat, 10 lbs of tea, 40 lbs of coffee, etc. = 20 yards of linen). This points the way for the emergence of the money form which is in fact identical with this general form except that gold now replaces the linen of our example. Thus has Marx traced the series of logical-historical transitions from the commodity form to the money form. Hence he is able to end this section (the third section of the opening chapter) thus: 'The simple commodity-form is therefore *the germ* of the money form' (Marx 1961: 70, emphasis added). The riddle of money is solved:

> Money is a crystal formed of necessity in the course of the exchanges, whereby different products of labour are practically equated to one another and thus by practice converted into commodities. The historical progress and extension of exchanges develops the contrast, latent in commodities, between use-value and value. The necessity for giving an external expression to this contrast for the purpose of commercial intercourse, urges on the establishment of an independent form of value, and finds no rest until it is

> once and for all satisfied by the differentiation of commodities into commodities and money.
>
> (Marx 1961: 86–87)

Only now is Marx able to understand the mystery of the commodity form which is treated in the famous section: 'The fetishism of commodities and the secret thereof'. He explains, after his investigation of the elementary form of value and its further development, that under capitalism: (a) the equality of human labour is expressed not as this equality but in the form of distinctly different commodities such as linen and overcoats; (b) the quantity of social labour time congealed in each commodity is not expressed in a direct comparison of time but in the *indirect* phenomenal form of equal quantities of value; (c) relations of people take the necessary appearance as relations between things; (d) the social character of labour, that is, its relation to total human output, appears as something else, as the value relation of a multitude of commodities to one universal equivalent (money).

Having established the genesis of the money form, Marx then shows how this can, under certain historical circumstances, lead to the emergence of *capital*: 'value ... suddenly presents itself as an independent substance, endowed with a motion of its own ... money in process, and, as such, capital' (1961: 154). This transition is reflected in the circulation schema which Marx discusses; under simple commodity production we have C–M–C (commodities–money–commodities) but under capital M–C–M (money–commodities–money). In the former we see that means of circulation, as a means of purchasing what one needs; in the latter it is turned into its opposite – now the owner of the means of production uses money to buy what he does not need to augment his capital, the driving force of production.

As we have several times said, the transitions involved in the movements from 'commodity' to 'money' were historical as well as logical movements. Marx makes this clear when examining the various value forms:

> It therefore follows that the elementary value-form is also the primitive form under which a product of labour appears historically as a commodity, and that the gradual transformation of such products into commodities, proceeds *pari passu* with the development of the value-form.
>
> (1961: 61)

But these developments should be not conceived of in a mechanical way; one can say that 'capital' is 'latent' within the 'commodity'. However, it is only under certain objective conditions, the outcome of long historical processes, that this potential can be realised. The circulation of commodities and the existence of money in one or other of its functions can and has pre-existed capitalism by many hundreds of years. It is quite otherwise with capital.

> The historical conditions of its existence are by no means given with the mere circulation of money and commodities. It can spring to life, only when

> the owner of the means of production and subsistence meets in the market with the free labourer selling his labour-power. And this one historical condition comprises a world's history. Capital, therefore, announces from its first appearance a new epoch in the process of social production.
>
> (Marx 1961: 170)

Why did Marx spend so much time on the problem of value. We should recall that this question finds much fuller treatment in *Capital* (1867) than it does in the *Critique* (1859) and was revised no less than four times, with the help of Engels, Kugelmann and others, between this latter date and 1872. He did so precisely because he wished to establish the link between the internal structure of the commodity and the heightened expression of the contradictions within the commodity form in the form of capital. Here was a decisive break with classical economy; because this latter had ignored the value form (in turn a reflection of its acceptance of capitalism as a 'natural' mode of production) it had failed to comprehend either the nature of money or of capital.[12] For classical economy, money was merely a means of overcoming the difficulties of barter; many of the early Utopian Socialists, criticised in *Theories of Surplus Value* had betrayed a similarly naive conception when they had proposed the abolition of money commodity production, equivalent to attempts, commented Marx, to retain Catholicism without the Pope. Similarly, as we have already noted, for Ricardo, capital was never seen as a social relation but merely as accumulated labour. Hence for Marx a presentation of the real nature of capital – not a thing but rather a definite social production relation – involved him in a *critique of* political economy.

Unless we accept the links between 'commodity'–'money'–'capital', then the unity of Marx's thought is immediately ruptured – and a fatal blow struck against historical materialism. We must repeat: Marx did not aim merely to demonstrate the exploitation of the working class – it can be said that this is implicit in Ricardo and certainly brought out by the Ricardian socialists long before Marx embarked upon his economic studies. Nor did Marx wish only to show that this exploitation was *endemic* to the system. What he had to establish was the manner in which the tendency to develop the productive forces came into increasing collision with the social relations of production. In other words, he had to show the relation between the contradictions of the accumulation process and the social relations of production, the basic expression of which was to be sought in the analysis of the relations between commodities. It was central to Marx's method to trace inner, undeveloped contradictions to their fullest expression. Speaking of the ever-increasing division of labour under capitalism he notes, 'the historical development of the antagonisms, immanent in a given form of production, is the only way in which that form of production can be dissolved and a new form established' (1961: 488).

Specifically: we do not accept that there is a separate Marxist 'theory of capitalist crisis' if this is taken to mean that the analysis of capitalism's contradictions can in any way be considered apart from the results of these contradictions as revealed in the process of capital accumulation. In this important respect, we must state that once more what might be called the 'Dobb school of political economy' is considerably inadequate. Not only do these writers fail entirely to deal with the question of the form of value,[13] but we actually find Dobb positively supporting those classical views which Marx was at pains to reject. Thus he writes, speaking of classical economy, 'money could be neglected in the determination of exchange-values, so for the same reason could the "amount of demand" (viewed as an absolute figure) be regulated as a factor determining the processes of production and exchange' (Dobb 1940: 42–43).

Equally serious is the manner in which this same group of writers has placed a rigid line between their exposition of 'crisis theory' and 'value theory'. Because of this, they must tend in the direction of some variant of Keynesianism. This latter theory starts from the conception of 'effective demand' (borrowed in its essentials from Malthus) treated in isolation from the structure of production. Sweezy's latest work (Baran and Sweezy 1966) is almost purely Keynesian in form.[14] Meek similarly accepts this division between what is conventionally viewed as the 'micro' as against the 'macro' problem when he attempts at one point to explain the relative lack of any creative work in the area of value theory in terms of the fact that the attention of Marxists has necessarily been turned on to other, 'theoretical problems (e.g. the problem of the "breakdown" of capitalism) which are of more direct and immediate relevance to the policy of the working class movement' (Meek 1956: 202–203).

At one blow, the unity of Marx's conception is broken and large concessions to vulgar economy are made. For here we see not merely a move in the direction of Keynes. There is also a tacit admission that whatever the strengths of 'Marxist political economy' (and from the argument of this chapter, it should be clear that this is a category that cannot be accepted) vulgar economy may be better able to analyse microscopic, short-run phenomena. This indeed has long been the explicit standpoint of a trend amongst Marxist commentators led principally by the late Oscar Lange. Once more the implications of this position are not confined to purely theoretical matters. For it implies that some form of marriage may be arranged between Marxian analysis and neo-classical 'price theory' (how there can be a price theory in the absence of a value theory is never explained) in the solving of 'economic problems' in all 'industrial societies' which are increasingly brought together by the imperatives of planning and state regulation of economic affairs.[15] Such ideas are only variants on the spurious sociological 'convergence' theory, a theory owing everything to Max Weber and nothing to Karl Marx.

The logic of many of the various positions we have analysed in the course of this chapter has demonstrated the crucial importance of a correct understanding of Marx's value theory and the implications of any distortions which lead it, via empiricism, in the direction of Ricardo, that is back to political economy. But it is not enough merely to show that Marxism cannot be reduced to some form of sociological 'model building'. We must go on to establish, against some increasingly fashionable ideas, that the completion of Marx's critique of political economy and his writing of *Capital* would have been impossible without the profoundest grasp of the Hegelian dialectic. We hope that on another occasion this aspect can be considered in much greater detail than has here been possible.

[This chapter was first published in *Economy and Society* (1972) 1 (3): 281–307. The version included here is one slightly amended by the author – ed.]

Notes

1

> Once for all I may here state, that by classical political economy I understand that economy which since the time of W. Petty, has investigated the real relations of production in bourgeois society, in contradistinction to vulgar economy, which deals with appearances only ... confines itself to systematising in a pedantic way, and proclaiming for everlasting truths, the trite ideas held by the self-complacent bourgeoisie with regard to their own world, to them the best of all possible worlds.
>
> (Marx 1961: 81)

It should be pointed out that it is not only those writing as Marxists who confuse Ricardo with Marx. Thus Schumpeter tells us that 'His [Marx's] theory of value is a Ricardian one' and of course 'Everybody knows that this theory is unsatisfactory' (1959: 23–24). A more recent writer is equally typical when he speaks of 'the labour theory of value which Marx takes over from Adam Smith and Ricardo' (Giddens 1971: 46).

2 Compare with:

> M. Proudhon, mainly because he lacks the historical knowledge, has not perceived that as men develop their productive faculties, that is, as they live, they develop certain relations with one another and that the nature of these relations must necessarily change with the change and growth of the productive faculties. He has not perceived that *economic categories are* only the *abstract expressions* of these actual relations and only remain true while these relations exist. He therefore falls into the error of the bourgeois economists, who regard these economic categories as eternal and not as historical laws which are only laws for a particular historical development, for a definite development of the productive forces.
>
> (Marx 1956: 45)

3 This remark by Engels has occasioned considerable controversy and we therefore feel obliged to comment upon some aspects of it. Engels, in the section in *Anti-Dühring* from which it is taken, clearly wishes to stress that whereas the distribution of social labour takes place *indirectly* within capitalism, that is through the exchange of commodities, under socialism this distribution will be achieved *directly*, in that sense 'simply'. Hence Engels should not be taken to mean that economic planning would represent no problems. Socialist economy would, for instance, need to arrange that a proportion of its output was used to maintain and extend the means of production. But this 'overproduction' of the means of production would take a form quite opposite to that under capitalism 'This sort of over-production is tantamount to control by society over the material means of its own reproduction. *But within capitalist society it is an element of anarchy*' (Marx 1957: 469, emphasis added). Thus we cannot mechanically translate the reproduction schema of the second volume of *Capital* into the analysis of a socialist society.

On the more substantial point concerning the disappearance of the law value under socialism: it was of course Joseph Stalin who terminated the discussion which had long continued in the USSR with his edict that the law of value did indeed continue to operate within Soviet economy, albeit in 'modified' form. This pronouncement still continues to form the basis for official Soviet thinking in this area. Stalin's statement threw writers like Meek into considerable difficulties. It was clearly in conflict with Marx's explicit statements that the law of value was a reflection of economic forces operating only under commodity production, and would disappear with socialism – which involved the elimination of such forms of production. On the other hand Stalin had also pronounced that the USSR was, by the 1930s, already 'socialist'. The real theoretical point is this: we have to distinguish, as Marx does in his letter, between 'economic laws' and 'natural laws'. Under capitalist commodity production, and under this form of production alone, the need to distribute labour in definite proportions takes the form of the creation of *values*. In other words, the labour process can take place only through the value creating process.

As we have already implied, Engels's statement can be supported by many drawn from Marx's own writings. In his *Critique of the Gotha Programme* (Marx 1971b: 16) he states:

> Within co-operative society based upon the common ownership of the means of production, the producers do not exchange their products; just as little does the labour employed on the products appear here *as the value* of these products, as a material quality possessed by them, since now, in contrast to capitalist society, individual labour no longer exists in an indirect fashion but directly as a component part of the total labour.

It is also often forgotten by those who wish to counterpose Engels's 'wrong' formulations to the 'correct' statements made by Marx that the whole of *Anti-Dühring* was read by Engels to Marx, partly written by the latter and published with his full knowledge (Engels 1977: 14).

4 It might seem that there is a paradox here. For on the one hand Ricardo defined the subject matter of political economy as one concerned primarily with the questions of distribution. It was this emphasis upon distribution which implicitly exposed the contradictions between the classes; thus while for Marx, Ricardo remained 'that most stoical opponent of the working class' for others, like the American Carey ('Mr. Ricardo's system is one of discords') he was denounced as the 'father of communism'. Yet Marx many times also sees Ricardo as the economist of *production, par excellence.* But as he explains (Marx 1971a: 201) this apparent contradiction only arose because Ricardo had 'instinctively treated the forms of distribution as the most precise expression in which the factors of production manifest themselves in a given society'. Yet Dobb's emphasis, when dealing with Marx's value theory is wrongly placed on distribution. Equally mistaken is Meek when he says: 'all economists, whether classical, Marxian or modern, have been largely concerned with the laws governing the distribution of the national cake between the main social classes' (1955: 232). For Marx, this was positively not his 'main concern'. What he did show was that relations of distribution and exchange cannot be understood 'in themselves' but only as a reflection of definite *social relations of production.* It almost goes without saying that vulgar economy treats 'production' and 'distribution' as discrete sectors. It was John Stuart Mill who made of this distinction a virtue; for him the laws of (capitalist) production were immutable while the laws of distribution might be capable of some modification in their operation. This trite idea later formed the basis for Fabian economics.

5 We can see how close Dobb, Mandel and others are to the most vulgar pragmatism when we read in Milton Friedman – amongst the most prominent apologists of *instrumentalism* – 'the only relevant test of the validity of a hypothesis is comparison of its predictions with experience' (1953: 8–9) and speaking of the 'adequacy' of hypotheses he says 'Whether they are sufficiently good approximations for the purpose in hand [is a question we can only answer by] seeing whether the theory works' (1953: 15). For Marx, in opposition to this conception, his categories were not 'chosen' according to pragmatic criteria, but were historical and social in character. Thus the category 'labour power' (the ability to work) was not arbitrarily 'selected'; it was a commodity brought into

being by the process of class struggle, in the manner described by Marx in the sections of *Capital* dealing with the forcible separation of the English peasantry from its land and its transformation into a class of wage labourers.

6

> The vulgar economist has not the faintest idea that the actual everyday exchange relations *cannot be directly identical* with the magnitude of value. The essence of bourgeois society consists precisely in this, that a priori there is no conscious social regulation of production. The rational and necessary asserts itself only as a blindly working average. And then the vulgar economist thinks he has made a great discovery when, as against the revelation of the interconnection, he proudly claims that in appearance things look different. In fact, he boasts that he holds fast to appearances, and takes it for the ultimate. Why, then, have any science at all?
>
> (Marx 1934: 74)

7 See Marx 1959, chs 13–15.

8 For the 'transformation problem' and its 'solution' see Marx 1959: 152–169.

9 Having defined the rate of profit as uniquely determined by the rate of surplus-value to variable capital ($p'=s{:}v$), Ricardo confined his discussion of changes in the rate of profit to a debate about changes in the value of labour power. Having accepted the infamous 'principle of population' as formulated by Malthus, which by pronouncing the supply of labour infinitely elastic assumes wages constant at subsistence level, Ricardo proceeded to limit the debate about the value of labour power to the question of the productivity of agricultural labour. He believed – also accepting the 'law' of diminishing returns – that agricultural productivity would decline over time and thus, by forcing up wages, bring about a reduction in profits. Hence his dictum: 'the interest of the landlord is always in opposition to that of every class in the community'.

10 The basic idea runs as follows; as capital accumulates, there is a tendency for the constant element (c) within the total capital to increase as a faster rate than the variable portion (v). The organic composition of capital is the ratio of constant capital to variable capital ($c:v$). If the rate of profit is represented by the relationship of surplus-value (s) to total capital ($c+v$), then, if the ratio $c{:}v$ is rising, the ratio $s{:}(c+v)$ must tend to decline on the assumption that there is no increase in the rate of exploitation, $s:v$.

11 A. Hussain (1972: 35–39) takes this position in attempting to show that Engels was wrong in the statement we quoted from *Anti-Dühring* above. He suggests, specifically, that Engels was guilty of confusing 'value' with its phenomenal form 'exchange-value'. We have already argued that there is a necessary connection between 'value' and its mode of appearance, which Marx shows is a function of the nature of the commodity itself. Hence his insistence on the primacy of the commodity as against any 'concept of value'. Second however, how does Hussain reconcile his position with Marx's insistence that the law of value of necessity can only operate in an unplanned, blind, way? It is from this understanding that Marx sees that 'value' and 'price' must diverge, a divergence demanded by the very law of value itself. Now if we accept that socialism involves not the blind, but the conscious regulation of production (that is, socialism involves the production of wealth, of use-values, not the production of 'values') then the law of value ceases to hold in such a mode of production.

12

> These gentry, the economists, have hitherto overlooked the extremely simple point that the form: *20 yards of linen = 1 coat* is only the undeveloped basis of *20 yards of linen = £2*, and that therefore the *simplest form of a commodity*, in which its value is not yet expressed as a relation to all other commodities but only as something *differentiated* from the commodity in its natural form, contains the *whole secret of the money form* and with it, in embryo, of *all bourgeois forms of the product of labour*.
>
> (Marx 1956: 228)

13 A notable exception is Blake (1939).

14 In this work (Baran and Sweezy 1966) we find virtually no reference to the theory of value in a study which purports to deal with the structure and dynamics of capitalism. Instead modern oligopoly 'price theory' is accepted without question and an almost purely Keynesian, underconsumptionist view of economic crisis elaborated. With the benefit of hindsight it is now possible to discern many of the seeds of this position in Sweezy's earlier and still popular work (Sweezy 1946) where again a near-Keynesian view of the functioning of capitalism is presented and no link whatsoever established between the exposition of value theory and the rest of the analysis.

15 A decade after the publication of his study of value theory (Meek 1956) which this chapter has criticised, Meek had moved to precisely this position. In a later work (Meek 1967) he had constructed extremely firm bridges towards the vulgar school. For now he was arguing for a reconciliation between Marxism and what no doubt he would earlier have called 'bourgeois economics'.

References

Baran, P.A. and Sweezy, P.M. (1966) *Monopoly Capital: An Essay on the American Economic and Social Order*, New York: Monthly Review Press.

Blake, W.J. (1939) *An American Looks at Karl Marx*, New York: Cordon Company.

Dobb, M.H. (1940, second edition) *Political Economy and Capitalism: Some Essays in Economic Tradition*, London: Routledge & Kegan Paul.

Dobb, M.H. (1955) *On Economic Theory and Socialism*, London: Routledge & Kegan Paul.

Engels, F. (1957) 'Preface' to Marx, K. *Capital*, vol. II, Moscow and London: Foreign Languages Publishing House and Lawrence & Wishart, pp. 1–19.

Engels, F. (1977) *Anti-Dühring*, Seventh Printing, Moscow: Progress Publishers. Progress Publishers 1947 edition, online available at: www.marxists.org/archive/marx/works/1877/anti-duhring (accessed 3 December 2011).

Friedman, M. (1953) *Essays in Positive Economics*, Chicago: University of Chicago Press.

Giddens, A. (1971) *Capitalism and Modern Social Theory: An Analysis of the Writings of Marx, Durkheim and Max Weber*, London: Cambridge University Press.

Hegel, G.W.F. (1929) *The Science of Logic*, London: Allen & Unwin.

Hussain, A. (1972) 'Marx's notes on Adolf Wagner', *Theoretical Practice*, 5: 18–39.

Lenin, V.I. (1934) 'Preface to the Russian translation of Marx's letters to Kugelmann', in Marx, K. *Letters to Dr. Kugelmann*, London: Martin Lawrence.

Mandel, E. (1968) *Marxist Economic Theory*, vol. 2, London: Merlin Press.

Marx, K. (1934) *Letters to Dr. Kugelmann*, London: Martin Lawrence.

Marx, K. (1956) *Marx Engels Selected Correspondence*, Moscow and London: Foreign Languages Publishing House and Lawrence & Wishart.

Marx, K. (1957) *Capital*, vol. II, Moscow and London: Foreign Languages Publishing House and Lawrence & Wishart.

Marx, K. (1959) *Capital*, vol. III, Moscow and London: Foreign Languages Publishing House and Lawrence & Wishart.

Marx, K. (1961) *Capital*, vol. I. Moscow and London: Foreign Languages Publishing House and Lawrence & Wishart.

Marx, K. (1969) *Theories of Surplus Value*, Part I, London: Lawrence & Wishart.

Marx, K. (1971a) *Contribution to the Critique of Political Economy*. Edited, with an Introduction by M.H. Dobb, London: Lawrence & Wishart.

Marx, K. (1971b) *Critique of the Gotha Programme*, Moscow: Progress Publishers. (*Marx/Engels Selected Works* (1970) vol. 3, Moscow: Progress Publishers, pp. 13–30. Online, available at: www.marxists.org/archive/marx/works/1875/gotha/index.htm (accessed 3 December 2011)).

Marx, K. (1972) 'Marginal notes on A Wagner's Lehrbuch der Politischen Okonomie'. Introduced by A. Hussain, *Theoretical Practice*, 5, Spring.

Meek, R.L. (1955) 'Professor Cole on Marxian economic theory', *Marxist Quarterly*, 2 (4), 230–236.

Meek, R.L. (1956) *Studies in the Labour Theory of Value.* London: Lawrence & Wishart.

Meek, R.L. (1967) *Economics and Ideology and Other Essays: Studies in the Development of Economic Thought*, London: Chapman & Hall.

Petty, W. (1690, third edition) *Political Arithmetick* Online, available at: www.marxists.org/reference/subject/economics/petty/index.htm (accessed 12 April 2012). (Originally posted on the Archive for the History of Economic Thought).

Ricardo, D. (1953, reprint of 1951 first edition) *The Works and Correspondence of David Ricardo*, vol. 1, *On the Principles of Political Economy and Taxation.* Edited with an Introduction by P. Sraffa, in collaboration with M.H. Dobb, Cambridge: Cambridge University Press.

Schumpeter, J.A. (1959) *Capitalism, Socialism and Democracy*, London: Allen & Unwin.

Smith, A (1976) *An Inquiry into the Nature and Causes of the Wealth of Nations*, R.H. Campbell and A.S. Skinner (eds) vols 1 and 2, Oxford: Clarendon Press.

Sweezy, P.M. (1946) *Theory of Capitalist Development*, London: Dobson.

4 Imperialism, trade and 'unequal exchange'

The work of Arghiri Emmanuel

Controversy in history and the social sciences still continues about the nature and meaning of the term 'imperialism'. Attitudes to this question have of course undergone considerable changes since the end of the last war and few writers, even the most orthodox, would now wish to deny that the term has a definite scientific content. It is not our intention to review this post-war work, but to examine a recent study which claims to derive from the Marxist tradition. Our treatment of Emmanuel's work (Emmanuel 1972a, 1972b)[1] will be focused not so much on the particular critique which he makes of other writers as on the wider questions of political economy which his work raises. It should also be made clear that it is not the aim of this chapter to present an alternative conception of imperialism to that which would appear to be implicit in Emmanuel's work. Nor are we primarily concerned with an examination of the empirical data which he employs. Instead we intend to try and show that Emmanuel's method and the categories he uses have little in common with those of Marx.

Emmanuel's principal thesis may be summarised as follows: the structure and functioning of the capitalist world market is determined by a definite law of price formation which has the effect of what he terms 'an unequal rewarding of factors' and notably the 'labour factor' which of necessity tends to produce an 'inequality in exchange' between 'rich' and 'poor' countries. This inequality in turn dictates an international division of labour which is detrimental to the interests of the latter group of countries. 'Unequal exchange', used in this sense, is thus Emmanuel's key theoretical category which is designed to convey the notion that on the world market the 'poor countries' are obliged to sell the products of a relatively large number of hours of labour (both direct and indirect) in order to obtain in exchange from the rich countries commodities incorporating a much smaller number of labour-hours.

More precisely, he argues that under capitalism prices are determined by what Marx called 'prices of production', which, according to Emmanuel, consist in part of wages. Given that wages are lower in colonial and semi-colonial countries, a product supplied thanks to a certain number of hours of labour on the part of these countries can be bought by the rich ones by giving in exchange a product that has cost a smaller number of hours of labour. For Emmanuel, these unequal trading relations are the root cause of the 'inequality between nations' as well as the cornerstone of imperialism.

This obliges him from the start to reject, albeit implicitly, any analysis of imperialism based upon the existence of capitalism as an international force, including Lenin's conception of imperialism as a stage in the development of capitalism dominated by 'finance capital'. Instead he prefers to begin from 'mercantile imperialism' which he takes as being logically and historically prior to finance capital.

Emmanuel's rejection of Lenin

The link between the group of Marxists – Lenin, Hilferding, Luxemburg and Bukharin – who analysed imperialism around the period of World War I was that they all treated it as a definite stage in the evolution of capitalism, and a stage moreover which had grown out of the contradictions of the capitalist system which Marx had analysed in the middle of the nineteenth century. Hilferding subtitled his work (*Das Finanzkapital*) 'the latest phase of capitalism' and Lenin went further, designating imperialism as the '*highest* stage of capitalism'. What Lenin wished to establish was that imperialism was no 'accident' or the result merely of reactionary policies on the part of a section of the ruling class. As against Kautsky, he set out to show that imperialism reflected the working out of trends which were endemic to *capitalism*:

> Imperialism emerged as the development and direct continuation of the fundamental characteristics of capitalism in general. But capitalism only became capitalist imperialism at a definite and very high stage of its development, when certain of its fundamental characteristics began to change into their opposites, when the features of the epoch of transition from capitalism to a higher social and economic system had taken shape and revealed themselves in all spheres.
>
> (Lenin 1964: 265)

In dealing with the general economic characteristics of imperialism, Lenin noted five principal and interconnected features: (1) The concentration of production and capital developed to such a high stage that it creates monopolies which play a decisive role in economic and political life. (2) The merging of bank capital with industrial capital and the creation on the basis of 'finance capital' of a finance oligarchy. (3) The export of capital, as distinct from the export of commodities, becomes of particularly great importance. (4) International monopoly combines of capitalists are formed which divide up the world. (5) The territorial division of the world by the great capitalist powers is completed.[2] Imperialism, for Lenin, was capitalism's *highest* stage in the sense that by the beginning of the present century the productive forces had developed to such a point that they were now in violent conflict with the restrictions imposed upon them by the social relations of production. Under imperialism there could be no smooth, even, all-round growth of the productive forces.[3] Lenin's work represents an attempt to understand the nature of the epoch which had announced its arrival with the outbreak of war in 1914.

It is necessary to stress that the features we have listed were seen by Lenin as closely *interconnected.* He was at pains to stress that no 'short-hand' definition of imperialism could suffice and he pointed to 'the conditional and relative value of all definitions in general, which can never embrace all the concatenations of a phenomenon in its full development' (1964: 266). For example, the tendency for the export of capital to replace the export of goods was a reflection of the downward pressure on the rate of profit associated with the process of capital accumulation; it was this tendency for the rate of profit to fall which in turn accelerated the trend towards the concentration and centralisation of capital. The growth of monopoly was similarly connected with the development of the banks into important sources of finance. It is therefore completely impermissible for Emmanuel, like so many before him, to lift out certain of these features which provided the framework for Lenin's analysis, and test them against a series of arbitrarily chosen data.

That Emmanuel proceeds in this way seems particularly clear in his treatment of trade. We should remember that Marx had in no way ignored this as an important aspect of his study of capitalism. Indeed, foreign trade was one of the major 'counteracting forces' which he lists as modifying the tendency of the rate of profit to fall. This it might do, Marx tells us (Marx 1959: 232–234), by raising the rate of surplus-value while at the same time both lowering the value of constant capital (through the cheapening of raw materials) and lowering the price of labour power (through the importation of cheap food in the country engaging in the trade). Capital invested in foreign trade was also likely to earn a higher rate of profit; this is so because it tends to be employed in more 'advanced' sectors and is thus able to produce commodities which undersell those of its competitors, but at prices which are still 'above value'. This means, says Marx, that labour power which has not been paid as of a higher 'specific weight' is sold as such. This process is likened to one where a firm introduces a new technique before it comes generally into use, is thereby able to undersell its competitors, but still at prices 'above value' thus earning a 'surplus profit'. It is important to note that Marx ends his brief discussion of foreign trade by noting that by assisting in the development of the productive forces, foreign trade in the long run tends to aggravate the contradictions involved in capital accumulation.

Thus our objection to Emmanuel's treatment of trade is not that this has no place in a discussion of imperialism. It is rather that he never starts from an all-round conception of imperialism as a definite stage in capitalist evolution, as the classical Marxist studies have done. Indeed, for him, the division of the world into 'rich' and 'poor' countries is not the result of economic forces which are endemic to imperialism, and notably its tendency to ever greater unevenness of development; he prefers instead to see this division in terms of 'mercantile imperialism'. He wishes, that is, to understand the structure of world economic relations, from the standpoint of forces which *pre-date* imperialism. In this respect we believe that his work rests upon a fundamental methodological error.

Marx actually warned his readers of the dangers of this very procedure (Marx 1971, particularly pp. 212–213) Nothing could be more 'natural' he says, than to take economic categories in the order in which they have evolved; this would have meant starting with the rent on landed property, then dealing with interest and only finally dealing with capital. But such a method, Marx says, would be 'erroneous'. For in every social formation a particular branch of production tends always to dominate, casting its special light on all other branches. For Marx capital was such a power, and therefore its analysis had to 'form the point of departure' for a study of bourgeois society.

In connection with the investigation of imperialism, Marx's method demands that every feature of world economy must be taken in its organic relation with the development of *capital*, not as a separate sphere, the development of which can be abstracted, to be treated in isolation from the rest. 'The anatomy of man is a key to the anatomy of the ape' (Marx 1971: 211). Emmanuel turns this around: the key to the present world capitalist economy (man) is to be sought in 'mercantile imperialism' (the ape) is what he in effect says.[4]

It is of course true that 'trade' has been one of the means by which state has dominated state in many periods of history. Trade was certainly an important factor in the emergence of industrial capital itself; as Emmanuel points out it was in trade that many of the fortunes were accumulated which were so decisive as sources of finance for the industrial revolution.[5] But a Marxist analysis of imperialism cannot be concerned with 'trade in general' but only trade in relation to 'the latest phase of capitalism'. In our view, it is impossible properly to investigate the role of trade in determining and perpetuating the structure of imperialism unless one starts with its concrete relations to an economic system which is dominated by the features to which Lenin and others have drawn attention. By treating the exchange circuit as separate from the relations of production, and particularly their uneven development on a world scale, he is unable to grasp the real meaning of the category 'unequal exchange'.

It is also the case that if, as Emmanuel argues, the source of 'economic inequality' resides not in the dominance of finance capital' but in 'mercantile imperialism' then he must tend to arrive at the conclusion that this inequality can be removed within the limits of the capitalist system.

> My subject is the 'exploitation' of one nation by another, not the exploitation of man by man. The former cannot exist without the latter, says Bettelheim, in effect. [This is a reference to Charles Bettelheim's comments on Emmanuel's work, printed as a series of appendices to Emmanuel 1972a – G.P.] Whoever dreams of denying this? The very fact that the indispensable condition of unequal exchange is the equalization of capitalist profits assumes capitalism as pre-supposed. But this does not mean that the former must *necessarily* exist if the latter exists, and this is important, for there is no guarantee that the 'exploited' countries will wait for the exploitation of man by man to come to an end in the dominant countries before they shake

> off the international 'exploitation' to which they are subject. They may seek other ways of getting rid of it before that happens.[6]
>
> (Emmanuel 1972a: 330)

It would appear that Emmanuel is arguing that 'unequal exchange' which he sees as the most important question in world economy, can be overcome while capitalist social relations continue in the metropolitan countries if not in the colonial and semi-colonial world. It seems, therefore, that 'unequal exchange' is not a necessary, but an incidental feature of world economic relations. It was precisely against such positions that Lenin's *Imperialism* was written. For Kautsky and his co-thinkers, World War I did not arise from the inescapable contradictions of modern capitalism, but resulted from the 'wrong policy' of a section of the ruling class. In a different form this is true for Emmanuel: the unevenness of capitalist development can, it would seem, be overcome independently of the future of capitalism in the metropolitan countries.

Second, in his rejoinder to Bettelheim, quoted above, Emmanuel assumes *capitalism* as given. Throughout his work, he tries to explain the mechanism of unequal exchange on the basis of the operation of *capitalism*; given the existence of foreign trade and disparities in wages between countries, then for Emmanuel 'unequal exchange' has existed from capitalism's birth, and is in no sense peculiar to *imperialism*.

It is also to be noted that Emmanuel places quotation marks around exploitation when speaking of the '"exploitation" of nation by nation'. When Marx employed the term he did so in a strict scientific fashion: capital represents a social power which is able to exploit labour on the basis of historically limited social relations of production. When we speak of 'economy' we speak of the antagonistic (class) relations which constitute its real foundation. The phrase 'exploitation of nation by nation' (Emmanuel's subject) is devoid precisely of this social and historical content. It reveals a method which Marx long ago castigated as 'vulgar' in that it is concerned only with the outward appearance of phenomena and not with an analysis of their internal contradictions which give them life and movement.[7]

Only by appreciating Emmanuel's *general* approach to the analysis of imperialism can we reply satisfactorily to some of the specific charges which he makes against Lenin's work. On this level, Emmanuel appears to have little new to say in so far as nearly all his points can be found in much anti-Marxist works over the last decade. (Kemp 1967, provides the best guide to this literature.)

To take first Emmanuel's treatment of capital exports. He quotes figures designed to show that capital has always tended to flow from highly developed capitalist country to highly developed capitalist country and imagines that Lenin's argument is thereby destroyed. Yet Lenin's *Imperialism* contains tables which illustrate exactly this point.[8] The direction of capital flows is determined not by the level of economic development but by the struggle between the capitalists for the largest possible share of the pool of available surplus-value. It is clear that there may be no strict correlation between the rate of profit earned on invested capital and the degree of development attained by the productive forces. Emmanuel's evidence that capital exports now play a less decisive role for the metropolitan countries than they did in the pre-1914 period similarly does no damage to Lenin's analysis. Capital exports in the last quarter of the nineteenth century were no doubt unusually high, their size influenced by Britain's near-monopoly and the predominant position attained by sterling. But the actual quantity of capital export is never the decisive question; the critical problem is the extent to which capital export, stimulated by the tendency of the rate of profit to fall, plays a decisive role in maintaining the momentum of extended reproduction of capital, in both the metropolitan countries and in the colonial and semi-colonial areas.

Perhaps an even more serious objection is that Emmanuel seems always to treat capital exports as a discrete factor. He pays little attention, for example, to the relationship between capital exports and the provision of raw material supplies, a matter which Lenin certainly considered. Recent work by Magdoff (1969) while unsatisfactory in many other important respects, does establish the dependence of the United States on the colonial countries for a range of vital raw materials concerned with its defence and space activities which, while small in a quantitative sense, are of considerable strategic importance. Nor does Emmanuel consider seriously the links between the export of capital and the export of goods, which is strange in the light of the fact that he tends to see capitalist crisis as one bound up with the need for markets and 'underconsumption'.

The discussion about capital exports raises in turn a more basic matter, namely the precise nature of the category 'capital' as employed by Marxists.

> When this dilemma [between overproduction and the consequent need for income redistribution – G.P.] does appear, it does not lead to the search for outlets for capital but for outlets for goods. Marx explained this very well when he said that over-production of capital ultimately meant nothing more than overproduction of goods. ... Nobody has ever had difficulty in placing his capital.
>
> (Emmanuel 1972b: 56)

A study of *Capital* indicates however that Marx went to great pains to distinguish clearly between 'commodity' and 'capital'. Indeed the aim of the opening chapters of the first volume of that work was to show how capital, given definite historical conditions, arises from the internal contradictions of simple commodity production (see Marx 1961: 170 where this is explained at some length; see also Pilling 1972 [Chapter 3 in this book – ed.]). Marx saw the root cause of capitalist crisis as an *overproduction of capital*, in relation to the available pool of surplus-value. Hence the essence of crisis is that it *destroys value* (stock exchange collapses, etc.) while quite often leaving the stock of commodities, as use-values, undisturbed.

Emmanuel's confusion on this point seems to be underlined when he uses figures in an attempt to show that Britain was actually a net capital importer in the years 1870–1914. He does this by reference to the balance of payments figures for this period, which indicate a net deficit. But this alone by no means establishes the fact that Britain on balance imported capital. As many studies have shown (Hall 1968, provides the main references) Britain, because of sterling's dominance, was able to force foreign governments in effect to hold the British payments deficit in the form of sterling balances, in much the same way that the Americans have been able to make Europe hold her payments deficit since the end of the last war. The pre-1914 gold standard was in reality a gold sterling standard.

Since Emmanuel has chosen to take the evidence of trends during the period as indications of the weakness of Lenin's analysis in other directions, we must also point out a number of salient facts. All the evidence from the last quarter of the nineteenth century would appear to reveal the closest possible links between the export of capital and the export of commodities. Britain was invariably able to make the capital importing countries place orders for British products. Second, there is little doubt that home and foreign investment tended to move in cycles against each other. A slackening of investment at home was likely to produce a boom in capital exports and vice versa (Cairncross 1953, is the classic study). This would appear to constitute prima facie evidence to support the argument that the export of capital is linked organically with pressure on the rate of profit at home.[9]

Emmanuel and the law of value

If the matters we have raised so far were the only ones with which Emmanuel deals his work would hardly be worthy of extended treatment. However, his work has the merit that it discusses at some length many of the key questions of political economy in its attempt to establish the conception of 'unequal exchange'. Emmanuel starts with an examination of Marx's law of value. He begins with the 'factors of production'. 'We recognise as such' he tells us (Emmanuel 1972a: 1) 'under the conditions of the production relations of commodity economy, whether capitalist or pre-capitalist, every established claim to a primary share in society's economic product'. And a few pages later (Emmanuel 1972a: 13) we are informed that 'according to my definition, and leaving rent and taxes aside for the moment, we have two factors, labour and capital'.

Here we see what proves to be perhaps the most persistent and glaring of Emmanuel's many theoretical errors. For we have here no mere criticism or modification of Marx, but a rejection of what the author of *Capital* took to be 'one of the two best points' of that work, namely the distinction between 'labour' and 'labour power'. Given that Marx was to base his rejection of many of the conceptions of political economy upon this distinction one might have hoped that Emmanuel would have explored the implications of his starting point. In his critique of political economy, Marx shows that the working class sells not its *labour*, as Ricardo had thought, but rather its ability to work, its *labour power*. It was this recognition that enabled him to solve the riddle which had so confused political economy: if labour is the measure of value, what determines the value of labour? In showing that it was labour power which exchanged against capital, Marx rejected the bourgeois notion that wages were the price of labour and profit and rent the rewards of capital and land for their participation in the production process.[10] He poured scorn upon the 'trinity formula' of vulgar economy which brought together as 'factors of production' 'land', 'labour' and 'capital'. Land and labour, he saw, are the prerequisites of production, in its material aspects, under all modes of production. Capital, however, is by no means merely the means of production, but the means of production under definite socio-historical forms – concentrated in the hands of a distinct class and facing the sellers of labour power (the working class) as an alien coercive power. Emmanuel rejects this materialist standpoint in favour of that of vulgar economy, a rejection emphasised when he states that in 'a pure competitive economy, the *reward of labour* and the profit on capital are fixed not by voluntary act, but by the market' (Emmanuel 1972a: 2, emphasis added).

Because this error is so fundamental it is not one which Emmanuel can 'leave behind' after the first pages, as it were. It necessarily reappears whenever he considers the operation of the law of value, both nationally and internationally. For we find that throughout he replaces Marx's law of value with a crude 'cost of production' theory derived from the type advanced by John Stuart Mill.[11] (Mill is wrongly characterised by Emmanuel as a 'classical economist' whereas in fact he was a writer who anticipated much of neo-classical economics.) According to this type of theory, prices are determined by an aggregation of the rewards of labour, rent and capital involved in the production of a commodity. 'It is the quantities of and rewards for these factors that determine prices, and not the other way round' (Emmanuel 1972a: 2); and later (Emmanuel 1972a: 368):

> My entire study of unequal exchange is based on the premise that in exchange it is not the incomes of the producers that depend on the relative prices, but the relative prices that depend on the incomes of the producers.

It is certainly wrong therefore of Bettelheim to accuse Emmanuel of operating at the level of 'political economy', rather than with Marxist categories. For it would be truer to say that Emmanuel adopts the standpoint of 'economics' rather than political economy. Economic theory is now in such great difficulties that it is being forced to go back to Ricardo over 100 years after Marx had gone beyond him. For economics has now discovered that it is impossible to measure capital, which is not a mere thing but a *value*. (Harcourt (1972) outlines the series of controversies which this recognition has produced.)

It was of course precisely because Marx insisted on starting from an analysis of value that he was able to understand price. Under capitalism Marx recognised, the exchange of the products of labour (wealth) took the form of the exchange of 'things' to which prices attached themselves. But these price relations could not be understood 'in themselves' but as a necessary manifestation of a value relation, that is, a social relation. More specifically, Marx aimed to show that the social relations of production determined the social relations of distribution and exchange. In other words he attempted to demonstrate the scientific validity of historical materialism. Now Emmanuel takes as his starting point one which is quite different from that of Marx. 'It is the quantities and rewards of these factors [that is the question of distribution – G.P.] that determine prices.' Emmanuel is thus quite explicit: *production is determined by distribution.*

Here Emmanuel places himself in a long line of critics of capitalism who start from the conception that it is possible to 'reform' the relations of distribution or exchange while at the same time leaving the social relations of production intact. We have seen already that this is the case in that Emmanuel believes it possible to overcome 'unequal exchange' within the capitalist system.

To underline the implications of Emmanuel's wrong conception of value theory we need only draw attention to a much later passage where he writes 'Once we assume the existence of private ownership it is not value that leads to exchange, but exchange that necessarily results in value.' He thus stresses once more: value arises not in production, but in exchange. Again, one might have expected a somewhat fuller defence of such a stand in the light of Marx's many explicit statements to the contrary. 'Our analysis' (Marx 1961: 60) 'has shown that the form or expression of value of a commodity originates in the nature of value, and not that value and its magnitude originate in the mode of their expression as exchange-value.'

Emmanuel goes even further in his distortions of Marx's law of value when he announces (Emmanuel 1972a: 326) 'I do not believe in absolute value.... The law of value is not a law of magnitude but a law of relations and the movement of relations'. It was however one of Marx's most serious strictures against the classical school, and Ricardo in particular, that they had continually confused the proper relationship between absolute value and surplus-value (which was almost completely ignored) and relative value and surplus-value.[12] And when surveying the decline of political economy following Ricardo's death, Marx paid particular attention to the work of Samuel Bailey (Marx 1972, notably ch. 20), pouring scorn on its shallow relativism. As Marx says many times: it is only possible to speak of relative value, because commodities consist of an *absolute* quantity of abstract labour-time.[13]

Wages theory

From the summary of Emmanuel's work already given, it is clear that he attaches central importance to his theory of wages: 'inequality of wages as such, all other things being equal, is alone the cause of the inequality of exchange' (Emmanuel 1972a: 61), a point many times repeated. Emmanuel goes on to link this inequality in wages to the process which Marx described as the transformation of values into production prices.

It is only possible to discuss Emmanuel's conception of wages in the light of his (mistaken) value theory. For him wages constitute an 'independent variable' in the functioning of the capitalist system [see particularly Emmanuel 1972a: 28 – ed.];[14] 'wages determine relative prices' (Emmanuel 1972a: 100). Here he would appear to be in conflict not only with Marx but also with Ricardo. The very opening of the first chapter of *The Principles* (Ricardo 1953: 11) is subheaded: 'The value of a commodity ... depends on the relative quantity of labour which is necessary for its production, and not on the greater or less compensation which is paid for that labour.' That is, exchange-value is independent of the value of labour power.

> This is precisely one of Ricardo's most important and most emphasised propositions, for otherwise the price of labour [power] would determine the prices of commodities which it produces, whereas, according to Ricardo, the price of labour [power] determines nothing but the *rate of profit*.
>
> (Marx 1972: 94)

And earlier, in connection with Smith we find:

> That commodities A and B exchange in proportion to the labour-time contained in them is in no way upset by the proportions in which the producers A and B divide the products A and B, or rather their value, between themselves.... The relation between the labour-time contained in commodities A and B is in no way affected by how the labour-time contained in A and B is appropriated by various persons.
>
> (Marx 1969a: 74)

As against this, Emmanuel argues that 'relative wages determine relative prices'. Evidently the source of his confusion is a misunderstanding about the nature of wages. In order to try and establish that wages are indeed an 'independent variable', institutionally determined, he lays great emphasis upon a quotation from *Capital* (Marx 1961: 171): 'Nevertheless, in a given country, at a given period, the average quantity of the means of subsistence necessary for the labourer is practically known.'

But in seeking Marx's authority, Emmanuel succeeds only in compounding his previous errors. For the key point here is that the value (and hence price) of labour power is determined not by the quantities of the means of subsistence which will enable the worker to maintain himself and his family and re-present himself on the market, but by their value (that is the socially necessary labour time required to produce these means of subsistence. 'The *quantity* of these necessaries is known at any given epoch of a given society, and can therefore be treated as a constant magnitude. What changes, is the *value* of this quantity' (Marx 1961: 519, emphasis added). In other words, assuming food to be the only subsistence item, the quantity of food incorporated in wages can be measured in a variety of ways – by weight, calorific content, etc. but this is quite independent of its *value*. This depends upon the productivity of labour, and changes in that productivity, not merely in agriculture, but throughout the economy.

Improvements in labour productivity in the tractor industry for example, will tend to reduce the value of wheat and hence, under normal circumstances, the value of labour power in all sectors. Emmanuel does not proceed in this manner (a method based upon Marx's value analysis) for to do so would force him back into an investigation of the social relations of production in *all* countries, which would in turn call seriously into question his division of the world into 'rich' and 'poor' countries.

This distinction between the *quantity* of means of subsistence (which Emmanuel wrongly takes as constituting the value of the wage) and the value of the wage has far wider implications for political economy. For lying beneath it is the more fundamental distinction between 'wealth' (the total of use-values) and 'value' (a social relation peculiar to commodity production). It is a distinction which provides the starting point for *Capital*. There Marx gives an example along the following lines: Assume that in a given period, *t*, either one ton of iron can be produced, or ten tons of wheat. Under normal circumstances, a ton of iron will exchange for ten tons of wheat. Let us now assume improvements in labour productivity in the iron industry which make it possible to produce two tons of iron in the same period of time, *t*. The *value* of iron, measured in terms of wheat, has *halved* (now a ton of iron will exchange for only five tons of wheat) whereas the *quantity of iron* (in tons) produced in time *t* has *doubled*.

Now the quantities of the products concerned constitute their respective use-values whereas the ratios in which they exchange against each other signifies their *exchange-value*, which is but the form of their value. Now if we follow Marx and recognise that 'value' is not a *thing*, but a *social relation*, we can see that Marx, in drawing the distinction between 'value' (a quality) and 'use-value' (a quantity) was pointing to the fact that as the productive forces grow, they tend to come into increasingly sharp conflict with the social relations of production. In other words, if we recognise the vital distinction between 'wealth' (a collection of use-values) and 'value' we cannot possibly hold that wages are an 'independent variable'. Nor can we accept that it is at all 'obvious' that wages in the colonial countries are necessarily lower than in the metropolitan countries. For, as we have seen, the value of labour power depends upon the amount of labour socially required for its production. It is determined by the productivity of labour of all sectors in the economy; it depends that is, upon the development of the productive forces. Unlike Bettelheim, we do not propose to engage in what is both a sterile and dangerous debate about whether the workers in the colonial countries are 'more' or 'less' exploited than their counterparts in the advanced capitalist countries. But clearly the issue cannot be resolved by mere reference to wage statistics, as Emmanuel seems to think (Emmanuel 1972a: 47).

When Marx briefly discusses 'National differences of wages' (Marx 1961, ch. 22) he shows that the matter is considerably more complicated.

> In the comparison of the wages in different nations, we must therefore take into account all the factors that determine changes in the amount of the value of labour-power; the price and extent of the prime necessaries of life

> as naturally and historically developed, the cost of training the labourers, the part played by the labour of women and children.
>
> (Marx 1961: 559)

And a page later (Marx 1961: 560) he does much to discredit Emmanuel's thesis

> it will be found, frequently, that the daily or weekly &c., wage in the first nation [the 'developed'] is higher than in the second [the 'underdeveloped'] whilst the relative price of labour, i.e. the price of labour as compared both with surplus-value and with the value of the product, stands higher in the second than in the first.

'Continental labour is' he adds 'in proportion to the product dearer than English' (Marx 1961: 561).

'Unequal exchange' and the transformation problem

Having dealt with Emmanuel's value and wage theory it will now be possible to deal more specifically with the manner in which he views the operation of 'unequal exchange'. He likens it to the process Marx referred to as the transformation of values into prices of production. In *Capital*, volume I, Marx works on the assumption that commodities exchange at prices which are identical with their values. Implicit in this assumption is the proposition that the organic composition of capital (the ratio of constant capital, *c*, to variable capital, *v*,) is uniform throughout the economy. Once this assumption is dropped (as it must be, particularly when we come to consider imperialism which tends towards increasing unevenness of development), then so also must the assumption that individual values will be equivalent to individual prices.[15] That this must be so can be seen if we look at two commodities incorporating equal values and equal rates of surplus-value. Commodity A comprises $10c+20v+20s=50$. Commodity B of $30c+10v+10s=50$. The rate of surplus-value ($s:v$) is the same in each case, 100 per cent. Their total values being identical, one might imagine that they would exchange for each other on a one-to-one basis. Yet were this to happen the capitalist producing A (the more 'backward' sector) would have a profit rate of 66.67 per cent while the capitalist in B (the more 'advanced' sector) would have one of only 25 per cent. Clearly this is both an unstable position and one which negates the basic principle of capital, namely the tendency towards a uniform rate of profit throughout the economy. Hence, say the critics, repeating Bohm Bawerk's 'discovery' there is a 'great contradiction' between volume I and volume III: either the assumption that a general rate of profit is established in all sectors is dropped or the law of value ceases to hold. Marx's reply to this line of attack is to be found in the famous 'prices of production' theory found in volume III.

Here he explains that commodities do not exchange at prices which are equivalent to their values, but to their 'prices of production' which consist of the value of both constant and variable capital advanced in their production, plus profit at the average rate on the *total* capital. In all the controversy surrounding the theory of prices of production, the decisive problem has always been: does the fact that prices never exchange at their values invalidate the analysis of volume I? Marx's critics have answered 'yes'; the law of value, while it might have applied to Adam Smith's 'rude and primitive' society ceases to hold under conditions of *capitalist* commodity production. We raise these points because Emmanuel appears to share this line of criticism when he writes (Emmanuel 1972a: 15) 'With the coming of capitalist relations the labour theory of value in its primitive form finds itself at a dead end, and a change in the original form of value becomes necessary'. Later he makes more clear his conception of this change in form:

> Since the French edition to this work appeared, a number of critics have alleged that there is a sharp break in my treatment of the transition from value to price of production. In my opinion – and I am going to try to prove the point – in so far as there is indeed such a break, it merely reflects a qualitative difference in reality itself.
>
> (Emmanuel 1972a: 387)

This is Emmanuel's position, and one which must be looked at in the light of Marx's statements on the nature of the transformation process. First it is clear that Marx realised that prices would never, whatever the stage of capitalist development, correspond directly with values. In other words Marx never held to a theory of relative prices. From evidence long before the publication of *Capital* volume I this is clear (see in this connection Marx's letter to Engels, 2 August 1862, where the essential features of the transformation process are set out: Marx 1956: 157–161). In any case, in volume I Marx already announces that commodities will not exchange directly at value:

> If therefore he [merchant or manufacturer – G.P.] thought about the matter at all, he would formulate the problem of the formation of capital ... on the supposition that prices are regulated by the average price, i.e. ultimately by the value of the commodities. *I say 'ultimately' because average prices do not directly coincide with the values of commodities, as Adam Smith, Ricardo and others believe.*
>
> (Marx 1961: 166, emphasis added)

Given that Marx held that commodity exchange would never take place at prices which were equivalent directly to values, why did he operate throughout volume I on the 'supposition' that they would? He provides the answer immediately above the footnote from which I have quoted and it is an answer which has a considerable bearing upon a critique of Emmanuel. 'The conversion of money into capital has to be explained on the basis of the laws that regulate the exchange of commodities, in such a way that the starting-point is the exchange of equivalents' (Marx 1961: 166). Marx was here insisting that one had to explain the accumulation of capital by starting from production relations and not relations of exchange.

It is not therefore the case that Marx's value theory found itself at a 'dead end' but rather that Emmanuel has failed to understand this theory or the method which lay behind its formulation. He seems to hold that the volume I analysis (what he refers to as 'Mark 1') became redundant when 'capital' as a factor of production enters the picture. Once the situation is 'complicated' in this way, then the 'Mark 2' analysis takes over. Marx however never saw the movement from 'value' to 'price of production' as a move from 'simple' to 'complex'. Rather it was a transformation which mirrored, in theoretical form, the development of the productive forces and particularly the socialisation of production which capitalist development involved.

> What competition, first in a single sphere, achieves is a single market-value and market-price derived from the various individual values of commodities. And it is competition of capitals in different spheres, which first brings out the price of production equalizing the rates of profits in the different spheres. *The latter process requires a higher development of capitalist production than the previous one.*
>
> (Marx 1959: 177, emphasis added)

It is because the organic composition of capital tends increasingly to vary between branches that values are transformed into prices of production and a redistribution of surplus-values takes place, through a deviation of prices of production from values. In other words, the regulator of capital accumulation, the establishment of an average rate of profit, demands this deviation, which is created by the very law of value itself.

But is quite misleading to speak of this transfer of surplus-value from sectors of low organic composition to those of high organic composition as constituting *'unequal exchange.' For what is involved first of all is a transfer of surplus value between the owners of capital themselves*, ('the capitalists become communists', says Marx) *such that each capital, whatever its composition, gets its aliquot share.*

Second, and perhaps even more crucial, while the transfer of surplus-value between branches necessarily takes place in the circuit of *exchange*, its *origin* lies in the sphere of production. Emmanuel's work tends continually to start at the end of the process (the realm of appearances) in the exchange circuit, and ignores almost entirely the social relations of production.

This is clearly evidenced in his treatment of the organic composition of capital. He distinguishes between two types of unequal exchange. First it can be conceived in its 'broad sense' where the organic composition of capital varies as between countries, but where wages are uniform (remembering that Emmanuel tends to use this category in a manner quite different from that of Marx). Second, there is unequal exchange in the 'narrow sense' where both the organic composition and wage tend to vary. It is this latter conception which receives most attention, being designated (Emmanuel 1972a: 160) as 'non-equivalence in the strict sense'.[16] Anybody familiar with the third volume of *Capital* will recognise immediately that this treatment is once more the reverse of that adopted by Marx. When he deals with the transformation of values into production prices, Marx always assumes that labour power is bought and sold at value, which is part of his general methodological approach. He then examines how production prices are modified when wages fall, making perfectly clear (Marx 1959: 199) that 'fall' must be taken to mean that either (a) wages have been forced 'below value' (that is below subsistence level) or (b) that they were previously 'above value'. He next shows that any fall in wages in this sense of the term will first tend to alter the rate of profit (via a change in the rate of surplus-value) and that prices of production will fall for capitals with a below-average composition and rise for capitals the composition of which is higher than the social average. If we follow Marx and assume that a fall in wages of this sort can only be an aberration from the 'normal' state of affairs (that is one in which labour power, like all commodities exchanges 'at value'), then this question is by its very nature of only relatively minor significance.

> In this entire chapter, the establishment of the general rate of profit and the average profit, and consequently, the transmutation of values into prices of production, are assumed as given. The question merely was, how a general rise or fall in wages affected the assumed prices of production of commodities. *This is but a very secondary question* compared with the other important points analysed in this part.
>
> (Marx 1959: 200, emphasis added)

It is worth noting that Marx adopts precisely the same analytical procedure when discussing the tendency of the rate of profit to fall.[17]

It was only a 'very secondary question' for Marx in that unless we work on the assumption (a theoretical assumption) that exchange takes place 'at value' then 'nothing can be explained at all'. It is for this very reason that prices of production do not, as Emmanuel thinks, constitute a qualitative break from values, but derive from the latter in both a logical and a historical sense. Production prices derive from values in that all that the former achieve is a *redistribution of already created* surplus-value between capitalists. This transformation writes Marx:

> does not affect the absolute size of this total surplus-value; but merely alters its *distribution* among the different spheres of production. The *determination of this surplus-value* itself, however, only arises out of the determination of value by labour-time. Without this, the average profit is the average *of nothing*, pure fancy.
>
> (1969b: 190)

Production, distribution and consumption

Here Marx is merely stressing a point which runs through *Capital*: that production relations *determine* relations of exchange. Indeed as we noted earlier it can be said that to establish the validity of this proposition was for Marx equivalent to establishing the scientific content of historical materialism.

For Marx the forms taken by the exchange relationships had to be understood in terms of the development of the productive forces. This is why the transformation of values into production prices must be seen as a result of the socialisation of production and the growing unevenness of the development of the productive forces, reflected in the ever-greater disparities between the branches of production, both nationally and internationally. It is for this reason that a consideration of the prices of production must be linked to an analysis of imperialism.

It is at this point that Emmanuel's division of the world into 'rich' and 'poor' countries (a procedure which in several respects many analyses of the 'Third World' share) directly cuts across this conception of capital as an international, social power. 'In each particular sphere of production', writes Marx (1959: 193):

> [it emerges that] the individual capitalist, as well as the capitalists as a whole, take direct part in the exploitation of the total working-class by the totality of capital and in the degree of that exploitation, not only out of general class sympathy, but also for direct economic reasons. For, assuming all other conditions ... to be given, the average rate of profit depends on the intensity of exploitation of the sum total of labour by the sum total of capital.

'In this form [that is the price of production – G.P.]' he notes earlier 'capital becomes conscious of itself as a *social power* in which every capitalist participates proportionally to his share in the total social capital' (Marx 1959: 191).

As against this conception, Emmanuel's attention is directed always to the sphere of exchange as the source of exploitation.[18] Under pressure from his critics he says in an appendix (Emmanuel 1972a: 329) '*Exploitation is not a fact of production but of appropriation*'. Whatever he means by the ambiguous 'a fact of' he is here heading towards Mercantilism which tried to explain the source of value 'upon alienation'. In his rejection of all those theories which attempted to explain profit by reference to a conception of 'force' or mere 'cheating' (as many of the Ricardian Socialists did for example) Marx had to show that in the exchange of wage labour and capital the law of value was upheld. It was in the sphere of production relations that exploitation had to be located, which in turn rested upon the ownership of the means of production by a class in the form of capital.

It soon transpires that Emmanuel does not confuse merely the relationship between 'production' (dealt with in the first volume of *Capital*) and exchange (the subject of the second volume) but also the relations between *production* and *consumption.* As in all works dealing with the nature of imperialism, there is implicit in Emmanuel's work a theory of capitalist crisis. In fact Emmanuel advances a somewhat naive *underconsumptionist* theory, that is one which locates the source of capitalist breakdown in a lack of 'effective demand'. 'What has especially shocked people in my thesis' he writes (Emmanuel 1972a: 378) 'is this idea that excessive unproductive consumption may not only not impoverish but may even enrich a capitalist country.' Nobody familiar with the economic writings of Malthus will be in the least 'shocked' by 'this idea'. For it was Malthus (that 'shameless sycophant of the ruling classes' as Marx dubbed him) who justified' excessive consumption on the part of the rich in that it raised 'effective demand' and thus overcame the contradictions of the accumulation process. Emmanuel's underconsumption is quite explicit: 'Since the prime problem for capitalism is not to produce but to sell, capital moves towards countries and regions where there are extensive outlets and expanding markets' (Emmanuel 1972a: 372). Or again:

> The capitalist world cannot show a single instance of a high wage country that has had to reduce wages owing to a failure to develop [perhaps he has 'forgotten' Nazi Germany after 1933? – G.P.] or a single instance of a country that has been able to develop while keeping wages low.[19]

These passages are entirely in line with the statement (Emmanuel 1972b: 56) that 'After 1870, the trade union struggle and the rise in salaries helped advanced capitalism out of this dilemma [the need for markets – G.P.] at any rate to a certain extent' as well as the proposition (Emmanuel 1972a: 379) that British investment obtained from plunder in India gravitated towards America because of the high wages obtaining in that country.

Perhaps little comment is required about these and Emmanuel's other statements along the same lines. We know of course that Marx always understood that for capitalism there was certainly a 'realisation problem'. He knew, that is, that capital had not merely to extract surplus-value, but to transform the value so created back into money so that the accumulation process could continue. It is also true that several Marxists, most notably Rosa Luxemburg, have tended to over-emphasise this side of the problem to the exclusion of others.

Emmanuel's position however has little in common with Rosa Luxemburg's. She would have treated with scorn the idea that 'high wages' – the result of successful trade union struggle – can overcome capitalist contradictions. Nor has Emmanuel's underconsumptionism anything in common with Marx's position:

> That commodities are unsaleable means only that no effective purchasers have been found for them, i.e. consumers. ... But if one were to attempt to give this tautology the semblance of a profounder justification by saying that the working-class receives too small a portion of its own product and the evil would be remedied as soon as it receives a larger share of it and its wages increase in consequence, one could only remark that crises are always

> prepared by precisely a period in which wages rise generally and the working-class actually gets a larger share of that part of the annual product which is intended for consumption. From the point of view of these advocates of sound and 'simple' (!) common sense such a period should rather remove the crisis.
>
> (Marx 1957: 410–411)

(Cf. Lenin 1964: 241–242, who is even harsher on the underconsumptionists.)

Few people would claim that all the problems involved in an analysis of imperialism have been resolved; few would wish to say that Lenin or indeed any Marxist, said the 'final word' on many of the questions taken up in this chapter. Our purpose has been to suggest that whatever new work still needs to be undertaken, it would be highly dangerous if it were to proceed with the theoretical conceptions advanced by Emmanuel.

Acknowledgements

I should like to thank G.B. Kay and D.S. Yaffe for a helpful discussion on an earlier draft of this chapter. They are of course in no way responsible for any weakness in its final form or content. A version of the chapter was originally read at a staff seminar in Middlesex Polytechnic, October 1972.

[This chapter was first published in *Economy and Society* (1973) 2 (2): 164–185 – ed.]

Notes

1 It should be pointed out that I am not here concerned explicitly with the points raised by Charles Bettelheim.

2 One can only be amused by Emmanuel's dismissal of Lenin's work, as 'a marginal work which never had any scientific pretensions' (1972b: 36) Certainly Lenin's work only aimed to be a 'popular outline' and the conditions of the censorship imposed severe constraints upon the form taken by the book. But anybody with a knowledge of the enormous data gathered and analysed by Lenin (1968) can only smile at Emmanuel's comment.

3 We should add that this did not mean that there was either a mechanical or absolute stagnation in the growth of the productive forces, as Lenin fully recognised (Lenin 1964: 276).

4 This same non-dialectical approach pervades the whole of Emmanuel's work. We will cite merely one example of the erroneous conclusions to which it leads. At one point he attempts to explain the 'acceptance' of imperialism by the trade union and labour leaders in Europe and North America in terms of the 'backwardness' of the workers of these countries, a 'backwardness' which he in turn ascribes to the high living standards prevailing in these countries. (Indeed he concludes at one point that the labour and trade union leaders are more 'enlightened' on colonial questions than are those in the ranks of the parties and organisations which they lead.) Now Lenin was the first to trace the connection between reformism as a political phenomenon and the emergence of an 'aristocracy' of skilled workers who to an extent shared in the superprofits derived from colonial exploitation particularly after 1850. But he also insisted that the continued existence and

strengthening of this reformist trend could not be understood merely from the standpoint of these historical divisions – between 'aristocracy' and 'non-aristocracy' – *within* the working class. The social and ideological basis of reformism cannot be grasped through an analysis of trends within the working class alone, but by understanding the relationship of reformism to imperialism and specifically to the *imperialist state*. The 'base' for reformism, according to Lenin, is increasingly not a privileged layer in the working class but this state and the role it plays in the 'latest phase of capitalism'. Therefore it is necessary to start not with the working class, but with the totality of class relations as they have developed to their highest point. Emmanuel here makes an error of the type which would appear to be common in much 'labour history'.

5 Even here his presentation is one-sided and therefore distorted. For while stressing 'colonial plunder' as a source of capital he ignores the role which the violent destruction of the English peasantry played in the preparation of the industrial revolution, a subject of great interest to Marx (1961, especially chs 27–31).

6 Emmanuel, it might seem, 'escapes' this criticism when he speaks of the 'socialist road' as a means of overcoming 'unequal exchange'. But the experience of the USSR was not that of a country which 'modified' its exchange relationships with the world economy, but one rather which virtually *ended* these relationships. For the industrialisation of Russia was carried out under the leadership of those who subscribed to the theory of 'Socialism in One Country' which involved the conscious isolation of the Soviet economy from the world market and division of labour, an isolation which brought enormous distortions in that industrialisation process. In other words the law of value was not 'modified' – as Emmanuel's thesis would lead one to imagine is possible, but *abrogated.* Had the monopoly of foreign trade been broken and the law of value been allowed to operate in an unfettered manner, the much higher productivity of labour in western Europe and America must have produced an exchange of commodities which would very quickly have undermined the planned basis of the Soviet economy.

7

> Colonial policy and imperialism existed before the latest stage of capitalism and even before capitalism. Rome, founded on slavery, pursued a colonial policy and practised imperialism. But 'general' disquisitions on imperialism, which ignore, or put into the background, the fundamental difference between socio-economic formations, inevitably turn into the most vapid banality and bragging.... *Even the capitalist colonial policy of previous stages of capitalism is essentially different from the colonial policy of finance capital.*
>
> (Lenin 1964: 260, emphasis added)

8 See specifically Lenin (1964: 243) where attention is drawn to the fact that French imperialism ('usury imperialism') invested heavily in Russia and that for Germany 'colonies are inconsiderable, and German capital invested abroad is divided most evenly between Europe and America'. The table given by Lenin actually lists capital in Europe and America as of greater importance than that invested in Asia, Africa or Australia.

9 Emmanuel ignores the dynamic of the relationship between home and foreign investment when he discovers (1972b) that the capital invested by Britain in 1870 'ought' to have grown at a much faster rate than the 1914 figures imply if there was in fact an export of capital in this period.

10 'The productivity of labour is merely the use-value of labour power' says Emmanuel (1972a: 418). The use-value of labour power is of course *labour.*

11 'Accordingly, exchange-value proves to be the sum of the workers' wages, plus the profit on the means of labour, plus the profit on wages.'

12 Marx deals with these matters at length, particularly in Marx 1969b, ch. 10, section 3.

13

> The relativity of the concept of value is by no means negated by the fact that all commodities, in so far as they are exchange-values, are only *relative* expressions of social labour-time and their relativity consists by no means solely of the rate in which they exchange for one another, but of the rate of all of them to this social labour which is their substance.
>
> (Marx 1969b: 172)

14 In this respect Emmanuel adopts the common 'model-building' approach to Marx's *Capital*. Thus he tells us that labour was 'chosen' as the measure of value because of its greater homogeneity than other 'factors'. This standpoint has been criticised in Pilling 1972 [see Chapter 3, this book – ed.].

15 From the fact that Marx's volume II analysis is presented in 'value' rather than 'price of production' terms, Emmanuel concludes that Marx was still 'uncertain' about the transformation process (Emmanuel 1972a: 391). We have already suggested that Marx's method obliged him to start with values and assume that commodities exchanged and circulated at value; only then could 'deviations' from this law be understood.

16 This being the case, and accepting Emmanuel's assumption that differences in wages internationally are at the base of 'unequal exchange' one would have imagined that as trade grew more rapidly between countries with similarly low wage levels (as against exchanges between 'rich' and 'poor' countries) then 'unequal exchange' would tend to become less pronounced and economic development more 'balanced'. Now it is the case that trade between colonial and semi-colonial countries has increased somewhat more rapidly than trade between these countries and those of Europe, North America and Japan (Magdoff 1969, provides a convenient summary of the figures). Yet the growing relative separation of the metropolitan countries from the colonial and semi-colonial countries is both an expression of and a cause of growing unevenness of development.

17

> Nothing is more absurd … than to explain the fall in the rate of profit by a rise in the rate of wages, although this may be the case by way of exception … The rate of profit does not fall because labour becomes less productive, but because it becomes more productive. Both the rise in the rate of surplus-value and the fall in the rate of profit are but specific forms through which growing productivity of labour is expressed under capitalism
>
> (Marx 1959: 234)

Here Marx implicitly rejects all 'explanations' for a decline in the rate of profit which rest upon conceptions such as labour's 'increased share' in the social product.

18 Compare with:

> The process of circulation is a phase of the total process of reproduction. But no value is produced in the process of circulation, and, therefore no surplus-value.… *If a surplus-value is realized in the sale of produced commodities, then this is because it already existed in them.*
>
> (Marx 1959: 274, emphasis added)

19 Emmanuel has to try and explain the case of Britain during the industrial revolution, a case where considerable evidence suggests that wages were certainly 'held down'. He does so by reference to the Corn Laws which, he tells us (1972a: 129), prevented surplus-value from escaping overseas. Land enjoyed a super-rent, 'this super-rent was automatically directed into capitalist accumulation and had from the standpoint of economic development, the same effect as that of a superprofit'. How Emmanuel would seek, on the basis of this analysis, to explain the long and bitter struggle on the part of the industrial bourgeois to repeal the Corn Laws we can only conjecture. The 'Manchester School' was quite right in regarding the operation of these laws as directly inimical to the process

of capital accumulation. For the restrictions on the import of corn, by keeping bread prices high, tended to keep wages up and therefore profits down. It was this same realisation that made many Chartists suspicious of the motives of the Anti-Corn Law League in the 1840s: they fully realised that 'cheap corn' could mean 'cheap wages'.

Apart from the example of Britain, Emmanuel's underconsumptionist position leads him to some rather startling conclusions. Thus, of South Africa he writes

> Let us suppose that tomorrow the South African whites were to exterminate the Bantus instead of employing them at low wages and replace them with white settlers receiving high wages ... the ultimate result would be a leap forward by South Africa, which would soon catch up with the more developed countries.
>
> (1972a: 125)

References

Cairncross, A.K. (1953) *Home and Foreign Investment, 1870–1913*, London: Cambridge University Press.

Emmanuel, A. (1972a) *Unequal Exchange: A Study of the Imperialism of Trade*, with additional comments by Charles Bettelheim, Translated from the French by Brian Pearce, London: NLB.

Emmanuel, A. (1972b) 'White-settler colonialism and the myth of investment imperialism', *New Left Review*, 1 (73): 35–57.

Hall, A.R. (ed.) (1968) *The Export of Capital from Britain, 1870–1914*, London: Methuen.

Harcourt, G.C. (1972) *Some Cambridge Controversies in the Theory of Capital*, London: Cambridge University Press.

Kemp, T. (1967) *Theories of Imperialism*, London: Dobson.

Lenin, V.I. (1964) 'Imperialism: the highest stage of capitalism', in *Collected Works*, vol. 22, Moscow and London: Progress Publishers and Lawrence & Wishart, pp. 185–304.

Lenin, V.I. (1968) 'Notebooks on imperialism', in *Collected Works*, vol. 39, Moscow and London: Progress Publishers and Lawrence & Wishart.

Magdoff, H. (1969) *The Age of Imperialism*, New York: Monthly Review Press.

Marx, K. (1956) *Marx Engels Selected Correspondence*, Moscow and London: Foreign Languages Publishing House and Lawrence & Wishart.

Marx, K. (1957) *Capital*, vol. II, Moscow and London: Foreign Languages Publishing House and Lawrence & Wishart.

Marx, K. (1959) *Capital*, vol. III. Moscow and London: Foreign Languages Publishing House and Lawrence & Wishart.

Marx, K. (1961) *Capital*, vol. I. Moscow and London: Foreign Languages Publishing House and Lawrence & Wishart.

Marx, K. (1969a) *Theories of Surplus Value*, Part I, London: Lawrence & Wishart.

Marx, K. (1969b) *Theories of Surplus Value*, Part II, London: Lawrence & Wishart.

Marx, K. (1971) *Contribution to the Critique of Political Economy*, Edited, with an Introduction by M.H. Dobb, London: Lawrence & Wishart.

Marx, K. (1972) *Theories of Surplus Value*, Part III, London: Lawrence & Wishart.

Pilling, G. (1972) 'The law of value in Ricardo and Marx', *Economy and Society*, 1 (3): 281–307; Chapter 3 in this book.

Ricardo, D. (1953 [1951 first edition]) *The Works and Correspondence of David Ricardo, vol. 1, On the Principles of Political Economy and Taxation*, Edited with an Introduction by P. Sraffa in collaboration with M.H. Dobb, Cambridge: Cambridge University Press.

5 A 'third industrial revolution'?

Marxism and the productive forces

This chapter will discuss a fundamental question in Marxist theory: the nature of the productive forces in the epoch of capitalism known to Marxists as imperialism. There is no doubt that this is a central question for Marxism. It is no exaggeration to say that our understanding of the prospects for socialism rest on our grasp of the nature of the productive forces and their fate in this epoch. 'Mankind's productive forces stagnate' wrote Trotsky (1963) in *The Transitional Programme*, the opening programmatic statement of the Fourth International written in 1938. Here Trotsky was basing himself on Lenin's contention that imperialism constituted the highest stage of capitalist development, the epoch where the productive forces and the social relations of capitalism came into a historical and insoluble contradiction. It is one of the fundamentals of historical materialism that the possibility of the overthrow of a social system arises only when its productive forces have outgrown the existing social relations in which they previously developed.

That the productive forces stagnate was for Trotsky an indication that just these objective conditions for the proletarian revolution existed: indeed he held that conditions for socialism were not ripe but even over-ripe. And only because the productive forces stagnated, that is only because the objective conditions for the transition to socialism existed, did the crisis of humanity reduce itself to the crisis of leadership in the working class. This proposition of Lenin and Trotsky has been vigorously disputed by many Marxists.[1] But how is the issue to be dealt with? The first thing to recognise is the nature of the task before us. For in struggling to reconsider some basic questions in world economy we do so against a specific background: the prostitution of Marxism in the service of a parasitic and counter-revolutionary bureaucracy for which Stalinism was responsible. It is only in the context of the struggle against this disastrous impact of Stalinism on the working class movement that we will be able not merely to defend the basic conceptions of Marxism, but to make a development in Marxist theory that will enable us to understand the changes in capitalism. But this development cannot be accomplished on the basis of textual exegesis alone. It is of course necessary to demonstrate that the Stalinist perversion of Marxism involved an attack on the spirit as well as the letter of all that Marx wrote. But more is required. Marxism is a living science or it is nothing. If it is not developed in a manner that can overcome every basic revision of Marxism it will perish and the working class will be disarmed.

Bernstein and Kautsky

The fate of Marxism in the period of the Second International is of relevance here. In the mid-1890s Eduard Bernstein began to publish a series of articles in *Die Neue Zeit*, the official journal of the German SPD. They were later expanded and published as the book *Presuppositions of Socialism and the Tasks of Social Democracy* [*Die Voraussetzungen des Sozialismus and die Aufgaben der Sozialdemokrati*, later published in English as *Evolutionary Socialism* – ed.].[2] Bernstein (1909) argued that the 'presuppositions of socialism' provided by Marx rested on the idea that a catastrophic economic collapse will automatically usher in socialism. While Marx, according to Bernstein, was correct in his general description of social evolution, he was mistaken in his contention that the end of capitalism was in prospect. Bernstein proposed that the material conditions of capitalism at the end of the last century meant that Marx's theory was no longer applicable: thanks to the growth of credit and cartels, a world market and 'democratic institutions' any notion that capitalism will break down is false. Instead capitalism tends towards a decrease in social conflict and crisis and towards the gradual elimination of contradiction. This refutation was accomplished by Bernstein with a presentation of much empirical material. It is the official response to Bernstein issued by Karl Kautsky (1925) that is of most interest here because in it can be seen the anticipation of the caricature of Marxism for which Stalinism was to be later responsible. *The Economic Doctrines of Karl Marx* (written in 1887) became the official commentary on Marx within the German movement. Kautsky advanced a unilinear notion of capitalist development, with depressions occurring with ever-greater severity until a 'final crisis'. The laws of capital analysed by Marx are presented in absolute form, not as laws of tendency. For Kautsky such laws are inexorably realised and empirically verifiable. Kautsky later dropped this notion in favour of an equally mechanical idea of 'chronic depression' based on the inability of the world market to expand rapidly enough to absorb society's growing productive forces. Later still Kautsky was to come round to Bernstein's view that a 'new capitalism' had achieved a permanent state of harmony.[3]

A comment on Kautsky's method should warn us how not to proceed. Kautsky adopts a mechanistic conception of the economy as an autonomous and isolated force in history and bases his notion of breakdown on this conception. Throughout his discussion of capitalism, Kautsky draws from the general analysis of *Capital*. He then supplements these analyses with large quantities of empirical data intended to meet the arguments of the revisionists and to establish a direct correlation between the laws and material conditions of capitalism. In this way Kautsky reinforces the revisionist tendency to view the conditions of capitalism as a series of 'facts', readily apparent and available for immediate utilisation (Hansen 1985: 47).

If for Bernstein and eventually for Kautsky also, it seemed clear that capitalism had entered a new crisis-free state, for many on the left today it seems equally obvious that the productive forces have developed over the last half century. The explosion of science and technology, ('the scientific and technological revolution') bringing with it new industries and a great increase in labour productivity,[4] together with the secular boom that the post-war economy experienced, could be adduced to support this proposition. To meet this theoretical challenge is no small task and is certainly not one to be accomplished in a single chapter. To repeat: it involves a considerable theoretical effort because in tackling it we are confronted with an equally obvious 'fact': the prostitution of Marxism associated with the degeneration of the Soviet state and the Communist International, a process stretching over more than six decades. And this prostitution affected not merely the ethos of the Stalinist parties but found its reflection in the working class movement, including those struggling to build the Fourth International. Stalinism distorted historical materialism beyond recognition when it presented history as a series of fixed stages through which each society would automatically progress. Relations of production would adjust mechanically to the level reached in the progress of the productive forces. And these forces of production were interpreted to mean techniques, or the implements of labour or natural forces subjugated by technology. Here Stalinism started where Kautsky and Bernstein had left off. This mechanical and teleological conception of history was no invention of Stalinism, just as it had been no invention of the 'orthodox' Marxists of the Second International. For involved here was a capitulation to bourgeois ideology at its most basic level – one that regards economic relations as natural, beyond human knowledge and control. To tackle the Stalinist distortion of Marxism thus means returning to the most basic questions that Marx himself had to establish in his fight against the bourgeois ideologists of his day.[5] In this chapter I propose to touch on just one aspect of this matter: the confusion of the relations between people and people on the one hand and those between people and nature on the other.

Technological revolution?

Over the last 50 years various theories have emerged amongst bourgeois apologists purporting to explain the 'transformed' nature of present-day society which rest precisely on this confusion or conflation. Thus theories of 'industrial society' claim that the imperatives of technical change in the post-war world have made it essential for the large corporations to plan their economic growth over a long term, ignoring the principles of profit maximisation. J.K. Galbraith (1967), for example, holds that technological advances have made the planning of the supply and marketing of goods and services, as well as their production by means of data-processing systems, a necessary component of management. From such conceptions Galbraith draws the conclusion that power now rests with a 'technostructure', a stratum engendered by the 'technological and scientific revolution' and one which shuns the traditional capitalist mentality. This layer plans production, seeking optimal profit in a manner that eliminates conflict between capital and labour.

The impact of this 'technological revolution' on the economic structure of society has undermined the Marxist thesis about the decisive role of the working class, argue the proponents of the theory of 'industrial society'. The specific weight of the working class has declined in the last half century because its share in the economy is diminishing as a result of the scientific and technological changes taking place over this period. Second, because in present-day 'consumer society' the working class acquire consumer durables and so develop into a propertied class which aims at conserving and multiplying its property, what was formerly the working class is transformed into a middle class whose relations with the owners of the means of production are no longer antagonistic. Here science and technology are separated from the social relations of which they are a part, transformed into disembodied, independent entities.

The productivity of capital

The theories advanced by writers such as Galbraith may appear new, they may adopt new terms, but they are in essence quite old, for in their technological interpretation of economic phenomena they continue a tradition that has been at the heart of bourgeois economics and social science generally for the past century and a half. While such theories have a definite apologetic content it would be wrong to let the matter rest there. As we know, Marx, in his most important work *Capital* set out to expose the class nature of what, with some contempt, he dubbed 'vulgar' political economy. But he simultaneously offered an explanation of the objective basis which enabled such political economy to mystify reality so as to veil the substance of capital's exploitative nature and at the same time prove that the principles of freedom and equality are realised in bourgeois society.

The final section of the opening chapter of *Capital* (Marx 1961) is entitled 'The fetishism of commodities and the secret thereof'. What is fetishism? It consists in the fact that natural objects assume properties which have nothing to do with their nature but are entirely the product of the social relations of which these things are a part. That 'things' do acquire such power is no mere illusion, no mere product of the inadequate thinking of individuals, and therefore not to be 'demystified' by the power of thought alone. Fetishism arises, held Marx, from the very nature of capitalist production itself – where the social relations between individuals take the form of, become attached to, inanimate objects.[6] As an example we can take the category of capital and its 'productivity': a question that is closely related to that of the nature of the productive forces. We know that capital appears, presents itself on the surface of society, in many material guises – buildings, machinery, raw materials, bank balances, stocks and shares. Now in what sense is machinery productive? It follows from Marx's theory that only labour creates value. But that in no way means that the objective factors of production such as machinery, or the application of science to industry, are to be denied any form of 'productivity'. To the degree that they contribute to raising the level of production they contribute to the production of use-values.

But this is not the end of the story, as it is for bourgeois economics as well as for those – Marxists and non Marxists – who believe that because the 'productivity of labour' has increased in the post-war world, the productive forces must have grown. What such people miss is that capital is productive in a quite different, even opposed, sense. As the ruling relation of bourgeois society, its 'great historical mission' consists 'in enforcing surplus labour'. The productivity of capital is measured not simply in its ability to raise the level of production of use-values (for it a nuisance although one it cannot escape) but in its ability to extract surplus labour. This is the key to the secret of capital's productivity: as an essential relation for the development of the social productive forces.[7] Capital was responsible for this development not because it constituted one of the 'factors of production' or because it 'furthered the application of science to industry' but because it was 'owned'. In other words, although always attached to things, capital is not in essence a 'thing' but rather an antagonistic social relation of a particular type – one based on an insatiable thirst for surplus-value, specifically for surplus-value in its relative form. Thus capital is productive 'insofar as it is a coercive force on wage-labour ... spurring on the productive power of labour to produce relative surplus-value' (Marx 1969a: 93). The contrast between past labour embodied in the means of production and living labour, of which the worker is the vehicle, lies at the basis of a technological interpretation of the productive forces.[8] While the power of capital, treated as a thing, is glorified, bourgeois economics regards the worker as merely one of the material 'factors of production' used by the owners of the instruments of labour as a component of the technological process, alongside machinery and raw materials. Of course it would be easy to set aside all this discussion of 'productivity' as a mere playing with words, a silly metaphysical game. After all what is the difference between a relationship between person and person and one between people and nature? For Marxism the social relations of production into which people enter to secure their material means of life constitute the foundation on which alone the whole structure of society can be explained. If these are confused with natural relations, after the manner of bourgeois political economy, then the very essence of capitalism must be lost sight of.[9]

The productivity of labour

Further, the nature of the productivity of capital leads, as it must, to the question of the productivity of labour which, as we have suggested, is a far from unambiguous concept. For bourgeois economics the matter is simple. By the productivity of labour it means only the rate at which the output of goods and services flows from the use of the 'factor of production' labour. This is a classic example of the confusion of things natural with things social. Here we reach the most fundamental issues in political economy: capitalism is not a mode of producing use-values to serve human needs. This would be to see it naturalistically and mechanically as a mere 'means' satisfying with a greater or lesser degree of irrationality a definite 'end' – the satisfaction of human needs. This is not the case, for the irrationality of capital is complete: the production of things to satisfy needs (use-values) is nothing but an inevitable but incidental break on capital's accumulation.

> The increase in the productive force of living labour increases the *value* of capital (or diminishes the value of the worker) not because it increases the quantity of products or use-values created by the same labour – the productive force of labour is its natural force – *but rather because it diminishes necessary labour.*
>
> (Marx 1973: 339, emphasis added)

Or again:

> The limit of capitalist production is the excess time of the labourers. The absolute spare time gained by society does not concern it. *The development of productivity concerns it only in so far as it increases the surplus labour-time of the working-class*, not because it decreases the labour-time of material production in general. It moves thus in a contradiction.
>
> (Marx 1959: 258–259, emphasis added)

Here is a crucial point. If the productivity of labour is understood as the rate at which labour produces products to satisfy human needs then its rise is unlimited, or at any rate limited by technical knowledge and its application, as well as by the bountifulness of nature. This idea is at the root of many who, basing themselves on the immediate outward appearances of bourgeois economy over the last decades, conclude that the productive forces have indeed developed. But if by productivity of labour under the specific conditions of capitalism we mean the production of surplus labour-time in the form of surplus-value, then there are definite social constraints on this process which arise from the very nature of capital itself.[10] Marx thus explains that the more capital accumulates, the more difficult becomes its task of raising the productivity of labour, that is of diminishing the 'necessary' part of the working day in favour of the 'surplus' portion falling to capital:

> the smaller the fractional part of the working day which forms the equivalent of the worker, which expresses necessary labour, the smaller is the increase in the surplus-value which capital obtains from the increase of productive force. Its surplus-value rises, but in an ever smaller relation to the development of the productive force.
>
> (Marx 1973: 340)

And on the same page we read:

> Thus the more developed capital already is, the more surplus labour it has created, the more terribly must it develop the productive force in order to realize itself in only smaller proportion, i.e. to add surplus-value – because its barrier always remains the relation between the fractional part of the day which expresses *necessary labour*, and the entire working day. It can move only within these boundaries.... The self-realization of capital becomes more difficult to the extent that it has already been realized.
>
> (Marx 1973: 340)

Industrial capital: the basic form

The general point Marx is making is this: capital rests on the extraction of surplus-value from the working class. This is its basis, one from which it can never escape, for were it to do so it would cease to be capital. But the development of machines and 'the power of the agencies set in motion during labour time' enables the production of wealth (use-values) on a scale out of all proportion to this narrow but, for capital, inescapable basis. '*The theft of alien labour time, on which the present wealth is based*, appears a miserable foundation in the face of this new one, created by large-scale industry itself' (Marx 1973: 705). In short, the more capital develops, the harder does it become for capital to extract relative surplus labour. The more successful is capital, the greater the contradiction between the social basis on which this process rests and its results – ever more use-values. In this struggle to raise the productivity of labour – to raise the rate of exploitation of the working class – capital demands two 'ideal' factors. According to Ricardo capital needed 'competition without restriction' and 'unhampered increase in products through industry'.[11] Commenting on Ricardo, Marx makes the following observation which is important in our theoretical conception of the epoch of imperialism.

> This means in other words nothing other than that the laws of capital are completely realized only within *unlimited competition* and *industrial production*. Capital develops adequately on the latter productive basis and in the former relation of production; i.e. its immanent laws enter completely into reality. Since this is so, it would have to be shown how this *unlimited competition* and *industrial production* are conditions of the realization of capital, conditions which it must itself little by little produce (instead of the hypothesis appearing here as merely that of the theoretician, who places free competition and the productive mode of capital's existence externally and arbitrarily into the relation of capital to itself as capital, not as developments of capital itself, but as imaginary presuppositions of capital for the sake of purity).
>
> (Marx 1973: 559–560)

Marx is suggesting that the industrial form of capital, operating on the basis of unlimited competition is the form in which the immanent laws of capital enter into reality. Why should the industrial form of capital be for capital the 'ideal' form?

> Industrial capital is the only mode of existence of capital in which not only the appropriation of surplus-value or surplus-product, but simultaneously its creation is a function of capital. Therefore with it the capitalist character of production is a necessity.
>
> (Marx 1957: 55)

Industrial capital is the basic form of capital because it is the foundation on which the extraction of relative surplus-value takes place, and relative surplus-value expresses the essential relations of capital.

As is well known, Marx distinguishes two forms of surplus labour. One Marx called absolute surplus-value, in which form surplus-value is increased via a prolongation of the working day, the productivity of labour remaining constant. The other is relative surplus-value where the productivity of labour increases, the length of the working day remaining constant. 'surplus-value in so far as it arises out of the growing productivity of labour' (Marx 1969b: 16); 'surplus-value arising from the curtailment of the necessary labour-time, and from the corresponding alteration in the respective lengths of the two components of the working-day' (Marx 1961: 315). It is surplus labour in its relative form that capitalism brings to dominance and this it does through machine production, through the factory system. It is not therefore in absolute but in relative surplus labour that 'appears the industrial and the distinguishing historic character of the mode of production founded on capital' (Marx 1973: 769). Here again, the distinction between what is 'natural' and what is 'social' is the key to understanding the critical distinction between these two forms of surplus labour. For Marx makes clear that absolute surplus labour depends on natural conditions. If nature did not provide the conditions for human beings to produce more than they required for their immediate subsistence there could be no surplus labour, surplus-value or surplus produce. 'This prerequisite of a certain level of productivity is based on the natural productiveness of land and water, the natural sources of wealth' (Marx 1972: 449). But it is quite other with relative surplus labour. While the same natural conditions that are necessary for the production of surplus labour in its absolute form also apply, the creation of relative surplus labour requires certain social conditions in which the productivity of labour can be progressively raised. And this involves the introduction of machinery. Thus: 'The basis for absolute surplus-value – that is, the real pre-condition for its existence – is the *natural fertility of the land*, of nature, whereas relative surplus-value depends on the development of the social productive forces' (Marx 1972: 449). In *Capital* Marx shows how the process during which the emergence of the economic form of relative surplus-value causes a growth in labour productivity, demands that capital replaces manual labour with machine labour and develops the technical basis of the production of surplus-value. It is also at the same time clear that it is the introduction of the machine itself that causes absolute surplus-value to be displaced by relative surplus-value as the dominant form of surplus-value production within capitalism. Relative surplus-value is in conformity with industrial capital precisely because this form is not merely a passive reflection, a parasitic outgrowth of the development of the productive forces, as it were, but is an active form exerting a strong reverse effect on industrial capital itself, that is on the very basis that produced it.

Here we take up an issue which flows from these observations of Marx. What are the implications of the erosion of industrial capital that has been such a feature of the older capitalist countries over the last 50 years? The answer to this question is connected with our understanding of the critical distinction between productive and unproductive labour within capitalism.

Productive and unproductive labour

There has been much confusion amongst Marxists about the substance of productive labour. As we have noted, for Marx productive labour was labour that produces surplus-value, and more than anything, labour that produces relative surplus-value, essentially labour employed in the factory system. There are two issues here which have a bearing on the nature of capitalism since the end of the last war. First, what is the significance of the growing number of state employees within the capitalist system? Second, how are we to view the growth in the service sector of the capitalist economy which, in the case of the more moribund capitalist economies such as Britain, has led to a marked process of 'de-industrialisation'? An answer to the first question involves an understanding of the distinction between productive and unproductive labour within the capitalist system.[12] The second appertains to a narrower question: the role of machine labour as that productive labour which creates surplus-value in its relative form.

Arising from the nature of capitalism, labour that is productive defines itself as exclusively that labour which, exchanging directly against capital, leads to the production of surplus-value. The usefulness, the material nature, of the product produced in the labour process counts here for nothing whatsoever, nor the fact that such labour may be necessary for social reproduction. Of course if capitalism is seen as an instrument for creating use-values, if the aim of production is regarded as consumption, then any labour paid for producing a useful good or service will be deemed productive. Thus all those receiving wages (or salaries) would be deemed productive workers. This latter definition is that of bourgeois economics and many would-be Marxists reject it – or appear to do so. Such Marxists accept the distinction between productive and unproductive labour but find the definition of productive labour as surplus-value creating labour too narrow. This latter group argues thus: many types of labour that do not produce surplus-value directly nonetheless make a vital contribution to the health service, to education, to scientific investigation, etc. Domestic work is likewise indispensable for the functioning of capital and to count it as non-productive is surely perverse. Similarly, say the same critics, productive labour should be defined as that labour which facilitates social reproduction and the rest – that employed in the manufacture of arms, in the provision of luxury goods for instance – should be deemed non-productive. Both these objections to the 'narrow' Marxist definition boil down to the same thing: they find the definition too restrictive because it refuses to take into account the material nature of the product concerned. In so doing these 'wider' definitions would take us back to the traditional bourgeois view outlined above. Here some very 'practical' questions are involved in the confusion of labour as merely a natural process and labour as a social process. For instance, many Marxists saw in state spending the key to capitalism's relative stability in the immediate post-war years. Here the influence of the Keynesian theory of effective demand was strongly felt. But if we understand the nature of productive labour as only that which produces surplus-value then it is clear that such state expenditure is expenditure on unproductive labour and as such far from assisting the creation of surplus-value constitutes a drain upon it. The rising share of state spending (and with it the level of taxation) in all the leading capitalist economies since the end of the war is an indication of the depth of the problem, and why there is a determined effort to cut down that share.

To turn briefly to our second question: the specific character of machine (factory) labour. Does it matter, from the point of view of capital, that ever increasing numbers are employed in the non-manufacturing sector of the economy: in the provision of services? Once more, if one conceives of productive labour as labour which is paid for a 'useful' product or service, the answer will be a negative one. But it is in just this sector that the limits to the creation of relative surplus-value are most obvious, for it is here that the possibilities for the mechanisation of labour are strictly limited. A retailer of hamburgers can squeeze more surplus-value from his staff by intensifying their labour (making them run and serve faster) by paying wages 'below value', as well as by lengthening the working day – extending hours, cutting meal breaks, etc. (that is increasing absolute surplus-value). But the scope for the extraction of such (absolute) surplus-value is objectively limited by nature. The working day cannot be extended beyond 24 hours – in practice of course a much lower limit is encountered. Second, the intensification of labour also has its limits: the strength and dexterity of the workers employed. So the more capital moves away from that form which gave it its historic specificity, the more is expressed its historic demise.[13]

The falling rate of profit

We have stressed that Marx, unlike bourgeois political economy, drew a clear distinction between the social relations of production and production as a material, technical process.[14] But this does not mean that he ignored these technical aspects. Quite the contrary: he understood for example that the labour process involved a unity of a material process (the struggle against nature) and a social process (which under capitalism involves the production of value and surplus-value).[15] In order to illustrate this point we can make a brief comment on the law of the tendency of the rate of profit to fall. This law is intimately linked with the development of the productive forces. If the *raison d'être* of capitalism is production for profit then its movement is decisive for the entire nature and functioning of the capitalist system. Thus the prospect of a secular decline in the rate of profit sent a 'shudder down the spine of that millionaire banker Ricardo'.

As Marx said: '[This law is] ... in every respect the most important law of modern economy, and the most important for understanding the most difficult relations. It is the most important law from the historical standpoint' (Marx 1973: 748).

And further:

> Simple as this law appears from the foregoing statements, all of political economy has so far had little success in discovering it. ... The economists perceived the phenomenon and cudgelled their brains in tortuous attempts to interpret it. Since this law is of great importance to capitalist

> production, it may be said to be a mystery whose solution has been the goal of all political economy since Adam Smith, the differences between the various schools since Adam Smith having been in the divergent approaches to a solution.
>
> (Marx 1959: 209)[16]

What is the basis of the law of the tendency of the rate of profit to fall? It is this: as capital accumulates, its composition alters. Capital is divided into two basic components: constant capital (buildings, machinery stocks of raw materials, etc.) and variable capital (that portion of capital advanced in purchase of labour power, equivalent to the wages bill).Thus the organic composition of capital is represented by the ratio c/v, where c is the expenditure on constant capital and v is the advances made in the purchase of labour power. Now if we assume that the division of the working day between capitalists and workers remains constant, that is if we assume that the surplus-value extracted from the working class (s) remains in the same ratio to variable capital (in other words, the rate of exploitation, s/v, remains stable) then the rate of profit, the surplus-value resulting from the advance of total capital, that is $s/(c+v)$, must decline as the organic composition of capital c/v, rises.[17]

This law has been the subject of vigorous attack not least from those claiming their allegiance to Marx. The nub of these objections is as follows. If capital can raise the rate of exploitation at a sufficiently rapid pace then why should this not counter-act completely the rising organic composition of capital?[18] If this were possible, then capitalism would in principle be crisis-free, for the tendency for the productive forces to develop would meet with no insurmountable barrier. But there are several objections to this position, the decisive one being the following: the possibility of raising or stabilising the rate of exploitation through an increase in the intensity of exploitation is not an abstract procedure. It concerns living workers in real situations. There are natural, physical, barriers to the amount of surplus-value that can be extracted from workers. First there are definite limits to the length of the working day. Second, the portion of the working day in which the worker has to reproduce the equivalent of the value of his labour power cannot be reduced to zero. As machinery is introduced workers are displaced ('technological unemployment') while the rate of exploitation of those remaining increases. The first tendency reduces the number of workers available for exploitation – that is the mass of surplus-value is reduced. The second tendency increases the rate of surplus-value, but as Marx points out:

> Two labourers, each working 12 hours daily, cannot produce the same mass of surplus-value as 24 who only work two hours, even if they could live on air and hence did not have to work for themselves at all. In this respect, then, the compensation of the reduced number of workers by intensifying the degree of exploitation has certain insurmountable limits. It may, for this reason, well check the fall in the rate of profit, but it cannot prevent it altogether.
>
> (Marx 1959: 242)

The purpose of this chapter has been to deal with a particular aspect of the analysis of the productive forces. We have suggested that without an understanding of the relationship between the natural and social aspects of the process of production it is impossible to clear up the confusions and distortions of various Marxists on this issue. The neglect of Marx's method, and its replacement with a shallow empiricism, the substitution of sterile dogma in place of genuine scientific enquiry, were the hallmarks of Stalinism's attack on Marxism. As we have shown, a fetishistic conception of the development of the forces of production was advanced in which productivity increases were seen as identical to the mere multiplication of use-values, of 'things', irrespective of the historically determined social relations through which those increases took place. On such a naturalistic foundation, the crucial theoretical developments made by Marx on key questions, such as the nature of productive and unproductive labour, are completely obscured. The development of the productive forces, within the mode of production based upon capital, rests not upon the mere creation of a surplus product, but upon its ability to overcome the barriers to a continual increase in the production of surplus-value, of profit, its whole *raison d'être*.

Notes

1 Amongst theories I would include as involving a rejection of Lenin and Trotsky's conception of the epoch are those associated with the theory of the 'permanent arms economy' as well as those of 'neocapitalism' and not least the Stalinist theory of 'state monopoly capitalism'.

2 For a discussion of Bernstein's work and the response of orthodox Marxism see F.R. Hansen (1985).

3 Thus Kautsky (1925):

> Indeed, we expected much more from the crisis at that time [1885].... Not only the revival of the socialist movement in Britain but the breakdown of capitalism throughout the world. This hope proved illusory. Capitalism survived the crisis, despite its considerable extension in space and time and its inordinate intensity. A new phase of capitalist prosperity ensued. But what emerged was an entirely altered capitalism. The older form of capitalism had been eclipsed.

4 Taking the decade 1949–1959, labour productivity rose at an average annual rate of growth of 5.9 per cent in Western Germany, by 4.8 per cent in Italy; even countries with the lowest rates of growth in western Europe – such as Britain and Belgium – experienced growth rates of around 2 per cent. As we shall see, the 'productivity of labour' is an ambiguous category.

5

> In our country no fundamental creative work has been done in Marxism-Leninism. Most theoreticians busy themselves with turning over and over again old quotations, formulas and theses. What is a science without creative work? It is not so much science as scholasticism, a pupils' exercise, not a science; for science is above all creation, creation of something new and not repetition of what is old.

Thus Mikoyan (1956) at the twentieth Congress of the CPSU in 1956, where the veil on some of Stalin's crimes was gingerly lifted.

6

> The categories of bourgeois economy consist of such like forms. They are forms of thought expressing with social validity the conditions and relations of a definite, historically determined mode of production, viz., the production of commodities. The whole mystery of commodities, all the magic and necromancy that surrounds the products of labour as long as they take the form of commodities, vanishes therefore so soon as we come to other forms of production.
>
> (Marx 1961: 76)

7 'The productivity of capital as capital is not the productive force which increases use-values; but rather its capacity to create value; the degree to which it produces value' (Marx 1973: 630). In other words capital produces and re-produces itself as a social relation of production in the form of the production and reproduction of things. To the extent that the capitalist system produces things in which surplus-value is not contained, to that extent it is involved in an expenditure of unproductive labour, however useful these 'things' may be.

8 The 'germ' of this fetishism lies in the commodity form itself. The commodity is a unity of two diverse aspects. In the first place a commodity is a means of satisfying a definite human want – it is a use-value. But at the same time the commodity is an exchange-value: it is the bearer of a social relation. Thus, uniquely under capitalism, social relations are expressed in the relations between objects. This is why empiricism, concerned with the immediate appearances of things will so easily confuse the natural – the relations between people and the material world – and the social: the relations between people.

9 Cf. the anarchist Bakunin: 'If the workers are to be free, then capitalism must be destroyed. But this does not mean the destruction of "capital", but rather its preservation.' Marx replied to such ideas: 'But capital … is the *capitalist*. Of course, socialists sometimes say, we need capital but not the capitalist. Then capital appears as a pure thing, not as a relation of production' (Marx 1973: 303).

10 'The productivity of capital consists in the fact that it confronts labour as wage-labour, and the productivity of labour consists in the fact that it confronts the means of labour as capital' (Marx 1969a: 394).

11 Marx thoroughly approved of these sentiments. Indeed it was here that Ricardo revealed a 'faint notion' of the 'historic nature of the laws of bourgeois economy'.

12 For an elegant note on the distinction between productive and unproductive labour see Geoffrey Kay (1979: 132–134), also I.I. Rubin (1972: 259–275).

13 The same is true of the disappearance of unlimited competition within the capitalist system. Its disappearance indicates that the laws of capital cannot be realised except in increasingly distorted forms which themselves build up the conditions for crises of increasing scope and depth.

14 In the same way, while it would be wrong to equate 'productive forces' with 'technique' the latter are an element in the former.

15 As another example we can take the question of Marx's theory of money. He stresses that money expresses a social relation and that this is the source of its power – not the fact that it is represented by a particular metal, say gold. But at the same time it is not an accident that gold emerges as the ideal money form. This is because its material properties – its durability, easy divisibility, the fact that its rarity means that a small amount represents considerable value (abstract labour) – make it the most suitable substance to act as the 'universal equivalent'.

16 Ricardo recognised the significance of the possibility of a long-term decline in the rate of profit. But, in line with our general theme, he had a naturalistic understanding of the problem. As cultivation extended to feed a growing population it was forced onto less fertile land. Because of this the value of subsistence goods (food) tended to rise and this produced a decline in the rate of profit. In explaining the decline of the

rate of profit via the fertility of the soil Ricardo 'flees from economics to seek refuge in organic chemistry' (Marx 1973: 754).

17 A simple example. In period 1 let the value of $c=100$, the value of v be = 50 and the surplus-value (s) extracted be also 50. Note that the rate of exploitation (s/v) is in the ratio 1 : 1 and the organic composition of capital (c/v) is in the ratio 2 : 1. Now, in period 2 as a result of technical change the following values apply: c is now 400; v is 120 and s is 120. The rate of exploitation (120/120 = 1 : 1) has remained constant (our assumption) but the organic composition of capital has now risen (400: 120). Now in period 1 the rate of profit ($s/c+v$) was 50/150 = 33.3 per cent, in period 2 it has fallen to 120/520 which equals 23.1 per cent.

18 To return to the numerical example given above. If in period 2 we assume that surplus-value, s, has risen to 175 – that is the rate of exploitation has increased sharply – then the rate of profit will have been stabilised, it will be given by 175/(400 + 120) = 33.6 per cent. (The same point is made in *Capital* volume I in the chapter where Marx discusses the 'rate and mass of surplus-value' – see in particular p. 305.)

References

Bernstein, E. (1909) *Evolutionary Socialism*, Independent Labour Party. Online, available at: www.marxists.org/reference/archive/bernstein/works/1899/evsoc/trans.htm (accessed 14 October 2011).

Galbraith, J.K. (1967) *The New Industrial State*, London: Hamish Hamilton.

Hansen, F.R. (1985) *The Breakdown of Capitalism: A History of the Idea in Western Marxism*, London: Routledge and Kegan Paul.

Kautsky, K. (1925) *The Economic Doctrines of Karl Marx*, London: A. & C. Black Ltd. Online, available at: www.marxists.org/archive/kautsky/1903/economic/index.htm (accessed 17 October 2011).

Kay, G. (1979) *The Economic Theory of the Working* Class, London: Macmillan.

Marx, K. (1957) *Capital*, vol. II, Moscow and London: Foreign Languages Publishing House and Lawrence & Wishart.

Marx, K. (1959) *Capital*, vol. III, Moscow and London: Foreign Languages Publishing House and Lawrence & Wishart.

Marx, K. (1961) *Capital*, vol. I, Moscow and London: Foreign Languages Publishing House and Lawrence & Wishart.

Marx, K. (1969a) *Theories of Surplus Value*, Part I, London: Lawrence & Wishart.

Marx, K. (1969b) *Theories of Surplus Value*, Part II, London: Lawrence & Wishart.

Marx, K. (1972) *Theories of Surplus Value*, Part III, London: Lawrence & Wishart.

Marx, K. (1973) *Grundrisse: Foundations of the Critique of Political Economy*, Harmondsworth: Penguin Books.

Mikoyan, A.I. (1956) *Speech at the 20th Congress of the CPSU*, Moscow: Foreign Languages Publishing House.

Rubin, I.I. (1972) *Essays on Marx's Theory of Value*, Detroit: Black & Red. Online, available at: www.marxists.org/archive/rubin/value/index.htm (accessed 16 December 2011).

Trotsky, L. (1963) *The Transitional Programme. The Death Agony of Capitalism and Tasks of the Fourth International*, London: New Park Publications. Based on 1981 Labor Publications printing, online, available at www.marxists.org/archive/trotsky/1938/tp/index.htm (accessed 13 December 2011).

6 The foundation of Keynes's economics

This chapter explores certain aspects of the relationship between the economic theories of Karl Marx and J.M. Keynes from one particular angle, that of the underlying methodologies and general conceptions of these two economic theorists. And because of its importance in current analyses of the Keynesian crisis, we intend to explore these matters from one specific angle: from the standpoint of those who wish to create a new political economy on the basis of a fusion of certain strands within Keynesian economics on the one hand, and some elements from the Marxist-classical tradition on the other. Such efforts involve two distinct, although related questions:

1 That concerning the relationship of the political economy of the classical school to that of Marx. Keynes himself certainly believed that his new economics would undermine what he called the Ricardian foundations of Marxism. In other words, he identified the classical political economy of Ricardo with Marx's critique of it. We have already commented on this issue and can therefore be brief. Marx's work involved a critique of political economy, one which understood that there were a series of flaws, fatal in the final analysis, associated with the work of even the best representatives of the school; it was these flaws which made it vulnerable to the attacks of the vulgar, commonplace writers who emerged in the period following Ricardo's death. (The best treatment of the transition from classical to vulgar economics is provided by Rubin 1979.) The collapse of Ricardian economics was not an event explicable in ideological terms only. That is to say, while Ricardo's doctrines were certainly attacked because of the subversive uses to which they were being put, not least by the various radical writers in the 1820s and 1830s, the fact remains that the opponents of the classical school did have definite weaknesses in Ricardo's economics at which to aim their fire and no amount of formal rearranging of the categories of that economics could protect it from its vulgar detractors. Only a fundamental reworking of classical economics which truly transcended it (that is, preserved its positive features while disposing of its negative aspects) could produce a real development of this tradition. It fell to Marx's lot to make precisely this advance. It is from this standpoint that those attempts made by certain post-Keynesians, as well as by several

Marxists, to conflate the work of classical economists and that of Marx are at base erroneous and must be rejected.

2 The second issue implicit in the efforts to reconstitute political economy along lines proposed by Kregel (1975) and others involves a certain view of the relationship of Keynes' work to the classical tradition.[1] In exploring the foundations of Keynes' economics we shall be concerned with this latter question. Briefly, to anticipate the line of argument, we shall suggest that at a fundamental level these two traditions have little in common and that Keynesian economics is, in the last resort, a continuation, under twentieth-century conditions to be sure, of the vulgar tradition in political economy. We intend to defend this proposition by means of an examination of the categories of *The General Theory*, suggesting that their subjective and psychological character expresses clearly that they do indeed derive from the vulgar school and not from that represented by Petty, Smith, Ricardo and others.

As we have already seen, the whole of the post-war period has witnessed something of a struggle for the soul of Keynes. On the one hand, in the case of the 'neoclassical synthesis' efforts were made to incorporate the teachings of Keynes into the body of neoclassical orthodoxy, producing what Robinson variously castigated as a 'bastard' or 'bowdlerised' Keynesianism. [In Chapter 1 (19–20) of *The Crisis of Keynesian Economics*, Geoff Pilling says of Joan Robinson:

> Standing at the crossroads of various strands in modern economic theory, she is representative of those working for a reconstruction of political economy which will overcome what she and her fellow thinkers see as the bankruptcy of neoclassical economics.... From 1950s onwards she has been attempting
>
> > to trace the confusions and sophistries of the neoclassical doctrine to their origin in the rejection of historic time in the static equilibrium theory of the neoclassical economics and at the same time to find a more hopeful alternative in the classical tradition revived by Sraffa, which flows from Ricardo through Marx, diluted by Marshall and enriched by the analysis of the effective demand of Keynes and Kalecki.
> >
> > (Robinson 1973: xii)

The current chapter sets out to show that the standpoint of Keynes is radically different from that of the classical economists (of whom Ricardo represents the highest point) and fundamentally different from that of Marx – ed.] From a quite different standpoint, equally persistent attempts have been made to bring together certain elements from Keynes's work with aspects of the classical-Marxian tradition. We shall be concerned not with those who sought to marry the work of Keynes to the prevailing neoclassical orthodoxy but with these latter efforts in order to examine whether, in principle, they are soundly based.

There is no doubt that the emergence of Keynesianism in the 1930s and its later rise to a position of almost unchallenged dominance in the post-war period exercised a decisive influence upon many Marxists operating within the field of economics. Because this is not our prime concern, the historical references will not be explored; but in brief the following can be asserted: under the impact of prevailing Keynesian orthodoxy many Marxists were inclined to read *Capital* and other of Marx's economic works from the standpoint of some version or other of an underconsumptionist theory of capitalist breakdown. That is to say they were inclined, as were certain of Keynes's followers, to see the principal problem for capitalism as lying in a tendency for consumption to fall below the level of that required to sustain investment and full employment, particularly the full employment of labour. The corollary of this position was that appropriate state action, particularly action associated with the state budget, could, by raising the level of consumption, overcome this deficiency.

A book such as Baran and Sweezy's *Monopoly Capital* (1966), is a striking case in point. In its overall approach this work is Keynesian, concentrating as it does on what the authors take to be the critical problem for capitalism in the post-war period: the disposal of a rising economic surplus. According to Baran and Sweezy, the big monopoly and near-monopoly concerns are able to fix the prices of their output in such a way as to ensure for themselves ever greater surpluses. This being so, the problem for capitalism boils down to finding ways to absorb this surplus. They see such things as increased advertising expenditures, the economic activities of the state and growing expenditure on arms as the principal means whereby capitalism disposes of its economic surpluses. For them the contradictions of capitalism, especially that between the capitalist class and the working class, no longer exist as they did in Marx's time. Capitalism is condemned not as a historical limited and inherently contradictory system but as one subjected to increasing irrationality. In this way Baran and Sweezy (1966: 72) find redundant the basic categories of Marx's political economy. Thus of the tendency for capitalism to generate a rising economic surplus they say:

> This law immediately invites comparison, as it should, with the classical-Marxian law of the falling tendency of the rate of profit. Without entering into an analysis of the different versions of the latter, we can say that all presuppose a competitive system. By substituting the law of rising surplus for the law of falling profit we are therefore not rejecting or revising a time-honoured theorem of political economy: we are simply taking account of the undoubted fact that the structure of the capitalist economy has undergone a fundamental change since that theorem was formulated. What is most essential about the structural change from competitive to monopoly capitalism finds its theoretical expression in this substitution.[2]

Their book, published in the middle of the inflationary boom, was an indication of the impact which the prevailing Keynesian orthodoxy had on Marxism.

But the seeds of this move towards Keynesianism had been laid long before – in fact in the 1930s, the decade when Keynes's major work first appeared. It is noteworthy that Maurice Dobb, for long undoubtedly the leading commentator on Marxist political economy in England, in introducing Sweezy's (1946) earlier and influential exposition of the principles of Marxian economics, *The Theory of Capitalist Development*, to English readers admits that he had himself moved closer to Sweezy's heavy emphasis on underconsumptionism as the major factor explaining capitalist crisis, a move which is reflected in much of Dobb's later writing.

In what is probably still the most satisfactory popular treatment of Marxist political economy, Sweezy had, in this earlier work, when speaking of Keynes as the leading representative of those arguing for liberal capitalist reform, proposed that the critique of such ideas should start, 'not from their economic logic but rather from their faulty (usually implicit) assumptions about the relationship, or perhaps one should say lack of relationship, between economics and political action' (Sweezy 1946: 346). Sweezy is making an important point here, namely, that the question at issue is not so much the economic theory of Keynes but rather the false conception which, as a liberal, he held about the relationship of the economic to the political sphere within the capitalist system. The implication is that Keynesian-type economics was sound in the abstract: the problem arose when one attempted to implement such economics in the 'real world' in the face of a state which was not impartial as between social forces and therefore not neutral about policy prescriptions. Keynes is to be rejected not on theoretical grounds, but from the point of view of pragmatism, namely that his 'solutions' to the ills of capitalism do not in fact work in practice.[3]

It should be noted in passing that this attitude of Sweezy towards Keynes is remarkably similar to that which Keynes himself took to the work of his predecessors: that it was the faulty assumptions rather than the internal logic of the Manchester School which fatally vitiated its work. Thus,

> Our criticism of the accepted classical theory of economics has consisted not so much in finding logical flaws in its analysis as in pointing out that its tacit assumptions are seldom or never satisfied, with the result that it cannot solve the economic problems of the actual world.
>
> (Keynes 1936: 378)

In our opinion, the position adopted by Sweezy marks a fundamental and wholly unwarranted concession to Keynes. In this chapter we shall suggest that, contrary to Sweezy's view, the 'economic logic' of Keynes was indeed faulty and fatally so; consequently a consideration of this 'economic logic' must form the starting point of any sustained Marxist critique of Keynesianism. And this in turn implies that those efforts on the part of 'left Keynesians' such as Joan Robinson, to effect some theoretical reconciliation between Marx and Keynes are at base misconceived. The critical distinction drawn by Marx between the classical and the vulgar schools in economics provides a decisive conceptual prism through which to examine certain aspects of Keynes's economics. For Marx (1961a: 81) what he dubbed the vulgar school was concerned only with the most superficial aspects of capitalist economy; at a certain point it was a school which degenerated into apologetics, attempting as it did to rationalise away the contradictions of the capitalist system.[4] In particular, Marx castigated the fetishism inherent in vulgar political economy: the tendency to ascribe social powers and functions to things: for instance to attribute the entrepreneur's ability to make a profit to the natural objects which make up the means of production.[5] We therefore propose to review the main aspects of Keynes's theoretical system from the point of view of Marx's distinction between classical and vulgar political economy.

We can start by pointing to certain key features of Keynes's work which have a direct bearing upon the philosophical and methodological bases of that work. From where, in general, does Keynes begin his analysis? He accepted the fact that capitalism in no way automatically guarantees full employment; there is no self-adjusting mechanism which generates a level of effective demand sufficient to ensure the full utilisation of resources. Keynes's argument runs along the following well-known lines. In the short run – for him the period of greatest concern, although not necessarily so for many of his post-war followers – the level of employment is a function of the level of output which is in turn a function of the level of effective demand. It is this concept, that of effective demand, which is in reality Keynes's key idea, a point widely accepted, certainly amongst his orthodox followers (e.g. Patinkin 1965). Effective demand is that demand backed by expenditure. Total expenditure and total sales (assuming no stocks) are the same thing as output. So output is determined by effective demand. Keynes proceeded to break down effective demand into two components – consumption and investment – and analysed each in turn. The basis of the distinction is that money spent on goods and services by individuals to satisfy their own wants is consumption; money spent by enterprises on buildings and machinery in order to produce goods and services in the future is investment. Or, regarding the matter from the standpoint of output, the division is one between investment goods (buildings, machinery, etc.) and consumer goods. To know what determines the level of output – and hence the level of employment – one needs to know what determines the level of consumption and the level of investment. In order to analyse fluctuations in the level of effective demand, Keynes makes use of his three fundamental operational categories – the propensity to consume, the marginal efficiency of capital, and the rate of interest. In combination, these three factors set the limits within which the capitalist economy oscillates, and we shall say more of them presently.

No attempt is made in what follows to provide a full and systematic critique of Keynes's work. Only a few aspects will be touched upon. It is intended to look briefly at certain of Keynes's key concepts, to explore their underlying assumptions, concentrating particularly on Keynes's notion of capital and its 'productivity'. In view of her central role in the interpretation of both Marx and Keynes, brief comment is made towards the end of the chapter about the work of Joan Robinson. But first the overall approach of Marx to the analysis of capitalism can be sketched out in order to highlight the quite different methodological premises from which his work commences.

For Marx the dynamics of capitalism, the search for the 'law of motion of modern society' ('and it is the ultimate aim of this work to lay bare the economic law of motion of modern society' – Preface to the First German Edition [of *Capital* I – ed.], Marx 1961b: 10) involves as one of its central tasks the investigation of the concept of capital. Despite the claims of empiricism to the contrary, every science has its own hierarchy of concepts; empirical research and individual theories always rest on certain fundamental ideas, forming the cornerstone of the particular department of knowledge concerned. This empiricism denies: it claims to commence from 'the facts', unmediated by any preconceptions. This is however pure illusion: all thought begins from definite concepts as to the nature of its object; in this case the capitalist economy. But whether this starting point is a conscious one or not is a matter not without its importance. For those who start with unconscious theoretical categories – that is, from categories which have not been arrived at on the basis of a real critical assimilation of all the past developments in the science concerned – inevitably start their operations from the most vulgar, commonplace definitions. Keynes was here no exception to this law of thought. As we shall see, he did in fact employ an implicit definition of capital and of capitalism, namely as a system of production which was aimed at the satisfaction of human needs. His objection to this system lay in the fact that in its twentieth-century form (where monopoly dominated) it was not doing this as effectively as it could.

There is no doubt that in the case of economic theory the most basic concept with which it deals is that of capital. One of Marx's most persistent criticisms of the classical school was that it had no real, worked-out, truly consistent concept of capital. Even for Ricardo, the best of the classical economists, capital was merely 'stored up labour', a notion which had the effect of making capital coeval with human existence in the sense that even the most primitive tool of the savage represents 'stored up labour', the result of past effort on his part, and therefore for Ricardo capital. The seeming universality and general applicability of such an idea was gained, Marx held, at the expense of any real concrete historical content. This is made clear in Marx's comments on the economists' conception of capital:

> Capital consists of raw materials, instruments of labour and means of subsistence of all kinds, which are utilised in order to produce new raw materials, instruments of labour and new means of subsistence. All these are component parts, are creations of labour, products of labour, *accumulated labour*. Accumulated labour which serves as a new means of production is capital.
>
> So say the economists.
>
> What is a Negro slave? A man of the black race. The one explanation is as good as the other.
>
> A Negro is a Negro. He only becomes a *slave* in certain relations. A cotton-spinning jenny is a machine for spinning cotton. It becomes *capital* only in certain relations. Torn from these relationships it is no more capital than *gold* in itself is *money* or sugar the *price* of sugar.
>
> (Marx 1977: 211)

According to Marx, the vulgar economists had an even shallower and fetishistic view of capital. Now the connection between capital and labour in the economics which emerged following the disintegration of the Ricardian school (*c.*1830) was entirely lost sight of: the reward to the holders of capital was hereafter held to be a reward for their abstinence or waiting. The unwritten assumption in this view was that capitalism was a system designed to produce wealth for consumption and that those who delayed such consumption had to be appropriately rewarded. Any historical analysis of capital, any inkling that it might express economic relations specific to certain periods and conditions only, fell quite outside the theoretical vision of neoclassical economics.

The commonplace view of capital

The outcome of this trend can be seen when we look at the contemporary idea of capital present in orthodox economics. As an example we take the definition of capital offered by the 1984 edition of the *Penguin Dictionary of Economics*, a summary of similar notions to be found in a hundred textbooks:

> The stock of goods which are used in production and which have themselves been produced.... The word capital in economics generally means *real capital* – that is physical goods.... Two important features of capital are (a) that its creation entails a sacrifice, since resources are devoted to making non-consumable capital goods instead of goods for immediate consumption, and (b) that it enhances the PRODUCTIVITY of the FACTORS OF PRODUCTION, LAND AND LABOUR; it is the enhanced productivity which represents a reward for the sacrifice involved in creating capital.
>
> (Bannock *et al.* 1984: 61)

Two points arise from this definition: (a) Capital is a 'thing' merely and not a social relation of production. As such it is presumably coeval with man, indeed perhaps even with the animal kingdom. This was a view which led to a series of strange conclusions and ones which gave Marx much pleasure;[6] (b) despite its seeming lack of social content, this definition does in point of fact carry a very specific conception of the capitalist mode of production. For the reward to capital, the sacrifice of owning it, arises from the fact that immediate consumption must be postponed. Here, implicitly, is the notion that capitalism is a system founded on the satisfaction of human requirements, a system dedicated to providing for the needs of 'the consumer'. Marx rejected such a petty bourgeois notion because it obscured the fact that under capitalism the aim of production is, and can only be, the self-expansion of capital, that is, its continual accumulation.

Now it is, of course, a truism to say that Keynes criticised certain aspects of the work of the neoclassical school of his day, just as others had done prior to him. But it is equally the case that such criticisms never achieved the rank of anything fundamental, never probed to the epistemological foundations of this school, never inquired into the historical and social conceptions which underlay it. On the contrary, it is apparent that Keynes's work was itself imbued with precisely the same anti-historical conceptions which predominated in neoclassical economics.

For as is well known, Keynes deliberately abstracts himself from any critical analysis of the social structure of society and its laws of development. In other words, he takes the capitalist system for granted, accepts its appearances as constituting its essence. His concern is exclusively with the functioning rather than the dynamics of capitalism. In his theoretical system he takes both the productive forces and the relations of production to be immutable elements, given once and for all:

> We take as given the existing skill and quantity of available labour, the existing quantity and quality of equipment, the existing technique, the degree of competition ... as well as the social structure including the forces, other than our variables ... which determine the distribution of the national income.
>
> (Keynes 1936: 245)

Elsewhere Keynes writes that he takes as given (that is, as fixed) the entire 'economic framework' of capitalism (Keynes 1936: 246).

Now, of course, the fact that Keynes took these factors as 'given' does not mean that he was innocent of the fact that, in the empirical sense, this was not the case. A far more serious issue is involved here. It reveals the fact that Keynes's work involved the conventional and essentially positivist process of model-building whereby, on the basis of a series of arbitrary assumptions, a model of the economy is constructed. That is, Keynes makes a series of assumptions in order to simplify the analysis of the economy – such that there is no technical change taking place, that the 'economic framework' of capitalism is fixed – and on the basis of these abstractions a coherent picture of the world is derived. But, as in the case of the traditional assumption of perfect competition, such abstractions are purely mental devices having no basis in the reality of the phenomena being investigated. And precisely because of this they must be arbitrary and subjective. Marx's analysis is of course based on abstractions ('In the analysis of economic forms, moreover, neither microscopes nor chemical reagents are of use. The force of abstraction must replace both' Marx 1961b: 8) but his are abstractions of a quite different order, reflecting as they do the real movement of capital. (For an excellent exposition of Marx's method of abstraction in *Capital* and the difference between his procedure and that employed by positivism, see Ilyenkov 1982.)

For Marx all real economic categories – capital, value, rent, interest, profit, etc. – reflect not a series of arbitrary mental assumptions but definite social relations of production. Consequently, they are not categories valid for all epochs and all societies. Let us take the example of capital. According to Marx, capital is no mere thing – raw materials, buildings, factories, etc. – but a social relation which finds expression in or attaches itself to many different things such as money or commodities. The central feature of capitalism, its *specifica differentia*, the quality which marks it off from past economic systems, is that the means of production are monopolised by a class and face another class, the working class, which is obliged out of necessity to sell its ability to work (in Marx's terminology, its labour power) to one or other owner of capital. This is why for Marx the essence of capital lies in the fact that it is a social relation and not merely a material thing. Just as the examination of a sack of wheat cannot disclose the social relations under which it was produced (in a feudal demesne, by slave labour, on a collective farm, etc.) so the natural properties of the means of production can never tell us whether they function as capital. A certain class of people may own things such as factories, financial assets and so on but only a definite social process transforms these things into instruments of exploitation, converts them into bearers of that social relationship which Marx designates by the term 'capital'. Capital is a specific, historically defined, social relation of production. By a fetishistic notion of capital Marx meant precisely that view which tended to ascribe to objects qualities which it was imagined flowed from the material properties of such objects but which in point of fact arose entirely and exclusively from the social role occupied by these things in the process of material production. The notion that things are productive by their nature rather than by virtue of the specific place they occupy in a definite network of social relations was precisely the fetishistic view of capital to which Marx objected. In its most general form (leaving aside its various types) capital is depicted by Marx in the schema M–C–C′–M′ (M representing the initial sum of money owned by the capitalist). Ignoring here its actual origin, this sum of money is thrown into production, being used initially to purchase commodities, C, including the commodity labour power. In the process of production these commodities are in turn transformed into ones involving a greater amount of (potential) value, C′ which are then sold for an equivalent sum of money, M′. It is from this latter sum of money, M′, that the capitalist meets his individual consumption needs but much more crucially it provides the means for the further accumulation of capital – the reconversion of the surplus-value embodied in M′ back into capital.

This schema, M–C–C′–M′, represents in conceptual form the only axis on which production within capitalism takes place. For Marx, capitalism can never be understood if it is seen merely as the production of things satisfying human needs. Were this the case, the limits to production would be purely technical, concerned with the best, most rational, most 'economic' allocation of certain material means to the satisfaction of a number of needs. But to envisage the process of production in this way is to ignore the crucial question of the social framework within which production takes place. For capital, its most vital need is to expand M into M′. As Marx says, this is like the law of Moses; should human needs be met in the process of the self-expansion of capital (as of course within limits they are) this is an incidental matter.

This sketch of Marx's concept of capital reveals, I believe, that he and Keynes approach the analysis of capitalism from quite distinct angles and with fundamentally opposed logics. For although Keynes and Marx both deal in aggregates (in this respect both stand opposed to the old neoclassical approach with its prime focus of interest being the individual), the nature of these aggregates is of a different order. Marx's principal concern is the total social capital (M–C–M′) and its subdivisions; Keynes's prime interest lies with effective demand and its chief components, investment and consumption.

If the examination of the capitalist process of production proceeds from the standpoint of Marx, it will be immediately evident that the size of the various revenues which in sum constitute the national income depends essentially upon the size of the total social capital and its rate of turnover in the production process. If, for instance, more capital is employed, if more money is transformed from money into commodities needed for production, more will, other things remaining equal, be advanced as variable capital; that is, as wages. In other words, it is the expansion of capital which increases the mass of labour power employed. The empiricist, because he merely records the 'facts' has no way of comprehending this process theoretically. The reverse of the real relationship could seem to hold: it could just as well be that if more money is spent on variable capital (wages) more capital will result. Indeed this is exactly how the matter does at first sight appear. 'It is these absolute movements of the accumulation of capital which are reflected as relative movements of the mass of exploitable labour-power, and therefore seem produced by the latter's own independent movement' (Marx 1961a: 620). And what is true of wages is true equally of all forms of income – profits, rent, interest, etc. The size of these revenues is limited (determined) by the accumulation of capital, and not the other way round. It is not the size of revenues that fixes the size of the total social capital but the latter which determines the former. To begin one's analysis with the conditions which determine the turnover of capital is to start from the inner determining source of the movement of the entire capitalist economy. This movement of social capital does of course reveal itself in the size and movement of the various forms of revenue. But to start with these revenues is to commence from a series of immediate, everyday phenomena as they present themselves on the surface of society. And this was just the central point of Marx's strictures against the school of vulgar economy, namely that it did start uncritically from the immediate economic relations as they appeared on the surface of society. There was no scrutiny of these phenomena to establish their origin, to demonstrate that their roots lay in the specific social relations of a definite economic system, capitalism. The procedure of the vulgar economist did, however, from the point of ideology, carry one advantage: it allowed all the revenues (wages, profits, interest) to be considered of the same status, as 'factor incomes' as they say.

To turn specifically to the case of Keynes: a fall in national income will, in the normal run of things, produce a drop in the level of employment; but this merely raises a deeper, more fundamental question: What brings about the initial fall in income? What is the inner (relatively hidden) source of this outer movement? It is this question which, says Marx, any serious analysis of capitalism and its crises must seek to answer. But it is a question which empiricism says does not admit of an answer – a search for the inner causes of phenomena is in the last resort deemed futile. According to Marx, the essence of capitalist crises, despite the many differing forms which such crises necessarily take, consists of a break in the conditions of capital turnover, a break in the circuit M–C–C′–M′. The movement of capital is the crucial thing from which all else derives and the laws, governing the movement of the aggregate capital are the fundamental laws of economics. That is why Marx held that confusion about the nature of capital must lead to confusion about all the other categories of the economy.

Revenue and capital

The point raised here, the angle from which an analysis of the capitalist economy should begin, is a matter which has continually concerned economics in the past. Let us take the case of Adam Smith. As is widely perceived, Smith held two contradictory theories of value. In places Smith holds to the idea that the value of a commodity is determined by one thing and one thing alone: the quantity of labour embodied in such a commodity. On many occasions, however, he proposed what Dobb and others have appropriately characterised as an adding-up theory of value in which the various forms of revenue (wages, profits, rent) were held, in their summation, to determine the value of the commodity. The conclusion of this latter conception of value is, as Marx puts it, 'that commodity value is composed of, or "resolves itself" into revenues of various kinds, so that the revenues do not consist of commodity values but the commodity values consist of "revenues"' (Marx 1957: 388). Here Marx is raising precisely the same fundamental question as that involved in a critique of Keynes: in the analysis of capitalism, does one begin from value and capital or from price and income (revenue)?

This duality in Smith constituted an unresolved contradiction in his theoretical work: on one hand the effort to discover the inner workings of the economy (here lay the truly classical element in his work), and on the other a mere registering or cataloguing of economic phenomena (here according to Marx are to be found the seeds of the vulgar strand in Smith). Marx attached considerable significance to Smith's confusion, of value and revenue.

> But it is this category of 'revenue' which is to blame for all the harmful confusion in Adam Smith. The various kinds of revenue form with him the 'component parts' of the annually produced, newly created commodity-value, while vice versa, the two parts into which this commodity value resolves itself *for the capitalist* – the equivalent of his variable capital advanced in the form of money when purchasing labour, and the other portion of the value, the surplus-value, which likewise belongs to him but did not cost him anything – form sources of revenue.
>
> (Marx 1957: 382)

And further:

> After starting by correctly defining the component parts of the value of the commodities and the sum of the value-product incorporated in them, and then demonstrating how these component parts form so many different sources of revenue, after thus deriving the revenues from the value, he proceeds in the opposite direction – and this remains the predominant conception with him – and turns the revenues into 'component parts' into '*original sources* of all exchangeable value', thereby throwing the doors wide open to vulgar economy.
>
> (Marx 1957: 372)

Again insisting that we must start from capital if we are to grasp the concept of revenue and determine its size, Marx says:

> If I determine the lengths of three straight lines independently, and then form out of these three lines as 'component parts' a fourth straight line equal to their sum, it is by no means the same procedure as when I have some given straight line before me and for some purpose divide it, 'resolve' it so to say, into three parts. In the first case the length of the line changes throughout with the lengths of the three lines whose sum it is; in the second case, the lengths of the three parts of the line are from the outset limited by the fact that they are parts of a line of given length.
>
> (Marx 1957: 383)

Keynes's key concepts

We have suggested that the departure points for the theoretical work of Marx and Keynes are of a diametrically opposed character: Marx insists that the crucial starting point for the examination of capitalism is the movement of capital, a movement which alone ultimately explains the nature and size of the various revenues or incomes in capitalist society. Keynes on the other hand starts his analysis from precisely this latter point, from income, or, to use his term, effective demand.

Keynes was concerned with one fundamental problem: the forms which determined the levels of investment and consumption. Now in the first place it is clear that these categories are not in any way unique or specific to capitalism. The consumption of wealth (as food, clothing, shelter) constitutes the material basis for life in all societies, whatever the specific conditions under which that wealth is produced and distributed. Similarly investment – the deployment of a portion of the current social wealth as a means of producing wealth in the future – is by no means an activity unique to capitalism but is present in all economies save the most primitive, where the low level of technique precludes the production of an economic surplus, at least on a regular and systematic basis. What we need to know is the specific form taken by that surplus and the manner in which it is extracted from those who produce it. Keynes here provides no answer, for the simple reason that such questions do not enter his horizon.

In this connection, many writers have drawn attention to a striking fact about Keynes's entire orientation: namely, that the aggregates of his system are not centrally concerned with the specific form taken by consumption and investment within capitalist economy. Thus one writer has said,

> One of the significant differences in the methodological character of the aggregate between Marx and Keynes lies in the direction in which *abstraction* is carried out. Marx's intention was to represent, as simply as possible, the specific interrelation of aggregates which is characteristic of capitalism, whereas Keynesian aggregates do not necessarily concern themselves with the specificity of capitalism. They are designed primarily to assist in accounting for the level of total employment under the simple assumption that it is proportional to the net national product.
>
> (Tsuru 1968: 193)

Marx does not commence his analysis from the standpoint of national income and its division but with the total social capital and its basic disaggregation into constant capital (equivalent to expenditure on machinery, raw materials), variable capital (equivalent to the wages bill) and surplus-value (in the form of profit, rent and interest).[7] Not only are these categories specific to capitalism but the contradictions which emerge between them are, according to Marx, an expression of a historically limited mode of production, capitalism. By comparison, the key concepts of *The General Theory* are abstract in the specific sense that they do not relate to the capitalist economic system as such. Keynes's theory is based on the proposition that three variables, the propensity to consume (consumption function), the inducement to invest (the marginal efficiency of capital) and the rate of interest (liquidity preference), in their interaction, determine the limits within which the national income fluctuates.

To take first the rate of interest: for Keynes this is determined by the quantity of money and 'liquidity preference'. (Liquidity preference Keynes defines as the 'natural' tendency of people to hold on to liquid assets in the absence of sufficient inducement – in the shape of interest – to relinquish this liquidity.) To understand the nature of liquidity preference it is necessary to know something of the 'psychological time preference' inherent in the propensity to consume. According to Keynes, each individual is confronted with two sets of time preferences on which he is obliged to act. First, the individual makes a decision about the proportion of his income to be spent now, and the proportion to be saved for future spending. Having decided the proportion to be saved, he must make a second decision: In what form are these savings to be held? As we know, Keynes proposed that there were three basic reasons for holding money, the speculative motive (the ability to take advantage of anticipated changes in prices) being the decisive one.

The rate of interest is the 'reward for parting with liquidity for a specified period', and is determined at the point where the desire to hold a certain amount of cash is just counterbalanced by the pull of the interest rate offered for that quantity of cash. Thus, as Keynes says, the interest rate is a 'highly psychological phenomenon' (Keynes 1936: 202). It is not a payment for waiting or for abstinence as with pre-Keynesian economics, but for not hoarding (Keynes 1936: 182), for parting with liquidity. Perhaps because Keynes became somewhat obsessed with the parasitic 'functionless investor', his theory ignores the fact that interest represents a return on money capital which is of the same general nature and origin as the return on all capital – in short, that interest is a segment of surplus-value. Keynes's theory, which proposes that interest is formed from forces quite independent of the production process, singularly fails to grasp this essential point. This is hardly surprising given that interest-bearing capital, where money seems to breed money, appears prima facie to be quite separate from the production process. As Marx puts it,

> Capital appears as a mysterious and self-creating source of interest – the source of its own increase ... the use-value of money ... becomes a property of money to generate value and yield interest, much as it is an attribute of pear-trees to bear pears.
>
> (Marx 1959: 384)

But economics did not always hold to the sort of fetishistic view of interest as proposed by Keynes. Adam Smith, for instance, says:

> It may be laid down as a maxim, that whenever a great deal can be made by the use of money, a great deal will commonly be given for the use of it; and that wherever little can be made by it, less will commonly be given for it. ... The progress of interest, therefore, may lead us to form some notion of the progress of profit.
>
> (Smith 1976: 105–106)

Interest, Smith implies, is merely part of the profit paid by the industrial capitalist to the money capitalist. Its limits are, therefore, fixed by the magnitude of profit. 'In any event, the average rate of profit is to be regarded as the ultimate determinant of the maximum limit of interest' (Marx 1959: 353). This position of Marx was also held by the best of the classical school for 'according to the Ricardians and all other economists worth naming, the rate of interest is determined by the rate of profit' (Marx 1972: 92).

It is for this reason, because profit and interest are both forms of one and the same category, namely surplus-value, that they normally move together in the same direction. The demand for liquidity only becomes a potent force in periods of acute economic crisis. The fact that the owners of capital as a whole wish suddenly to transform their capital from its commodity into its money form is itself a graphic expression of a serious rupture in the turnover of capital. According to

Keynes's liquidity preference theory, money assumes the form of a hoard and interest is the reward for not hoarding. In point of fact, however, the function of money as a hoard is but one of its several functions and all of them must be studied in their contradictory unity before we can group the real role of money within the capitalist economy.[8] For instance, one function of money, as everybody recognises, is as a means of payment. But this is a contradictory function, a fact by no means universally recognised. For when payments balance each other, money functions only nominally, as money of account, as measure of value. But when actual payments must be made, money no longer acts as a mere intermediary in the process of social metabolism but as the incarnation of wealth in the abstract, as the universal commodity. When, for whatever reason, there is a generalised disturbance in the developed system of payments, money ceases to play its hitherto merely nominal role as unit of account but now becomes the embodiment of social wealth as such. Previously the owners of capital had declared money to be an imaginary creation, and only commodities to constitute real value. Now, in times of sharp crisis, a different cry is heard and 'as the hart pants after fresh water, so pants the soul after money, the only wealth' (Marx 1961a: 138). It is thus in times of crises that the demand for money rises sharply and along with it the rate of interest which may now move quite out of line with the rate of profit. Thus:

> If we observe the cycles in which modem industry moves ... we shall find that a low rate of interest generally corresponds to periods of prosperity or extra profit, a rise in interest separates prosperity and its reverse, and a maximum of interest, up to the point of extreme usury corresponds to the period of crisis.
>
> (Marx 1959: 353)

And a little later Marx says:

> The rate of interest reaches its peak during crises, when money is borrowed at any cost to meet payments. Since a rise in interest implies a fall in the price of securities, this simultaneously offers a fine opportunity to people with available money-capital, to acquire at ridiculously low prices such interest-bearing securities as must, in the course of things, at least regain their average price as soon as the rate of interest falls again.
>
> (Marx 1959: 354)

In other words, it is in a crisis, when the rate of profit collapses, that the rate of interest may rise by leaps. It is under conditions of crisis that the rush for liquidity to meet obligations contracted during the phase of prosperity may become a controlling factor. As the pressure for liquidity becomes more generalised, a money famine may occur and bring about a sharp increase in interest rates as the price of other assets falls equally sharply. Many obligations cannot be met and a spate of bankruptcies ensues. It is under these conditions that the demand for liquidity for immediate means of payment becomes so pronounced that to the theoretically untrained eye it may seem to assume an entirely independent existence, such that it can be elevated into the determining cause of the crisis and not seen for what it is, as one of the symptoms of the crisis itself.

The last passage quoted from Marx is interesting in that it suggests that a theory of interest of the type proposed by Keynes took certain phenomena which emerge under conditions of crisis – when, by definition, all monetary and credit relations become violently disrupted – and generalised them into universal principles. As we have already pointed out, for Marx, interest is a return to money capital. It is, from this standpoint, of the same fundamental nature as the return on capital as a whole – it is the payment made out of surplus-value earned on the entire capital for the use of a particular portion of that capital. Loan capital depends for its reward on its being successfully employed in the sphere of production. Thus Marx says, 'Loaning money as capital – its alienation on condition of its being returned after a certain time – presupposes, therefore, that it will be actually employed as capital, and that it actually flows back to its starting point' (Marx 1959: 343). One entrepreneur (involved, let us suppose, in vehicle production) shares his total profit with another owner of capital (a banker, let us say) in return for a loan which is to be used with the aim of expanding his capital and surplus-value. Returning to the most general form of capital, depicted by the circuit M–C–C′–M′, an entrepreneur wishing to expand his capital must be prepared to do several things. First, he must part with his money capital, M. He must turn it into capital having a different form, C, by transforming it into labour power, materials and production equipment. Our entrepreneur must then put these various commodities through a process of production which will turn them into different commodities, C′ which can (hopefully) be sold for an equivalent sum of money, M′. Thus has M been 'metamorphosised' as Marx puts it.

Now this initial parting with liquidity occurs quite independently of the proclivities of the owner of capital. Only on condition that capital is initially transformed from M into C can it continue to exist. Marx took great care to stress that in this process capital should not be viewed one-sidedly, as either M or C: it was in point of fact the unity of both these forms, forms which continually passed into each other. Capital was 'value in motion'. The process of capital accumulation arises not from the inclinations or preferences of the owner of capital: its imperatives stem from the very nature of capital itself and it is precisely because of this that the laws of its accumulation impose themselves upon the individual capitalist, indeed upon the owners of capital as a whole.

On this point, Keynes takes a radically different view. For according to him, the willingness of the owner of money to part with it is at root a psychological matter, not a reflection of the intrinsic needs of capital itself. Here Keynes is quite wrong in that money is always thrown into circulation on definite conditions, ones which are in the final analysis rooted in the realisation of a definite rate of profit. Should such conditions not be met, should there be a sudden collapse in the profit rate, then not only will money capital cease to be committed to circulation but as we have already suggested, the exact opposite can well occur: there will be a general rush for liquidity which will serve both to aggravate the crisis and to force up the rate of interest. (Naturally, miscalculations can be made by the owners of capital as to future profit prospects and under the appropriate circumstances this can clearly aggravate the problems of capital as a whole. But such miscalculations cannot, of themselves, form the basis for an explanation of a crisis.)

In the Keynesian scheme of things the rate of interest and the money supply are abstracted from the process of capital turnover; that is, from the very process in which they alone originate. Keynes's standpoint is that of the isolated individual who, given certain dispositions, makes a series of decisions about how to hold his wealth. There is here no concrete analysis of how money functions specifically within the capitalist system, and this notwithstanding the fact that Keynes rejected the idea present in some versions of neoclassicism that money was merely a veil, having no independent role. For the money from which the turnover of capital commences in the schema M–C–C′–M′ is not money merely but money functioning as capital – in short, money capital. In other words it can be understood only from the point of view of a worked-out scientific conception of capital and it is just this which is lacking in Keynes. Further, the existence of money playing the role not of money but of capital obviously implies the existence of capitalism but also capitalism at a point in its evolution where a differentiation between the various forms of capital has occurred – industrial capital, money capital, commodity capital, etc. If these specific relations are kept in view then the question of liquidity and the rate of interest will be approached in a manner quite different from that of Keynes. Whereas for Keynes the decision whether to hold one's assets in liquid form depends on expectations about future price movements and the rate of interest, for Marx the investigation of whether the owner of money capital will actually commit such capital to production depends upon the prevailing conditions of production, and critically upon the conditions under which surplus-value is being extracted.

A final point in connection with the Keynesian theory of the rate of interest can be made. As we have already noted, for Keynes the rate of interest is determined by the psychology of creditors and by the lending policy of the banking system. To take this second factor, the amount of money in circulation: Here Keynes's theory is deceptive, confusing as it does the quantity of money and the amount of loan capital. But these two are by no means the same thing ('the mass of this loanable money-capital is different from, and independent of, the mass of circulating money' (Marx 1959: 488)). The former functions as capital, as a necessary initial phase in the circuit of capital. In the event of inflation, given a growth of paper money in excess of the requirements of commodity turnover and prices, an increase in the supply of loan capital which will occur as a result of a growth of temporarily free funds in the bank, will be counteracted by a depreciation of loan capital resulting from inflation. Consequently, in these circumstances there might be no increase in the real supply of loan capital. Here again is revealed the fact that the phenomena of capitalism cannot be judged on the basis of their immediate appearances but require real theoretical analysis if they are to be grasped.

Keynes and the falling rate of profit

In Marx's opinion, the tendency of the rate of profit to fall – a much discussed and disputed question amongst the classical economists – was the single most important law of political economy. This was so because it was understood that it was the rate of profit which effectively regulated the process of capital accumulation. In other words, profit was important not merely as one of several forms of income within the capitalist system but as the source from which the means for the further accumulation of capital could alone come. In commenting on Ricardo, Marx demonstrates the central importance which he attaches to the profit rate and its tendency to decline, a tendency which Ricardo had himself sensed, if not fully grasped:

> The rate of profit is the motive-power of capitalist production. Things are produced only so long as they can be produced with a profit. Hence the concern of the English economists over the decline in the rate of profit. The fact that the bare possibility of this happening should worry Ricardo, shows his profound understanding of the conditions of capitalist production ... What worries Ricardo is the fact that the rate of profit, the stimulating principle of capitalist production and driving force of accumulation, should be endangered by the development of production itself.
>
> (Marx 1959: 254)

The issue is also important in a consideration of the relationship between the economic theory of Keynes and that of Marx in so far as many writers have in the past likened Keynes's declining marginal efficiency of capital to Marx's theory of the tendency of the rate of profit to fall.[9]

Before dealing with Keynes's treatment of this matter, we can briefly set out, in somewhat formal terms, Marx's general notion of the falling rate of profit. Marx divides the total social capital into three broad categories: (1) constant capital (c), equivalent to expenditure on machinery, raw materials and heat, light and power. This capital was deemed constant in that it merely transfers the value embodied in it and cannot be the source of new value. (2) variable capital (v), the expenditure by capital on the purchase of labour power, variable because it is the only source for the expansion of value. (3) surplus-value (s), the increment in value accruing to the owners of capital. The rate of profit is given by surplus-value over total capital: $s/c + v$. Now as capital accumulates, there is a tendency for the constant capital to grow more rapidly than the variable portion of capital: this is the expression in value terms of the improvements in technology associated with capitalism throughout its history. The relatively rapid increase in constant capital as compared with the variable element of capital Marx refers to as the tendency for the organic composition of capital (c/v) to rise. Although an increase in the organic composition of capital will normally produce an increase in the rate of surplus-value (s/v), or at least its mass (s), there are definite objective limits to such an increase, not least amongst them the actual physical limit to available working-time. But unless s/v does rise with sufficient rapidity to compensate for the increasing organic composition (c/v), then the tendency for the rate of profit to fall will assert itself in an actual fall.

This is the simplest possible outline of what is in reality a complex law, an outline which ignores both those many counteracting forces to its operation to which Marx drew attention, as well as to the long-standing disputes amongst Marxists about its proper interpretation. But the point to be stressed here is that, as far as Marx is concerned, the tendency for the rate of profit to decline was a product of forces intrinsic to capital. The essential quality of capital is that it is driven to expand and one result of this was the tendency for the rate of profit to fall. Now Keynes, no doubt in an effort to sharpen the impact of his own work, tried to create the impression that all orthodox writers throughout the nineteenth century had subscribed to the notion of a crisis-free capitalism. This was far from being the case; but what did characterise virtually all discussions of the problems associated with capital accumulation was that they were almost invariably seen as being located in disturbances emanating outside the actual social relations of capitalism. (Such was the case with Jevons' celebrated 'sunspot' theory of the trade cycle.)

Bearing this point in mind, we can consider Keynes's treatment of the movement of the marginal efficiency of capital. By capital Keynes means a thing, a 'capital asset' that yields an income. In interpreting capital as a series of assets that produce income, Keynes distinguishes two of its principal forms: 'instrumental capital' (a materialised form of capital engaged in the process of production, as in the case of a machine) and 'consumption capital' (a material form of capital operating in the sphere of consumption, like, for example, a house) (Keynes 1936: 226). If we apply this definition to production, it would mean that by capital we have only means of production, that is, employing Marx's term, constant capital, and not the whole of capital which comprises both constant and variable elements. But in any event, the train of Keynes's overall argument indicates that by capital he means only its materialised elements, that is the means of production (a view shared by his radical followers, notably Joan Robinson). So it turns out that the marginal efficiency of capital is not to be equated with the Marxian rate of profit, as many appeared in the past to have assumed, since here profit is taken only in connection with constant capital rather than with the whole of capital.

According to Keynes's theory, any investment which is as yet unutilised will be carried out on one condition, that the anticipated rate of return over the cost of investment exceeds the rate of interest. Given that entrepreneurs aim at profit-maximisation, new investment will be carried on to the point at which the marginal efficiency of capital is equal to the interest rate. The marginal efficiency is determined by two factors: (a) the expected return from an income-yielding asset, and (b) the supply price, or replacement cost of the asset which is the source of that prospective yield. Such a yield takes the form of a flow of income over a period of time, a series of annuities over the anticipated life of the investment; if this stream of yields is then compared with the cost of supplying the assets necessary to produce these yields we have the marginal efficiency of capital, defined by Keynes thus:

> More precisely, I define the marginal efficiency of capital as being equal to the rate of discount which would make the present value of the series of annuities given by the returns expected from the capital asset during its life just equal to the supply price.
>
> (Keynes 1936: 135)

The prospective yields on an asset are undoubtedly for Keynes the key element in determining the marginal efficiency of capital. They are prospective rather than actual because at the moment the investment takes place they are nothing but expectations on the part of the investor. Because of the nature of capital assets, especially those of a long-term durable type, large immediate outlays are required before any returns are available to the investor. In Keynes's view capital assets are a link between the known present and an uncertain future.

Now why should the marginal efficiency of capital decline in the long run? Because, ran Keynes's argument, as more capital is invested it becomes more abundant (less scarce) and therefore produces a lower yield. Subscribing to the scarcity theory of capital, Keynes argues that the returns from capital assets exceed their supply price only because they are scarce (Keynes 1936: 213). Every increase in investment brings an increase in output which competes with the output of existing capital. The growing volume of output tends to lower prices and hence to lower too the expected yields from future plant capacity. Keynes of course argued that if the interest rate was kept below the (declining) marginal efficiency of capital schedule then investment could continue unchecked. With ongoing investment, capital would at a certain point cease to be scarce and its return, or marginal efficiency, would then be reduced to zero, a prospect which might be realised within the space of one generation, Keynes felt. (Quite how capitalism could function with a zero rate of return to capital can only remain a sheer mystery from the point of view of the Marxist understanding of such a system. Keynes was in effect proposing the existence of capital without the existence of profit, not a very tolerable state of affairs for the owners of capital one might think!)

A familiarity with the history of economic theory reveals that in Keynes's explanation for a secular decline in the marginal efficiency of capital is to be found more than an echo of Adam Smith's theory of the falling rate of profit advanced some 150 years earlier. For it was Smith, following David Hume on this point, who sought to explain the decline in the rate of profit as a result of increasing competition amongst capitals consequent upon accumulation. In *The Wealth of Nations* Smith says:

> The increase of stock, which raises wages, tends to lower profit. When the stocks of many rich merchants are turned into the same trade, their mutual competition naturally tends to lower its profit; and when there is a like

> increase of stock in all the different trades carried on in the same society, the same competition must produce the same effect in them all.
>
> (Smith 1976: 105)

And speaking of the decline of profits in the towns, Smith says

> The stock accumulated in them comes in time to be so great, that it can no longer be employed with the antient profit in that species of industry which is peculiar to them. That industry has its limits like every other; and the increase of stock, by increasing the competition, necessarily reduces the profit.
>
> (Smith 1976: 144–145)

Marx rejected such explanations for the decline in the rate of profit which were centred on competition. We can assume that the 'forces of competition' fix the rate of profit at 15 per cent, but the question still remains: Why is this figure 15 per cent? Why not 150 per cent? To ascribe the determination of the rate of profit to competition was, Marx held, to indulge in supply and demand explanations which left unexplored those forces which lay behind supply and demand. It led to a circular argument: the 'forces of competition' determined the rate of profit while at the same time the intensity of this competition was measured by precisely the self-same rate of profit. Naturally nobody denies the palpable fact of competition between capitals; Marx's point however was that this competition is merely the external, outer form in which the inner contradictions of capital expressed themselves. Competition is the realm in which the laws of capital are executed, but such laws are not *generated* in this sphere.

Keynes's explanation of the decline in the rate of profit, despite the fact that it is decked out in what superficially appears to be a new terminology, in the last resort rested upon the old neoclassical law of diminishing returns. Marx poured scorn on this 'law', first formulated in a clear manner by the eighteenth-century economist, Turgot, as being nothing more than a tautology, based on static assumptions, and in this respect little different from the Malthusian 'theory' of population which was also implicitly founded on the assumption of a static technology.

Keynes's theory of the marginal efficiency of capital was a law which purported to deal with a fundamental secular trend in capitalist economy, an economy characterised by just those forces from which the law abstracts, namely a tendency constantly to revolutionise the techniques of production. It is for this reason that Keynes has been attacked on the lack of realism attaching to this aspect of his theory, a criticism by no means confined to those sympathetic to Marxism. As Schumpeter (1952: 283), for instance, rightly pointed out about Keynes's theoretical devices: 'All the phenomena incident to the creation and change in this apparatus [industry], that is to say, the phenomena that dominate the capitalist process, are thus excluded from consideration.'

This quite artificial assumption of a 'given' technology has direct consequences for the Keynesian multiplier theory. This theory deals with the fact that consumption grows as a result of the expansion of production. The growth of Department I production (that producing means of production) actually creates an additional demand for machinery, raw materials, etc. as well as for the means of consumption of workers employed in this department. This in turn implies a growth of output in the other department – Department II, producing means of consumption. But the more rapid growth of the production of means of production signifies the growth of the productive power of social labour and is merely another way of expressing the fact that the organic composition of capital (the ratio of constant to variable capital) is increasing. An increase in the organic composition of capital finds expression in the relative, and in certain cases the absolute, decline in the demand for labour power. The accumulation of capital means the expansion of production on a new, higher level of technology. And this growth in the relative weight of constant as against variable capital will take place in both departments of the economy. The results of this increase in the organic composition depend upon the precise nature of the rise, but one thing does follow: although the accumulation of capital (for the Keynesian, an increase in investment) may bring about an absolute increase in the numbers employed, it will cause a relative lowering of employment. Consequently there is no precise relationship between an increase in investment and an increase in employment; although it might be possible to obtain such a relationship for previous investment, it is one disrupted every time new investment takes place in so far as such investment almost invariably takes place at a new, higher level of productive technique. So here again Keynesianism abstracts from the features specific to capitalism, namely that the development of the productive forces takes the form of a rising organic composition of capital and that production does, in the final analysis, depend on the level of consumption.

There is one final consequence of Keynes's assumption of a given technology which is worthy of note: namely, that it cannot offer any adequate explanation for the cyclical movement of the rate of profit. If, as capital accumulates and it becomes 'less scarce' such that its marginal efficiency declines, then the rate of profit can move in one direction only: downwards. It implies that the fundamental problem of capitalism is one not of the cyclical alteration of booms and slumps but of stagnation and steady decline, as we have noted, precisely the direction in which a number of Keynes's followers, such as Alvin Hansen (1951) in the United States, did indeed interpret his work. Here again it must be emphasised that Marx's view was of a quite different order. For despite interpretations to the contrary, there is no element of mechanicalism in his conception of the tendency of the rate of profit to fall. Precisely because this law reflected the clash of both objective and subjective factors (which latter included the strength of the working class, its degree of consciousness, the quality of its leadership, etc.), its empirical unfolding could never be known in advance. Capital makes continual efforts to overcome the effects of the operation of this law, but in so doing only raises ever greater obstacles to the smooth, crisis-free expansion of the productive forces: such is the contradictory nature of the capitalist system:

'Capitalist production seeks continually to overcome these immanent barriers, but it overcomes them only by means which again place these barriers in its way and on a more formidable scale' (Marx 1959: 245).

Keynes on consumption

We can consider briefly the final component of Keynes's system, namely consumption. Here again the overall tendency of his work, to abstract from the social relations specific to capitalism, is all too evident. (It is noteworthy that orthodoxy on the whole deals with 'the consumer' as one of the central actors, if not the central actor, on the economic stage. Naturally, such a person is an empty abstraction, torn from all social and class relations. The fact that 'everybody is a consumer' is a proposition which serves to hide the antagonistic divisions which characterise capitalist society.)

Keynes's propositions about consumption have already been mentioned, are well known, and thus require no more than a brief outline. First, he held that because of the existence of the marginal propensity to consume – according to Keynes a fundamental psychological law – the gap between income and consumption would grow, and unless this gap was appropriately bridged the level of income would fall below that needed to sustain full employment. Various measures were available to raise the level of income including a certain degree of income redistribution, although Keynes was careful to insist that this should be of only 'moderately conservative' proportions.

For Keynes 'consumption' is the consumption of all individuals in society, each individual being subject to the basic psychological law which he believed determined the relationship between income and consumption. This is far from being Marx's approach. He drew a distinction between individual consumption on the one hand and industrial consumption on the other. An analogous distinction is that between buyer and consumer. The buyer for Marx is someone who uses up something for his own needs whereas the act of consumption involves using up something in the process of labour. The purchases carried out by the majority of the population within capitalist economy excludes the greater part of the commodities produced in such an economy. For workers buy no instruments of labour, no raw materials; they buy only articles of subsistence, that is, commodities which enter into individual as opposed to 'productive' consumption. Marx explains the significance of this point when he says:

> This also shows the ambiguity of the word consumer and how wrong it is to identify it with the word buyer. As regards industrial consumption, it is precisely the workers who consume machinery and raw materials, using them up in the labour-process. But they do not use them up for themselves and they are therefore not *buyers* of them. Machinery and raw material are for them neither use-values nor commodities, but objective conditions of a process of which they themselves are the subjective conditions.
>
> (Marx 1969: 518)

Marx is here in effect insisting that it is not possible to deal with the level of consumption in the abstract, a-socially, explaining it by reference to a supposed universal psychological disposition on the part of each separate individual. Within the capitalist system consumption takes place always within definite economic (class) relations and it is only by starting with these quite objective relations that the real nature of consumption and its limits can be analysed. As far as the capitalist system is concerned the essential features of these economic relations, as they affect consumption, are (1) the majority of the producers (the working class) are non-consumers (non-buyers in Marx' terminology) of the greater part of their products, namely the means of production and raw materials, and (2) the majority of producers can consume the equivalent of their product on one condition: that they create surplus-value. In short, the level of consumption of the working class cannot be deemed to be determined by the psychological proclivities of a large number of disparate individuals, but by the amount of variable capital (the equivalent to the wage bill) which in turn depends upon the rate of capital accumulation. If this is so then we have but a further illustration of the fact that it is impossible to understand any aspect of capitalist economy unless one starts from the nature of capital and its turnover.

Once again on the nature of capital: the case of Joan Robinson

We have deliberately concentrated on the conflicting conceptions of capital in the work of Marx and Keynes. This we have done, given that the problem of the essence of capital affects the innermost nature of the production of wealth in contemporary society. We have suggested that Keynes's treatment of capital is amongst other things characterised by a desire to divorce it from its real relation to production: 'It is much preferable to speak of capital as having a yield over the course of its life in excess of its original cost, than as being productive' (Keynes 1936: 213). So says Keynes, thus in effect reducing the matter to one of semantics only. His sole concern is not with the source of the 'yield from capital' but the grounds on which an asset as capital brings a yield in excess of its 'supply price'. As we know he finds these grounds in the scarcity of such assets.

This chapter has spoken of the decisive importance for Marxists of a theoretically sound critique of Keynes, given the efforts of a number of writers to construct a bridge between Marx and Keynes (albeit a suitably interpreted Keynes). Joan Robinson has here been the decisive figure for such attempts. It goes without saying that Robinson for long occupied a central position in the economic theory of the twentieth century. A member of the famous 'Cambridge Circus' which helped Keynes formulate the ideas which produced *The General Theory*, she has been a leading defender of the Keynes tradition in the years after his death, against both his 'friends' as well as his declared enemies. No Marxist, she has nevertheless always claimed considerable sympathy for the ideas of Marx. Politically, throughout the post-war years she identified herself with a number of radical causes. Given these several facets to her work, her views are of considerable interest in the context of the issues raised in this chapter. She has of course also been in the vanguard of those criticising some of the cherished propositions of neoclassical economics, particularly those which deal with the alleged 'productivity' of capital. We have not been concerned here with the nature of these criticisms as such. They stem essentially from the work of Sraffa, first begun in the 1920s. The Cambridge school has persistently drawn attention to those problems which orthodox neoclassical theory has encountered in connection with the theory of capital [see Sraffa 1960 – ed.]. They can be summarised as follows. This theory contains no prerequisites for aggregating capital goods, that is for discovering the true basis that unites things to form capital and determine its size. Second, in any theory linking the origin and returns on capital with the matter of time a vicious circle ensues: the size of capital is determined by capitalising future revenues, but to establish this method a rate of interest is required; this is however a magnitude the size of which depends upon the amount of capital. This is the nub of the criticisms of orthodox theory made by those in the Sraffa school. (For Marxists it can be said that these problems are the reflection of a decisive confusion, one involving the lumping together of the socio-historical substance of capital with its material form, and in particular one that entails the confusion of 'capital' with 'means of production'. This confusion persists throughout Keynes's work.)

Now the question is: has the Cambridge school really got to the bottom of the issue in their criticisms of the neoclassical notion of capital? Joan Robinson outlines her idea of the problem of the productivity of capital when she says:

> Whether we choose to say that capital is productive or that capital is necessary to make labour productive, is not a matter of much importance [here, as with Keynes, the matter is reduced to that of a purely semantic problem – G.P.]...
>
> Indeed, a language that compels us to say that capital (as opposed to the ownership of capital) is not productive rather obscures the issue. It is more cogent to say that capital, and the application of science to industry, are immensely productive, and that the institutions of private property, developing into monopoly, are deleterious precisely because they prevent us from having as much capital, and the kind of capital, that we need.
>
> (Robinson 1942: 21–22)

Now, unless one takes the view that, like value, capital is 'just a name' the issue as to whether capital is productive, and if so in what precise sense, is by no means a matter of word definitions, but a central, indeed the central question for economic theory. This is demonstrated by amongst other things the history of economics, which has been forced continually to grapple with the mystery presented by capital.[10]

It follows from the standpoint of Marx's theory of capitalism that only labour (more precisely abstract labour) creates value. But it is by no means a consequence of this view that in the opinion of Marxism the 'objective factors of production' (machines, etc.) are to be denied any form of 'productivity', as Robinson (1960a: 19) suggests ('Thus Marx's refusal to treat capital as a factor of production seems well founded.') Quite the opposite is the case: to the extent that such factors raise the level of labour productivity they most certainly contribute to the production of wealth, that is to use-values. The word 'productivity' however here carries two distinct meanings. First, it can be used to denote the production of use-values; it can also indicate that definite social relations are being produced and reproduced. When Marx stressed that capital is productive he did so from a definite angle: as the predominant social relation of capitalist society. And its productivity is from this standpoint quite specific: it is productive of surplus labour which takes the form of interest, profit, etc. And capital was in a position to extract such labour not at all because it involved 'waiting' because 'risk' was involved, was 'scarce', functioned as a 'means of production' or furthered the 'application of science to industry' (Robinson 1942: 22). Capital is productive precisely because it was an essential historical relation for the extraction of surplus labour and far more 'productive' in this sense than was feudalism or any other pre-capitalist form of economy. A steam engine in a mine is productive of use-values (or rather the labour materialised in such an engine is productive) but this has nothing whatsoever to do with its being capital. It would be equally productive of wealth were it owned by the workers at the mine rather than the entrepreneur. We are dealing here not at all with a matter of words but with a central question: Do we derive the meaning of the word productivity from the relations of man to nature or from the relations of man to man? In other words is there a distinction to be made between productivity in the abstract and something which is productive specifically for capital? In Marx's opinion not only is there a distinction here but a profound and ever-deepening contradiction: that which is productive for human beings (particularly the working class and other oppressed people) is increasingly positively unproductive (unprofitable) for capital.[11] (Robinson's distinction between capital and the ownership of capital confuses precisely the essence of the matter: that capital being a social relation cannot exist apart from definite relationships of ownership. Like those utopian socialists of the nineteenth century criticised by Marx, she wants to get rid of the capitalists while retaining capital. But of course to eliminate the one is necessarily to eliminate the other.) When Keynes advanced his scarcity theory of the return to capital he was clearly 'explaining' its productivity from the former point of view; that is, from the point of view of the relationship of man to nature: capital is productive because it exists in only limited quantity, just as land yields a rent because it is 'scarce'. And so with Robinson who conflates capital with 'the application of science to industry', a purely natural phenomena.[12]

The concept of equilibrium

One persistent theme amongst many of the radical Keynesians is their hostility to the notion of equilibrium. Now one thing Marx and Keynes certainly shared in common was their rejection of Say's law, the notion that capitalism was an automatically self-equilibrating economic system. But their agreement on this point in fact hides more than it tells us because the grounds on which Marx opposed Say were fundamentally different from those of Keynes. We have suggested that in his characterisation of the development of nineteenth-century economic thought, Keynes attached far too much weight to Say's law of markets. Indeed, as we have noted, in his redefinition of classical economics, Keynes went so far as to make the acceptance of Say's law the distinguishing criterion for membership of that school, a solecism which enabled him to include not only Ricardo (for Marx the last of the classical economists) but all those who followed Ricardo down to and including Keynes's contemporary, Pigou.

There is no doubt that the widespread support given to Say's contention that disequilibrium within capitalist economy is in principle impossible was a significant expression of the increasingly apologetic nature of nineteenth-century economics, as well as a reflection on the part of sections of the middle class for social peace and stability. But it does not follow from this that the denial of any long-run disequilibrium within bourgeois economy marked the real essence of the vulgar school of which Say is the true father. Nor does it follow either that the rejection of the notion of equilibrium, after the fashion of post-Keynesianism, constitutes a sound basis either for the criticism of neoclassical economics or for the establishment of a theory which grasps the real movement of capitalism. We have argued that the degeneration of classical economics resided not in its acceptance of Say's law (Ricardo had, after all, accepted Say's proposition in opposition to Malthus)[13] but arose from a deeper, more universal source: in the conscious removal of a consideration of the social relations of production from the province of economics. It was this turn away from an analysis of the (antagonistic) relations of bourgeois economy, a justification of the capitalist system as one based on a natural and eternal harmony of interests, that transformed the science of political economy into the ideology of the vulgar school. In this respect Keynes was far from justified in lumping together Say and Ricardo on the grounds that they shared a common belief in the inherently stable nature of capitalist production, however convenient this device might have been for the pedagogic purposes of *The General Theory*.

We have attempted to demonstrate that at the level of his basic categories Keynes adopted the standpoint of the vulgar school which started its analysis not from the objective social relations of capitalist economy but from the immediate reflection of those laws in the consciousness of the participants in bourgeois production. Thus when Marx criticised Say's assertion that capitalism assured the conditions for equilibrium, and automatically so, Marx pointed out that Say was able to reach this (false) conclusion only by ignoring precisely those features which were specific to capitalism. Concretely, when Say proposed that 'supply creates its own demand' (Marx called this 'childish babbling' and 'unworthy' of Ricardo when he repeated it) he had in fact assumed the conditions not of capitalist production but of elementary barter. 'The conception ... adopted by Ricardo from the tedious Say,... that *overproduction* is not possible, or at least that no *general glut of the market* is possible, is based on the proposition that *products* are exchanged *against* products' (Marx 1969: 493).

Marx objected to Say's proposition – that supply and demand would always exist in a state of equilibrium – because it was an empty tautology, emptied, that is, of any social and historical content. Naturally the categories of supply and demand exist within capitalist economy, just as the categories which are the basis of Keynes's system (investment, consumption, savings, etc.) certainly exist in an empirical sense. But in order to analyse concretely supply and demand within such an economy one had to understand that the production of wealth takes on a specific social form – the production of commodities for the market, and that the supply and demand for commodities was shaped by the feature which dominates in this economy – its division into the two great classes, one which monopolises the means of production and another dependent entirely on the sale of its labour power. In connection with commodity production, a commodity, as something meeting a specific human need is a use-value; but at the same time it has a definite exchange-value, signifying the fact that it constituted a proportion of total social labour. Marx objected to Say's empty proposition because in effect it obscured the contradictory nature of all wealth produced within the capitalist economy.

The gist of Marx's argument on this point runs as follows. Let us take the case of a manufacturer supplying steel. He supplies in a given period of time an amount of steel of a definite use-value; say ten tons of the metal of a certain quality. At the same time he supplies steel of a specific exchange-value, signified by its price, £500. But between these two sides of the commodity there is a profound difference which formal thought obscures. For on the one hand the manufacturer places steel with a definite use-value on the market which, because of its physical characteristics, is capable of supplying definite needs. At the same time the exchange-value of this steel exists only ideally in the shape of a price for the steel which has still to be realised. The seller of the steel is interested in one thing and one thing alone: the exchange-value of his steel. He supplies a use-value but he is concerned only with the exchange-value he will thereby obtain (in money). It is, of course, quite possible for the exchange-value of the steel to be expressed in quite different quantities of the metal and indeed this will be the case when there are changes in the productivity of labour in steel-making. The supply of the use-value and the supply of the exchange-value to be realised are thus by no means identical, since quite different quantities of use-value can be represented in the same quantity of exchange-value. And just because the exchange-value of the steel supplied, but yet to be realised, and the quantity of steel do not coincide, there can be no grounds, a priori, for assuming that there will be no contradiction between these two polar opposites.

The point here is that Marx did not object to Say because he employed the notion of equilibrium as such but because in the proposition that supply and demand always necessarily balance the specific social relations lying behind these abstractions were not considered and nor therefore was the possibility of a contradiction arising between them. Say, in short, reached his conclusions on the basis of empty, purely formal abstractions.

> It must never be forgotten, that in capitalist production what matters is not the immediate use-value but the exchange-value and, in particular, the expansion of surplus-value. This is the driving motive of capitalist production, and it is a pretty conception that – in order to reason away the contradictions of capitalist production – abstracts from its very basis and depicts it as a production aiming at the direct satisfaction of the producers.
>
> (Marx 1969: 495)

And further:

> ...since the circulation process of capital is not completed in one day but extends over a fairly long period until the capital returns to its original form, since this period coincides with the period within which market-prices equalise with cost prices, and great upheavals and changes take place in the *market* in the course of this period, since great changes take place in the productivity of labour and therefore also in the *real value* of commodities, it is quite clear, that between the starting point, the prerequisite capital, and the time of its return at the end of one of these periods, great catastrophes must occur and elements of crisis must have gathered and develop, and these cannot in any way be dismissed by the pitiful proposition that products exchange for products. The *comparison* of value in one period with the value of the same commodities in a later period is no scholastic illusion ... but rather forms the fundamental principle of the circulation process of capital.
>
> (Marx 1969: 495)

An analysis of capital must take not only the specific social relations of this mode of production into account but must grasp its movement as a whole – in all its interconnected and contradictory moments. The essence of eclecticism is to take bits and pieces from what is a unified process and combine them into a series of empty abstractions. However flexible this may appear to be, however seemingly 'undogmatic' such eclecticism seems to the untrained mind, Marx rightly insists upon a different method: in this instance one that aims to grasp capital as a whole in the course of its real development. And if this is the aim of science it becomes impossible to separate out the moments of equilibrium from those of disequilibrium in any absolute sense; this is so because the conditions for the equilibrium of bourgeois economy grow out of the conditions of its disequilibrium, and vice versa. Here the formal method of economics is quite lost. During the period of boom the vulgar eye is directed exclusively to those indices – production figures, growth of trade, expansion of investment – which mirror only the surface outward forms of the capitalist economy. Such empirical 'facts' can be compared in any number of ways, and many economists spend their time doing little but just this. In a slump all such indicators tend to be transformed into their opposite. Again, following the prescription of positivism, the indicators can once more be compared in an effort to explain the transformation. But because bourgeois economics does not penetrate beneath the surface of immediate economic 'data' (declaring such efforts to be impossible or to involve 'metaphysics') this transformation, while it may be recorded empirically, can never be understood theoretically. To understand any phenomena theoretically, scientific concepts are essential. And just because these are lacking in orthodox economics, neither the periods of upswing nor the periods of slump which grow organically out of boom conditions can ever be comprehended.[14]

Marx's analysis of the production of individual capitals could perhaps give rise to the false impression that the sole object of capitalist production – the creation of value and above all the creation of surplus-value – is one in which the role of use-values can be left out of account. When Marx comes to study the production and reproduction of social capital, that is capital considered as a whole, this is shown not to be the case, for it transpires that this production of value and surplus-value is indeed constrained by a barrier which was not taken into consideration in the earlier analysis, namely the barrier constituted by use-value on a social scale. In order to reproduce its capital, society must not only have a total fund of value available but it has to find these values ready to hand in a particular useful form; that is, in definite material shape (as machines, raw materials, means of subsistence, etc.). And all these various things must present themselves in proportions determined by the technical requirements of production, proportions which, because methods of production are undergoing continual change, must alter over time.

At the same time, however, Marx's basic proposition – that capitalism is a system founded on the production and reproduction of surplus-value, and a process in which the satisfaction of human needs is an entirely incidental matter – still holds. That is to say, human needs are only met to the degree that satisfying them is a means to the accumulation of surplus-value. It is this ever-present growing and developing contradiction between use-value and exchange-value which lies at the heart of the contradictions of capitalism.

Marx in no way denies the possibility of a solution to this contradiction. But it is the nature of this solution which must be carefully considered.[15] The 'Reproduction Schemes' of volume II of *Capital* provide the key to grasping this contradiction and manner in which capitalism deals with it. Marx divides social production into two large departments, that producing means of consumption for both the basic classes (Department II), and that producing means of production out of which the existing stock of capital is replaced and extended (Department I). Marx shows how each department is obliged to work for the other, thus establishing a series of complex reciprocal relationships between them. Each department can replace its necessary elements of production only on condition that it obtains a fraction of these elements from the other department and in a suitable material form. On the other hand, each department only comes into possession of the use-values it needs if it obtains them from the other department by means of the exchange of equivalent values. In these schemata of reproduction, Marx aims to establish not only the manner in which all the components of the annual value product of society ($c+v+s$) mutually replace each other. For he also demonstrates how a proportion of the total surplus-value produced can be devoted to the further expansion of capitalist production, which naturally presupposes the regular exchange of these value components and their realisation on the market. In this sense the schemes of reproduction in *Capital* are an aspect of Marx's solution to the realisation problem.

It should be noted that this division of the capitalist economy into two basic sections was for Marx no arbitrary one. The product of Department I is, in physical terms, machinery and equipment, materials of various kinds such as fuel and electricity which are consumed productively. The products of Department II (food, clothing, housing) can only be used for personal, non-productive consumption. Marx's central aim, following the example of Quesnay, was to portray the many individual acts of circulation which appear on the surface of society in their characteristic movement, that is in the light of 'the circulation between the great functionally determined economic classes of society' (Marx 1957: 359). Here Marx's distinction between productive consumption and personal consumption is of a quite different nature from the consumption/investment distinction of Keynes. Whereas Marx's analytical separation is in the last resort a reflection of the basic class division of society, that of Keynes is devoid of real social content in that for him the distinction between consumption and investment is confined essentially to the question of time.

As we have already indicated, a number of economists – James Mill, Ricardo and Say amongst them – in fact 'solved' this problem of the relationship of production to consumption, but only in a superficial manner. They did so by confusing capitalist production (M–C–M′) with simple commodity production (C–M–C) and the latter with barter (C–C).

Any act of production, according to this view, creates its own demand, and since, in the last analysis, products are by definition exchanged for products there is an automatic equilibrium of sellers and buyers. But it is a conclusion established not through an investigation of the actual processes of production and circulation in capitalist economy but one arrived at through arbitrary and quite unrealistic assumptions. If the assumptions proposed by Say are accepted the only source of capitalist breakdown will occur if, for whatever reasons, commodities are not produced in the right proportions. In other words, the crisis of capitalism would be one of disproportionality.

Sismondi took a diametrically opposed position on the question of equilibrium within the capitalist economy. Unlike the English classical economists he regarded the commodities appearing on the market not merely as the products of labour but as the products of capital. He believed that capital is able to generate an increase in value; that is, create the conditions for its own self-expansion, because the owner of capital does not pay the full production costs and essentially because he gives the worker an insufficient wage in return for his labour. For him it is precisely this increase in value which provides the source for the accumulation of capital. But then the question must arise: How can the surplus product be sold if the worker who has produced it cannot buy back the portion of the product corresponding to his labour, and if the capitalists themselves do not consume this surplus product (a proposition which follows if a part of it has been capitalised)? Sismondi regarded this as creating an insurmountable problem. He believed that in the final analysis the realisation of surplus product was impossible, unless, that is, it was disposed of, and thus realised, abroad.

Marx rejected both Malthus' and Sismondi's 'solutions' as being equally one-sided and therefore ultimately false. He did not wish to deny that the realisation of surplus-value was a real problem for the capitalist economy. He did however reject Sismondi's doubts as to the possibility of realisation under capitalism. According to Marx, capitalist production does in fact create its own market and in this way it is able to 'solve' the problem of the realisation of surplus-value. But it does so not in a metaphysical manner (by abolishing the problem) but in a truly dialectical sense. It solves it, that is to say, by raising this problem to an ever higher and wider – in short, more universal – level. Or, to be more concrete, the realisation problem is resolved only to the extent that the capitalist mode of production advances, only to the extent that it constantly expands its internal and external markets. In this regard, extended reproduction of capital is neither purely impossible, nor can it proceed forever, uninterruptedly, without breaks, without discontinuities, as the classical economists imagined to be the case. Capitalism 'solves' the problem of realisation by taking its internal contradictions to an ever higher level, by continually producing and reproducing them on an ever wider basis until the point where they engulf the whole of society and create the possibilities for the transition to socialism.

For Marx, phases of expansion and of relative equilibrium lead inexorably to their opposites and it is through the form of crises that the contradictions accumulated during the phase of expansion are finally and violently resolved by means of a destruction of capital; this serves to bring the total social capital once more into an appropriate relationship with the total pool of surplus-value. Speaking of the many influences which are at work during the period of expansion, Marx says:

> These different influences may at one time operate predominantly side by side in space, and at another succeed each other in time. From time to time the conflict of antagonistic agencies finds vent in crises. The crises are always but momentary and forcible solutions of the existing contradictions. They are violent eruptions which for a time restore the disturbed equilibrium.
>
> (Marx 1959: 244)

It is clear that Marx objected to the notion of equilibrium advanced by Say. But one should not conclude from this that such a concept has no place in his analysis. He certainly criticised Say and other economists for having abstracted the notion of equilibrium from the social relations which constitute the real foundation of capitalist economy. This allowed the apologists to make this category absolute. And they were thereby able to declare that equilibrium was a 'natural', 'normal' condition while movement away from it was but a temporary, passing aberration.

But, we stress, this should not lead us to the conclusion that Marx excludes the concept of equilibrium from his work. Let us consider this from the point of view of the law of value. If we assume that two products of labour exchange at their labour value we assume an equilibrium exists between the two given branches of production. Changes in the labour value of a product destroy this equilibrium and cause a transfer of labour from one branch of production to another, thereby bringing about consequent redistribution of the forces of production in the economy. It is changes in the productive powers of labour which cause changes in the amount of labour needed for the production of given commodities, setting in motion corresponding increases or decreases in the value of commodities.

The above mechanism Marx sees as an expression of the functioning of petty commodity production. Under the conditions of capitalist production the process through which equilibrium is simultaneously shattered and established is of a different, higher order. Under capitalism the organisation of production no longer resides in the hands of individual, petty producers, but is now organised by industrial capitalists. Capitalists invest their capital in the sphere of production which is most profitable. The transfer of capital to a given sphere of production creates increased demand for labour power in that particular branch of the economy. As a result, assuming other things to be equal, this brings about an increased price of labour power (wages). This draws living labour into this expanding sector. The distribution of the productive forces amongst the various spheres of the economy and the establishment of conditions of relative equilibrium between them takes the form of the distribution of capitals amongst them. It is the movement of capital, the decisive element of bourgeois production, which is the source of stabilisation and destabilisation alike. Wage labour must move in response to the needs of capital. In short, 'Wage labour subordinated by capital … must submit to being transferred in accordance with the requirements of capital and to being transferred from one sphere of production to another' (Marx 1959: 191). Specifically it is the movement of capital from those areas with low profit rates to those with higher rates which brings about a tendency towards equilibrium and the establishment of a general rate of profit.

But again this tendency must be seen as a process which is realised not in any mechanical manner. Like all laws it can never appear in unadulterated form. That is, it never produces a situation in which there is actually a general rate of profit throughout the economy. As in the case of all laws, we are faced with a tendency, a contradictory movement towards a never attainable equilibrium, and a movement which must take the form of necessary and constant disruptions. It is this contradictory movement Marx is speaking of when he refers to the 'incessant equilibration of constant divergences' (Marx 1959: 192).

Now the neo-Keynesians rightly object to the fact that orthodox neoclassical theory treats capitalist economy as though it were a machine, tending by its very nature towards equilibrium. This does not mean however that the whole notion of equilibrium should be consigned to the rubbish bin, as Kaldor and others tend to suggest.[16] The fact is that there is a certain tendency within capitalism towards equilibrium but this is a tendency not to be treated as absolute, nor as a state in which capitalism 'naturally' exists but as one attained through just that incessant equilibrium of constant divergences of which Marx speaks. If we consider the movement of the rate of profit and, we repeat, it is this movement which is most significant in the functioning and development of bourgeois economy, it is the existence of the tendency for the establishment of a general rate of profit which serves to pull supply and demand into balance, only to disrupt that equilibrium in the very course of its establishment. Those who see in capitalism only an equilibrating mechanism do of course take a one-sided (and usually an apologetic) view of the capitalist system. But equally one-sided are those who see capitalism as one based exclusively on disequilibrium.

The necessary laws of any series of phenomena find their way, establish themselves, through a maze of deviations. Superficially, such deviations appear as contingent occurrences; yet it is only though such apparent accidents that the law, necessity, establishes itself. At the same time, because it is in such deviations that the tendency is expressed, there are also introduced into the process many new aspects which do not flow from necessity but are conditioned by external circumstances. Take as an instance the Marxist law of value. This holds that there is a necessary relationship between the prices of commodities and their values – the amount of socially necessary labour for its production. This connection manifests itself, and can only manifest itself, in the shape of constant divergences of value from price, first in one direction and then another. Such deviations are, as already indicated, precisely the mechanism through which the general rate of profit is established under conditions where the organic composition of capital – the ratio of constant to variable capital – is not uniform throughout the various branches of the economy. To underscore the point that Marx recognised that the concept of equilibrium was a necessary abstraction – that is to say, a necessary moment in the real path of capitalist development – we can refer to a passage in which he discusses the function of the general rate of profit. He starts by saying that if we assume that the forces of supply and demand are in equilibrium, we have then to explain the phenomena in which we are interested (in this case price) by means of forces other than those of supply and demand:

> If supply equals demand, they cease to act, and for this very reason commodities are sold at their market-values. Whenever two forces operate equally in opposite directions, they balance one another, exert no outside influence, and any phenomena taking place in these circumstances must be explained by causes other than the effect of these two forces. If supply and demand balance one another, they cease to explain anything, do not affect market-values, and therefore leave us so much in the dark about the reasons why the market-value is expressed in just this sum of money and no other.
>
> (Marx 1959: 186)

Marx then proceeds to explain why it is necessary to assume, for the purposes of analysis, that supply and demand coincide, even though in reality this is not the case. Such a procedure was necessary 'To be able to study phenomena in their fundamental relations, in the form corresponding to their conception, that is to study them independently of the appearances caused by the movement of supply and demand' (Marx 1959: 186). And there is an additional reason. This was to allow thought to:

> ...find the actual tendencies of their movements and to some extent to record them. Since the inconsistencies are of an antagonistic nature, and since they continually succeed one another, they balance out one another through their opposing movements and their mutual contradiction. Since, therefore, supply and demand never equal one another in any given case, their differences follow one another in such a way – and the result of a deviation in one direction is that it calls forth a deviation in the opposite direction – that supply and demand are always equated when the whole is viewed over a certain period, but only as an average of past movements, and only as the continuous movement of their contradiction.
>
> (Marx 1959: 186)

In examining Keynes's basic theoretical conceptions we have argued that far from marking any advance on the work of his classical predecessors they constitute a serious degeneration, for whereas Smith, Ricardo and others set out to establish the objective laws of capitalism, Keynes's work is deeply imbued with the subjectivism which characterises bourgeois thought as a whole in the twentieth century. In the first place, as we have tried to show, his work was highly eclectic, drawing on elements from the neoclassical school for its explanation of the laws of distribution, yet at the same time calling on Malthus for the explanation of the poverty of the 1930s. It was for this reason, because Keynes's work resembled a rag-bag, that anybody could dip in and choose what they wanted. This is certainly connected with Keynes's view of the state as a supra-class institution, a point examined in the previous chapter ['The significance of the Keynesian revolution' in Pilling 1986: 27–58) – ed.]. The state was an institution to be used to direct the economy according to one's ideas. But this must leave open the question of precisely which policies are to be pursued. Sismondi and Proudhon [on the relationship of the economics of Keynes and Proudhon see Dillard 1942 – ed.] employed an analysis not unlike that of Keynes to advocate utopian socialist ideas; Malthus used his underconsumptionism to defend the position of feudalism within a rapidly advancing capitalism; in the twentieth century (under quite different historical conditions when capitalism had ceased to be a force for progress) both Fascism and social democracy have operated economic policies which can claim legitimate parentage in Keynes. That such conflicting ideologies are able to find some degree of support in Keynes's economic theory is no accident given that (a) it was confined to the sphere of circulation (taking the relations of production as given), and (b) it operated with subjective psychological categories.

Keynes's three independent variables (Keynes 1936: 246–247) do not even mention profit which for Keynes took back-seat to the gambling instinct which was supposedly inherent in human nature, for 'If human nature felt no temptation to take a chance, no satisfaction (profit apart) in constructing a factory, a railway, a mine or a farm, there might not be much investment as a result of cold calculation' (Keynes 1936: 150). And what are we to make of an economic theory, which after all claimed to explain some of the fundamental problems of twentieth-century capitalism, which could declare: 'In estimating the prospects of investment, we must have regard, therefore, to the nerves and hysteria and even the digestions and reactions to the weather of those upon whose spontaneous activity it largely depends' (Keynes 1936: 162)?

Despite its obvious weaknesses, Keynesianism was certainly an important strand in post-war bourgeois ideology. It was the theory which legitimated government spending and the creation of the Welfare State...

[This chapter was first published in Pilling, G. (1986) *The Crisis of Keynesian Economics: A Marxist View*, London and Sydney: Croom Helm, pp. 59–102 – ed.]

Notes

1

> The Keynesian [theory], on the other hand, is more closely linked to Ricardo and Marx of the classical tradition, of the analysis of value in physical terms, the analysis of quantities in terms of some type of measure based on labour, and of the analysis of a system undergoing change through historical time.
>
> (Kregel 1975: 33)

2 One issue involved in the critique of Baran and Sweezy is their notion of economic surplus. As part of their disposal of the categories of Marx they substitute the notion of economic surplus for that of surplus-value. These terms are, of course, by no means the same; all societies, save the most primitive, generate an economic surplus. Only under capitalism does this surplus take the form of surplus-value.

3 Keynes was certainly not as accommodating to Marx. He asserted that Marx's ideas were 'characterised ... by mere logical fallacy', and he believed that 'Marxian Socialism must always remain a portent to the historians of opinion – how a doctrine so illogical and dull can have exercised so powerful and enduring an influence on the minds of men, and through them the events of history' (Keynes, 'Laissez-faire and Communism', quoted in Hunt 1979: 377). Elsewhere Keynes could say,

> How can I adopt a creed which, preferring the mud to the fish, exalts the boorish proletariat above the bourgeoisie and the intelligentsia who, with whatever faults, are the quality in life and surely carry the seeds of all human advancement?
>
> (Keynes 1972: 258)

And this from a man who on the one hand had failed to make even a cursory inspection of Marx's ideas but nevertheless knew that his own work would destroy its foundations.

4

> Once for all I may here state, that by classical political economy, I understand that economy which, since the time of W. Petty, has investigated the real relations of production in bourgeois society, in contradistinction to vulgar economy, which deals with appearances only, ruminates without ceasing on the materials long since provided by scientific economy, and there seeks plausible explanations of the most obtrusive phenomena, for bourgeois daily use, but for the rest, confines

> itself to systematising in a pedantic way, and proclaiming for everlasting truths, the trite ideas held by the self-complacent bourgeoisie with regard to their own world, to them the best of all possible worlds.
>
> (Marx 1961a: 81)

5 Here empiricism is quite useless as a means to scientific knowledge. Every individual views the world, including its economic phenomena, through social eyes, as an integral part of a definite network of social relations formed historically on the basis of human labour. And because this is so,

> Socio-historical properties of things very often merge in the eyes of the individual with their natural properties, while transitory properties of things and of man himself begin to seem eternal properties bound up with the very essence of things. These fetishistic naturalistic illusions (commodity fetishism is only one example) expressing them cannot therefore be refuted by mere indication of things given in contemplation.
>
> (Ilyenkov 1982: 127)

6

> Political economists have laid it down as an axiom that Capital, the form of property at present predominant, is eternal; they have tasked their brains to show that capital is coeval with the world, and that it has no beginning, so it can have no end. In proof of which astonishing assertion all the manuals of political economy repeat with much complacency the story of the savage who, having in his possession a couple of bows, lends one of them to a brother savage, for a share of the produce of the chase. So great were the zeal and ardour which economists brought to bear on their search for capitalist property in prehistoric times, that they succeeded, in the course of their investigations, in discovering the existence of property outside the human species, to wit amongst the invertebrates: for the ant, in her foresight, is a hoarder of provisions. It is a pity that they should not have gone a step farther, and affirmed that, if the ant lays up stores, she does so with a view to sell the same and realise a profit by the circulation of her capital.
>
> (Lafargue 1975)

7 Strictly speaking variable capital is equivalent to the total wage bill of productively employed workers, that is workers producing surplus-value, and not to that of all workers. So figures such as that for the share of wages in the national income cannot tell us anything directly about such things as the rate of exploitation. The distinction between productive and unproductive labour will be discussed in the next chapter [refers to Chapter 4 of Pilling's *The Crisis of Keynesian Economics* (1986); also discussed in Chapter 5 of this book – ed.]; but there is an indication that the categories of Marx's *Capital* do not correspond immediately to empirical data.

8 Economists continually argue amongst themselves about the essential qualities of money. It is conventional to say that money has four functions: (a) as a means of exchange; (b) as a standard of value; (c) as a means of payment; and (d) as a store of value. It was Keynes who laid particular stress on this latter function, making it the basis for his theory of interest: interest was the payment for not hoarding. On the other hand, adherents to the quantity theory of money place their prime emphasis on money's role as a medium of exchange. Efforts to arrive at the essence of money by means of registering its functions are bound to fail in that they actually stand the real issue on its head. Its functions turn out to be not the manner in which the essential quality of money appears but, on the contrary, the condition from which its nature is deduced. The point is that money manifests several related but contradictory aspects within the capitalist system; to take one aspect, as expressed in one particular function, is bound to lead to an abstract and erroneous conception of money. Thus in the

case of Mercantilism, an absolute was made of money's function as a store of wealth and this paved the way for the identification of money with gold and silver. In recent years, at the time of mounting criticism of the position occupied by the dollar in the world monetary system, economists such as Jacques Rueff (1973) in France advocated the restoration of the gold standard, forgetting that this Standard operated under specific historical conditions during the last century which were incapable of resurrection in the present. On the other hand, those theories which hold that money is purely a convention, employed as a means of fixing relative prices, are equally one-sided. They lead to the conclusion that paper money, rather than the precious metals, are the ideal money-form. Paper money is, however, but one specific form of money and one which arises from its function as means of exchange. The point is that the various functions of money cannot merely be listed but must be considered in their real interconnection.

9 An early example of this was John Strachey (1938), who saw a close analogy between Marx's theory of the declining rate of profit and Keynes's notion of the declining marginal efficiency of capital.

10 The mystery of capital consists in the following: How can things (stocks of raw materials, bank balances, machinery and equipment, etc.) so different in appearance be united under the same head as 'capital'? And second, what is the secret of capital's ability to expand in value? For a historical account of the various, ultimately futile, efforts on the part of orthodox economics to answer these questions, see Shemyatenkov (1981).

11 At one point Joan Robinson rightly observes that 'Technical and physical relations, between man and nature, must be distinguished from social relations between man and man' (Robinson 1960b: v). This is indeed the nub of the issue, but it is clear from what she says elsewhere that the real significance of the distinction has eluded her.

12 Joan Robinson suggests that Keynes had a quite new and revolutionary view of capital: 'The whole elaborate structure of the metaphysical justification for profit was blown up when he pointed out that capital yields a return not because it is productive but because it is scarce' (1962: 75). That income arises in connection with a good or service which is naturally or artificially scarce is one of the central features of orthodox rent theory and in this respect Keynes was saying little new. Just as land yields a rent not because it is in scarce supply but because it is privately owned, so the return to various instruments of production reflects not their scarcity but their private ownership as capital. On the similarities between Joan Robinson's views on capital and those of Proudhon, see Rosdolsky (1977).

13 Given the time that he was engaged in his polemics with Malthus (the early years of the nineteenth century) Ricardo was to an extent justified in assuming that capitalism could develop the productive forces in a smooth crisis-free manner. Such an assumption became far less tenable as the century progressed.

14 The point is that while the world is given to man in sensation it cannot be comprehended through sensation. Empirical material is a necessary component of knowledge and in this sense Marxism is in no way hostile to the study of empirical material; indeed, such study is essential. Marx's *Capital*, for instance, involved the exhaustive study of a mass of factual material over a period of some 25 years. But the study of empirical material requires concepts and categories which have to be consciously developed. Those who imagine that they are dealing with 'the facts' and the facts alone, invariably operate with the most crass categories of thought which have been uncritically assimilated from bourgeois thought.

15 This involves a conception of the idea of contradiction. In general it can be said that positivism sees in contradiction an error in thought and views the development of thought as always involving the elimination of contradiction. Marxism, on the contrary, sees contradiction as the most vital property of the object itself, and the

essential task of scientific thought to be not the elimination of contradiction through the redefinition of terms but as the uncovering of real contradictions and an analysis of their real solution. On this question, see Pilling (1980).

16 Joan Robinson appears not to take this extreme position for 'The concept of equilibrium, of course, is an indispensable tool of analysis' (1962: 81).

References

Bannock, G., Baxter, R.E. and Rees, R. (1984) *Penguin Dictionary of Economics*, Harmondsworth: Penguin.

Baran, P.A. and Sweezy, P.M. (1966) *Monopoly Capital: An Essay on the American Economic and Social Order*, New York and London: Monthly Review Press.

Dillard, D. (1942) 'Keynes and Proudhon', *Journal of Economic History*, 2 (1): 63–76.

Hansen, A.H. (1951) *Business Cycles and National Income*, New York: Norton.

Hunt, E.K. (1979) *History of Economic Thought: A Critical Perspective*, Belmont: Wadsworth Publishing Company.

Ilyenkov, E.V. (1982) *The Dialectics of the Abstract and the Concrete in Marx's Capital*, Moscow: Progress Publishers, online, available at: www.marxists.org/archive/ilyenkov/works/abstract/index.htm (accessed 14 May 2012).

Kaldor, N. (1978) *Further Essays on Economic Theory*, London: Duckworth.

Keynes, J.M. (1936) *The General Theory of Employment, Interest and Money*, London: Macmillan.

Keynes, J.M. (1972) *The Collected Writings of John Maynard Keynes, vol. ix, Essays in Persuasion*, London and Basingstoke: Macmillan for the Royal Economic Society.

Kregel, J.A. (1975, second edition) *The Reconstruction of Political Economy*, London: Macmillan.

Lafargue, P. (1975) *The Evolution of Property: From Savagery to Civilization; and, Social and Philosophical Studies*, London: New Park. Swan Sonnenschein & Co., London 1890 edition, online, available at: www.marxists.org/archive/lafargue/1890/property/index.html (accessed 13 December 2011).

Marx, K. (1957) *Capital*, vol. II, Moscow and London: Foreign Languages Publishing House and Lawrence & Wishart.

Marx, K. (1959) *Capital*, vol. III. Moscow and London: Foreign Languages Publishing House and Lawrence & Wishart.

Marx, K. (1961a) *Capital*, vol. I, Moscow and London: Foreign Languages Publishing House and Lawrence & Wishart.

Marx, K. (1961b) 'Preface to the first German edition' in *Capital*, vol. I, Moscow and London: Foreign Languages Publishing House and Lawrence & Wishart.

Marx, K. (1969) *Theories of Surplus Value*, Part II, London: Lawrence & Wishart.

Marx, K. (1972) *Theories of Surplus Value*, Part III, London: Lawrence & Wishart.

Marx, K. (1977) 'Wage labour and capital', in *Karl Marx and Frederick Engels: Collected Works*, vol. 9, Moscow and London: Progress Publishers and Lawrence & Wishart, pp. 197–228.

Patinkin, D. (1965) *Money, Interest and Prices: An Integration of Money and Value Theory*, New York: Harper Row.

Pilling, G. (1980) *Marx's 'Capital': Philosophy and Political Economy*, London: Routledge. (Pilling, G. (2009), *Marx's 'Capital' (Routledge Revivals): Philosophy and Political Economy*, London: Routledge).

Pilling, G. (1986) *The Crisis of Keynesian Economics: A Marxist View*, London: Croom

Helm, pp. 27–58, online available at: www.marxists.org/archive/pilling/works/keynes/index.htm (accessed 14 May 2012).
Robinson, J. (1942) *An Essay on Marxian Economics*, London: Macmillan.
Robinson, J. (1960a) *Collected Papers*, vol. 2, Oxford: Basil Blackwell.
Robinson, J. (1960b) *Exercises in Economic Analysis*, London: Macmillan.
Robinson, J. (1962) *Economic Philosophy*, London: Watts.
Rosdolsky, R. (1977) *The Making of Marx's 'Capital'*, London: Pluto Press.
Rubin, I.I. (1972) *Essays on Marx's Theory of Value*, Detroit: Black & Red. Online, available at: www.marxists.org/archive/rubin/value/index.htm (accessed 16 December 2011).
Rubin, I.I. (1979) *A History of Economic Thought*, London: Ink Links.
Rueff, J. (1973) *La Réforme du Système Monétaire International*, Paris: Librairie Plon.
Schumpeter, J.A. (1952) *Ten Great Economists*, London: Allen & Unwin.
Shemyatenkov, V. (1981) *The Enigma of Capital: A Marxist Viewpoint*, Moscow: Progress Publishers.
Smith, A. (1976) *An Inquiry into the Nature and Causes of the Wealth of Nations*, vol. 1. Edited by R.H. Campbell and A.S. Skinner, Oxford: Clarendon Press.
Sraffa, P. (1960) *Production of Commodities by Means of Commodities*, Cambridge: Cambridge University Press.
Strachey, J. (1938) 'Mr. J.M. Keynes and the falling rate of profit', *Modern Quarterly*, 1: 337–347.
Sweezy, P.M. (1946) *The Theory of Capitalist Development*, London: Dobson.
Tsuru, S. (1968) 'Keynes v. Marx: the methodology of aggregates', in D. Horowitz (ed.) *Marx and Modern Economics*, London: MacGibbon & Kee, pp. 176–202.

7 On disinterring Karl Marx

Cyril Smith, *Marx at the Millennium*, Pluto Press, 1996

This is one of a profusion of books that aim to re-consider the state of Marxism in the aftermath of the collapse of the regimes of Eastern Europe and the Soviet Union. In the main most of this output comes, not unpredictably, to the conclusion that the demise of such regimes spelt the definitive 'death of socialism' and Marxism. The book under review takes a somewhat different line. It proposes that in the light of these recent events a thorough-going re-examination of Marx's ideas must be undertaken and one that involves making the sharpest distinction between 'Marxism', and the actual ideas of Karl Marx, for the one bears little, if any, relationship to the other. For our author finds that long ago Marx was buried by his would-be or self-proclaimed followers, 'the Marxists'. Systematic and deep digging is needed if Marx is to be rescued, and one of the main aims of the book is to engage in the necessary unearthing of the 'real' Marx. Of those who took part in the interment of Marx, the Stalinists were culprits-in-chief. But this is not the end of the story, for the Stalinist bureaucracy 'erected its falsifications on the basis of a body of doctrine which had already distorted the essence of Marx's work' (Smith 1996: xii). Here Kautsky and Plekhanov were the people principally responsible for misinterpreting the work of Marx, but the tale did not stop there. For those who founded the Third International (1919) – including Lenin – accepted these (mechanical) distortions of Kautsky and Plekhanov. Clearly, for the author, the work of all the outstanding thinkers who made up this 'Marxist' canon constitutes a barrier to discovering what Marx was actually getting at.

In this respect for Cyril Smith there has been a sort of continuity within the 'Marxist' movement. For since the time of Marx's death, if for the moment we leave Engels aside, every prominent figure who claimed the name Marxist in fact ripped out the heart of Marx's original work. For all of them saw in Marx the founder of an 'economic doctrine' which was simply a variant of classical political economy; all of them, to one degree or another, understood Marxism as a philosophy of fatalism in which human beings were simply the playthings of history, at the mercy of its 'objective laws'; in short all returned to a form of pre-Marx mechanical materialism. Hence the author's need to go back to Marx and find out what he was really up to.

My fundamental objection to this view is as follows: while no doubt the various interpretations of Marx suggested by Cyril Smith were present in the movement that took his name, and at times may have constituted a decisive element, it is also true that throughout the history of the movement there has been a fight against such interpretations and the politics that accompanied them. In other words, the Marxist movement has been profoundly contradictory. It is a sense of this contradiction that I find quite absent from Cyril Smith's work. He has, in effect, started with his hypothesis – that the movement has throughout been characterised by a mechanical, inhuman, interpretation of Marx's work – and has proceeded to cast around for the evidence to sustain this view. In so doing he has, I believe, provided a highly tendentious account of the history and nature of both Marxism and the Marxist movement. To show that this is so will be the main purpose of this review.

Before embarking on its account of the sad history of 'Marxism', the book starts with a short sketch of the world today. Cyril Smith finds it to be in something of 'a mess'. After his survey of the work of 'Marxism' our author then turns to Marx, whose achievement, he now discovers, 'was primarily concerned with grasping the nature of human beings and the way that present-day society is alien to that nature' (Smith 1996: xii–xiii). From there the book turns to some aspects of current academic fields of study and how they treat of this human nature. In the light of his re-discovered Marx, the final chapter is an attempt by the author to look at 'some of the problems of the present time' (Smith 1996: xiii).

Although a fairly short book, it ranges over a wide variety of topics – among them Marx's conception of 'science' and 'theory', and the role of technology at the end of the century. Here I have concentrated on what I believe are the most important aspects of the book – those that deal with the relationship of the work of Marx (and Engels) to that of their predecessors and followers alike, as well as the connection between the development of Marxism and the struggle of the working class. It is here, on this latter point, that I find myself in the strongest disagreement with *Marx at the Millennium*, as I shall attempt to elucidate.[1]

'Marxists' on the charge sheet

The author informs us that there were two principal reactions to the collapse of the regimes in Eastern Europe and the Soviet Union. (He talks, somewhat inaccurately, about 'the collapse of the Soviet Union and its satellite states'.) Some declared socialism dead. 'Others', he tells us, carried on as though nothing had happened, or said that they had always predicted as much.[2] Our author has, he seems to think, avoided the pitfalls involved in what he tells us were these two reactions to the downfall of the Stalinist bureaucracy. He has taken a different path, which, if we are to believe him, avoids the twin dangers of despair or dogmatism. For he has concluded from this experience, together with his long time in the Trotskyist movement, as well as from his latest 'diggings',[3] that the real problem is to be located in the fact that nearly all the 'Marxists' of the past – no doubt their current equivalents are no better – managed to get most things wrong about the work of Karl Marx. In so doing they buried Marxism (Smith 1996: 19).

If this is in need of spelling out, we find later:

> What I am trying to show is that the philosophical bases of Marx's thought, lost in the days of the Second International, were never rediscovered in the Third [International]. Even before Stalin began his 'revision' of Marxism – not with the theoretician's pen but with the heel of the GPU – the fundamental ideas of Marx had been buried.
>
> (Smith 1996: 48)

This book is part of the efforts by Sexton Smith to exhume 'the real' Marx in the hope that the Moor may, perhaps, still be alive. In any event he is clearly set upon trying to put the rest of us luckless 'Marxists' right, although one suspects he is not very hopeful about the likely success of his project.

The use of quotation marks around Marxist is the author's, not mine, and occurs throughout the book. Indeed it is one of Smith's central contentions that the strictest separation between Marx and those who subsequently presumed to speak in his name, the 'Marxists', is now imperative.

> Some readers might think that in the course of these pages I have exaggerated the gulf between the ideas of Marx and the body of doctrine called 'Marxism'. If so, please excuse me, but I am convinced that it would have been a far more serious error to understate this gap … it began to dawn on me that keeping Marx and 'Marxism' *quite separate from each other* provided the chance to see the world more clearly.
>
> (Smith 1996: xi, emphasis added)

The list of those belonging to this hapless band of error-committing 'Marxists' is dauntingly long. It includes many figures, apart, obviously, from Stalin and his epigones. Kautsky (as the founder of 'Marxism' he is culprit-in-chief), Plekhanov, Rosa Luxemburg, Lenin and Trotsky all come under the 'Sexton's' sedulous eye, all are present on his charge sheet – to one degree or another each and every one consigned to the dreaded inverted commas.[4]

We shall come back to some specific ways in which these Marxists – for, unlike our author, I consider them all, whatever their various deficiencies, to have made a contribution to the cause of the working class and the development of Marxism and therefore have no need of inverted commas – are here treated. But just to give a taste:

Plekhanov (perhaps with a bit of unintended help from Engels (1977) via certain passages in *Anti-Dühring* which lacked Engels's 'usual clarity') invented the 'myth' (but one accepted by Lenin) of 'dialectical materialism' – a mechanical combination of 'materialism' and 'dialectics'; Kautsky, according to Smith, was a thoroughly mechanical materialist, who, poor dear, thought that Marx had simply written a book on economics. It seems (Smith 1996: 61) that Kautsky from the outset might even have been attracted to the Marxist movement precisely because he thought that Marxism equalled mechanical materialism.[5]

(How's that for the doctrine of original sin?) Even more seriously, Rosa Luxemburg, despite her 'brilliant' demonstration that revisionism represented 'an opportunist adaptation to bourgeois society', proved unable to approach the philosophical basis of the problem of opportunism in the Second International. Why not? Because, sad to say: 'The truth of "Marxism" was taken for granted as a body of doctrine by her as much as Kautsky' (Smith 1996: 36). Turning his blunderbuss in another direction, Smith aims next at Lenin, finding that unhappily he was dominated for much of his political life by the false conceptions of Kautsky ('his leader') as well as by those of Plekhanov. And because of this his book *Materialism and Empirio-Criticism* (1977), was a crucial text that provided an important basis for the further vulgarisation of Marxism.[6] If that wasn't a hanging offence, Lenin's notion of the formation of ideology in *What is to be Done* (1973) – here he followed Kautsky explicitly – had nothing in common with the position of Marx and Engels. And while Lenin appeared to be making some modest progress in his reading of Hegel after the outbreak of war in 1914, unfortunately the progress came rapidly to an end, the work was put aside and that terrible beast 'Marxism' reasserted itself. On the Smithian scale – obviously our author is one of the few teachers who has refused to lower his marking standards – poor old Lenin would be lucky to get a Beta minus. Trotsky and his followers fare even worse, for, hapless dears, they 'never had the theoretical resources to penetrate to its [Stalinism's] philosophical core' (Smith 1996: 25). That is why 'Trotsky] could not escape being affected by it [the orthodoxy of Stalinism]'. The best that Trotsky and his comrades could do – naturally they get a pat on the back for their efforts – 'was to show that Stalinist policies and distortions were contrary to the decisions of Lenin's party and the teachings of "Marxism"' (Smith 1996: 25).

In connection with the problems associated with the dominance of 'Marxism' the most important thing our author has to say is the following: 'it became *impossible* to view Marx's work unless it was first refracted through the distorting lens of this [Stalinist] tradition' (Smith 1996: 25, emphasis added).[7] So Trotsky's contention that the laws of history (the class struggle) would prove more powerful than the Stalinist apparatus turned out to be without foundation.

Let us consider Cyril Smith's last statement carefully, and in particular ponder its methodological implications. To me it expresses very well the passive, contemplative stance of its author.[8] In the first instance it invites an obvious question: if all Marxism was perforce distorted by Stalinism, if all would-be Marxists got virtually everything wrong, how did it come to pass that one C. Smith made his escape? Or that he even *knows* that he has escaped, and that, like Kant, has awoken from his 'dogmatic slumbers'? Posed in this (abstract) manner, there can be no answer to such a question. Knowledge can never be an individual thing, whatever illusions a particular thinker might have. To be competent in any field of science means to know the history of that science, to be familiar with the record of the disputes within it and the major landmarks that have marked its progress. It is impossible to grasp the tasks facing Marxists today and to consider the so-called 'crisis of Marxism' without reviewing critically the history of the Marxist movement, a history that can be fully understood only in connection with the life and history of the working-class movement.

Second, just what *is* this 'Stalinist tradition' through which all Marxism was, according to Cyril Smith, of necessity refracted? We presumably 'all' know what it was? But do we? *And to the extent that we do, how, in what process, in the struggle against which political and ideological enemies, was this knowledge won*? The truth is that the degeneration of the Soviet state, the destruction of the Bolshevik Party, the nature of the 'Stalinist tradition' have been the most hotly contested and bitterly fought-over issues in the labour movement since 1917. The divisions on the 'Russian Question' have been amongst the most important ones ever since 1917. This 'Stalinist tradition' as Smith calls it, did not drop from the sky ready-made. It developed, came into being over a longish period of time, in the last resort the product of the pressure of imperialism on a backward, workers' state. The product of this isolation, it itself became a powerful force in ensuring the continuation of just that isolation. As is well known, Trotsky took issue with those of his supporters (such as C.L.R. James) who tended to see the Stalinist bureaucracy as present from day one of the revolution. Yes, a bureaucracy was there from the beginning but only over time did it become a *Stalinist* bureaucracy. That is, a transformation took place – from a bureaucracy that constituted a privileged caste into one that became a *counter-revolutionary* privileged caste resting on the property relations brought into being by 1917 and simultaneously serving the needs of imperialism.[9] But how did Trotsky grasp this process? *Only in the long-drawn-out fight against it.* It was only in the process of this real, living struggle, that not only did the specifically Stalinist bureaucracy emerge, *but the knowledge of what it was that was emerging was won.* It was a fight that went through definite stages, during which an increasingly concrete knowledge of what the Stalinist bureaucracy was becoming was won. When, at the time of the Germany tragedy of 1933, some of Trotsky's erstwhile supporters said: we warned you what was going to happen, you should have left the Comintern long ago, Trotsky replied with a shrug of the shoulders and in effect said: I'm sorry you are obviously cleverer than I and knew more than I did. The point being that neither Trotsky nor anybody else could have known in advance what the outcome of the emergence of the Stalinist bureaucracy would be, and whether it was a process that could or could not be reversed. It had to be tested out, fought out, in life – in the clash of real, living forces.

The struggle to comprehend what was involved in the degeneration of the Soviet state and the Bolshevik party necessitated the struggle for a *development* of Marxism, and not at all simply an insistence that the politics of Stalin diverged from the politics of Lenin, as Cyril Smith, re-inventing the history of the Left Opposition, pretends is what happened. (And surely a gratuitous insult to Trotsky and his comrades.) In taking up the fight against the coming-into-being of the Stalinist bureaucracy, Trotsky was dealing with something quite *new*. There were no exact precedents to guide him. He designated the bureaucracy as a 'caste', but realised that this analogy with Indian society had its strict limits; indeed given the unprecedented character of the Stalinist bureaucracy all analogies were bound to be severely limited. At the same time Trotsky always ruthlessly opposed those who claimed that Stalinism was a natural emanation of Bolshevism, something rooted in the very 'being' of Lenin's party. He was also obliged to take issue with those who wanted to elevate this bureaucratic caste to the status of a new class (although the bureaucracy certainly had features in common with a class) and this in turn called for a *development* of historical materialism. But to repeat, there was no precedent for what was happening in the Soviet Union: the establishment, by proletarian revolution, of a workers' state that tragically remained isolated. This involved the struggle for new concepts, for new definitions, for fresh theoretical conquests. That is what makes Trotsky's *Revolution Betrayed* (1972a) without doubt the outstanding contribution to Marxist theory and politics of the last six decades.

The essential point to be made here is one concerning the theory of knowledge. Cyril Smith refers to the 'Stalinist tradition'. At the same time he is of the opinion that *all* 'Marxism' was refracted through this very tradition. But he puts himself into a vicious circle from which there is no escape. For if all Marxism had to see the world through Stalinism's spectacles how was it possible to get a scientific understanding of these very spectacles? Presumably, if Trotsky was tainted by this Stalinist tradition (as Smith says) then he could not in principle have understood it! From the standpoint of Marxism (sans inverted commas) the matter cannot be posed in Smith's way, but only from the standpoint of 'revolutionising practice' (Marx). If today part of the theoretical capital of the working-class movement is the understanding of the class nature of that force, the Stalinist bureaucracy, that betrayed the 1917 revolution this is so *only* because of the fight conducted – principally by Trotsky and his followers – against its emergence. It was *only* in this fight that the working class won its 'definition' of the Stalinist bureaucracy. And that is how, in all sciences, definitions are arrived at – in the course of practice. It was only in this fight that the thoroughly anti-Marxist nature of this (emerging) bureaucracy – its social character, its politics, its ideology – could be grasped. And, while we're on the subject we should stress that this is not of merely historical interest, something for the record books, giving past figures in the movement their due. (Although none of these things are unimportant.) For it is only on the basis of a knowledge of what this bureaucracy was, the counter-revolutionary role that it played in the class struggle over several decades, that the real meaning and consequences for the working class of its collapse can be truly understood *for today, for what we must now do*. Thus is the 'past' and the 'present' inseparably bound together. That is why Marx and 'Marxism' cannot be metaphysically separated, as this book proposes.

And we must add that this fight against Stalinist politics and ideology in the working-class movement did not end with the assassination of Trotsky in 1940. For the fact is that within the Trotskyist movement there *was* a battle against those who claimed that the Stalinist bureaucracy had a 'dual nature' that it could be 'reformed' and that the process of what was at the time fashionably known as 'de-Stalinisation' could be successful. (Where do such people stand today? They are completely silent.) Those who took up that fight did so against the idea that the world was divided into three camps – that of imperialism, that of the so-called 'Third World' and finally that of the 'Workers' States' – with the last mentioned being able to develop more or less independently of the first two sectors. This view, propounded chiefly by the late Ernest Mandel and his followers, was in fact a clear concession to the Stalinist theory (and practice) that it was possible to build 'socialism in one country'. And painful though it may be for Cyril Smith to be reminded, it must be recorded that the struggle did not stop there: for there *was* an attempt to probe to the philosophical basis of the positions that Mandel and others adopted, and this involved 'a return to Lenin', especially the work of Lenin carried out after 1914.[10]

And they also served...

One further point should be made in connection with Cyril Smith's ill-founded claim that all would-be Marxists were trapped, more or less completely, within the limits of the ideological categories of Stalinism. We have already pointed to the fact that Trotsky and his comrades carried out not simply a political fight against Stalinism but a theoretical-philosophical struggle. We can say with confidence that it was Trotsky and his comrades in the Left Opposition that most profoundly understood the roots of the degeneration of the Soviet state. (István Mészáros although not a Trotskyist, considers that Trotsky's analysis of 'actually existing socialism' was 'the most devastating critique' offered (see *Beyond Capital* 1995: xxii). Incidentally, this book, the product of a lifetime's endeavour, is itself a critique of the Stalinist orthodoxy that reigned in left circles for such a long time.) But others, non-Trotskyists, were also involved – albeit in many cases inconsistently and episodically – in the effort to combat the influence of Stalinism. Smith makes mention of Karl Korsch and his early disputes with the Stalinist bureaucracy. But he forgets that after being expelled from the Comintern Korsch wrote a number of works which, whatever their defects, can certainly be classed as anti-Stalinist. Thus his book *Karl Marx* (1963) remains a valuable exposition of Marx's critique of classical political economy and one that in particular avoids the errors that Smith detects in the work of the whole of 'Marxism'. For what it is worth, it was a book which certainly had an important formative influence on the present reviewer. And what about the criticism that Antonio Gramsci launched in the 1920s against the mechanical materialism of Bukharin? Despite the fact that much later the 'Euro-communists' could – I think with good cause – find in Gramsci's writings much to sustain their reformism, his critique of Bukharin's attempt at a 'popular Marxism' still deserves our attention (in Gramsci 1971). And what of the work of figures such as Roman Rosdolsky? His brilliant exegesis on Marx's *Grundrisse* (*The Making of Marx's 'Capital'*, 1977) stands as but one testimony to those who were able to take their distance from the influences of Stalinism. (What a pleasure it was at the time to read his devastating critique of the work of 'neo-Marxist' and for a time fellow traveller of Maoism Professor Joan Robinson and her efforts to marry Marx and classical economics!) Other names could be mentioned in this context. That of

Paul Mattick, for example, who, for my generation at any rate, provided many fresh insights into Marx's *Capital* and especially its incompatibility with the standpoint of J.M. Keynes (see his *Marx and Keynes*, 1969). Likewise Henryk Grossman's (1992) work on questions of capital accumulation.

Or take the celebrated dispute among philosophers in the Soviet Union in the 1920s mentioned by Cyril Smith, namely the argument between those led by Deborin (later condemned, on the basis of their regard for Hegel, as 'Menshivising idealists') and the 'mechanists' (who generally supported the by then out of favour Bukharin). Stalin brought a brutal halt to the discussion in 1931, denouncing and often killing members of both parties in the dispute. But was that the end of the matter? Did the ideas of Stalinism – especially, in connection with this dispute, which centred on the mechanical debasement of Marxism – triumph *completely*, even in the Soviet Union, as Smith's account would suggest? Did *all* traces of Marxism disappear? No they did not, for there is no doubt that the emergence in the recent past of figures such as the late E.V. Ilyenkov (who committed suicide in 1979 as a result of his treatment at the hands of the Stalinist bureaucracy, and of whom more later) and Felix Mikhailov was bound up with this earlier struggle against just that mechanical materialism which came to dominate with the victory of the Stalinist bureaucracy. Ilyenkov's work, including his defence of Lenin's *Materialism and Empirio-Criticism* (Ilyenkov 1982) against just the sort of criticisms made in the book under review – namely that it was an example of mechanical materialism – as well as his writings on the logic of *Capital* and his essays on the history of logic are, I suggest, important contributions to the renewal of Marxism. Just so with F.T. Mikhailov's *The Riddle of the Self* (1980), which is likewise centred on the repudiation of the mechanical Stalinist 'Marxism' and especially the notion that there could ever, even in principle, be a 'thinking machine', as the proponents of the idea of 'artificial intelligence' believe. (When he comes to deal with the question of artificial intelligence (Smith 1996: 115–117) the book under review makes no mention of Mikhailov. There is the same silence about Ilyenkov's work. One can but wonder why. Could it be that what they have written fits ill into the Smithian fatalistic thesis – that 'we' are 'all' labouring under the distortions of Stalinist 'theory', and inevitably so, given that 'Marxism' could not but view the world except through the distorting spectacles of the Stalinist bureaucracy?)

The work of each of the thinkers noted above – and many others – must, I contend, be carefully reconsidered. None of them meekly accepted the prevailing 'Stalinist orthodoxy' and their work must be critically re-examined in the light of a situation where history itself has passed its definitive judgment on Stalinism and its horrendous 'Marxism'.

A personal note

If I may at this point enter a personal note which has a bearing on the question of the continuity of Marxism and the ideological struggle against Stalinism. One of the oft-repeated charges of Cyril Smith is that the dreaded 'Marxists' treated Marx's work as a variety of 'economics'. Thus,

> The 'Marxist' notion that Marx had developed a new kind of political economy, a set of 'economic doctrines', including a 'theory of value' got it all wrong.
>
> (Smith 1996: 129)

Or again, 'In the "Marxist" tradition, it was assumed that he [Marx] was trying to provide a better, "Marxist" socialist economics' (Smith 1996: 75). (We were all no doubt operating along the wrong line that Karl Kautsky had established.) Here again, one has to say that some of the things said in the book, while true, are seriously vitiated by an unwarranted one-sidedness and exaggeration. Thus there is no doubt that the theoreticians of the Stalinist movement *did* fundamentally distort Marxism by presenting it as a variant of classical political economy. This trend was especially marked in Britain where Communist Party intellectuals such as Maurice Dobb (*Political Economy and Capitalism*, 1940) and Ronald Meek (*Studies in the Labour Theory of Value*, 1956) were anxious to show that Marxism was no 'German import' but something soundly rooted in the good old Anglo-Scottish tradition of political economy established by Adam Smith (1976) (and brought to its apogee by David Ricardo in his *Principles*, 1953). But what Smith (Cyril, not Adam) chooses to 'forget' is that there *was* a fight against just this distortion. (I've already cited the case of Korsch; that of W.J. Blake's, *An American Looks at Karl Marx* (1939) should also be recalled.) More than this: a fight against the attempts to reduce Marx's *Capital* to some form of political economy came from within the movement to which Cyril Smith at the time belonged, and indeed a fight which he helped carry out.

Thus in 1972 the present reviewer wrote an article ['The law of value in Ricardo and Marx', *Economy and Society*, 1, (2); see Chapter 3 of this book – ed.] which took Dobb and Meek to task. In particular it argued strongly that Marx had never held to a 'labour' theory of value, as they suggested, and in the course of so doing it tried to spell out the philosophical implications of their wrong view. (The work was developed in a later study, Pilling 1980, *Marx's Capital: Philosophy and Political Economy*.) Not only did the article produce a weak, plaintive response from Meek; more important it led to work by a series of writers (unfortunately I was not among them) in which the relationship between Marx and classical political economy was further explored and critically re-assessed. I recall this episode here only to stress that the idea that 'we' were 'all' imprisoned within Stalinist categories doesn't stand up to serious scrutiny. And, as a postscript to this incident, let me say that the inspiration to write a piece which suggested that Stalinism had for long seriously misread Marx's work in political economy and in particular had mis-interpreted his law of value came from none other than … V.I. Lenin – the self-same man who, if Smith's account is to be believed, proved incapable of ever breaking free in any real sense from the baleful influences of the 'Marxists' K. Kautsky and G.V. Plekhanov. For it was while reading an edition of the Marx–Kugelmann letters (the one issued by Martin Lawrence in the 1930s) that I came across a Preface that Lenin (Lenin 1934: 12) had earlier written to this correspondence. It was there to my considerable surprise that I found Lenin's reference to Marx's '*so-called*' labour theory of value! It was this that convinced me that my gropings towards a similar conclusion were perhaps a bit more than gropings. But if Smith is correct – namely that, despite some episodic, even laudable, attempts to break away from a Marxism dominated by mechanical conceptions, Lenin remained entrapped within 'Marxism' – how to explain Lenin's insight? One simply cannot.

An idealist view of history

Before coming to some specific points that I believe will substantiate this charge – that our author is distorting, sometimes wilfully, the history of the Marxist movement – it is worth noting Smith's general approach to history that all this implies. No doubt all the individuals whom he has in his sights had weaknesses (who hasn't?). And no doubt some of these weaknesses were graver in some than in others. But they must be put into their concrete historical context. The inadequacies of Plekhanov, Kautsky and others (including for that matter Eduard Bernstein, whom Engels did after all make his literary executor) can be understood only in light of the fact that they lived in the period of transition from the relatively peaceful period of 'classical' capitalism to that of imperialism. Poor dears, they proved unable to make the daunting leap across these two epochs.[11] The problems of Kautsky *et al.* lay *here* – problems that in some cases were compounded by long years of exile and thereby relative isolation from the day-to-day struggles within the working class movement.

Turning to the history of the Fourth International this latter point must surely be underlined, and more than once. The problems of the Fourth International cannot be understood simply, or even mainly, from the point of view of how adequately its leaders grasped the work of Karl Marx. For that 'understanding' and its level, have to be placed against a real historical background, must be investigated in connection with the contradictory development of the class struggle. The long years in which the movement was largely marginalised, the bitter years during which many of its leading cadres were wiped out by Stalinism's death squads, the years during which it was forced to defend the heritage of Marxism against the gangsters of Stalinism in relative isolation from the working class, obviously left their mark *not simply on the Marxists, but on the working class as whole.* But, critically, the continuity of the movement was indeed preserved; Marxism was *not* expunged from the working class movement, whatever the terrible damage that both Marxism and the working class suffered at the hands of Stalinism. If anything is amazing it must be that Marxism was kept alive in that period. (As Dr. Johnson said of his dog: the wonder wasn't that it could walk so well on its hind legs but that it could walk on them at all.) The work, its many shortcomings notwithstanding, carried out in these long and difficult years against Stalinism is quite indispensable in preparing for the tasks of today and of tomorrow. (And I would certainly want to include the past work of Cyril Smith in this contribution. In any event he was someone who in the past taught the writer of this review a great deal.)

In short, the problems of the movement do not simply, or even predominantly, reside in the fact that Kautsky and company had 'misread' their Marx. If this really were the case we would have a quite bloodless, bookish, history, of the type dished up in this present work, one where it is all too easy for some – well at least C. Smith – now to be wise after the event. And this in a book that is replete with the sternest strictures against any mechanistic materialism as well as calls for 'ruthless objectivity' on theoretical matters!

Contrast the attitude of Lenin towards Plekhanov – who, let us not forget, went over to the camp of imperialism after 1914 – with the sort of lifeless approach Smith would have us adopt to his collection of poor old 'Marxists'. Not only did Lenin make the principal speech by way of tribute at Plekhanov's funeral (1919) but he strongly urged all young party members to make a detailed study of the whole of Plekhanov's voluminous writings. Otherwise, they could not hope to become real communists, could not hope to assimilate the theoretical treasures of the past to which Plekhanov, at his best, had contributed mightily:

> Let me add in parenthesis for the benefit of young Party members that you *cannot* hope to become a *real* intelligent Communist without making a study – and I mean a *study* – of all Plekhanov's philosophical writings, because nothing better has been written on Marxism anywhere in the world.
> (Lenin 1965a: 94)

I believe that this had nothing to do with Lenin's inability to recognise Plekhanov's limitations in the field of philosophy. Nor was it a piece of sentimentalism in the immediate aftermath of Plekhanov's passing. What it did indicate was that Lenin was profoundly aware that he was dealing with a real living movement, not one that can be reduced simply to 'texts', to the exchange of this 'position' against another 'position'. Plekhanov remains one of the finest of his generation who were won to the cause of the working class, who made a decisive contribution to the foundation of Marxism on Russian soil and who, whatever his subsequent evolution, made an imperishable contribution to Marxism and the cause of the working class that endures to this day.

Noting this attitude of Lenin towards Plekhanov, Smith sees in it proof positive that 'Lenin was unable to talk about philosophy without invoking the name of Plekhanov' (Smith 1996: 48). Why, our tut-tutting author reminds us, the captivated Lenin even proposed that an edition of Plekhanov's works be published, and with an index forsooth! Dare I say it, but I find little materialism in such a desiccated attitude, and just about as much human feeling.[12]

The questions raised here don't simply concern our approach to history. For only if we can understand that the problems of the movement must, in the most fundamental sense, be considered from the standpoint of the development of the class struggle, and not from the point of view of the weaknesses, even grave ones, of this or that individual, will it be possible to grasp the significance of the period we are now in. The collapse of the Stalinist bureaucracy has brought a new situation in the class struggle, one that is favourable for the working class, and therefore one that makes possible and requires a further development of Marxism, a process that will certainly involve the struggle to overcome the limitations, even the mistakes, of the past.

Lenin before *Materialism and Empirio-Criticism*

What the book says about the relationship between Lenin and Plekhanov I find disingenuous. For Cyril Smith deliberately obscures certain features of that relationship which would have thrown a somewhat different light on matters. He is keen to peddle the old tale: in 1908 when *Materialism and Empirio-Criticism* was being written Lenin was still a mechanical materialist, philosophically speaking still in the pocket of Karl Kautsky and G.V. Plekhanov. By the middle of World War I, when he was studying Hegel (in fact he was *re-studying* him),[13] Lenin began to break (sadly inconsistently) with this mechanical standpoint and to that extent from the tutelage of Plekhanov. I cannot accept this tale.

Let us deal briefly with two initial points: first the relationship between 'philosophy' and the 'inner party struggle' and second the standpoint from which we should approach the question of differences over philosophy in a movement. As to the first point, Cyril Smith, like many before him, wants to portray Lenin as one who 'used' philosophy pragmatically to exaggerate differences with opponents. In this case Smith wants to present Lenin as one who adopted extreme positions in philosophy to establish his radical credentials. (See for instance the points made in the book (Smith 1996: 43) about the theory of 'hieroglyphs' in *Materialism and Empirio-Criticism*.) In fact Lenin was as scrupulously objective in this field as he was in all others. When he came to tackle Bogdanov (Bolshevik who was one of the chief Russian proponents of 'Machism' or 'empiriocriticism') and company he was willing to join hands with Plekhanov in the defence of Marxism even though (a) Plekhanov was by that time the de facto leader of the Mensheviks and (b) Lenin was already aware that there were important limits to Plekhanov's defence of Marxism.[14] Lenin vigorously opposed those who wanted to reject what Plekhanov had rightly said on matters philosophical on the grounds that in politics he was moving rapidly to opportunism. Writing in *Marxism and Revisionism* in 1908, just before his *Materialism and Empirio-Criticism* appeared, Lenin had the following to say:

> [T]he only Marxist in the international Social-Democratic movement to criticise the incredible platitudes of the revisionists from the standpoint of consistent dialectical materialism was Plekhanov. *This must be stressed all the more emphatically since profoundly mistaken attempts are being made at the present time to smuggle in old and reactionary philosophical rubbish disguised as a criticism of Plekhanov's tactical opportunism.*
>
> (Lenin 1987: 33–34,[15] emphasis added)

Turning to the second point: in studying the history of the Marxist movement the danger is that we try to consider such matters merely by a comparison of 'texts' forgetting that the development of Marxism is bound inseparably with the concrete life and development of the working class.[16] I believe that Cyril Smith is guilty of just this mistake. He presents the history of the Marxist movement almost exclusively as a dispute over philosophical questions.[17] We cannot possibly consider Lenin's work of 1908, and the time he began his renewed study of Hegel without remembering that during these years Lenin went through some of the richest experiences of a rich life, culminating in the shock he experienced at the betrayal of the working class by almost every prominent leader in the Second International.

Likewise, we must not overlook the fact that Lenin brought to his writing against the empirio-critics a wealth of theoretical struggles in defence of Marxism that stretched right back to the 1890s, when he had first joined the movement. It is quite erroneous to believe that before 1908, when he engaged with the latest form of positivism, Lenin had confined himself to a series of works that were narrowly socio-economic. Thus his very first struggles against the Narodniks involved a deepening of the early theoretical struggles of Marx and Engels to establish that the working class was the only consistently revolutionary class.[18] This necessitated a return to another of Marx and Engels's earlier fights – namely against the idea that society could be divided into 'heroes' and 'the mob', a division based on the distinction between 'critically minded' people and the working masses.[19] These early polemics against the Narodniks are, among other things, also brilliant examples of a concrete study of the relation between 'freedom' and 'necessity'. While insisting that social development is governed by laws which are independent of will and consciousness, Lenin simultaneously rejected the Narodnik charge that Marxism was 'economic materialism,' that is fatalism:

> The idea of determinism which postulates that human acts are necessitated and rejects the absurd tale about free will, in no way destroys man's reason or conscience, or appraisal of his actions. Quite the contrary, only the deterministic view makes a strict and correct appraisal possible instead of attributing everything you please to free will.
>
> (Lenin 1972a: 159)

It was on the basis of his fight against the Narodniks that Lenin was able to tackle the emergence of 'Bernsteinism' in the movement. In Russia this found its reflection in the 'legal Marxism' of Struve, Tugan-Baranovsky and others. This was the school that, in opposition to the Narodniks, stressed the 'progressive' character of capitalism and tried to convince the workers that their interests should be completely subordinated to those of the bourgeoisie. What should be stressed here is that this involved Lenin in a systematic repudiation of 'objectivism', that standpoint that sees history as unfolding automatically outside of human intervention and consciousness. I say that this should be stressed because it is precisely this objectivist standpoint which Cyril Smith believes dominated the life of the Second International. Lenin showed the connection between the fight against objectivism and the struggle to embrace the standpoint of the working class. Thus in *The Economic Content of Narodism and the Criticism of it in Mr Struve's Book*:

> The objectivist speaks of the necessity of a given historical process; the materialist gives an exact picture of the given socia -economic formation and of the antagonistic relations to which it gives rise. When demonstrating the necessity for a given series of facts, the objectivist always runs the risk of becoming an apologist for these facts; the materialist speaks of the class which 'directs' the given economic system, giving rise to such and such forms of counteraction by other classes.... Thus, on the one hand, the materialist is more consistent than the objectivist, and gives profounder and fuller effect to his objectivism.... On the other hand, materialism includes partisanship, so to speak, and enjoins the direct and open adoption of the standpoint of a definite social group in any assessment of events.
>
> (Lenin 1972a: 400–401)

Nor is that much-maligned work *What is to be Done?* (published in 1902) concerned simply with political strategy and tactics. It involves a profound consideration of the relationship between the spontaneous element in the struggle for socialism and the conscious fight for the Marxist world outlook. This work is often presented as one in which Lenin was over-anxious to stress the *conscious* element in the struggle for socialism as against the spontaneous movement of the working class. It is presented by Cyril Smith in this familiar way, but, even allowing for the concrete circumstances under which it was written, it is not possible to sustain this interpretation. However much he might have 'bent the stick' in a particular direction Lenin certainly did not draw a completely hard and fast line between 'spontaneity' and 'consciousness', as many have suggested. Thus he specifically rejected the notion that the 'spontaneous' was something taking place outside and independently of human consciousness, a blindly acting force. For him 'the spontaneous element' was nothing more nor less than consciousness in '*embryonic form*'. It is of course well known that Lenin held that the theory of socialism initially arose,

> altogether independently of the spontaneous growth of the working-class movement; it arose as a natural and inevitable outcome of the development of thought among the revolutionary socialist intelligentsia.
>
> (Lenin 1973: 375–376)

But Lenin also knew that the very emergence of the world outlook of Marxism, a world outlook based on the negation of all the principal conquests of bourgeois thought, had, at its very centre, an understanding of the world historical role of the modern working class as that force which alone could free mankind from exploitation. So while the theory of socialism may have *initially* arisen independently of the spontaneous strivings of the working class, its further development was bound up inseparably with the struggle and fate of the working class. That is to say, the very coming-into-being of Marxism involved a transformation in the relationship between 'theory' and 'practice', as Marx and Engels very well knew.

Lenin's *Materialism and Empirio-Criticism*

E.V. Ilyenkov in his work *Leninist Dialectics and the Metaphysics of Positivism* paints a somewhat different picture of the relationship between the work of Lenin and Plekhanov than that proffered by Cyril Smith. In what follows I rely heavily on Ilyenkov's account. Naturally Lenin was profoundly influenced by Plekhanov's work in philosophy and had normally deferred to him in this field. There is nothing remarkable, and certainly nothing sinister, in such a situation; among other things it involves the question of generations within a party. But with the revival of positivism within the Bolshevik Party Lenin felt it was necessary to make an independent study of some new questions, and especially the use which the positivists were making of the 'latest developments' in science, physics in particular.[20] This was so because he felt that Plekhanov's response to the positivists was deficient *in just this area.* Plekhanov, with his unrivalled learning, was able to show in detail that this new positivism (it went under a variety of pretentious names, including 'empirio-criticism' and 'empirio-monism') in fact involved a return to either the idealism of George Berkeley or the scepticism of David Hume. And Plekhanov did so in a generally biting and dismissive way. Lenin sensed that however much he might agree with what Plekhanov had said, this was inadequate, especially when Plekhanov's opponents answered him with a: 'so what?' And they further challenged Plekhanov: the world's greatest scientists – Ernest Mach, Poincaré and others – are embracing the standpoint of empirio-criticism or one of its variants. They are world-ranking scientists after all, and if science is being guided by this 'new philosophy' who are we, humble non-scientists, to challenge them? And for good measure, they added: Marxism isn't dogma, suggesting to Plekhanov that Marx would have been the first to realise that in the face of these developments in the natural sciences and the 'philosophy of science' the 'old materialism,' indeed materialism as a whole, had to be ditched. In such manner were the 'empirio-critics' able to brush aside Plekhanov's otherwise withering remarks.

Lenin's chief criticism of Plekhanov was that he had not paid sufficient attention to the developments in physics on which Bogdanov and others were so heavily reliant. It is clear that Lenin attached the greatest importance to this, to such an extent that, himself no natural scientist, he embarked on the most thorough study of the 'crisis in physics' that his access to the literature allowed. He actually set out to turn the tables on the 'God builders' in the Bolshevik Party by showing that what they thought their strong card – namely that the latest developments in science were leading to the inescapable conclusion that materialism was now old hat – was in reality their weak point. Here Lenin aimed to establish two inter-related points: (1) That the developments in science, physics in particular, far from showing that materialism was out of date were underlining the fact that a purely mechanical materialism was proving to be redundant. In short, the development of science was revealing the fact that the only consistent materialism was a truly *dialectical* materialism. Here lay the significance of the discovery that the atom was not the 'ultimate' particle of matter, but, like nature as a whole, was infinite. (2) Lenin also set out to show not simply that with each new important development in the natural sciences 'materialism had to change its form'. (Cyril Smith notes *this* point.) He wanted to establish something *in addition*. Namely that the very form that physics was taking itself laid the basis for the emergence of idealist philosophies of science among some of science's leading practitioners. He had in mind the increasing mathematisation of physics where the latter was more and more working with symbols and formulae whose connection with the material world was not immediately apparent. It was this that led some of the outstanding scientists astray when it came to philosophical matters, for they took their symbols as the 'only reality'.[21] Matter had 'disappeared' they announced. As Lenin wryly remarked of such people: they were often brilliant scientists but somewhat less than brilliant philosophers.

Here we can see the dialectician Lenin at work. He was not satisfied simply to 'defend' the 'old orthodoxy' (if one may be permitted the phrase.). He did not rest content with Plekhanov's demonstration that what Bogdanov and company were saying did not accord with what Marx and Engels had written on philosophical matters, however correct 'the father of Russian Marxism' might have been. Lenin set out to demonstrate that the new forms of idealism that were being encountered amongst scientists – and ones seized upon by elements in the Bolshevik Party in the aftermath of the defeat of the 1905 Revolution – were themselves engendered by the very development of science, its changing forms in particular. In other words, he set out to defend and develop 'materialist dialectics', and not simply to defend 'materialism', as was Plekhanov's penchant. So when, in his re-reading of Hegel in 1915, Lenin drew attention to the absence of any writings on dialectics in Plekhanov's considerable philosophical output this was by no means an entirely new criticism – although no doubt Lenin now saw matters more clearly and attached greater significance to this lacuna than he had done at an earlier stage.

It is in the same spirit, surely, that we must approach Lenin's remark in the middle of World War I: 'Half a century later, none of the Marxists understood Marx!!' Lenin did not mean, as Smith implies, that the Marxists at that time were *absolutely wrong about everything* that Marx had written. (Naturally, given his initial thesis about Marx and 'Marxism' our author is forced in this silly direction.) Such an interpretation would be sheer childishness. Lenin meant something else, and something far more important: that the conditions of the war had forced a re-examination of many 'old' questions and at the same time made imperative not simply a *defence* of Marxism conceived as a fixed body of knowledge, but a *development* of Marxism. His differences with Plekhanov and others resided here – and they did not start in 1914 either.

The critique of political economy

Before coming to where I consider that Smith's digging has landed him, I feel that his persistent remarks about political economy and Marx's critique thereof warrant some attention. Because I believe they show that he has not at all grasped the relationship between Marx's theoretical endeavours and the nature and tasks of the working class.

Let us start though with a piece of carelessness. I draw attention to it if only because it comes from a man who is always speaking in the sternest terms about the need for 'ruthless objectivity' and the like, as one who charges all the 'Marxists' of having been mistaken about virtually everything. Drawing a distinction between the classical economists and those who followed, members of the vulgar school, he tells us that while the latter was 'inane' '[Adam] Smith, Ricardo and James Mill were tremendously helpful' for Marx for:

> Unlike their successors, they were striving to find an objective explanation of the huge social and economic developments unfolding in Europe during their lifetimes.
>
> (Smith 1996: 76)

Now it is quite impermissible to lump James Mill (father of J.S. Mill) together with Smith and Ricardo. The latter two were leading members of the classical school. James Mill, a close friend of Ricardo, was also his great populariser. But when James Mill was writing (in the early 1820s at around the time of Ricardo's death) the working class was just beginning to emerge. It was this emergence that had brought forth in Ricardo's work a series of contradictions, which were not located just in his thought but were a reflection of objective contradictions. In particular Ricardo was increasingly doubtful about a position he had held in the first edition of his *Principles* (1817), namely that the development of machine production would automatically benefit the young working class. Feeling these contradictions his populariser, Mill senior (1821) tried to overcome them in a purely verbal way, through the re-definition of terms and the like. Thus, with Mill the 'disintegration' of scientific political economy really started, says Marx.[22]

Nor is it correct to say that vulgar economics was simply 'inane'.[23] By vulgar economy Marx meant the work of those economists who were content to rest simply within the realm of how the social relations of capital appeared directly on the surface of society. They took such appearances to be the same as the essence of the relations of 'modern society'. For this Marx rightly condemned them and contrasted their work with that of Ricardo ('the master') who in particular had sought to penetrate to the 'economic anatomy' of the antagonistic class relations of present-day society. But Marx at the same time recognised that in dealing with the 'appearances' of bourgeois society the economists were dealing with real things, 'damned real' things, said Marx. That the social relations appeared to be relations between things (money, etc.) was precisely because under capitalism this is what they really were. In other words, this was no 'illusion' that could be got rid of by the 'critical critic', however 'critical' he might be (and the author of *Marx at the Millennium* is more critical than most). The task of science was to find that force that in life, in practice, would overcome, destroy, really 'smash up' – as Marx put it in a letter to Engels of 1868 – these appearances; that could demonstrate *in reality* that they were historically limited forms of appearance and by no means 'natural', as vulgar thought contended. And Marx discovered that it was in the arena of the *class struggle* that this 'smashing up' would take place. In short, 'the weapons of criticism' must be replaced by 'the criticism of weapons'.

Thus:

> At last we have arrived at the *forms of appearance* which serve as the *starting point* in the vulgar conception.... But from our point of view the thing is now seen differently. The apparent movement is explained.... Then – the whole movement takes place in this form of appearance. Finally since these three (wages, ground rent, profit (interest)) constitute the respective sources of income of the three classes of landowners, capitalists and wage labourers, we have, in conclusion, the *class struggle*, into which the movement and the smash up of the whole business resolves itself.
>
> (Marx 1956: 250)

This is *not* the standpoint of Cyril Smith. He informs us that

> The aim of Marx's 'critique of political economy' is to exhibit and to challenge the assumptions, common to all schools of economics, that there have to be social forms like these [that is capital] distinct from and in opposition to the lives of the people who live within them.
>
> (Smith 1996: 87)

But Marx was far from being the first to grasp that the present social relations of production were not the only ones possible. Utopian socialists such as Robert Owen saw that the great wealth unleashed during the industrial revolution contained the possibility of a society freed from classes and exploitation. And on this basis they tried *in practice* to overcome the relations of capital with the various communities that Owen and others established. That is why Marx and Engels regarded someone such as Owen as a genius. What Owen and his fellow Utopians could not grasp (they came too early) was the force that could bring about this transformation – namely the working class. That is why the Utopians saw themselves as 'educators' of the rest of society. But how the educators themselves were to be educated was a question beyond their (theoretical) purview.

Marx saw in this new class one that in life, out of its inner necessity, was driven to 'criticise' capital and its political economy. His task was *not* as proposed by Cyril Smith but a different one: to give theoretical, conscious, expression to this unconscious struggle of the working class, to demonstrate scientifically that in the struggle of the working class and the owners of capital was concentrated all the contradictions of the capitalist system. That is why Trotsky (*In Defence of Marxism*, 1966) was right when he called Marxism the 'conscious expression of an unconscious process'.

And if Cyril Smith gets it wrong about vulgar economy, he does so equally about Ricardo and the classics: he says (Smith 1996: 129) that Ricardo and Smith were obliged to 'maintain the story that the relations of bourgeois society are the expression of "human nature", that the exchange of equivalents is necessary for human freedom'. 'That was why Marx valued the work of these writers so highly', he adds.

But Marx did not praise Ricardo for equating the human nature produced under capitalism with some supposed universal human nature. (In any case there was nothing particularly new there, for such a prejudice was common to all forms of bourgeois ideology.) On the contrary, as even a beginning student knows, that was one of the serious *limitations* Marx saw in their work. What he *did* value in their achievements was the fact that they marked a decisive stage *along the road* to a scientific understanding of the relations of bourgeois society. There was a profound objectivity in their work – made possible by the fact that it was conducted when the capitalist class still had the real leadership of the nation in its hands, when its battle with the remnants of the feudal order and with the landed aristocracy necessitated a scientific understanding of the laws of modern society. And, within limits, this is what Smith, Ricardo and others achieved. Their work was a step beyond Mercantilism as well as French Physiocracy, just as the work of these latter two schools marked an advance over the economic thought of the Middle Ages (the Schoolmen, etc.). Without it Marxism would have been impossible.

And finally, on this matter of political economy. Throughout the work Cyril Smith repeatedly tells us that the relations of capital are 'mad' (he doesn't approve (Smith 1996: 76) of the older translation of the German *verrückte* as 'absurd'). Indeed the exchange relationship, the fact that human activities are exchanged for 'things' is itself mad, he says. This all sounds very radical in some circles, I suppose, but it is plain wrong – once again because matters are not approached *historically* and *concretely*. Capital is a definite historically-formed social relation which while certainly older than capitalism is not at all coeval with human existence. It may be 'old-hat Marxism' but for a decisive period in its history capitalism was a progressive social force, within limits a force for reason (the growth of science which it encouraged, the emergence of humanism, the Enlightenment as a whole) as against medieval obscurantism. It led to a great socialisation of production, eventually bringing into being a world market. The fact that under the rule of capital the relations through which human beings produce wealth was not a *direct* one, but became a relationship *mediated through things* (money and the like) meant not that a 'crazy' situation existed but something else: that the social relations of production were assuming an ever-more *universal* character. Direct, unmediated relations between producers (as in the primitive commune, or, at a higher level, in the shape of barter) have in the past been a measure of the narrowness, the poverty, of such relations.

Let us take, as an example, Marx's understanding of the law of value. As capitalism develops, the law of value ceases to operate 'directly' as it does in the simple exchange of commodities. The uneven development of capital – reflected amongst other things in the growing unevenness in the organic composition of capital – finds its reflection in the fact that the value of a commodity no longer coincides *immediately* with its price. Rather the latter is determined by the price of production. But this increasing indirectness in the operation of the law of value signifies that there has been a development of socialised production. And likewise with the rate of profit. In *Theories of Surplus Value*, and elsewhere, Marx explains that due to the operation of the law of value, the rate of profit is not determined by the amount of surplus-value that the capitalist extracts through use of his own capital, but by the relationship between capital as a whole and wage labour as a whole.

> It is a matter of indifference to the capitalist whether his commodity contains more or less unpaid labour than other commodities, if into its price enters as much of the general stock of unpaid labour, or the surplus product in which it is fixed, as every other equal quantity of capital will draw from that common stock. In this respect the *capitalists are 'communists'*.
>
> (Marx 1972: 83)

Contra Cyril Smith, Marx was interested not so much in the absurdity (if I may be old-fashioned) of capital as in its *contradictions*, because it was only to the extent that those contradictions could be discovered and their growth and development traced that it was possible to locate those forces that could take humanity beyond the confines of capital. And Marx and Engels found that force in the modern working class. That is why I say that Cyril Smith has not understood at all the relationship between Marx's work on *Capital* and the historical significance of the existence of the working class.

Where must the struggle for the development of Marxism today start from?

Let us ask another question that I believe goes to the very core of this book and its anti-Marxist stance. If we are to separate rigidly Marx from those who sought to defend and extend his work in the manner recommended by Cyril Smith, from what standpoint do we, or can we, commence our re-examination of Marx's work? With an 'open mind' that carries out an unproblematic 're-reading' of the Marx texts? Such a procedure is of course quite impossible and to believe otherwise would be to relapse into the crudest empiricism. Every re-examination of the past, including the past of Marxism, starts from some conceptions or other, not from some imaginary 'clean sheet'. The only question is: *which* conceptions? Are they good ones, based on the highest development of knowledge? Or are they out-dated ones, and therefore merely prejudices in the heads of isolated individuals? (Thus Cyril Smith's book starts from the proposition that everything has gone wrong, generations of 'Marxists' have misled the working class, and this explains the sorry state 'we' are now in.)

Let me start from where I think that the struggle for the re-conquest, the further development, of Marxism must begin and then contrast this with Smith's starting point. Any re-examination of the achievements of Marx today, it seems to me, must commence from what is now new, or becoming new, in the class struggle and what tasks this means for the working class. Only in this way – by starting from 'the standpoint of labour' – can Marxists orient themselves and avoid the meanderings and despair that fill the pages of a book such as this.

From this standpoint our first consideration must be the global, structural, crisis of capital that has been emerging for something like the past two decades. The nature of the crisis, the new features that it has brought to the surface, means that we must not, and cannot, simply 'go back' to Marx's *Capital*, but, naturally on its basis, set out to *go beyond it* – as István Mészáros has insisted. For it is this global-structural crisis of capital that lies behind the collapse of social democracy, reflected in the politics and role of the Labour Party in Britain, and indeed the politics of social democracy throughout Europe. But I want to emphasise something just as crucial, and this against Smith's conception: the task of 'going beyond' Marx, in this case in trying to grasp what is new in the crisis of capital today, must be solidly based not only on Marx's own work *but also on that of all those who attempted, adequately or otherwise, to develop it* – including for instance those such as Lenin, Trotsky, Bukharin, Luxemburg and Hilferding. These figures were prominent among those who set out to grasp the new features of capital (the epoch of imperialism) that coincided approximately with the start of the present century. Every development in science, no matter what the sphere of knowledge, takes place only through a critique of what has gone before, and the outstanding figures in the past knew this to be so (Hegel and Marx in particular). By 'critique' is meant not a simple 'criticism' but a truly concrete negation of the past that preserves all that is valuable from it while at the same time discarding all that has become, or maybe always was, out-dated. We cannot hope to make a development in Marxism that matches up to the new needs of the working class if we start from the presumption that since the days of Marx virtually everything has been wrong, that what has happened in the meanwhile must be divorced from Marx's own work.

In light of this consideration, let us take the book's opening chapter, 'The way we [!] live now'. It draws attention to some features of world capital today that are obvious and to which no Marxist would want to take exception: for instance the dominant role assumed by speculative, parasitic capital. But in a reference to the Gulf War we find the following:

> [it] was explained from many points of view, but always in unexamined terms from the past like 'imperialism', 'democracy', 'North–South divide', and so on. But what was happening could not be captured *by these old phrases.*
>
> (Smith 1996: 13, emphasis added)

Leave aside that empty terms ('democracy', 'North–South divide') – empty because devoid of social content – are lumped together with that of 'imperialism' (a scientific term): *is* the latter simply an 'old phrase' drawn from the past? Well maybe it is. But this has to be *demonstrated*, not simply asserted in this sort of casual, light-minded manner – one that might occasion not a little surprise given the book's ringing call for 'ruthless objectivity' in our treatment of the work of past 'Marxists' (Smith 1996: 62). In any event it is my firm contention that Lenin's analysis of world economy (together with Trotsky's theory of Permanent Revolution) remains indispensable for the analysis of contemporary capitalism. Yet it seems quite in order for this most fastidious scholar to make use of Lenin's work when he wants to but on other occasions when it fits his bill to treat it as something quite redundant. For it was Lenin after all who more than anybody else drew attention to capital in the present century as increasingly 'moribund', as more and more dominated by speculation and other forms of parasitism – and this in a polemic against his 'leader' and philosophical guru Kautsky![24] What a strange world we do live in.

I am suggesting that here, in Smith's attitude to the work of past Marxists on imperialism, is an example of a thoroughly non-dialectical approach, but one I find running through this whole work, its calls for a rejection of mechanical material notwithstanding. I shall attempt to demonstrate this further, in particular when below I come to look at the author's attitude to the history of political economy.

Second, any development of Marxism today must also start with the profound implications for the class struggle of the collapse of the Stalinist bureaucracy. (This is not of course separate from our first point, the deepening crisis of world capital.) Not only was it the politics of this counter-revolutionary bureaucracy that allowed capitalism to survive long after its shelf life was passed (with all that meant for the lives of countless millions of people); it was the Stalinist bureaucracy that was principally responsible for the degradation of Marxism in the period after 1917 – although in its onslaught on Marxism it was undoubtedly able to lay hold of and build on certain weaknesses present in the 'Marxism of the Second International'. The disappearance of this counter-revolutionary bureaucracy has now removed the main barrier between the working class and Marxism. In so doing it has opened up a new stage in the work of Marxists. But, continuing the point made above, Marxists will be able to grasp what new tasks confront them and the working class only if they engage in a thorough re-working of the history of the struggle – political and theoretical – against this Stalinist bureaucracy, taking into account all the deficiencies, even errors, that it involved. And in considering the history of the fight against Stalinism the experiences of the working class – especially at all the great turning points in this fight, such as 1953–1956, culminating in the Hungarian Revolution, Czechoslovakia in 1968 – must be thoroughly analysed from the standpoint of today's tasks. But in any event it is quite false and reactionary to hold that it was impossible to grasp Marxism except through the lens of the Stalinist bureaucracy. To accept this would be to grant the Stalinist bureaucracy victory in its struggle to destroy Marxism completely. It would be to admit that the continuity of the struggle for Marxism was definitively broken and that bourgeois ideology (for Stalinism was a form of such ideology) has scored a complete victory. If this really were so, then the deep pessimism now gripping much of 'the left,' and reflected so clearly in this book, would be well-founded.

Where has the working class gone?

From where does Cyril Smith start in his digging operations to exhume the long-ago buried Marx?

Let me give a series of quotations from his opening chapter. (All emphases are mine.)

> Chapter 1 is a brief sketch of the world today, showing what a mess it is in. This may be pretty obvious, but what is more interesting is that *everybody* seems to find it inconceivable that there can be any other way to live.
>
> (Smith 1996: xii)

> This is a world which becomes less and less comprehensible to its *inhabitants*.
>
> (Smith 1996: 3)

> it has now become *almost unthinkable* that *we* might possibly live in any other way, or even that *we* should try.
>
> (Smith 1996: 3)

> Stalinism had convinced *large numbers* of people that bureaucratic control – this was the *generally accepted* meaning given to the words 'socialism' or 'communism' – was the only alternative to the power of capital.
>
> (Smith 1996: 4)

> three-quarters of a century after the October Revolution, *the belief is widespread* that, however bestial its forms of appearance, the existing social order is the only one possible.
>
> (Smith 1996: 4)

> I have pointed to some features of the world at the end of the century – that people have no control over their own lives, that they are unable to comprehend the consequences of their own actions, that social life is fragmented – and to *the widespread belief that no other way of life is possible.*
>
> (Smith 1996: 4)

> Even *before* [NB] the collapse of the Soviet bloc, the international labour movement, the only force which could [?] challenge the power of capital,

> was on the retreat. During the 1980s, trade unionism shrank in size and influence in every one of the older industrial nations. While the relocation of industry to newly industrialised countries led to the emergence of a new trade unionism, it is significant that, in both old and new movements, the idea of socialism is rarely talked about.
>
> (Smith 1996: 4)[25]

> More and more *thought* is dominated by the certainty that there is no way out.
>
> (Smith 1996: 15)

This is where his 'return to Marx' has brought our author: with the most helpless and hopeless ruminations cast in the most non-theoretical manner about the sorry 'state' 'we're' in. (I mean 'non-theoretical' in the sense that they are based on mere impressions.) The working class hardly features in all this, except that he tells us, significantly, it was in dire shape 'even' before the Stalinist bureaucracy disintegrated.[26] His position is little different from those 'on the left' who in Britain for example have long moaned that Thatcher definitively defeated the working class, that the right-wing lurch by the Labour leaders has left us with no alternative to the Tories. But it was above all the collapse of the Stalinist bureaucracy that was the biggest blow to such lefts, sending them into headlong retreat, with reams on 'midnight at the century' and the like. Here is a measure of the illusions that the 'progressive' intellectual had in the Stalinist bureaucracy and in 'really existing socialism', which, while it might not be perfect, was a step in the direction of socialism. As we have noted similar views were widespread among those claiming to be Trotskyists. This was the meaning of the contention of Ernest Mandel and others that the Stalinist bureaucracy had a 'dual character' and that the development of Soviet economy could take place in isolation from world economy, that this was a process that would extend over centuries. (Pablo's 'centuries of degenerated workers' states [for an exposition of these views see Pablo 1951 – ed.].)

Highly characteristic of the manner in which the book opens is its thoroughly abstract nature. No names are mentioned: we seem to be 'all' in the same leaking boat and heading rapidly for the rocks. I don't know who all these unnamed forces who believe there is no alternative to society as presently constituted are. Certainly the ruling class and its ideological representatives never tire of telling us that 'there is no alternative'. Not by accident did Baroness Thatcher earn the sobriquet TINA so many times did she tell 'us': there is no alternative. But the problem is that there is one force in society which simply cannot reconcile itself to society 'as it is'. That is the working class. Whatever its 'beliefs' or 'moods' may at any moment be, this remains the case. Marxists start not from these moods of the working class – although of course they are not unimportant – but from what the working class must *do*, that by its nature the working class is a class forced to 'help itself'. Or is this yet more 'Marxism' which must now be ditched?

If the book opens from the standpoint of hopelessness, it certainly ends on the same note. Look, for instance, at what Smith says about slavery:

> Marx's contribution was to grasp how the horrors of modern slavery and the African slave trade were the inhuman outcome of the activities of humans.
>
> (Smith 1996: 163)

I'd always thought that slavery involved the enslavement of one group of 'human beings' by another group of human beings, the slave masters who were looking for a quick profit. At least this is what I found in Marx's *Capital*. But no doubt, like all 'the Marxists' down the years I've clearly got it wrong.

But even worse is to follow:

> Under all conditions, while humanity survives, its conflict with its inhuman forms goes on. Since the obscenities of the concentration camps are the work of human beings, albeit dehumanised ones, human beings can erase them. That, it seems to me, is the way that Marx's conceptions can show us the way forward.
>
> (Smith 1996: 163–164)

So this re-examination of Marx has brought us to this sorry and reactionary pass. 'Human beings' were responsible for fascism! This is the worthless hand wringing that liberals are so fond of and one that always serves to obscure the issues at stake. Human beings never exist as such: they always confront nature through definite social relations, in this period of history the antagonistic relations of capital. Fascism was not a sudden outbreak of 'madness' or 'craziness' on the part of 'depraved' people but the working out of the brutal logic of capital in its death throes. The employers found that millions and millions of human beings were 'surplus to requirement', that is the requirement to make profits. And it wasn't 'humanity' 'in general' that paid the price for this crisis: in the main its victims were the working class and persecuted groups scapegoated by capitalism. (Reading passages like this recalls *Private Eye*'s celebrated columnist, the Reverend J.C. Flannel, who ends every comment on the various agonies of our times with the plaintive: 'Ultimately we're all guilty.')

Some conclusions: intellectuals and the working class

This chapter has concentrated on Cyril Smith's view of the history of the Marxist movement, a view which for reasons I have tried to explain, I find quite false and abstract. It is a movement in which the main activity is presented as the exchange of ideas, not one that was bound up intimately with the life and development of the working class. It is just because Smith sees the problems of 'Marxism' as something separate from the problems of the working class that his history is thin and empty. It is this standpoint that leads him to such profound misjudgements about the work and achievements of Plekhanov and others, not to mention Lenin and Trotsky.

The book starts by saying that with the collapse of the regimes of Eastern Europe and the USSR many intellectuals concluded that Marxism was dead. But hasn't Cyril Smith come to precisely this conclusion? His story is this: there was a man called Marx who developed a revolutionary theory that pointed the way to a communist future. All his followers, with the (possible) exception of Engels abandoned his ideas. To one degree or another, Stalinism came to represent 'Marxism'. But if this was the sad fate of Marx's ideas, if they failed for a period of a century and more to get *any* grip in the working-class movement then what are we to say about their strength, their explanatory power? *Why* should we believe Cyril Smith when he tells us that the 'real' ideas of Marx, once uncovered, have much to say for the world we live in today? From the very manner in which he has approached the matter we can have no basis for that assertion.

We must, I believe, start from a quite different angle. Marx's standpoint was the standpoint of 'labour' the standpoint of the working class. The capitalist social formation developed according to strictly objective laws. But Marx uncovered the contradictions of this formation which found their highest expression in the conflict between capital and labour, the class with the future in its hands. This, I believe, constituted the greatest theoretical achievement of the founders of Marxism, and explains why revisionism has always concentrated its attack on this conception. Having arrived (by strictly scientific means) at this conclusion about the world-historical significance of the appearance of the working class in the 1840s, Marx set out to deepen the content of his conclusion, and this produced *Capital.* The fundamental aim of this (incomplete) work was to demonstrate that the working class was destined to overthrow the rule of capital and in so doing lay the basis for socialism, a truly human society founded on the 'free association of the producers'.

Marx's confidence in the working class was not a *personal* matter. It was based on the profoundest theoretical conquests, on the negation (transcending) of the highest achievements of the bourgeoisie and its intellectuals. The world outlook which Marx, together with Engels, established developed in the closest proximity to the struggles of the working class. Marx and Engels were involved in every major struggle of the working class during their long years of exile in Britain – from the Chartist movement, through the days of the First International (whose effective leader was Marx himself) down to the formation of the Second International at the end of Engels's life. It was in the course of this participation, in the struggle to represent in the existing movement its real future, that the theoretical foundations of the movement were enriched and developed. Marx and Engels set out to combat every form of bourgeois ideology that appeared in the working-class movement.

'The world is in a mess' Cyril Smith tells us. But this is not science. To give it its proper name it is *impressionism*. What is the fundamental contradiction of this messy world? Is it that between the 'inhumanity' of the world as it exists today and its potential humanness? To pose the matter in this way provides no way of *really* going beyond capital. Is the working class the only force that can take us beyond capital? If so, our investigations must start not from a catalogue of the disasters, potential and actual, that we face but from the impact that the decaying capitalist system is having on the structure, organisation and consciousness of the working class. These I believe are the tasks that Marxists must now be turning to, and knowing that they do so in a period when the main force that perverted and in large measure discredited Marxism in the working class (Stalinism) is no more. Certainly, in the course of carrying out this task we will deepen our understanding of Marx's work. But this 'return to Marx' has little if anything in common with the route that *Marx at the Millennium* has taken.

[This chapter was first published in *Workers International Press* (1997) 3, June: 11. The version published here was revised by the author – ed.]

Notes

1 Having said this, and unlike most MPs, the present reviewer, must, as they say, 'declare an interest'. I have known Cyril Smith for some 30 years and more, and worked closely with him for a good number of years in the same Trotskyist group: the Socialist Labour League that later became the Workers Revolutionary Party. Cyril Smith made what I still consider an invaluable contribution to the work of these organisations, not least in his defence of the principles of Marxism. So it is with some sadness that I have here to record a series of basic theoretical and political differences with him today, and ones reflected in the book under review.

2 One of the more irritating aspects of this book is that it is littered with references to unnamed 'others,' to 'some people,' to the 'majority of people' and the like. One only wishes that he would have been less coy and have had the courage to 'name names'. But you don't have to be a member of Mensa to surmise that we in the Workers Revolutionary Party and the Workers International number high on this particular list of 'others'.

3 One of the first results of this 'digging', he tells us, was the small book, *Communist Society and Marxist Theory* (Smith 1988). He says that as a result of the book people he had worked with for years stopped talking to him. I can only reply that he has a very selective memory. I for one reviewed the book in a favourable manner, while at the same time pointing to some of the mistakes I thought it made, especially in connection with the relationship between Marx and the classical German philosophical tradition. See *Workers Press*, 17 December 1988.

4 Engels, you will notice, is not formally on the wanted list, not yet at any rate. But he comes perilously close to being sought as a member of the unsavoury gang that helped bury Marx. 'It is quite common to hear Engels blamed exclusively [!] for the vulgarisation of Marx's ideas, but I think this is too easy [!] an option' (Smith 1996: 48). And while it must be admitted that Engels was more than a little guilty of fostering the idea that Marx's *Capital* was a book about 'capitalist economics', 'compared with the later perversions of Marx's work', Engels's errors, you will be relieved to learn, were 'insignificant'. But there again, it was the weaknesses in Engels's writings that were used as part of the material for the later construction of 'Marxism'. So hardly a clean bill of health for The General, who may soon be awarded his inverted commas. This is more than likely when we discover that Engels shared what for Cyril Smith was one of Plekhanov's cardinal errors, namely the belief that Marxism constituted a 'world outlook'. (See Engels's Foreword to the 1888 edition of *Ludwig Feuerbach and the End of Classical German Philosophy*. Referring to the 11 theses that Marx had 'hurriedly scribbled down' Engels (1970) says they were nonetheless invaluable as the 'first document in which is deposited the brilliant germ of the *new world outlook* (emphasis added).)

5 In our haste to denigrate Kautsky, unlike our zealous hunter for the infidel, we should not forget that he was the author of *The Foundations of Christianity*, 1972, and many other important works [e.g. *The Economic Doctrines of Karl Marx*, 1925 – ed.]. A glance at Engels's letters to Kautsky underlined that they were both dealing with the living problems of a movement and that while Engels clearly detected weaknesses in Kautsky he by no means had the wholly negative attitude displayed by Cyril Smith. But there again, unlike some of us, Engels did not live in 1996.

6 This is of course not a new story. That *Materialism and Empirio-Criticism* represents 'kindergarten materialism' (as the French anti-Marxist Roger Garaudy – a one-time prominent 'theoretician' in the French Stalinist movement once put it – see Ilyenkov 1982) and only when he came to a re-study of Hegel did Lenin become interested in 'dialectics' is a fairy tale told by anti-Marxists for generations. E.V. Ilyenkov's *Leninist Dialectics and the Metaphysics of Positivism*, 1982, is a powerful rejoinder to this sort of argument and therefore to the ideas defended in the book under review. We shall return to this work below, as well as to work from comrades in our ranks who also took exception to the sort of tale retailed by Garaudy and others. See particularly C. Slaughter 1963, *Lenin on Dialectics*.

7 'A thinker of the stature of Jurgens Habermas' is cited as exemplar of this sad fact! [Refers to Habermas 1989 – ed].

8 This is an important point if only because Cyril Smith makes much play of the fact that bourgeois science, or rather the bourgeois philosophy of science, tries to present the world as something standing quite apart from the activities of human beings. In his approach to Stalinism I believe that our author shares just this viewpoint.

9 This distinction is absent in Smith's treatment of the bureaucracy.

10 See, for example, C. Slaughter, *Lenin on Dialectics*, 1963.

11 In an analogous way there are those today unable or unwilling to appreciate that the collapse of the Stalinist bureaucracy poses qualitatively new theoretical, political and organisation tasks for Marxists, as well as posing new tasks for the working class. (More specifically their view as to what a 'party' is cannot get beyond the sects to which they are habituated.)

12 Compare the attitude of Cyril Smith with that of Trotsky towards Plekhanov shortly after his death:

> COMRADES! We are living in an epoch when a particular man's life seems nothing or almost nothing in the colossal whirlpool of events. During the war millions perished and died, and hundreds of thousands perished during the revolution. In such a movement and such a struggle of the human masses an individual personality is insignificant. Nevertheless even in a period of the greatest mass events there are those particular deaths which do not permit passing by in silence without attention. Such is the death of Plekhanov…
>
> Plekhanov belonged to that generation of the Russian revolution and to that stage in its development when only small bands of intellectuals had joined the revolutionary struggle…
>
> It was he who 34 years before the October proved that the Russian Revolution would only triumph in the form of a revolutionary movement of workers. He strove to place the fact of the class movement of the proletariat at the root of the revolutionary struggle of the first circles of intellectuals. It is this that we learnt from him and in this lies the foundation not only of Plekhanov's activity but also of the whole of our revolutionary struggle. To this we have remained true right up to the present day. In the subsequent development of the revolution Plekhanov abandoned that class which he had so excellently served in the grimmest period of reaction…
>
> But now when the fact that Plekhanov is no longer among the living has stabbed our consciousness we can sense in ourselves alongside an irreconcilable revolutionary hostility to all those who stand in the way of the working class,

> sufficient ideological breadth to recall Plekhanov now not as the one we fought against with every firmness but as the one from whom we learnt the alphabet of revolutionary Marxism. Plekhanov did not place in the weaponry of the working class a single sword he had sharpened or a single spear that does not mercilessly strike home ... [W]e shall go on making use of the best part of the spiritual legacy which Plekhanov has left to us. He is dead but the ideas which he forged in the best days of his life are immortal just as the proletarian revolution is immortal. He is dead but we, his pupils, are living and fighting under the banner of Marxism, under the banner of the proletarian revolution. And before we turn to today's struggle against oppression and exploitation, against lies and slander, I call on all of you to silently and solemnly honour the memory of Plekhanov and stand up.
>
> (Trotsky 1972b: 94–95)

And while Trotsky did not praise Kautsky in quite the same terms, he did start from a consideration of the period in which Kautsky had lived and worked. Thus:

> Kautsky was without doubt the most outstanding theoretician of the Second International and over the major part of his conscious life he represented and generalized the *better* sides of the Second International. Kautsky the propagandist and vulgarizer of Marxism saw his principal theoretical mission in reconciling reform and revolution. But he himself took shape ideologically in an epoch of reform. For him reform was the reality. Revolution was a theoretical generalization and a historical perspective.
>
> (Trotsky 1972b: 65)

13 We have the testimony of Krupskaya that Lenin was studying Hegel while in exile in Siberia in the early 1890s. One of Lenin's comrades in the League for the Struggle for the Emancipation of the Working Class, also exiled alongside him in Siberia wrote:

> I remember, for instance, that at the time he studied *Science of Logic* by Hegel. And he enthusiastically told us, his comrades, of the wealth of thought contained in this treatise, without noting, it seems, that many of us (I can boldly assert this for myself anyway) were not yet ready to understand the ideas of Hegelian philosophy.
>
> (*Reminiscences of Lenin* (1969) vol. 2, Moscow: 69 (in Russian), quoted in Suvorov 1981: 15)

14 Before he came to write *Materialism and Empirio-Criticism* Lenin had pointed out the limited nature of Plekhanov's criticism of the Machists. In connection with the preface to a Russian edition of Engels's *Ludwig Feuerbach and the Outcome of Classical German Philosophy* published in 1905 Lenin wrote: 'How petty are his sallies and "pinpricks" against the Machists. For me this is the more to be regretted since Plekhanov's criticism of Mach seems to me to be essentially correct.' As Lenin (1977: 355) also pointed out in a footnote in *Materialism and Empirio-Criticism*: 'Plekhanov in his criticism of Machism was less concerned with refuting Mach than with dealing a factional blow at Bolshevism. For this petty and miserable exploitation of fundamental theoretical differences, he has already been deservedly punished.'

15 It is clear that Lenin repudiated the idea that movements should split on the basis of philosophical differences. This does not of course mean that a sharp struggle on the 'theoretical front' is not at all times necessary.

16 'Our struggle cannot be understood at all unless the concrete circumstances of each battle are studied. But once that is done, we see clearly that development does indeed proceed dialectically, by way of contradictions' (Lenin 1965b: 411).

17 Dare I say it but I find here something of an echo of the days of the Healy (Workers Revolutionary) party with its obsession with 'philosophy' (here the inverted commas are imperative) to the exclusion of virtually all other theoretical questions.

18 This produced Lenin's first major work, *What the Friends of the People are and How they Fight the Social-Democrats* (1972b, first published in 1894).

19

> On the one side is the Mass as the passive, spiritless, unhistorical, *material* element of history. On the other is *the* Spirit, *Criticism*, Herr Bruno and Co. as the active element from which all *historical* action proceeds. The act of transforming society is reduced to the *cerebral activity* of Critical Criticism.
>
> (Marx and Engels 1975: 86)

20

> To analyse Machism and at the same time to ignore this connection [between Machism and a trend in the new physics] – as Plekhanov does – is to scoff at the spirit of dialectical materialism, i.e. to sacrifice the method of Engels to the letter of Engels.
>
> (Lenin 1977: 251)

21 'The crisis in physics lies in the conquest of the realm of physics by the mathematical spirit' (Lenin 1977: 307).

22

> With the master [Ricardo] what is new and significant develops vigorously amid the 'manure' of contradictions out of the contradictory phenomena.... It is different with the disciple [James Mill]. His raw material is no longer reality, but the new theoretical form in which the master had sublimated it. It is in part the *theoretical disagreement of opponents of the new theory* and in part the *often paradoxical relationship of this theory to reality* which drive him [Mill] to seek *to refute* his opponents and *explain away* reality. In doing so, he entangles himself in contradictions and with his attempt to solve these he demonstrates the beginning *disintegration of the theory* which he dogmatically espouses.
>
> (Marx 1972: 84–85)

23 There is another confusion in the treatment of the history of political economy. Cyril Smith pours scorn on present-day economics – not a difficult job. But he makes a mistake in characterising present day textbook economics as simply 'vulgar'. In the evolution of economics Marx notes that vulgar economy – that which confines itself simply to recording uncritically the categories of bourgeois economics – gives way to *apologetics*. That is a school of economists who appear to set out *deliberately* to defend the existing social order. Thus Nassau Senior invented the 'theory' that all value was created in the last working hour of the day, just at the moment when the working class was coming forward with a powerful campaign for the reduction of the working day! Similarly profits and interest are explained either in terms that some people are prepared to *wait* before they enjoy the consumption of wealth, and profit is therefore the reward for waiting; or they *abstain* from such consumption and profit is the reward for such abstinence. This is a step beyond vulgar economics for now any concern with science has been abandoned; the economists are now merely 'prize fighters' for the owners of capital. For an example of Marx's scrupulous treatment of the history of economics, of his demonstration of the degeneration of even vulgar economy see *Theories of Surplus Value*, Part III, 500–503. Marx always sets out to grasp these developments from the standpoint of the sharpening contradictions of capital, and not from the stupidities of the individuals concerned.

24 It perhaps should be added that one of the important challenges that we, that is those of us in the Socialist Labour League at the time, took up in defence of Lenin against his detractors (I have Michael Kidron principally in mind) concerned just this question of the dominance of finance capital in this epoch. It was Kidron (1974) and others who told us that Lenin was old hat, that in the functioning of contemporary capitalism industrial capital was as decisive as finance capital, if not more so. But alas perhaps this too was just another piece of 'Marxism' that we must now junk?

25 It never seems to occur to Cyril Smith that the collapse in levels of employment was a reflection of capital's intensifying crisis, nor that in this situation the 'old' trade unionism was increasingly inadequate.

26 There is a general point about the place of 'class' in Marx's analysis (historical materialism) that is at issue in the book under review. Not least among the many things that the 'Marxists' got wrong was their understanding of class. 'The place of classes in Marx's view of history is not as simple as "Marxists" have often supposed' (Smith 1996: 92), Cyril Smith tells us and he proceeds to remind us that the famous Preface to the *Critique of Political Economy* (Marx 1987) does not mention classes at all. Drawing attention to the fact that Ricardo's work starts with the notion that modern society is divided into three fundamental classes, distinguished by their different 'revenues', and, implying that this is how 'Marxism' has normally viewed classes he says: 'But what Marx wants to know is how the social relation, capital, shapes our lives, and how the division into classes and sub-classes helps to hide and constrict humanity' (Smith 1996: 93). I suggest that this was *not* the nature of Marx's criticism of classical political economy. While praising Ricardo's concentration on the analysis of classes and their relationships, he chastises him for taking these classes for granted, as simply 'given' 'by nature'. In short he takes exception to Ricardo's fundamental standpoint, that of capital.

As to the absence of a reference to 'class' in the Preface to the *Critique.* Unfortunately Cyril Smith does not spell out what he thinks are the implication of this lacuna. But it does *not* mean that Marx had abandoned his contention (in the *Manifesto*) that all (written) history had been the history of class struggle. Although the root of the contradictions of capitalism lay in that between the development of the productive forces and the social form (capital) in which these productive forces were increasingly being entrapped, the *resolution* of that conflict lay in the class struggle, specifically in the sphere of politics 'where men become conscious of that conflict *and fight it out*' (Marx 1987: 263).

References

Blake, W.J. (1939) *An American Looks at Karl Marx*, New York: Cordon Company.

Dobb, M. (1940, second edition) *Political Economy and Capitalism: Some Essays in Economic Tradition*, London: Routledge & Kegan Paul.

Engels, F. (1970) Foreword to 'Ludwig Feuerbach and the end of classical German philosophy', in *Selected Works in One Volume*, Second Printing, Moscow and London: Progress Publishers and Lawrence & Wishart, pp. 584–585.

Engels, F. (1977) *Anti-Dühring*, Seventh Printing, Moscow: Progress Publishers. Progress Publishers 1947 edition, online, available at: www.marxists.org/archive/marx/works/1877/anti-duhring (accessed 3 December 2011).

Gramsci, A. (1971) *Selections from the Prison Notebooks*, London: Lawrence & Wishart and New York International Publishers. Online, available at: www.marxists.org/archive/gramsci/prison_notebooks/selections.htm (accessed 15 August 2011).

Grossman, H. (1992) *The Law of Accumulation and Breakdown of the Capitalist System*, London: Pluto. Translated from1929 publication, online, available at: www.marxists.org/archive/grossman/1929/breakdown/index.htm (accessed 12 August 2011).

Habermas, J. (1989) 'The reconstruction of historical materialism' in *Habermas on Historical Materialism*, Bloomington: Indiana University Press.

Ilyenkov, E.V. (1982) *Leninist Dialectics and the Metaphysics of Positivism*, London: New Park Publications. Online, available at: www.marxists.org/archivey/ilyenkov/works/positive/index.htm (accessed 18 August 2011).

Kautsky, K. (1925) *The Economic Doctrines of Karl Marx*, London: A. & C. Black. Based on 1936 edition re-published by NCLC Publishing Society, online, available at: www.marxists.org/archive/kautsky/1903/economic/index.htm (accessed 17 October 2011).

Kautsky, K. (1972) *Foundations of Christianity: A Study in Christian Origins*, New York: Monthly Review Press. Russell and Russell 1953 edition, online, available at: www.marxists.org/archive/kautsky/1908/christ/index.htm (accessed 18 August 2011)

Kidron, M. (1974) *Capitalism and Theory*, London: Pluto.

Korsch, K. (1963) *Karl Marx*, New York: Russell & Russell. Original 1938 edition, online, available at: www.marxists.org/archive/korsch/1938/karl-marx/index.htm (accessed 18 August 2011).

Lenin, V.I. (1934) 'Preface to the Russian translation of Marx's letters to Kugelmann', in Marx, K. *Letters to Dr. Kugelmann*, London: Martin Lawrence.

Lenin, V.I. (1964) 'Imperialism, the highest stage of capitalism', in *Collected Works*, vol. 22, Moscow and London: Progress Publishers and Lawrence & Wishart, pp. 185–304.

Lenin, V.I. (1965a) 'Once again on the trade unions, the current situation, and the mistakes of Trotsky and Bukharin', in *Collected Works*, vol. 32, Moscow and London: Progress Publishers and Lawrence & Wishart, pp. 70–107.

Lenin, V.I. (1965b, second edition) 'One step forward, two steps back', in *Collected Works*, vol. 7, Moscow and London: Progress Publishers and Lawrence & Wishart, pp. 203–425.

Lenin, V.I. (1972a) 'The economic content of Narodism and the criticism of it in Mr Struve's book', in *Collected Works*, vol. 1, Moscow and London: Progress Publishers and Lawrence & Wishart, pp. 333–507.

Lenin, V.I. (1972b) 'What the friends of the people are and how they fight the Social Democrats', in *Collected Works*, vol. 1, Third Printing, Moscow and London: Progress Publishers and Lawrence & Wishart, pp. 129–332.

Lenin, V.I. (1973) 'What is to be done? Burning questions of the moment', in *Collected Works*, vol. 5, Third Printing, Moscow and London: Progress Publishers and Lawrence & Wishart, pp. 347–529.

Lenin, V.I. (1977) 'Materialism and empirio-criticism', in *Collected Works*, vol. 14, Fourth Printing, Moscow and London: Progress Publishers and Lawrence & Wishart, pp. 17–388.

Lenin, V.I. (1987) 'Marxism and Revisionism' in *Collected Works*, vol. 15, Fifth Printing, Moscow and London: Progress Publishers and Lawrence & Wishart, pp. 29–39.

Marx, K. (1956) *Marx Engels Selected Correspondence*. Moscow and London: Foreign Languages Publishing House and Lawrence & Wishart.

Marx, K. (1957) *Capital*, vol. II, Moscow and London: Foreign Languages Publishing House and Lawrence & Wishart.

Marx, K. (1959) *Capital*, vol. III, Moscow and London: Foreign Languages Publishing House and Lawrence & Wishart.

Marx, K. (1961) *Capital*, vol. I, Moscow and London: Foreign Languages Publishing House and Lawrence & Wishart.

Marx, K. (1972) *Theories of Surplus Value*. Part III, London: Lawrence & Wishart.

Marx, K. (1987) Preface to 'A contribution to the critique of political economy', in *Karl Marx Frederick Engels Collected Works*, vol. 29, Moscow and London: Progress Publishers and Lawrence & Wishart, pp. 259–265.

Marx K. and Engels, F. (1975) 'The Holy Family, or critique of critical criticism. Against Bruno Bauer and company' in *Karl Marx Frederick Engels Collected Works*, vol. 4, Moscow and London: Progress Publishers and Lawrence & Wishart, pp. 5–211.

Mattick, P. (1969) *Marx and Keynes: The Limits of the Mixed Economy*, London: Merlin.

Meek, R.L. (1956) *Studies in the Labour Theory of Value*, London: Lawrence & Wishart.

Meek, R.L. (1973) 'The law of value in Ricardo and Marx. A reply to Mr. Pilling', *Economy and Society*, 2 (4): 499–506.

Mészáros, I. (1995) *Beyond Capital*, London: Merlin.

Mikhailov, F.T. (1980) *The Riddle of the Self*, Moscow: Progress Publishers. Online, available at: www.marxists.org/archive/mikhailov/works/riddle/index.htm (accessed 22 August 2011).

Mill, James (1965 [1821]) *Elements of Political Economy*, third edition revised and corrected, New York: A.M. Kelley. Online, available at: www.econ.uba.ar/www/institutos/economia/Ceplad/HPE_Bibliografia_digital/James%20Mill.pdf (accessed 22 August 2011).

Pablo, M. (1951) 'On the duration and the nature of the period of transition from Capitalism to Socialism'. Online, available at: www.marxists.org/archive/pablo/1951/06/stalinism.htm (accessed 11 December 2011).

Pilling, G. (1972) 'The law of value in Ricardo and Marx', *Economy and Society*, 1 (3): 281–307.

Pilling, G. (1980) *Marx's Capital: Philosophy and Political Economy*, London: Routledge and Kegan Paul. (Pilling, G. (2009), *Marx's 'Capital' (Routledge Revivals): Philosophy and Political Economy*, London: Routledge).

Plekhanov, G. (1976) *Selected Philosophical Works*, Moscow: Progress Publishers.

Ricardo, D. (1817) *On the Principles of Political Economy, and Taxation*. (Ricardo, D. (1953, reprint of 1951 first edition) *The Works and Correspondence of David Ricardo*, vol. 1, *The Principles of Political Economy and Taxation*, Edited with an Introduction by P. Sraffa, in collaboration with M.H. Dobb, Cambridge: Cambridge University Press.)

Rosdolsky, R. (1977) *The Making of Marx's 'Capital'*, London: Pluto.

Slaughter, C. (1963) *Lenin on Dialectics: An Introduction to the Philosophical Notebooks of Lenin*, London: New Park Publications. Labour Press, 1962 edition, online, available at: www.marxists.org/reference/subject/philosophy/works/en/cliff.htm (accessed 13 December 2011).

Smith, A. (1976) *An Inquiry into the Nature and Causes of the Wealth of Nations*, R.H. Campbell and A.S. Skinner (eds) vols 1 and 2, Oxford: Clarendon Press.

Smith, C. (1988) *Communist Society and Marxist* Theory, London: Index Books.

Smith, C. (1996) *Marx at the Millennium*, London: Pluto Press. Online, available at: www.marxists.org/reference/archive/smith-cyril/works/millenni/index.htm (accessed 13 December 2011).

Suvorov, L.N. (1981) *Marxist Philosophy at the Leninist* Stage, Moscow: Progress Publishers.

Trotsky, L. (1966) *In Defence of* Marxism, London: New Park Publications. Online. available at: www.marxists.org/archive/trotsky/idom/dm/index.htm (accessed 22 August 2011).

Trotsky, L. (1972a) *The Revolution Betrayed. What is the Soviet Union and Where is it Going?* New York: Pathfinder. 1937 first edition, online available at: www.marxists.org/archive/trotsky/1936/revbet/index.htm (accessed 22 August 2011).

Trotsky, L. (1972b) *Political Profiles*, London: New Park Publications. Online, available at: www.marxists.org/archive/trotsky/profiles/index.htm (accessed 22 August 2011).

8 A very peculiar capitalism

Some reflections on the 'decline of Britain'[1]

> The country which is more developed industrially only shows, to the less developed, the image of its own future.
>
> (Preface to the first German edition of *Capital*, Marx 1961a: 8–9)

Discussion about the causes and consequences of the 'decline of Britain' shows little sign of flagging (for a recent survey see Gamble 1994). Indeed such discussion threatens to become something of a national pastime, perhaps stimulated over the recent past by the growing recognition that the 'Thatcher experiment' did little to arrest this decline. But if today's debate is intense, it is far from new. Indeed discussion about the 'British disease' can be traced back to a period when the symptoms of the illness were hardly visible. Thus in 1844 Frederick Engels, that young and recent arrival to Manchester, was even then anticipating the challenge to the 'workshop of the world' that was to come from North America.

> German manufacture is now making great efforts, and that of America has developed with giant strides. America, with its inexhaustible resources, with its unmeasured coal and iron fields, with its unexampled wealth of water-power and its navigable rivers, but especially with its energetic, active population, in comparison with which the English are phlegmatic dawdlers, – America has in less than ten years created a manufacture which already competes with England in the coarser cotton goods, has excluded the English from the markets of North and South America, and holds its own in China, side by side with England. If any country is adapted to holding a monopoly of manufacture, it is America.
>
> (Engels 1975a: 579–580)

Some 40 years later a Royal Commission, appointed to examine the depressed state of trade and industry, was equally concerned with the threat from abroad, although in this case the principal challenge was seen as coming from Germany:

> We are beginning to feel the effects of foreign competition in quarters where our trade formerly enjoyed a practical monopoly. In every quarter of the world the perseverance and enterprise of the Germans are making themselves felt.
>
> (Quoted in Hutchison 1951: 19)

At the end of the twentieth century signs of the decline that agitated nineteenth-century commentators are even more evident: the collapse of large swathes of industry; the chronic weakness of the once mighty pound sterling, long ago unable to look the dollar in the face and incapable of preserving its place in the European monetary system; heavy and persistent unemployment, concentrated especially among young people; the loss of world markets, even where British industry in the past enjoyed a monopoly.

(The so-called 'recovery' of the British economy after 1992 was due entirely to the sharp fall in the value of sterling after ejection from the Exchange Rate Mechanism and the consequent boost this gave to exports. But even this 'recovery' proved short-lived, for as the value of the pound rose against the D-mark and the French franc, exports were immediately hit while at the same time inflationary pressures began to mount, requiring steep rises in the cost of borrowing money.)

If the evidence of decline is palpable and pervasive and if discussion about the malaise has been long drawn out it is as yet an inconclusive discussion.[2] In a short space it is difficult to classify the various, often contradictory, explanations for Britain's loss of industrial and commercial power but broadly speaking we can group them under three heads (Dintenfass 1992 provides a good survey.)

The most frequently encountered explanation for Britain's inability to compete with the economies of Japan, the United States and Western Europe is the failure of manufacturers to replace at an adequate rate those tools and techniques that enabled Britain to rise to pre-eminence towards the end of the eighteenth century. Whatever can be said of such an explanation, it is far from new, for it first emerged when Britain was still undisputed 'Workshop of the World'. Its corollary is that when the right sort of machinery is put in place and there is a labour force trained to operate it Britain has little problem in competing successfully in the world market. Closely allied to this point is the criticism of the inadequate British educational system that, unlike the German system in particular, is insufficiently concentrated on technical and vocational training. (This was undoubtedly one of the major concerns of the report of the Great Britain National Committee of Inquiry into Higher Education (Dearing Report) that appeared in 1997.)

In explaining Britain's poor economic performance others have pointed to what they regard as the persistent 'bias of British capital'. The nub of the argument here is that the British ruling class has for decade after decade invested disproportionately abroad at the expense of investment at home. According to this view, for a long period the City is seen as having established a separate and privileged niche for itself in the British class structure; uninterested in industry the

City is principally concerned with lending abroad to the detriment of investment in domestic industry.

Proponents of this view point to the undeniable fact that the decades when the competitiveness of British industry started manifestly to wane – that is from the 1870s onwards – coincided with the export of a considerable volume of British capital. This lead to the notion, sharply expressed in the recent past among the advocates of an 'alternative economic strategy', that the huge outflow of funds from Britain for a century and more, by diverting capital from domestic industry and trade is largely responsible for Britain's decline and for her 'de-industrialisation' in particular. This, it is claimed, has been especially true of new hi-tech industries – for here the indifference of the City of London to the needs of domestic industry has been especially injurious in the face of high initial capital requirements.

This raises a question that is illustrative of the argument of this chapter as a whole – namely did British experience here *anticipate* the path that capital as a whole was to take in the twentieth century? Or, putting the matter another way: was the export of capital a necessary feature of the development (more strictly the decline) of capital as a whole that was first witnessed in Britain? For Lenin (1964), unlike Kautsky, the features of imperialism did not arise from 'policy options' and this was true of the increasing tendency of the metropolitan capitalist powers to export capital on an ever-larger scale, with Britain in the vanguard. The drive to find outlets for 'surplus' capital arose as a result of the operation of 'the most important law of political economy' (Marx 1973: 748) – the tendency for the rate of profit to fall. If Britain began to export capital on a considerable scale some quarter of a century before her major rivals this surely anticipated that parasitism that was to afflict capital as a whole in the present century. As we shall note later, Germany – the country usually held up as the model by many who deplore the role of the City of London, especially its neglect of 'home industry' – is now beginning to export capital on a scale far greater than Britain, this under the impact of a mounting domestic crisis.

Connected to the view that the export of capital and the privileged place occupied by the City of London has had a deleterious effect on British economy is the contention that it is in British institutions and culture that the root cause of Britain's decline, the decline of her industry in particular, is to be located. Two recent writers have expressed the matter thus:

> Entrenched institutional structures – including the structures of industrial relations, industrial organization, educational systems, financial intermediation, international trade, and state-enterprise relations – constrained the ability of individuals, groups, or corporate entities to transform the productive system.
>
> (Elbaum and Lazonik 1984: 568)

Sir Keith (later Lord) Joseph – the major ideological influence in the early phases of 'Thatcherism' – expressed a similar point of view:

> Unlike some countries in Europe and the New World, e.g. Holland and the United States, Britain never had a capitalist ruling class or a stable *haute bourgeoisie.* As a result, capitalist or bourgeois values have never shaped thought and institutions as they have in some countries.
>
> (Joseph 1976, quoted in Ingham 1984)[3]

Related to this standpoint is the argument that the British middle classes have a deep antipathy to industry in favour of the pursuit of leisure and political service. Power in the state, it is claimed, has always rested firmly in the hands of those drawn from the gentry or from those of humbler origins educated in its mores. Industrialists have themselves been persistently excluded from the seats of power in Whitehall and consequentially decision-making has invariably exhibited if not an outright hostility then certainly an indifference to industry's needs. British manufacturers, it seems, have long envied the knights of the shires; and those who could abandon industry and trade for a life of gentility have eagerly done so. Those obliged to remain have continued to harbour 'anti-business values'. Thus it has been this gentrification of the English middle classes that has created a 'dampening of industrial energies'. (Weiner 1981, provides a good account of this view.)

(Not least among the virtues of 'Thatcherism', according to supporters of the Iron Lady, was that she set out to reverse this situation. But whether the culture her administrations encouraged did anything to revitalise British industry, or whether it simply stimulated graft and corruption among a new breed of money-makers is a moot point.)

How are we to evaluate this manifest decline of Britain? Is it, as many hold, simply the retribution meted out by history to the British ruling class for having dared to be first in the field?[4] Or is this decline, whatever its roots, symptomatic of a more universal crisis for capitalism as a historical system? If this latter is the case then the decline of Britain can be examined only from the standpoint of trends in world economy. In this sense, is Britain's development peculiar only in the sense that it exhibits trends within the capitalist system as a whole in their most extreme, 'pure' form? In which case is Britain at last holding up a mirror for the rest of the world, as Marx said it would? Other matters are involved: how are we to evaluate the decline of British industry, a fact much bemoaned by many commentators? Is the de-industrialisation of Britain the result of long-term policy mistakes? Or is it symptomatic of something else: namely the decline of capital as such, and therefore not something peculiar to Britain?

The 'Anderson–Nairn thesis' and its criticism

Given the vastness of the literature and the many questions, including those referred to above, it is proposed to concentrate what follows around a neglected contribution by the Canadian Marxist, Ellen Meiksins Wood (1991). I do so because this author has set out to provide a synthesis of recent work in this field that, although written from an explicitly Marxist standpoint, eschews the sort of slavish adherence to 'orthodoxy' which in the past has vitiated much of the work of Marxists. Her contribution, I believe, allows us to look afresh at issues that many have long regarded as settled. Although her work cannot be seen as original in the conventional sense of that term – in that, like the present writer, she has not consulted primary sources, as would a historian – her work *is* original in that it departs strikingly from many of the conventional accounts of the roots of Britain's supposed backwardness, including many of those proffered by the left.

As we have suggested, most explanations of the decline of British capital are content to confine their attention to the last century or so. One striking exception to this was the work of Perry Anderson and Tom Nairn that sought much deeper roots to the 'English malaise' (see especially, Anderson 1968). Further, their account of the peculiar trajectory of English history was cast in Marxist terms while simultaneously drawing on elements from the three broad approaches to the decline of Britain indicated above. First appearing in the 1960s (Anderson 1964), it was caustically, and many believed successfully, challenged by the late E.P. Thompson (1965). Anderson (1987) was to return to his arguments a decade later, presenting his case in a somewhat modified form which took into account Thompson's trenchant criticisms.

What was the 'Anderson–Nairn' thesis? [See Ellen Meiksins Wood 1991 for a more detailed account than presented here, especially pp. 11–17 – ed.] In its original form it can be summarised as follows: because the capitalist economy in England originated in the countryside, dominated by a landed aristocracy, it is an impure capitalism, 'improper', immature, inadequately modern and, above all, peculiar – a sort of 'bastard capitalism' burdened with a pre-modern state and a correspondingly impoverished ideology, empiricism. British capitalism, first in the field, was a feeble, deviant, capitalism, confined to small scale-production typified by the Lancashire textile industries. This was in marked contrast to the experience of Other Countries where a 'proper' bourgeoisie made a much cleaner and decisive, albeit belated, break with the (pre-modern) past, where a powerful heavy industry was developed, assisted throughout by a strong capitalist state. This peculiar British history, which also involved a 'wrong' relationship between the City and industry, leaves its mark right down to today – not simply in the parlous state in which British industry finds itself and the continuing impoverished thought that has traditionally marked the British intelligentsia, but also in the shape of a working class dominated by a pusillanimous 'Labourism' – and now by 'new Labourism'.

As Looker (1988) has shown, Anderson was to modify his position somewhat. There are two points to be made about this change. Whereas the chief barrier to the 'proper' capitalist development of Britain had, in the first version, been principally the interests of the landed aristocracy,[5] Anderson's later position laid more stress on the role of the City and merchant capital as forces which had arrested British development.[6] In the second place, Anderson tended to widen the scope of his original argument, for he now seems to believe that the failure to complete the bourgeois revolution can be extended to France and other countries. It is noteworthy that this thesis seems, prima facie, to contradict the ideas of 'postmodernism', the notion that we live in an epoch where, precisely because so-called 'liberal capitalism' has completed its work of modernisation, and under conditions where 'socialism' in Eastern Europe and the former Soviet Union has collapsed, it is no longer appropriate to speak of 'society', no longer possible to engage in the 'grand narrative', no longer feasible to speak meaningfully of 'ideology'; everything is reduced to the contingent, the small scale, to the local.

But I believe that these two positions are two sides of the same coin in so far as both hold that capitalism has a long future ahead of it. For some (Anderson) capitalism has yet to complete its work; for others that work is already completed, liberal capitalism is firmly in place, and the 'end of history' is upon us. Neither accepts that the contradictions of the present economic system make possible and indeed necessitate the transition to a newer, and higher, form of society.

Following Thompson's lead, many have of course challenged the view that Anderson initially advanced. It would be fatuous to contest the Anderson–Nairn claim that British economic development, and indeed her overall historical evolution, has been highly peculiar. Given Britain's place as the first industrial capitalist nation in the world, the first to experience what, before the arrival of the currently fashionable 'new economic history', used to be known as an 'industrial revolution', this is hardly surprising. It is obvious that there were series of features uniquely associated with the origins and development of capitalism in Britain that were not replicated exactly anywhere else in the world. But the question remains: what meaning and character are to be ascribed to these peculiarities? Are they deviations from a Weberian-like 'ideal type' of capitalism? Or are these self-same peculiarities to be regarded, as Meiksins Wood and others are inclined to do, from just the opposite angle – as indications that the penetration of capitalism in Britain was more thorough-going than anywhere else in the world, as expressive of the fact that Britain may be suffering not from any 'backwardness' but from the fact that it is the most capitalistically-developed country in the world?[7]

Much rides on the answer to this question, no less for an understanding of the nature of capitalism as for an interpretation of the unique path taken by social relations in Britain.

The state and the supposed weakness of British capital

As we have noted, one of the complaints of writers such as Anderson is that the British state has never undergone a complete process of modernisation: the nineteenth-century doctrine of laissez-faire and the existence of a 'minimalist state' expressed just this precocity of British capitalism in contrast to the Continent where a series of thorough-going bourgeois revolutions created modern, centralised and rational states that were thereby equipped to take a decisive hand in economic development and management.

It is, to put it no more strongly, at least arguable that the very facts adduced here to establish the supposed weakness of the British state testify not at all to the absence of a thorough-going transformation of social relations in this country. Quite the opposite may well be the case: the fact that for much of the last century the state in Britain played a relatively minor role in economic matters could just be an indication of the extent to which capitalist social relations had been established in this country, in contrast to the situation in much of the rest of Europe.

Here, lurking below the surface of discussions about the peculiar development of British state and economy are arguments about the very nature of capital itself. What is the *specifica differentia* of capitalism? For Marx the distinction between one social system and another turns on the manner in which the economic surplus is pumped out of the direct producers.

> The specific economic form, in which unpaid surplus-labour is pumped out of direct producers, determines the relationship of rulers and ruled, as it grows directly out of production itself and, in turn, reacts upon it as a determining element. Upon this, however, is founded the entire formation of the economic community which grows up out of the production relations themselves, thereby simultaneously its specific political form. It is always the direct relationship of the owners of the conditions of production to the direct producers – a relation always naturally corresponding to a definite stage in the development of the methods of labour and thereby its social productivity – which reveals the innermost secret, the hidden basis of the entire social structure, and with it the political form of the relation of sovereignty and dependence, in short, the corresponding specific form of the state.
>
> (Marx 1959: 772)

According to Marx, the uniqueness of capitalism resides in the fact that this surplus – in the form of surplus-value – is extracted from the direct producers not, as in previous modes of production, through political force, not by dint of 'custom and practice', but by *economic* means. This gives the state a particular economic function within the capitalist system, at least in 'normal' times. (We say 'normal' times because clearly in situations of war, for instance, or acute political and social conflict, the state adopts different methods and even forms of rule in its efforts to defend the interests of the ruling class.) In the normal run of events, and certainly in its heyday, capitalism is regulated *spontaneously*, by the market, that is by competition. The economic surplus (surplus-value) arises on the basis of the buying and selling of commodities, including critically the commodity labour power.

The more decisive role in economic affairs played by the state in countries such as France, Germany and Japan in the last century was a reflection, not of a mature capitalism but of something quite different: of the survival of powerful pre-capitalist relations. It was this immaturity that had earlier led to a situation in France, for instance, where the state became a major primary instrument of appropriation, in which peasant-produced surpluses were appropriated in the form of taxes. In other words the state in France and Germany had a far more powerful 'economic' function than did the English state, but in the latter case this indicated the near-complete penetration of capitalist relations in the agricultural sphere, a situation found nowhere else in the world.

The uniqueness of British agrarian relations

What about the claim that one source of the weakness of capitalism in Britain was that it was established first in the agrarian sector? Here the Anderson–Nairn thesis stands in marked contrast to the position of many other writers. Tom Kemp, for instance, writing about the conditions for capitalist development in this country, draws very different conclusions from this fact:

> It is not incorrect to regard the way in which these conditions were prepared in Britain, especially in England, as being the classic case. It was also a unique one; nowhere else were the conditions precisely reproduced; *nowhere else did agrarian relations, by the eighteenth century, conform so exactly with the requirements of industrial capitalism*.... In England the transformation of feudalism began early and conditions rapidly became favourable for the strengthening of the forces of the market and individual possessiveness. Partly owing to the changes which the feudal class underwent through its internecine conflicts and its ability to strengthen its power in relation to the Crown, it adapted itself to the commercial possibilities which opened up in the sixteenth century. The disintegration of the peasant community began early and its position steadily weakened while the lords were extending their control over their estates and viewing them increasingly as a commercial proposition.
>
> (Kemp 1985: 38, emphasis added)

The same author indicates that the evolution of agrarian relations elsewhere in Europe was 'distinctly different'. There many landlords were absentees, the product of the estates was siphoned off in the old forms through surplus labour services or by other servitudes exacted from the peasantry, which meant that the lords' privileges, and their income, arose from their monopoly of coercive power in society.

A similar position to that of Kemp is expressed by another writer (Saville 1969: 248) in the following terms:

> Above all, the experience of Britain in respect of the transformation of her social structure prior to industrialisation has not been paralleled in the history of any other industrialising society. Nowhere save in Britain was the peasantry virtually eliminated before the acceleration of economic growth that is associated with the development of industrial capitalism, and of the many special features of early industrialisation in Britain none is more striking than the pressure of a rapidly growing proletariat in the countryside.[8]

The establishment of what were thorough-going capitalist social relations and the relative unimportance of the economic functions of the state that this implied did not mean, as Meiksins Wood reminds us, that the English ruling class was uninterested in sinecures and offices of state – after all the Old Corruption of the eighteenth century plundered the national-state wealth on a scale perhaps unparalleled until recent times. But, and here lies the crucial point, by the eighteenth century the state in Britain was not itself a direct instrument of surplus extraction; rather it creamed off a part of the gains generated, by capitalist means, in the non-state sphere of the economy. In short, to the extent that the subordination of the state to the economy marks one of the defining characteristics of 'classical' capitalism, one that separates it off from other forms of society, it can be truly said that capitalism emerged in its most complete and pure form in Britain.

If in French and especially German ideology there was a greater concentration on the need to establish a truly 'modern state' this was, once more, a sign of the *immaturity* of capitalist relations, and not their ripeness. Thus Hegel's aim to create such a state was a response to the weakness of the scattered German principalities in contrast with the unity and power of the Napoleonic state. In similar vein, along with Meiksins Wood, we can take issue with Nairn's contention that the retention of the Monarchy in Britain, the obsession with matters of status, what Nairn refers to misleadingly as 'class' – as distinct from capitalist class relations without the inverted commas – are an indication of British backwardness, of the ability of the ruling class to suppress class consciousness. The following comment (Meiksins Wood 1991: 37) is surely justified:

> No doubt the survival of 'class', its superimposition on class in the capitalist sense, can be explained, again, by the fact that the emergence of capitalist class relations was organic and spontaneous, the outcome of a process internal to the social relations of pre-capitalist England. Thus here too there was a greater likelihood that social transformation would take the form of new wine in old bottles. But here again it is misleading to focus on the old bottles at the expense of the new wine, if the consequence is that qualities belonging to capitalism are attributed to pre-modern residues.

Proceeding along the same lines, she takes up issues of sovereignty and law, again aiming to show that the very features that Nairn and Anderson point to as indicators of backwardness ought properly to be interpreted in a quite different, indeed opposite, way – as significations of the advanced character of the social relations in Britain. She notes that there is a striking absence of any clear conception of sovereignty in English political thought; unlike the French, the English were content to make do with untidy ideas of political authority, with 'mixed constitutions'. Meiksins Wood also draws a contrast between French and English political theory; without entering into all the details, we can summarise her as saying that the concentration in France on the need for an undivided sovereignty reflected the absence of just such a phenomenon in a country where power remained parcelled out among numbers of nobles who competed for domination with the monarch. In Britain the relative indifference to these theoretical matters pointed not to the weakness of 'English ideology' but rather to the fact that the capitalist class had already concentrated economic power firmly into its own hands.

Classical political economy and English backwardness

One of the persistent complaints of the New Left has concerned the supposed ideological 'mediocrity' and 'inertness' of English culture stemming, we are led to believe, from the incomplete development of capitalism in this country. It is a charge difficult to take very seriously. After all Britain did produce figures such as Bacon, Hobbes and Locke whose influence on European thought as a whole was considerable. Seventeenth-century British empiricism certainly involved a narrowness of outlook. But this was born, not of a weak capitalism, not out of backward *social relations* in Britain, but, essentially, out of the limited level of development of the *natural sciences* at that time. Given the lack of knowledge of evolution, of the earth sciences, etc. there was as yet no scientific basis for a historical view of nature; all change appeared due to the work of the mind. But despite its undoubted one-sidedness, empiricism did mark a step forward in human knowledge, did represent a break from the dominance of theology that had characterised the Middle Ages.

The series of articles Engels contributed to *Vörwarts* in September–October 1844 – at the time he was at work on his classic text, *The Condition of the Working Class in England* – is worth reading as an antidote to Anderson and others who fail to discern any revolutionary content in either British thought or British history. Here Engels emphasises that English thought cannot be conceived apart from that in France and Germany. Thus:

> The Germans, the nation of Christian spiritualism, experienced a philosophical revolution; the French, the nation of classical materialism and hence of politics, had to go through a political revolution; the English, a nation that is a mixture of German and French elements, who therefore embody both sides of the antithesis and are for that reason more universal than either of the of the two factors taken separately, were for that reason drawn into a more universal, a social revolution.
>
> (Engels 1975b: 471)

And if we are considering the contribution made by Britain to the development of European thought how can we possibly forget what was perhaps its greatest contribution, classical political economy? Arising in Scotland and England, this not only exercised a deep influence on the thought of Hegel but did after all form one of Lenin's 'three sources and component parts of Marxism'. One of the most regrettable features of the work of Anderson and Nairn is that its effect is to sunder the unity of European thought. Marxism would have been impossible without developments in each one of the major capitalist countries. These gave us French conceptions of history and society, the investigation of the anatomy of capitalist economy, for which Anglo-Scottish political economy was responsible, and classical German philosophy, from Kant through to Feuerbach. Each contribution was equally decisive. The three 'schools' were in any case closely inter-linked: think of Hegel's indebtedness to the Scottish enlightenment, not to speak of the impact of the French revolution on his thinking; consider Smith's study of French Physiocracy, as well as the obligations of this latter school to Smith.

In connection with this charge of British backwardness and insularity the history of political economy in Britain is of particular interest and significance. While the term may have been introduced first in France (it seems by the Mercantilist Montchértien) its decisive development was to take place in England and Scotland. The point can be looked at in this way: the eighteenth-century French Physiocrats, greatly influenced by the social relations of English agriculture, developed the notion of 'natural law', the conception that the economy worked according to a set of universal and objective principles. Here was undoubtedly an important step forward in the establishment of political economy as a science focused on production and not confined exclusively to trade – as was the case during the period when Mercantilist conceptions dominated. But the advances made by the French Physiocrats in reality marked only a half-step forward. For French economic thought could not break entirely free from the earlier conception that in matters concerning the economy the state was all-important.

Thus the French Physiocrats warned that should those in charge of state economic policy institute measures that violated natural law then the progress of the economy could be seriously arrested. Francois Quesnay, for instance, while firmly holding to the idea of 'natural right' at the same time held that any positive legislation contradicting this right would bring ruin to the country and the degradation of its economy. In other words, economic progress or regression depends on whether the imperatives of natural right are carried out or thwarted by bad law.

Here the contrast with the work of Adam Smith is striking, and one not at all supportive of the charge of British 'backwardness'. For Smith took over the idea of 'natural law' from the Physiocrats but gave it a much more powerful and advanced interpretation. The *Wealth of Nations* (first published 1776) enshrines the belief that, whatever governments may or may not do, natural law will prevail, will force a way for itself.

In other words Smith gives to legislation a far more modest role than did Physiocracy. 'Mr. Quesnai', he wrote,

> seems to have ... imagined that [the political body] would thrive and prosper only under a certain precise regimen, the exact regimen of perfect liberty and perfect justice. He seems not to have considered that in the political body, the natural effort which every man is continually making to better his

> own condition is a principle of preservation capable of preventing and correcting, in many respects, the bad effects of a political economy, in some degree, both partial and oppressive.
>
> (Smith 1976: 674)

In Smith's 'political economy' the emphasis is on the 'economy' rather than the 'political'. In this sense economic policy is of relatively minor account. And in placing this emphasis where he did Smith was reflecting the maturity of social relations in mid-eighteenth-century Britain, compared with their relatively underdeveloped state in France. Apart from this it should not be forgotten that for Marx at any rate it was 'backward' Britain, not 'advanced' France that produced, in the shape of Ricardo, the supreme economist of production-distribution.

A good summary of the point at issue is provided by the Russian historian of economic thought, I.I. Rubin (1979):

> The explanation for this marked difference in the views of Quesnay and Smith lies in the differing economic conditions of France and Britain in the eighteenth century. In France capitalist agriculture was not so much an actually-existing phenomenon as a Physiocratic slogan that had still to be put into practice. Given France's feudal survivals and absolute monarchy, the extensive development of capitalism was genuinely impossible without a fundamental social and political revolution and the implementation of the 'natural law' of bourgeois society. This accounts for the extreme importance of natural right in Quesnay's system. England in the eighteenth century found itself in a different situation. Despite the continuing dominance of the landowning oligarchy, the basic social preconditions for the development of capitalism were already present. The capitalist economy was developing rapidly, either breaking or bypassing the separate guild or Mercantilist restrictions which, despite slowing down the former's growth, could not halt it – hence Smith's view that economic progress is continuous, even where legislation is bad and contradicts the principles of natural right.

British decline and the place of Keynes

The present-day followers of Keynes have occupied an important place in recent discussions about the decline of Britain, evidenced recently in the huge success and influence of Will Hutton's best-selling, *The State We're In* (Hutton 1995). Whatever differences there may be among the Keynesians, in general they assume that a return to Keynes's (1936) teachings is the key to restoring the health of British capitalism, with the corollary that it is the monetarism and neo-liberalism of the Thatcher years that is the proximate source of our current economic woes. Whether such views can be sustained – indeed whether any central role can be attributed to 'economic policy' as a whole in accelerating or reversing Britain's decline – is highly problematic. But what is of more interest here is the high regard that Anderson displays for Keynes – not simply as economic statesman but as a contributor to English thought as a whole. In an essay that appeared fairly soon after his first formulation of the roots of the British crisis, Anderson (1968) exempted Keynes from the general charge levelled against the English intelligentsia. One of Anderson's complaints is that in the present century the British have been obliged to import their leading intellectuals – Wittgenstein, Popper, Malinowski *et al.* – rather like our leading football clubs increasingly buy their star players from overseas.[9] Keynes, in contrast was home-grown,

> Retrospectively Keynes magnitude has grown. He was perhaps the last great social thinker produced by the English bourgeoisie, with all the largeness and generosity of once confident liberalism. His theoretical system was validated practically.
>
> (Anderson 1968: 35)

These are indeed remarkable claims; in the light of what has happened since this was written they were at best grossly-inflated ones. Whether Keynes did effect a 'revolution' in economics is open to serious doubt (see Pilling 1986, ch. 2): his system was derived, eclectically, from a wide variety of sources including the Mercantilists, Malthus and the English underconsumptionist, J.A. Hobson. For some, Keynes simply patched up a disintegrating neo-classical structure; for others it was the introduction of uncertainty into economics that marked his contribution. Whatever the merits of these interpretations, Keynes's theory relied heavily upon psychological factors, not to say 'animal spirits' as explanations for the depth and longevity of the inter-war slump. And far from his ideas having been 'vindicated' they have singularly failed to answer capitalism's problems; indeed the weight of opinion among today's professional economists has swung against Keynes as it becomes ever clearer that the globalisation of capital makes it increasingly impossible for any state to fashion its 'own' socio-economic policy, especially so in the case of a severely debilitated British capitalism.

As one commentator (Commission on Social Justice 1994) has recently put it, what is now fashionably referred to as the 'globalisation' of world economic relations has

> effectively created an international market in government policies. Speculators who doubt the ability of a national government to maintain a particular exchange rate can destroy the government's position by betting against the currency, as one individual, George Soros, did to great effect in 1992. The search for market credibility has already imposed a deflationary straightjacket on European economies, led by high interest rates across Europe in the last 15 years, and the power of individual economies to buck these trends is severely restricted.

And yet the establishment of conditions that would enable Britain to pursue its 'own' economic and social policy was at the very centre of Keynes's concerns for much of his life. Thus his opposition in the 1920s to the retention of the gold standard and his (unsuccessful) efforts to establish a world monetary system at the end of World War II that would serve British interests were inspired by just this aim. When a Labour government in the mid-1970s did try to implement a classical Keynesian programme to counter rising unemployment it proved a short-lived experiment and that same government embarked on measures – especially cut-backs in state spending – which were to point the way for the Thatcher government after 1979.

Given these obvious deficiencies, how can one explain the particular praise that Anderson reserved for Keynes? Undoubtedly because it was Keynes, more than anybody else in the 1930s, who saw that the 'end of laissez-faire' had arrived. It was Keynes who led the way in demanding a changed role for the state; it was Keynes who questioned the nostrums of neo-classical economics, including belief in the universal benefits supposedly attaching to free trade. These are very much in line with the spirit of Anderson's claim that, despite Keynes's efforts, the British state remains archaic, and as such unable to tackle the roots of Britain's decline. Further, it was Keynes who denounced the rentier class, confidently predicting its demise in the not-too-distant future. (What a prediction that turned out to be!) Here again this fits well with Anderson's thesis, especially in its revised version, namely that the ills of British capital are down to the dominant position occupied by the City.

Keynes in effect called for an alliance between the industrial capitalists and the labour movement, against the financiers. In so doing he provided important ideological tools which were far from progressive; indeed they helped provide the conceptual basis for the extreme right in British politics in the 1930s, including the fascist Oswald Mosley.

As Mosley's biographer (he also happens to be the biographer of Keynes) has pointed out:

> [C]uriously enough Keynes did not include the class struggle [between capitalists and workers] in his account of interest conflicts. He tended to assume an identity of interest between workers and manufacturers against their common enemy – the rentier and the banker. The notion of the conflict of interest within the capitalist community and the identity of interest between the workers and one section of that community – the manufacturers – was to have profound influence on Mosley's thought. It was to give him both a strategy and a philosophy quite different from the standard socialist conception in which the workers were all on one side, and the wicked capitalists all on the other. Henceforth the producers' state would be the goal; and finance the enemy.
>
> (Skidelsky 1975: 141)

Keynes's abandonment of the doctrines of free trade and laissez-faire and his acceptance of the need for greater state supervision of the economy are hardly expressive of a 'confident liberalism'. Rather they point to the crisis of that very liberalism that has marked the present century as a whole. Here the warm reception afforded to Keynes's *General Theory* in Germany in the 1930s is not without interest. (Not without reason have some historians of economic thought seen Keynes as representative of the 'New Mercantilism'.)

The case of the industrial revolution

The explanation offered by Anderson for Britain's decline involves an underlying conception about British history as a whole, namely that it has never experienced the type of revolutionary upheavals that have characterised Other Countries, with France here being the archetypal case. There are perhaps two periods in British history to which the term 'revolutionary change' could be applied: the transformation wrought by the English civil war of the seventeenth century and its aftermath; and second, the 'industrial revolution' of the eighteenth and nineteenth centuries.

It is Anderson's contention that a 'classical' commercial class's overwhelming dominance left Britain a semi-industrialised nation; in any case what industry there was in Britain was puny, small-scale stuff, and centred largely on the consumer goods sector – in contrast to the Continental situation where large-scale, capital-goods industries predominated.

In his denial of the revolutionary character and consequences of what used to be widely known as the 'industrial revolution' Anderson is not alone, for it has become increasingly fashionable among economic historians to deny any validity to this term [see Pilling 1996a; Chapter 9 of this book – ed.]. The 'new economic history' arrives at this conclusion with highly dubious statistics that are confined largely to discussions about 'rates of growth' at the end of the eighteenth century and early part of the nineteenth century. But, of more pertinence, the matter cannot be settled by simple resort to statistics, even if the data were readily available and reliable. For involved in the industrial revolution was a *qualitative* transformation of conditions in Britain, and one that was *social* in character.

It was Britain's early start that in part lent her industry its peculiar character. The 'industrial revolution' occurred first in the sphere of textiles. Capital requirements here were relatively modest, not needing the considerable long-term investments that heavy industry was later to demand. As we have noted, for some this is a sign of weakness. But to assume that heavy industry, producing capital goods, had no place in British economic development would surely be a travesty. Steel, locomotives, machine tools, textile machinery, and shipbuilding, for instance, formed powerful sectors of the British economy in the last century and in many cases provided the wherewithal for the Continent's industrialisation. From the opposite point of view, the differences with the Continent should not be exaggerated, as Anderson and other commentators tend to do. Thus the family firm, largely financed out of its own resources, was not confined to Britain; even enterprises in the capital goods sector, such as Siemens, Krupps, or de Wendel did not draw closer to the banks until the steel-making process of the late nineteenth century required great amounts of capital outlay. Likewise the German chemical industry initially grew with little support from the banks.

As one recent writer (Gibbard 1996: 42) has noted:

> [T]he evidence does not support a picture of the role of banking capital as the key to German industrial success. As late as 1928 the lion's share of bank credit in that country was being channelled into the older staple industries, the two biggest recipients being textiles with 11.8 per cent and food with 11.2 per cent, against only 3.6 per cent for the chemical industry and 2.9 per cent for engineering and automobile construction.

With developments in Britain, the decisive question is that the changes being introduced into the Lancashire cotton textile industry towards the end of the eighteenth century – which had at their centre the creation of a modern factory-based working class – were, as Engels realised on his arrival in Manchester in the early 1840s, of world significance (Engels 1975a: 302). And the creation of this new class of factory-based wage workers was in turn possible only because of the thorough-going nature of the changes in the agrarian sector of the economy to which we earlier drew attention.

While too many Marxists have in the past relied on 'authority' to settle arguments it is nonetheless instructive to consider the position of Anderson and Nairn in the light of what Engels wrote in the early 1840s about the industrial revolution and British 'backwardness':

> The century of revolution has to all appearances passed England by, causing little change. While on the Continent an entire old world was shattered, while a twenty-five year war cleared the air, in England everything remained calm, neither state not church were in any way threatened. And yet since the middle of the last century *England has experienced a greater upheaval than any other country* – an upheaval which is all the more momentous the more quietly it is brought about, and it will therefore in all probability attain its goal more readily in practice than the political revolution in France or the philosophical revolution in Germany. The revolution in England is a social one and therefore more comprehensive and far-reaching than any other. There are no fields – however remote – of human knowledge and no conditions of life which have not contributed to it and which in turn have not been affected by it.
>
> (Engels 1975b: 469, emphasis added)

or again

> Sixty, eighty years ago, England was a country like every other, with small towns, few and simple industries, and a thin but *proportionally* large agricultural population. Today it is a country like *no* other, with a capital of two and a half million inhabitants; with vast manufacturing cities; with an industry that supplies the world, and produces almost everything by means

> of the most complex machinery; with an industrious, intelligent, dense population of which two-thirds are employed in trade and commerce and composed of classes wholly different; forming, in fact, with other customs and other needs, a different nation from the England of those days. The industrial revolution is of the same importance for England as the political revolution for France, or the philosophical revolution for Germany; and the difference between England in 1760 and 1844 is at least as great as that between France under the *ancien régime* and during the revolution of July.
>
> (Engels 1975a: 320)

Nor does the view of the New Left correspond to the manner in which contemporary English thinkers saw the transition to capitalism. For John Locke – whose work embraced both philosophy and political economy – in considering the rise of capitalism the relevant distinction was not between town and country, bourgeois and aristocrat, but between passive rentier property and agricultural 'improvement', between a class of landlords who simply lived off their rents as against those who developed agriculture along commercial lines in response to the needs of the market. And here 'improvement' did not simply mean the use of superior techniques on the land – however important the introduction of new crops and their better rotation, for example, might be – but essentially *enclosure*, that is the scrapping of the open field system. (Here is another example of the fact that social processes cannot be reduced to the techniques of production.) By the end of the eighteenth century the peasantry in England had all but disappeared: from then on the distinction was no longer between freeman and peasant but between owners and non-owners. While the enclosure movement, and with it the concentration of land into the hands of a comparatively small number of families, took place over a long time the revolutions of the seventeenth century were nonetheless decisive turning points. The outcome of the great changes in that century decided the supremacy of these new property forms, recognised the dominance of individual ownership and laid the basis for the final elimination of the English peasant. The English landlords from then onwards were able to take full advantage of these new legal possibilities and integrate their estates into the structure of capitalism. The issue was not simply that of the ownership of the land (that is property relations) but *the social relations of production* that existed in the countryside; nor was it decisive that the new breed of commercial landowners retained many of the trappings and style of a feudal aristocracy. (Not the least merit of Meiksins Wood's work is that she reminds Marxists that the terms 'property relations' and the 'social relations of production' are not at all synonymous.) In other words we should not be misled by immediate appearances, as Anderson–Nairn so often are. As one writer (Kemp 1985: 41) has put it:

> Because of its concentrated nature, because of the ancient lineage of many of the landowning families and because of the extensive administrative and juridical powers which landowners conserved, landownership retained a kind of feudal shell, even when it had been thoroughly transformed on lines entirely congruous with capitalism.

Locke was among those who saw the property relations that were emerging in the England of his day not simply as an extension of age-old commercial practices but as involving quite new social relations based on the improvement of the productivity of labour generated by the imperatives of competition.

This being so it is quite natural that one of the pre-occupations of classical political economy in Britain from at least the middle of the eighteenth century onwards was the distinction between 'productive' and 'unproductive' labour. Smith, and later Ricardo (1953), despite many ambiguities and inconsistencies, saw productive labour as '*labour productive of capital*' while unproductive labour was labour that, however useful it might be 'in general', constituted a drain on capital accumulation. It is true that the Physiocrats had also distinguished between productive and unproductive activities, but for them this distinction coincided with that between the 'productive' agricultural sector and the rest of the economy, which was deemed 'sterile'. Even here, this distinction was made with conditions in British agriculture very much in mind.

Anderson's more recently emphasised charge that the British were over-concerned with commerce, to the detriment of industrial activities is also misplaced As Meiksins Wood among others has pointed out, the commercial activities of the British ruling class, in the period when capitalist social relations were being established, were far from being of a traditional kind. Indeed England lacked many of the classical instruments of a conventional commercial power: those concerned with money-changing operations, public banks dealing with state finances and currency regulations and the mechanisms for financing long-distance trade. There was little need for money changers of the normal type because, unlike any other nation state, England already possessed a single unified coinage. Nor were there anything like the great merchant bankers of Italy in the fourteenth century or of Germany in the sixteenth. The banking system that did develop was, however, unique in one respect: it was concerned with the domestic market, the domestic market in agricultural commodities in particular. This commercial system rested on superior productivity and not on geopolitical or military power, although naturally the colonial ventures of the English landed class vastly increased its wealth. By the eighteenth century the imperial drive was no longer the old pre-capitalist drive for land and wealth – as it was classically with the Spanish conquistadors in South America – but an expansion in search of markets that could absorb the growing output of British industry. In this regard the exploitation of the colonies by 'backward' Britain was more advanced, more thoroughly ruthless *in a capitalist sense*, than in the Spanish but also the later French and German cases.

Capitalism as a specific social system

Behind many of the attempts to prove that British history has seen little in the way of fundamental ruptures or dis-continuities and that its decline has been a process stretching back for centuries is a view of capitalism that would seek to eliminate, that is to ignore, the laws of motion peculiar to this social system. As we have suggested, it is this view that is implicit in those attempts to reduce the industrial revolution to a series of changes in the techniques of production, and one that thereby plays down the social significance of that revolution. This involves a view of capitalism as something historically always present, coeval with human existence, if only embryonically so. (As implied above, much of this approach depends upon the acceptance of an abstract 'model' of how capitalism 'ought' to have developed; reality is then measured against this model, with the reality of British capitalist development found severely wanting.) This ahistorical view of capitalism is deeply rooted in bourgeois thought. It was a view advanced long ago by Adam Smith who regarded the essence of human nature as lying in the tendency to 'truck, barter and exchange'; this ever-present human nature had finally found its full realisation with the arrival of capitalism, a system founded on just this trading activity, and one therefore involving the ever-greater division of labour. (In defence of the classical political economists it can be said that, though accepting the social relations of capitalism as natural, they did nonetheless seek to establish the anatomy of modern society from the point of view of these social relations. Such a defence cannot be extended to those present-day historians and economists in whose work the social relations of production have little or no place.)

There is no doubt that certain Marxists have also, to one degree or another, been influenced by such views, especially those Marxists whose work was vitiated by a technological determinism, that, for example, understood 'productive forces' as little more than the techniques of production; that regarded 'industrialisation' as an autonomous technical process; that conceived of capitalism as simply a stage in the general improvement of productive forces. I would include here all those who believed that the period after 1945 witnessed a 'new industrial revolution' based on technical developments stimulated by the war. Here again is a confusion between the *technical* and the *social*, and one, I would argue, that lies at the root of much confusion in the social sciences. (Meiksins Wood has charged that even those Marxists who in Britain pioneered the study of the transition from feudalism to capitalism – Maurice Dobb, Rodney Hilton and others – are not entirely exempt from traces of this standpoint, even though she clearly admires much of their work.) Meiksins Wood (1991: 9) gets it right when, again stressing the uniqueness of relations in the agrarian sector, she remarks: 'A certain level of productive forces was certainly a necessary condition for the breakthrough to industrial capitalism, but it was sufficient only in the context of English property relations.'

If I read this right, what is being objected to is a mechanical notion that history involves a process whereby productive forces come into conflict with (passive) social relations and thereby create the conditions for social revolution. By analogy, it is as if those 'social relations' were a jug, being filled up by water (expanding productive forces) to the critical moment where a (revolutionary) overflow of liquid occurs. The point here is that productive forces must always be considered in their inner connection with the social relations in and through which they alone have their existence; further, the social relations never play a passive role as means for the development (in some epochs the stagnation) of such forces. It is not as though the social relations of production sit around waiting for the forces of production to reach a certain point in their maturation before they take a hand in the shaping of history. Such would be a caricature of historical materialism but sadly the sort of 'straw man' that opponents of Marxism often set up in their ideological operations.

Another aspect of this mechanical approach to the transition to capitalism is the contention that it was the growth of 'the market' that constituted the essential precondition for the emergence of capitalism. Such a view, heavily influenced by the work of Henri Pirenne, has a long history, and was the subject of the celebrated discussion among Marxist historians (Maurice Dobb, Christopher Hill, Paul Sweezy, *et al.*) that began in the 1950s about the nature of the transition from feudalism to capitalism (Hilton 1976). Following Meiksins Wood it is necessary to draw a distinction between 'the market' viewed as an abstract entity (which, as in the case of present-day neo-classical economic theory, is usually seen as the means whereby freedom is attained) and the specifically *capitalist* market that is an instrument of coercion. Here again she suggests that the work of many Marxists has been more than a little tinged with an abstract conception of the market and its role in the establishment of capitalism (on this see Meiksins Wood 1994).[10]

Some conclusions

British experience was unique in that it was the British economy that brought the world market into being while simultaneously being profoundly affected by the growth of that very market. Many of those commenting on the roots of the 'British disease' are apt to treat the development of the economy and the class relations that were its foundation as though British capitalism can be understood apart from the world economy of which it is in reality an integral part. The peculiar historical path taken by capitalism in any one country can be understood in a truly concrete manner only from a study of the way in which the forces of world economy (and politics, ideology, etc.) were uniquely combined in the country concerned.

We have already noted that Engels grasped the world significance of what was happening in Manchester in the 1840s – then a city of some 400,000 people in the north-west of a tiny island off the coast of the continent of Europe. Engels realised that the emergence of modern industry and its 'first born son', the working class in the mills of Manchester and its environs, was a process that could not stop there. Even though the critique of political economy that he and Marx were to make was not yet completed, he realised that capital was a relation that by its very nature had continually to expand, to go beyond itself. Further, capital existed only in the shape of 'many capitals' in competition with each other. Although capitalism necessarily took on somewhat different forms when it began to establish itself on the Continent and in North America it was Britain that had paved the way in the development of industrial capitalism.

It was Ricardo who argued that the best, most adequate conditions for the development of capitalism were ones in which (a) it developed in its industrial form and (b) where the forces of competition were strongest (see Marx's *Grundrisse*, 1973 and Ilyenkov 1982).[11] Marx fully accepted Ricardo's position. For he came to understand that it was industrial capital that was the form in which relative surplus-value was best created (rather than its more primitive form, absolute surplus-value) and second, that it was in the realm of competition that the laws of capital were 'executed'.[12]

In this sense we can say that it was in eighteenth- and nineteenth-century Britain that the conditions for capitalist development were most fully realised. But if Britain at that period held up a mirror to the rest of the world, is this not true today? In other words, are not all the features of a weak, decadent British capitalism *features of the system as a whole*?

We know that in the last quarter of the nineteenth century British capital anticipated many of the features that were to be common to the capitalist system as a whole in the present century. Thus the dominant position attained by financial institutions; the increasing importance of the export of capital; the acquisition of a vast empire; the development on the basis of such an empire of a 'labour aristocracy' that was to be critical for the path taken by the working-class movement – all these phenomena emerged first in Britain. But her competitors were, willy-nilly, albeit belatedly, forced along the same path. Capitalism at the end of the twentieth century is one dominated by financial institutions – by the banks, insurance companies, pension funds, etc. These are not features unique to Britain, nor do they represent constraints simply on economic policy in Britain, as, for example, the short-lived 'Mitterrand experiment' at Keynesian-style reflation in the early 1970s illustrates.

Let us consider just two facts about the nature of contemporary capitalism and the point it has reached on the edge of the next millennium:

1 The fact is that there has been a huge increase on the part of all the major capitalist powers in the export of capital over the last two decades. By the end of the 1980s, direct investment made by the capitalists of all countries outside their national borders had reached $1.5 trillion. But what is significant is not so much the sum involved as the speed of its growth over the last two decades. For the figure almost tripled in the 1980s alone. Put another way: for the period 1983–1989 the outflows of direct investment to other countries rose by almost 29 per cent each year, whereas world exports rose much more slowly – at about 9 per cent a year – and world domestic product even more slowly. And the investment involved went far beyond manufacturing and the extraction of raw materials. To an ever-greater extent it involved such areas as finance, real estate, insurance, advertising and the media. In the 1950s and early 1960s most foreign investments came from US corporations, although Britain, which was able to re-invest earnings from previous investments, was also important in this respect. But, as part of her relative loss of power, the United States had to face increasing

competition from other countries in the field of foreign investment. Thus whereas in 1960 almost half of all direct foreign investment originated from the United States, by the end of the 1980s this had dropped to under 30 per cent. The figure for Japan had risen from under 1 per cent to over 11 per cent during the same period.

Thus whether or not the export of capital has the deleterious consequences for the development of 'domestic' industry that some claim, one thing is certain: this is not simply a 'British phenomenon' but one common to all the leading capitalist powers. Indeed, at the time of writing (January 1996 [the version published in *Thames Papers* – ed.]) there is more capital flowing out of Germany (the result of high labour costs and the rising costs of re-unification with the eastern Länder) than of any other European country.

2 There has been an astronomical growth of bank lending across national frontiers. In the past such activity was regarded as abnormal. As recently as the mid-1960s the volume of international banking reached only approximately 10 per cent of the combined national incomes of the capitalist countries. By the mid-1980s that figure had doubled. The comparison with world trade is even more striking. A normal function of international banking is to facilitate world trade and some 30 years ago the volume of banking activity across national borders came to about 10 per cent of world trade. Over the last two decades that volume has swollen out of all proportion with world trade, and by the middle of the last decade it actually exceeded the volume of trade of the capitalist countries. This is how one leading financial institution (Morgan Guarantee Trust 1991) sums up these trends:

> The [economic and financial instability of the 1970s] engendered government deficits and external imbalances that required financing on a scale unprecedented in peacetime and that exceeded the capacity or willingness of the traditionally fragmented financial markets to cover. These financing needs joined with the advances in technology and communications to spawn a host of innovations ranging from securitisation in place of intermediated bank credit to new derivatives including swaps. Taken together these financial innovations have helped overwhelm traditional and regulatory segmentation of national markets and thereby have contributed much to the effective integration of financial markets globally.

Or as another writer (Drucker 1986: 782) puts it:

> [World trade in goods and services] amounts to around \$2.5 trillion to \$3 trillion a year. But the London Eurodollar market, in which the world's financial institutions borrow and lend to each other, turns over \$300 billion each working day, or \$75 trillion a year, a volume at least 25 times that of world trade. In addition, there are foreign exchange transactions in the

> world's money centres, in which one currency is traded against another. These run around $150 billion a day, or about $35 trillion a year – 12 times the world-wide trade in goods and services. Of course, many of these Euro-dollars, yen, and Swiss francs are just being moved from one pocket to another and may be counted more than once. A massive discrepancy still exists, and there is only one conclusion: capital movements unconnected to trade – and indeed largely independent of it – greatly exceed trade finance.

Thus the last two decades have seen an astonishing growth in the funds devoted purely to speculation. This period witnessed the appearance of quite new exotic financial instruments that have the most tenuous connection with the production or even circulation of commodities but which both extended greatly the credit base while at the same time opening wide the gates for speculation. For instance, financial futures markets – where bets are laid on what interest rates will be at a specified date in the future – first emerged in the early 1970s and are now reckoned to total over $1 trillion world-wide, although in truth nobody really knows their magnitude. There has been an even faster growth in interest and currency swaps. These consist of swaps between two parties who possess interest-bearing securities or future-currency contracts, the purpose being to hedge and/or seek additional speculative gains. There are now over $2.5 trillion worth of such contracts outstanding in the financial markets, yet they were almost unknown before 1980. [For a discussion of the significance of these trends see Pilling 1996b; Chapter 2 of this book – ed.]

It seems clear, even from these figures, that the central role of financial institutions is not something today confined to 'backward' Britain – if it ever was. The fact that these trends are more and more obviously common to all countries, or at any rate the big capitalist countries, surely tells us something about the overall nature of capital and the point it has reached. In so far as financial institutions retain great specific weight in the functioning of capital in Britain – as they do – this is part of a universal trend and not an expression of some peculiarly parasitic capital confined to this country.

In the same way, the 'British disease' – the decline of traditional industries; the consequent low rates of economic growth; the persistence of heavy structural unemployment; chronic budgetary imbalances; the decay of the inner cities, etc. – are manifestly becoming European, not simply British, questions.[13] Germany, the 'strong man' of Europe is today experiencing almost exactly the same sort of crisis that emerged earlier in Britain. It is a crisis that obviously has implications far beyond the borders of Europe, placing as it does a serious question mark over the possibility of European monetary integration, perhaps over the European Union itself. The crisis in Germany is now producing the same sort of cry that we have long heard in Britain: too much capital is being invested abroad as German employers seek to avoid high labour costs at home; that the banks must be more 'responsible' and direct their investment to German firms especially to the small business sector, the *Mittlestand*; that too many of the country's resources are being absorbed in the payment of welfare benefits that are no longer sustainable, etc. A similar story could be told in the case of France. To the extent that in these countries big business calls for a Mrs. Thatcher to tackle their problems points to the fact that 'Thatcherism' was not uniquely British, called into being to modernise a backward economic and social structure, but was something that speaks to the needs of capital and its crisis in a far more general sense.

If the problems of the leading capitalist countries today begin to appear in similar *forms* this is hardly sustaining evidence for the supposed 'exceptionalism' of British capitalism. It rather suggests that in examining the roots of the British crisis our starting point must be the nature of the capitalist system as a whole, a system that exists and can exist only on a world scale. If what has been written here helps in the re-orientation of future work in this direction it will have more than served its purpose.

[This chapter was first published in 1996, *Thames Papers in Political Economy*, School of Social Sciences, University of Greenwich. The version published here was revised by the author – ed.]

Notes

1 This chapter is dedicated to the memory of Tom Kemp, who knew a lot more about these things than I do. I must thank Susanne MacGreggor and John Lea, Department of Sociology and Social Policy, University of Middlesex, for helpful comments on an earlier draft [of the version published in *Thames Papers* – ed.] My thanks also to Keith Gibbard, Department of Economics and Economic History, Metropolitan University of Manchester, for references to Marx's *Capital.* Given the controversial nature of the issues dealt with, the usual disclaimer, that sole responsibility for any deficiencies in this chapter rest with me, should not be taken as a formal statement.

2 The lack of any agreement about the sources of the British crisis is underlined by the fact that the very 'Gentlemanly Capitalism' based on the City of London that some see as the source of British economic decline is regarded as the strength of British capitalism. (See Cain and Hopkins (1989) *British Imperialism: Innovation and Expansion, 1688–1914*, for a defence of this position.)

3 Rupert Murdoch provides a more vulgar view of this position. Speaking at the 1989 Edinburgh Festival he said: 'The socially mobile are portrayed as uncaring; businessmen as crooks; money-making is to be despised. British television has been an integral part of the British disease.'

4 It is far from clear why Britain, as first in the field, should *necessarily* have been overtaken by newer arrivals onto the world market. Why an initial lead should not have been self-sustaining and why any penalty should have attached to having been first in the field is never really made clear by the advocates of the idea that a penalty is of necessity attached to the country that was first in the field. The fact is that the problem is wrongly, and abstractly, posed. Gamble (1992: 82) is surely correct when, in opposition to such a fatalist view, he argues that Britain's early start was not as such *the cause* of the later failure to keep up with foreign competitors. Rather that failure is to be understood in terms of the very social relations that made an early start on the road to capitalist industrialisation possible, social relations that remained intact and were strengthened by the very success of that start. In other words, the unique social relations of production that emerged in this country from the end of the sixteenth century onwards made capitalism possible. The strengthening and development of these relations as capitalism in Britain grew further came to constitute the essential *barrier* to

the smooth development of the productive forces. Contradictory, but true! It is just this emphasis on 'technology', methods of industrial organisation, etc. at the expense of a concrete analysis of the development of the social relations of production that vitiates much of the work on the 'decline of Britain'.

5 This was always a difficult thesis to sustain. The 'compromise' effected between the rising industrial capitalists and the 'landed interest' (this was not at all the same thing as a feudal aristocracy) was arrived at very much on terms dictated by the former. The Corn Laws, which Ricardo had rightly seen as representing one of the chief barriers to the growth of industrial capital, were after all repealed in the 1840s. And the victory was final. As Saville (1994: 5) notes,

> Laissez-faire and free trade soon became articles of faith for most politicians; when the dramatic fall in agricultural prices occurred from the mid-1870s onwards – affecting especially the arable areas – no one seriously contemplated the return of protectionism for the agricultural interest.

We should add that today this 'agricultural interest' is bound up completely with capital. British agriculture is now among the most capitalistically organised in the world.

6 It may be correct to characterise the City of London today as parasitic. But it is parasitic only as part of capital as a whole. When Lenin referred to the stage reached by capital at the start of the century (like other Marxists he used the term 'imperialism' to characterise this stage) as 'parasitic' he did so in a precise sense. For Lenin finance capital was parasitic because it lived off and dominated the whole of capital. There is however another point at issue. It is necessary to understand the *historical* relationship between the City and the rest of the economy in the development of British capitalism. The City's wealth was not in the past based simply upon passive rentier property and the drawing of 'invisible' earnings from abroad. From the end of the seventeenth century onwards the City was at the centre of an extensive network of colonial relations, including rubber and cotton plantations, tea estates, etc. This was property based on the *extraction* and not merely the *circulation* of value. It is of course true that at a later stage, as Britain began to emerge as the leading capitalist nation, London became the principal centre for money capital from around the world. But this was not a mark of exceptionalism. Marx (1961b: 755–756) saw these relations in this way:

> [T]he villainies of the Venetian thieving system formed one of the secret bases of the capital-wealth of Holland to whom Venice in her decadence lent large sums of money. So also was it with Holland and England. By the beginning of the eighteenth century the Dutch manufacturers were far outstripped. Holland had ceased to be the nation preponderant in commerce and industry. One of its main lines of business, therefore, from 1701–1776, is the lending out of enormous amounts of capital, especially to its great rival England. The same thing is going on today between England and the United States. A great deal of capital, which appears today in the United States without any certificate of birth, was yesterday, in England, the capitalised blood of children.

The idea that the various forms of capital can be rigidly separated out some being deemed 'reactionary' – is wrong. Cf. Marx (1961b: 754): 'Today industrial supremacy implies commercial supremacy. In the period of manufacture properly so called, it is, on the other hand, the commercial supremacy that gives industrial predominance.'

7 We should not make the issue a black and white one. Thus in Britain the ruling class never operated a *pure* policy of laissez-faire, a fact long recognised among economic and social historians. As early as the middle of the last century liberals such as John Stuart Mill were arguing for limited state involvement in social and economic matters in a manner that anticipated much of Fabian doctrine towards the end of the century.

Where the state did intervene – through legislation that made the violation of private property a capital offence, through the introduction of the New Poor Law, through laws that attempted to suppress Chartism and trade unionism – it did so in a manner that was decidedly in tune with the needs of capital.

8 Above all, Marx understood that in British history over three centuries the relationship between the growth of a capitalist agriculture, with its accompanying social changes, was integrally involved with the changes in industry and trade in the rest of the economy (Saville 1994: 3).

9 In any event this presumed inertia and insularity of English thought inspired Anderson's project of introducing, through the pages of the *New Left Review*, a series of Continental Marxists to Britain – Althusser, Colletti, etc. – whose mission was presumably to raise the British intelligentsia to a more exalted level. A consideration of the fate of such thinkers over the last couple of decades – most of the imports proved to be five minute wonders, with some, such as Colletti, renouncing any adherence to Marxism – provides a salutary lesson about the worth of this project.

10 Marx himself seems to have been clear enough on this point about the role of the market and merchant capital in the transition from feudalism. He certainly never underestimated its role, in that he knew that merchant capital was the means by which money wealth was concentrated and second it was responsible for stimulating production for trade, for encouraging the growth of selling on a large scale and not simply to this or that customer. 'Yet its [merchant capital's] development, as we shall presently see, is incapable by itself of promoting and explaining the transition from one mode of production to another' (Marx 1959: 322).

Or again, speaking of the role of commerce:

> It will subordinate production more and more to exchange-value by making luxuries and subsistence more dependent on sale than on the immediate use of products. Thereby it dissolves the old relationships. It multiplies money circulation. It encompasses no longer merely the surplus of production, but bites deeper and deeper into the latter [production – G.P.] and makes entire branches of production dependent upon it. *Nevertheless this disintegrating effect depends very much on the nature of the producing community.*
>
> (Marx 1959: 325, emphasis added)

And again:

> In the ancient world the effect of commerce and the development of merchant's capital always resulted in a slave economy ... However, in the modern world, it results in the capitalist mode of production. *It follows therefrom that these results spring in themselves from circumstances other than the development of merchant's capital.*
>
> (Marx 1959: 326–327, emphasis added)

It is clear from these passages that, of itself, merchant's capital, however developed, could not effect the transition to capitalism. It required something else: deep-going changes in the social relations of *production.*

Summing up this point in the discussion about 'British exceptionalism', we can say that it was not the expansion of trade *as such* or the growth of productive forces *as such* that made possible the transition to industrial capitalism that took place uniquely in this country, but the thorough-going nature of capitalist social relations (especially in agriculture) in which these productive forces had developed. If this is so, the charge that backwardness and immaturity have predominated in English social and economic history ought properly to be stood on its head.

11 This is Ilyenkov's (1982: 121–122) comment on the importance for the capitalist system of the introduction of machine production and the connection between this and the dominant position assumed by the relative form of surplus-value: 'It is clear ... it

is the appearance of machines that is the real cause of the absolute form of surplus-value being ousted by its relative form.'

Relative surplus-value clearly becomes the dominant form of surplus-value exactly for the reason that it is in better conformity with machine labour than absolute surplus-value, which is increased by a simple lengthening of the working day, labour productivity remaining unaltered.

> The whole point is, however, that the correspondence itself between the economic form of a stage in the development of a productive force is, in its turn, a dialectical correspondence. Relative surplus-value conforms to machine production exactly because it does not remain a passive form with which machines work but rather becomes an *active form* exerting a very strong reverse effect on machine production, that is on its own basis that gave rise to it, developing this basis and thereby creating a new incentive for its own movement.

This is why the decline of 'machine production' in Britain and the growing importance of the absolute form of surplus-value marks a decline, a degeneration even, in capital. But this trend is European-wide, and therefore says something about the general character of capital as a whole, and not simply British capital.

12 An interesting feature of capitalism in its decline is the manner in which it exhibits tendencies that characterised it in its youth. Thus in its early days capitalism relied heavily upon the extraction of surplus-value in its absolute form. This involved the intensification of labour, the lengthening of the working day, etc. In its classical, heroic phase, it develops mainly through the drive for relative surplus-value – that is, through the raising of the productivity of labour by means of the application of machinery to the productive process. Today capitalism reverts increasingly to its older forms of exploitation, involving the cutting of wages, the lengthening of hours and the intensification of labour – the 'low wage economy'. This is a general tendency throughout Europe and the world – an expression of the decline of capital as a whole. Looking at this question from another angle, it is noteworthy that in its rise capital relies heavily on the state to protect its interests (expressed in the policy of Mercantilism, for example). In its decline it tends to revert to similar policies, expressed in the present century [this refers to the twentieth century – ed.] not simply in Keynesianism (which some have dubbed 'the new Mercantilism') but in fascist economic policies. Likewise the early capitalism is characterised by the powerful role that *monopoly* occupied within it, a feature which reappears from the start of the present century onwards. Again we are dealing not with trends confined to Britain, but with a characteristic common to capitalism as a whole.

13 For trends in long-term unemployment at work throughout Europe see OECD, *Economic Outlook* table quoted in Dicken (1992), p. 426. [Similar figures are available in Ljungqvist, L. and Sargent, T.J. (1997) *The European Unemployment Dilemma*, Table 1. Online, available at: http://swopec.hhs.se/iuiwop/papers/iuiwop0481.pdf (accessed 12 December 2011) – ed.]

References

Anderson, P. (1964) 'Origins of the present crisis, *New Left Review*, 23: 26–53.

Anderson, P. (1968) 'Components of the national culture', *New Left Review*, 50, 3–57.

Anderson, P. (1987) 'The figures of descent', *New Left Review*, 161, 20–77.

Cain, P.J. and Hopkins, A.G. (1989) *British Imperialism: Innovation and Expansion, 1688–1914*, London: Longman.

Commission on Social Justice (1994) (The Borrie Report) *Social Justice: Strategies for National Renewal*. London: Vintage.

Dicken, P. (1992, second edition) *Global Shift: The Internationalization of Economic Activity*. London: Paul Chapman Publishing.

Dintenfass, M. (1992) *The Decline of Industrial Britain: 1870–1980*. London: Routledge.

Drucker, P.F. (1986) 'The changed world economy', *Foreign Affairs*, Spring.

Elbaum, B. and Lazonik, W. (1984) 'The decline of the British economy: an institutional perspective', *Journal of Economic History*, 44 (2): 567–583.

Engels, F. (1975a) 'The condition of the working class in England. From personal observation and authentic sources', in *Collected Works*, vol. 4, Moscow and London: Progress Publishers and Lawrence & Wishart, pp. 295–596.

Engels, F. (1975b) 'The condition of England. I. The eighteenth century', in *Karl Marx and Frederick Engels: Collected Works*, vol. 3, Moscow and London: Progress Publishers and Lawrence & Wishart, pp. 469–488.

Gamble, A. (1994, fourth edition) *Britain in Decline: Economic Policy, Political Strategy and the British State*. Basingstoke: Palgrave Macmillan.

Gibbard, K. (1996) 'The decline of British capital', in J. Lea and G. Pilling (eds) *The Condition of Britain: Essays on Frederick Engels*, London: Pluto Press, 38–57.

Great Britain, National Committee of Inquiry into Higher Education (Chairman Sir Ron Dearing) (1997) *Higher Education in the Learning Society; National Committee of Inquiry into Higher Education*, London: HMSO.

Hilton, R. (ed.) (1976) *The Transition from Feudalism to Capitalism*, London: New Left Books.

Hutchison, K. (1951) *The Decline and Fall of British Capitalism*, London: Archon.

Hutton, W. (1995) *The State We're In*, London: Jonathan Cape.

Ilyenkov, E.V. (1982) *The Dialectics of the Abstract and the Concrete in Marx's Capital*, Moscow: Progress Publishers. Online, available at: www.marxists.org/archive/ilyenkov/works/abstract/index.htm (accessed 12 May 2012).

Ingham, G. (1984) *Capitalism Divided? The City and Industry in British Social Development*, Basingstoke: Macmillan.

Kemp, T. (1985, second edition) *Industrialization in Nineteenth-Century Europe*, London: Longmans.

Keynes, J.M. (1936) *The General Theory of Employment, Interest and Money*, London: Macmillan.

Lenin, V.I. (1964) 'Imperialism, the highest stage of capitalism', in *Collected Works*, vol. 22, Moscow and London: Progress Publishers and Lawrence & Wishart, pp. 185–304.

Looker, B. (1988) in C. Barker and D. Nicholls (eds) *The Development of British Capitalist Society: A Marxist Debate*, Manchester: Northern Marxist Historians Group.

Marx, K. (1959) *Capital*, vol. III, Moscow and London: Foreign Languages Publishing House and Lawrence & Wishart.

Marx, K. (1961a) 'Preface to the first German edition' in *Capital*, vol. I, Moscow and London: Foreign Languages Publishing House and Lawrence & Wishart.

Marx, K. (1961b) *Capital*, vol. I, Moscow and London: Foreign Languages Publishing House and Lawrence & Wishart.

Marx, K. (1973) *Grundrisse*, Harmondsworth: Penguin.

Meiksins Wood, E. (1991) *The Pristine Culture of Capitalism: A Historical Essay on Old Regimes and Modern States*. London and New York: Verso.

Meiksins Wood, E. (1994) 'From opportunity to imperative: the history of the market', *Monthly Review*, 46, 3.

Morgan Guaranty Trust Company (1991) *World Financial Markets*, April.

Pilling, G. (1986) *The Crisis of Keynesian Economics: A Marxist View*, London and

Sydney: Croom Helm. Online, available at: www.marxists.org/archive/pilling/works/keynes/index.htm (accessed 16 December 2011).

Pilling, G. (1996a) 'Frederick Engels and the industrial revolution', in J. Lea and G. Pilling (eds) *The Condition of Britain: Essays on Frederick Engels*. London: Pluto, pp. 58–83.

Pilling, G. (1996b) 'Globalisation and the British working class: an essay in economic analysis and political prognosis', in T. Brotherstone and G. Pilling (eds) *History, Economic History and the Future of Marxism: Essays in Memory of Tom Kemp*, London: Porcupine Press, pp. 13–50.

Ricardo, D. (1953 [1951 first edition]) *The Works and Correspondence of David Ricardo*, vol. 1, *On the Principles of Political Economy and Taxation*. Edited with an Introduction by P. Sraffa, in collaboration with M.H. Dobb. Cambridge: Cambridge University Press.

Rubin, I.I. (1979) *A History of Economic Thought*. London: Ink Links.

Saville, J. (1969) 'Primitive accumulation and early industrialisation in Britain', *Socialist Register*, 6, 247–271.

Saville, J. (1994) *The Consolidation of the Capitalist State, 1800–1850*. London: Pluto.

Skidelsky, R. (1975) *Oswald Mosley*. London: Macmillan.

Smith, A. (1976) *An Inquiry into the Nature and Causes of the Wealth of Nations*, vol. 2. Edited by R.H. Campbell and A.S. Skinner, Oxford: Clarendon Press.

Thompson, E.P. (1965) 'The peculiarities of the English', *Socialist Register*, 2, 311–362. (Reprinted in Thompson, E.P. (1978) The *Poverty of Theory and Other Essays*, London: Merlin.)

Weiner, M.J. (1981) *English Culture and the Decline of the Industrial Spirit 1850–1980*. Cambridge: Cambridge University Press.

9 Engels and the industrial revolution

It is a commonplace amongst historians, sociologists, political scientists and others that English history is unique, characterised as it is by a lack of sharp turning points and violent disjunctures. Such a view is held not simply by writers of a conservative disposition. Thus Perry Anderson and Tom Nairn have for long argued that it is the incompleteness of the bourgeois revolution, the lack of a thorough-going modernisation of the state in this country, that marks British history off from that of Continental Europe [see Chapter 8, 'A very peculiar capitalism' – ed.].

Whatever can be said for such a position, it was not one shared by Frederick Engels. Coming to England as a young man in his early twenties he witnessed a social transformation taking place that he regarded as far more profound than the changes then taking place in France and Germany. In the industrial revolution he saw something of far greater significance than for the city of Manchester and its surrounding towns; it was an event with truly universal implications. For the industrial revolution brought into being a quite new social class – the modern working class, and it was this that, more than anything interested Engels. It was in *The Condition of the Working Class in England* (afterwards referred to in this chapter as *The Condition)* that Engels demonstrates that this class was not simply a hopeless, trampled-down class but one that was forced to fight against the conditions into which it had been plunged. In so doing Engels made a decisive contribution to the development of the materialist conception of history.

This chapter takes up this question of the nature and the consequences of the industrial revolution as part of a wider project: the rescuing of Engels, and Marx, from the fate that befell them after their deaths. Their creative work became distorted beyond belief, in part in the lifetime of the Second International but above all in the period when the Stalinist bureaucracy ruled the Soviet Union and controlled a significant sector of the world's labour movement.

For most writers the 'industrial revolution', assuming the term retains any validity, has, especially in the recent past, been reduced to a series of technical changes in the sphere of production; either that, or to a discussion about rates of 'economic growth' in the late eighteenth/early nineteenth centuries. In this respect the social character of the revolution is lost sight of. What follows lays no claim to be a historiography of the industrial revolution. Rather it sets out to consider certain methodological issues which are felt to be crucial if the real character of the changes that were taking place in England 150 years ago are to be understood. It attempts to rescue Engels's conception of the industrial revolution from a narrow, mechanistic misreading; for it was precisely because the changes Engels witnessed on his arrival in Manchester were part of a profound social upheaval that he was obliged to study how the consciousness of the working class was developing and would develop.

Looking back some 50 years after the first publication of *The Condition*, Engels had the following to say in the preface to the 1892 edition:

> It will hardly be necessary to point out that the general theoretical standpoint of this book – philosophical, economical, political – does not exactly coincide with my standpoint of today. Modern international socialism, since fully developed as a science, chiefly and almost exclusively through the efforts of Marx, did not yet exist in 1844. My book represents one of the phases of its embryonic development; and as the human embryo, in its early stages, still reproduces the gill-arches of our fish-ancestors, so this book exhibits everywhere the traces of the descent of modern socialism from one of its ancestors, German classical philosophy.
>
> (Engels 1990a: 313–314)

Engels was drawing attention to the fact that his work was part of that 'pre-history' of Marxism during which time both he and Marx were still developing the foundations of their new, revolutionary, world outlook. Any theoretical limitations in *The Condition* lay essentially in the fact that the critique of bourgeois economy ('Marxist economic theory') was still to be completed. This limitation is reflected in the first place in the fact that, at certain points, Engels asserts that the doctrine of Communism transcends the contradictions between labour and capital, an idea which, in effect, stands in opposition to the thrust of the entire work. Engels came to this conclusion principally because certain members of the bourgeoisie were coming to realise the inevitability of socialism and were siding with the working class. Thus he writes towards the end of the work:

> as Communism stands above the strife between bourgeoisie and proletariat, it will be easier for the better elements of the bourgeoisie (which are, however, deplorably few, and we can look for recruits only among the rising generation) to unite with it than with purely proletarian Chartism.
>
> (Engels 1975a: 582)[1]

Similar traces of the standpoint of utopian socialism are to be seen in Engels's Hobbesian-like contention that society consists of a war of all against all. He tended to see the basic contradiction underlying this war in a manner not unlike that of the utopian socialists, namely as:

> [a] glaring contradiction between a few rich people, on the one hand, and many poor on the other, a contradiction which has already risen to a menacing point in England and France and is daily growing sharper in our country too.
>
> (Engels 1975b: 244)

These limitations notwithstanding, Engels's work represented a decisive step in the direction of Marxism, above all because it saw in the modern working class, that force created by the industrial revolution, not merely a suffering class, but one that was forced to fight its oppression, one that was obliged to 'help itself'.[2] Thus says Engels about the work in the new factory:

> It offers no field for mental activity, and claims just enough of his [the worker's] attention to keep him from thinking of anything else. And a sentence to such work, to work which takes his whole time for itself, leaving him scarcely time to eat and sleep, none for physical exercise in the open air, or the enjoyment of Nature, much less for mental activity, how can such a sentence help degrading a human being to the level of a brute? Once more the worker must choose, must either surrender himself to his fate, become a 'good' workman, heed 'faithfully' the interest of the bourgeoisie, in which case he most certainly becomes a brute, or else he must rebel, fight for his manhood to the last, and this he can do only in the fight against the bourgeoisie.
>
> (Engels 1975a: 415–416)[3]

The entire book is focused on the emergence of this new class and the historical significance of that emergence. Thus although Engels set out to survey the conditions of the working class as a whole, rather than confining himself to a particular industry, as many previous studies had, his book is nonetheless not simply such a survey. Nor is *The Condition* merely a statement and systematisation of the facts that Engels so carefully recorded. His conclusions went far beyond the particular historical situation which provided the factual basis for his study: his main conclusion was that the working class is not simply capable of fighting its capitalist oppression but of establishing the basis for a new society. 'The condition of the working class is the real basis and point of departure of all social movements of the present because it is the highest and most unconcealed pinnacle of the social misery existing in our day.' This allowed Engels to speak of the world-historical significance of the transformation he studied (Engels 1975a: 302).

The Condition is, above all, a general analysis of the development of industrial capitalism and the social impact of that development, the most important feature of which was the emergence of the modern labour movement. That is why Engels tells us that he does not intend to write a history of the industrial revolution but to conduct his study from the point of view of grasping the nature of the English working class:

> We have not, here and now, to deal with the history of this [the industrial] revolution, nor with its vast importance for the present and the future. Such a delineation must be reserved for a future, more comprehensive work. For the moment, we must limit ourselves to the little that is necessary for understanding the facts that follow, *for comprehending the present state of the English proletariat.*
>
> (Engels 1975a: 307, emphasis added)

Engels's conclusion about the nature of the working class was arrived at on the basis of a most detailed and conscientious study of the conditions in which the working class was obliged to live. He not only drew on a wide range of literary sources (Peter Gaskell, John Wade, George Richardson Porter, Edward Baines, Andrew Ure, Thomas Carlyle, amongst others)[4] but he made full use of the official reports of the parliamentary commissioners, factory inspectors and statisticians. Reports from workers were obtained from the Chartist newspaper *The Northern Star* which published regular articles and letters from workers and Engels attended many workers' meetings. Last but not least Engels made extensive visits to working class districts in Manchester ('the first manufacturing city of the world' (1975a: 355)) and surrounding towns, often accompanied by his companion, the young Irish woman, Mary Burns.[5] In this respect Engels's work remains a powerful refutation of the still-existing prejudice that Marxism is based on empty speculation and that Marxists are perforce hostile to empirical investigations.[6] This was the charge of the Young Hegelians who, accused Marx and others of producing speculative constructs of world history.[7] The fact is that long before the appearance of 'empirical sociology' Marx and Engels engaged in a series of concrete social studies, of which *The Condition* is an outstanding early example.

What marks *The Condition* is its recognition that something unique was taking place in England in general and in particular in the industrial towns of the north where work for his book was undertaken. The year before he wrote *The Condition* Engels had spoken thus about the profound developments occurring in England:

> The century of revolution has to all appearances passed England by, causing little change. While on the Continent an entire old world was shattered, while a twenty-five-year war cleared the air, in England everything remained calm, neither state nor church were in any way threatened. And yet since the middle of the last century England has experienced a greater upheaval than any other country – an upheaval which is all the more momentous the more quietly it is brought about, and it will therefore in all probability attain its goal more readily in practice than the political revolution in France or the philosophical revolution in Germany. The revolution in England is a social one and therefore more comprehensive and far-reaching than any other. There are no fields – however remote – of human knowledge and no conditions of life which have not contributed to it and which in turn have not been affected by it.
>
> (Engels 1975c: 469)

He makes a similar point in *The Condition*:

> Sixty, eighty years ago, England was a country like every other, with small towns, few and simple industries, and a thin but *proportionally* large agricultural population. Today it is a country like *no* other, with a capital of two and a half million inhabitants; with vast manufacturing cities; with an industry that supplies the world, and produces almost everything by means of the most complex machinery; with an industrious, intelligent, dense population of which two thirds are employed in trade and commerce, and *composed of classes wholly different*; forming, in fact, with other customs and other needs, a different nation from the England of those days. The industrial revolution is of the same importance for England as the political revolution for France, and the philosophical revolution for Germany; and the difference between England in 1760 and 1844 is at least as great as that between France under the *ancien regime* and during the revolution of July.'
>
> (Engels 1975a: 320,[8] emphasis added)

In the series of articles that Engels contributed to *Vorwärts* in September–October 1844 he says:

> The Germans, the nation of Christian spiritualism, experienced a philosophical revolution; the French, the nation of classical materialism and hence of politics, had to go through a political revolution; the English, a nation that is a mixture of German and French elements, who therefore embody both sides of the antithesis and are for that reason more universal than either of the two factors taken separately, were for that reason drawn into a more universal, a *social* revolution.
>
> (Engels 1975c: 471, emphasis added)

> The history of the proletariat in England begins with the second half of the last century, with the invention of the steam-engine and of machinery for working cotton. These inventions gave rise, as is well known, to an industrial revolution, a revolution which altered the whole civil society; one, the historical importance of which is only now beginning to be recognised. England is the classic soil of this transformation, which was all the mightier, the more silently it proceeded; and England is, therefore, the classic land of its chief product also, the proletariat. Only in England can the proletariat be studied in all its relations and from all sides.[9]
>
> (Engels 1975a: 307)

For Engels these fundamental changes were summed up in the notion of an 'industrial revolution'. He was not the first to employ such a term. In England it is one associated with the name of Arnold Toynbee (1852–1883) whose posthumously-published *Lectures on the Industrial Revolution of the Eighteenth Century in England* (1884) seems to have been the first book to use the term in its title.[10] But despite the widespread belief to the contrary, Toynbee and his followers did not invent the term. Understandably it originates with French writers in the 1820s and 1830s where a parallel between the technical changes then taking place in the major cotton manufacturing centres and the revolutions of 1789 and 1830 was drawn (Bezanson 1922: 342–349). It was these references that Engels almost certainly had in mind when at the very opening of his book he spoke of the 'industrial revolution' as being something 'well known' (Engels 1975a: 307). But if Engels was not the first to deploy the term, he was the first to invest it 'with the full force of a revolutionary event'.[11] Whereas others 'knew' that an industrial revolution was underway, Engels was the first to grasp its true, world-historical, significance, that is its profound social meaning.

In connection with his conception of the industrial revolution, Engels has been subject to a variety of attacks.[12] In the first place the notion of an 'industrial revolution' has been derided as a piece of German Romanticism, a product of the baleful influence exercised over him by Hegel and Moses Hess in particular. In the second place, the whole idea of an industrial revolution ever having taken place has been increasingly questioned by economic historians. Here the object of criticism is not simply Engels but a long line of historians that would include Toynbee, the Hammonds, Paul Mantoux and others. We will look at these two lines of criticism in turn. It was Engels's supposed romanticism, so the story goes, that allowed him to depict the industrial revolution as a 'transcendent historical process', to be set side by side with other sorts of revolution in France and Germany, and carrying inevitable implications for the future. This conception was clearly 'a child of Romanticism' (Coleman 1992: 7).[13] In similar vein, Engels is accused of presenting the industrial revolution as a 'social catastrophe', something that destroyed a state of pre-lapsarian bliss. There are certainly passages in *The Condition* which, if torn out of context, might give rise to such an impression. Thus:

> Before the introduction of machinery, the spinning and weaving of raw materials was carried on in the working-man's home. Wife and daughter spun the yarn that the father wove or that they sold, if he did not work it up himself. These weaver families lived in the country in the neighbourhood of the towns, and could get on fairly well with their wages, because the home market was almost the only one, and the crushing power of competition that came later, with the conquest of foreign markets and the extension of trade, did not yet press upon wages.
>
> (Engels 1975a: 307–308)

And a little further on:

> So the workers vegetated throughout a passably comfortable existence, leading a righteous and peaceful life in all piety and probity; and their material position was far better than that of their successors. They did not

need to overwork; they did no more than they chose to do, and yet earned what they needed.... They were, for the most part, strong, well-built people, in whose physique little or no difference from that of their peasant neighbours was discoverable.

(Engels 1975a: 308)

But this is far from all that Engels has to say about conditions in pre-industrial England. For on the very next page we find:

> But intellectually, they were dead; lived only for their petty, private interest, for their looms and gardens, and knew nothing of the mighty movement which, beyond their horizon, was sweeping through mankind. They were comfortable in their silent vegetation, and but for the industrial revolution they would never have emerged from this existence, which, cosily romantic though it was, was nevertheless not worthy of human beings. In truth, they were not human beings; they were merely toiling machines in the service of the few aristocrats who had guided history down to that time. The industrial revolution has simply carried this out to its logical end by making the workers machines pure and simple, taking from them the last trace of independent activity, and so forcing them to think and demand a position worthy of men. As in France politics, so in England manufacture and the movement of civil society in general drew into the whirl of history the last classes which had remained sunk in apathetic indifference to the universal interests of mankind.
>
> (Engels 1975a: 309)[14]

Comparing the lot of the modern worker, living under conditions of 'hypocritical slavery', with the serf, Engels says:

> But the hypocritical disguised slavery recognises the right to freedom, at least in outward form; bows before a freedom-loving public opinion, and herein lies the historic progress as compared with the old servitude, that the *principle* of freedom is affirmed, and the oppressed will one day see to it that the principle is carried out.
>
> (Engels 1975a: 474)

Or again:

> In the patriarchal relation that hypocritically concealed the slavery of the worker, the latter must have remained an intellectual zero, totally ignorant of his own interest, a mere private individual. Only when estranged from his employer, when convinced that the sole bond between employer and employee is the bond of pecuniary profit, when the sentimental bond between them, which stood not the slightest test, had wholly fallen away, then only did the worker begin to recognise his own interests and develop

> independently; then only did he cease to be the slave of the bourgeoisie in his thoughts, feelings, and the expression of his will.
>
> (Engels 1975a: 419)

In other words, the industrial revolution was a profoundly contradictory event: it brought misery and degradation for the working class but simultaneously, through the creation of just such a class, it laid the basis for a newer, truly human form of society. Criticising the Owenites for their attitude to the working class he says of such socialists:

> While bemoaning the demoralisation of the lower classes, they are blind to the *element of progress in the dissolution of the old social order* and refuse to acknowledge that the corruption wrought by private interests and hypocrisy in the property-holding class is much greater. *They acknowledge no historic development* and wish to place the nation in a state of Communism at once, overnight, not by the unavoidable march of its political development up to the point at which this transition becomes both possible and necessary. They understand, it is true, why the working-man is resentful against the bourgeois, but regard as unfruitful this class hatred, which is after all, the only moral incentive by which the worker can be brought nearer the goal.
>
> (Engels 1975a: 525, emphasis added)

Thomas Carlyle is the man most often accused of providing Engels with his Romantic view of the industrial revolution.[15] There is no doubt that Engels greatly admired Carlyle's work.[16] Carlyle had 'sounded the social disorder more deeply than any other English bourgeois' (Engels 1975a: 578); his *Past and Present* was 'the only one which strikes a human chord, presents human relations and shows traces of a human point of view' (Engels 1975d: 444). Carlyle had condemned the British ruling class for having plunged the English people into unprecedented impoverishment, degradation and moral evil. And Engels found Carlyle's criticisms of capitalism all the more valuable because they were admissions wrung from a member of the ruling class. Engels also quotes with approval Carlyle's exposure of bourgeois democracy:

> The notion that a man's liberty consists in giving his vote at election-hustings and saying, 'Behold, now I too have my twenty-thousandth part of a Talker in our National Palaver; will not the gods be good to me?' – is one of the pleasantest.
>
> (Engels 1975d: 455)

But to imply that this involved an uncritical acceptance of Carlyle's viewpoint is patently absurd. For Carlyle's class standpoint made it impossible for him to take a scientific approach to the problems of doing away with the evils he had so eloquently and passionately described. Carlyle saw the evils produced by the development of capitalism as rooted not in capitalism itself but in atheism and the self-seeking supposedly connected with it. Accepting that there can be no return to the past, he has visions of a new religion based on pantheism and the cult of labour, a position that Engels rejects as a reactionary utopia. Whereas according to Carlyle, society must be saved from the social evils stemming from capitalist civilisation by a 'true aristocracy,' for Engels it is in the working class that 'the strength and the capacity of development of the nation' reposes (Engels 1975a: 529). Only the workers,

> are really respectable, for all their roughness and for all their moral degradation. It is from them that England's salvation will come, they still comprise flexible material; they have no education, but no prejudices either ... they still have a future.
>
> (Engels 1975d: 445–446)[17]

It is on this basis that Engels condemns the reactionary conception of 'heroes' and 'the mob' which Carlyle sought to justify on the basis of the failure of democracy.

As we have stressed, the fundamental point for Engels about the industrial revolution was that its 'mightiest result' (Engels 1975a: 320) was the creation of a new class, the working class, a class that was forced to fight against its conditions of oppression. In other words for him this was a social revolution, not something to be reduced to narrowly technical matters such as the inventions that occurred in this period, important though these were. It is from this angle that Engels sees the importance of the introduction of the spinning jenny: 'While the industrial proletariat was thus developing with the first very imperfect machine, the same machine gave rise to the agricultural proletariat' (Engels 1975a: 311). Or again,

> Having already seen what a transformation in the social condition of the lower classes a single such clumsy machine as the jenny has wrought, there is no cause for surprise as to that which a complete and interdependent system of finely adjusted machinery has brought about.
>
> (Engels 1975a: 312–313)

It is this aspect of the industrial revolution – as something marking a fundamental change in British economic and social structure that has been subject to increasing attack over the recent past. The attack has gained such ground that some historians are now obliged to talk in terms of the need to rehabilitate the industrial revolution.[18] This is no doubt part of the more general claim that British history has been free of sharp turning points, free of violent interruptions, a history characterised by Fabian gradualness. In this respect the attack is not confined to Engels but is directed at a long line of economic and social historians from Arnold Toynbee onwards.[19] Although gaining pace in recent years, the repudiation of the idea of an industrial revolution marking a unique turning point in British history was first evidenced in the 1920s and 1930s in the work of people such as Clapham, Redford and Ashton. These writers stressed the long tap-roots of industrialisation, its unevenness and incompleteness. Their work marked a turn away from the social character of the great changes taking place from the middle of the eighteenth century onwards in favour of a study of the technical changes occurring in industry which went hand-in-hand with a concentration on 'growth rates'. But even then, the majority of historians retained the idea that something that could properly be called an 'industrial revolution' had taken place.[20]

In this respect recent work has taken a step forward, or more accurately a step backwards, in that the very idea of the existence of an industrial revolution in Britain is increasingly rejected, or where the term is accepted it is drained of its social content.[21] Much of this research – the 'new economic history' – has concentrated on statistical work which seeks to show, for instance, that the rate of growth during the period of the industrial revolution was much slower than had previously been thought, and that much of the economy remained unaffected by the technical changes that were taking place in the cotton textile industry. Some writers have laid great stress on the fact that recent estimates of national income over the period concerned show far slower rates of growth than the earlier estimates of Deane and Cole. [A useful recent account of the critique of Deane and Cole's estimates by C. Knick Harley and Nick Crafts is given in the introduction and Chapter 2 of Emma Griffin's *A Short History of the British Industrial Revolution* (2010). Griffin points out that Crafts himself did not reject the notion of an 'industrial revolution' but saw it rather in terms of a structural shift in the economy in terms of getting human labour out of agriculture and into industry, rather than in terms of rapid economic growth. Griffin says that while we may agree with Crafts that Britain underwent 'an event of great historical significance' we are left with many questions about what that event was. This chapter indicates the significance of 'the event' in terms of a profound transformation of social relations – ed.] According to the latest calculations growth was particularly slow in the last four decades of the eighteenth century. The problem here is not so much the fragile data on which these 'estimates' are made but the meaning to be attached to them. For what is crucial is not the quantitative rate of growth of national income but the *qualitative* transformation of social relations in Britain in the century up to 1850. This raises important theoretical problems. No economic system, least of all the capitalist economy, can be understood as a series of 'sectors' which stand side-by-side in some passive relationship. It is the *interaction* of its various sectors that determines the real dynamic of an economy. Thus in the case of the world economy: its momentum is determined by the real, changing relationships between its various national components. Its movement cannot be understood by resort to simple arithmetical entities – for instance average growth rates, even average growth rates of the manufacturing sector. Such statistics can disclose little about the real forces which either impel forward or retard its development. Naturally no economic historian is unaware of the fact that there were marked disparities in the growth rates of the different sectors of the economy both during the pre-industrial period and then during the industrial revolution itself. But the matter is not simply one of quantities, as many seem to believe.[22]

The manner in which Trotsky set out to grasp the peculiarities of Russia's economic development in the period before 1917 is here instructive from the point of view of method. Could, for example, the dynamic of economic relations in pre-1917 Russia be understood from the smallness of the working class as a proportion of the total population? This sort of question, Trotsky makes clear, can only be approached concretely, from the standpoint of the real inter-relations within the economy – as they had arisen historically. The working class, although a tiny proportion of a population comprising largely peasants, was a relatively new phenomenon. Thanks to Russia's belated economic development, because industrialisation took place on the basis of techniques and forms of organisation already developed in the west, the working class was concentrated in some of the most advanced factories in Europe. This gave it a specific weight which no simple averaging of the population could disclose; on the contrary, such averaging could lead only to the conclusion that the working class was a relatively powerless class.

Thus Trotsky says

> But it is just in the sphere of economy ... that the law of combined development most forcibly emerges. At the same time that peasant land-cultivation as a whole remained, right up to the revolution, at the level of the seventeenth century, Russian industry in its technique and capitalist structure stood at the level of the advanced countries, and in certain respects even outstripped them. Small enterprises, involving less than 100 workers, employed in the United States in 1914, 35 per cent of the total industrial workers, but in Russia only 17.8 per cent.
>
> (Trotsky 1980: 10)[23]

The same methodological questions that are involved in grasping the nature and dynamic of the industrial revolution in Britain arose in the dispute in the 1920s about whether socialism in a single country, Russia, was feasible. It was Bukharin who argued that because the correlation between the working class and the peasantry in the USSR corresponded to the 'average' figure for the world economy, this meant that the conditions for building socialism in the Soviet Union were no less or no more favourable than anywhere else. Replying to Bukharin's 'scholastic casuistry' Trotsky made the following remark (if 'industrial revolution' is substituted for 'world revolution' and 'national revolution', Trotsky's point has more than a little relevance for the present discussion):

> In the first place, it is quite probable that the correlation of forces between the proletariat and the peasantry on the world scale is not very much different from the correlation within the USSR. But the world revolution is not accomplished in accordance with the method of the arithmetic mean, and, incidentally neither is the national revolution. Thus the October Revolution

> occurred and entrenched itself first in proletarian Petrograd, instead of choosing such a region where the correlation between the workers and peasants would correspond to the average for the whole of Russia. After Petrograd and later Moscow had created the revolutionary government and the revolutionary army, they had to overthrow the bourgeoisie in the outlying country, in the course of several years; and only as a result of this process, called revolution, was there established within the boundaries of the USSR the present correlation between the proletariat and the peasantry. The revolution does not occur in accordance with the method of the arithmetic mean. It can begin in a less favourable sector, but until it entrenches itself in the decisive sectors of both the national and the world frontiers, it is impermissible to speak about its complete victory.
>
> (Trotsky 1974: 46)[24]

A general issue is involved in this discussion about recent trends in economic history, namely the tendency to separate out narrowly 'economic' question from wider social processes.

According to an earlier comment by one writer

> it is now unusual for economic historians in Britain to refer in their specialist or their general writing to historical categories or types of societies, and any discussion of change, of early industrialisation, for instance, is set in generalised terms relating to 'the industrial revolution,' or to the period of 'take off,' without reference to the broader context of society in which these events occurred. There has come about a narrowing of interest from society at large to the more limited problems of economic growth and change. Social questions are nearly always considered separately from economic development; political matters are left entirely alone.
>
> (Saville 1969: 248)[25]

It is one of the contentions of the 'new economic history' that the development of the industrial sector during the 'industrial revolution' was far less rapid than has hitherto been thought. But here again two matters arise. In the first place, it must again be stressed that simple averages cannot disclose the real relationship of forces at work. Landes makes a telling point which is worth quoting at length:

> In sum one must not mistake the appearance for the reality. The census returns and other numbers [are] … without the virtue of wholeness to compensate for their lifelessness … numbers merely describe the surface of society and even then in terms that define away change by using categories of unchanging nomenclature. Beneath this surface, the vital organs were transformed and though they weighed but a fraction of the total … it was they that determined the metabolism of the entire system. We have seen that, in so far as small-scale enterprise continued to flourish, it did so largely because of demand derived from the growth of concentrated manufacture:

> the demand of the large producers themselves; of their employees; and of the urban agglomerations that grew up around them. But not only small industry was tied in this way to the modern sector. Agriculture, trade, banking – all came increasingly to depend on the needs, the products, the bills of exchange, the investments of Lancashire, the Midlands, and the other nodes of British factory industry.
>
> (Landes 1969: 122)[26]

The fact is that it was a qualitative breakthrough in one branch of textiles – cotton spinning – that was decisive.[27] And we stress 'qualitative' because the 'breakthrough' was not simply a quantitative matter. It was the development of the *factory system*, the development of *industrial capitalism* in that sphere that is the vital issue. In other words it was not merely, or primarily, changes in the techniques of production that led to a development of the productive forces during the period of the industrial revolution, but a transformation of the social relations of production, albeit initially in one sector.

Second, and just as important: we can say that while the 'breakthrough' was made in cotton textiles, such a development would have been impossible without the fundamental changes that took place in English agriculture in the 300 years, 1500–1800. Unless the relationship between the industrial and agricultural sectors is grasped then the origins of the industrial revolution in England will be lost. In the last resort it will be impossible to answer the question: why was it that that 'primitive machine' (Engels) introduced into one sector of one branch of production (textiles) could set in motion such a profound social transformation of England? Clearly not because of the material qualities of the machine per se but because the social conditions were ripe in England in a way that they were not elsewhere. (We will return shortly to this question of the 'natural' and the 'social'.) And in grasping this 'ripeness', the revolution brought about in agriculture holds the key.

As Saville puts it:

> Above all, the experience of Britain in respect of the transformation of her social structure prior to industrialisation has not been paralleled in the history of any other industrialising society. Nowhere save in Britain was the peasantry virtually eliminated before the acceleration of economic growth that is associated with the development of industrial capitalism, and of the many special features of early industrialisation in Britain none is more striking than the pressure of a rapidly growing proletariat in the countryside.
>
> (Saville 1969: 250)[28]

The major theme of this chapter has been the defence of the notion of the industrial revolution as above all a social phenomenon, as against those who see the revolution (assuming they think that such a term has any validity) in narrowly technical terms. This issue has wider implications than merely an appreciation of the character of the industrial revolution. It is to these wider implications that we briefly turn. For those who wish to see in the industrial revolution simply the application of new inventions to the productive process, who wish to concentrate their attention on increases in labour productivity and 'growth rates' are in fact guilty of confusing the 'technical' with the 'social', of fetishising science.[29]

It was the so-called 'scientific and technological revolution' that supposedly occurred after 1945 that led many to talk about the 'transformation' of capitalism, and some to speak in terms of a 'new' industrial revolution. Thus the once-fashionable notion of 'industrial society' is based on claims that the imperatives of technical change in the post-war world have made it essential for large corporations to plan their economic growth over long periods of time, ignoring profit maximisation. The claim was that advances in technology had made the planning and the marketing of goods and services, as well as their production by means of data-processing systems, a necessary component of management. The conclusion drawn by Galbraith (1967) and others was that power now lies in the hands of a 'technostructure', a stratum engendered by the 'technological and scientific revolution' and one that shuns the traditional capitalist mentality, a social group that seeks optimal profit in a manner that attenuates or even eliminates the traditional conflict between capital and labour. In the 'new world order' (in fact it is a world of chaos) such ideas seem positively antediluvian when compared with what Engels wrote 150 years ago.[30]

But it is not simply the apologists for capitalism who have contended that, thanks to the development of science and technology, there has been a decisive change in contemporary capitalism. It is here that important questions about the degeneration of Marxism in the present century must be referred to. The enormous damage done to the theoretical heritage of Marxism by its Stalinist perversion is now widely recognised. It was Stalinism that distorted historical materialism almost beyond recognition when it presented history as a series of fixed stages through which each society would automatically progress. Relations of production would adjust semi-automatically to the level attained in the ever-upward progress of the productive forces. And these forces of production were in turn interpreted narrowly to mean productive techniques, or the implements of labour or natural forces brought under control by technology: with the 'working class' sometimes 'added on' as one of the productive forces. These mechanical conceptions reached their nadir with the writings of Stalin – or rather the writings that were issued in his name

But it is clear that this degeneration was by no means confined to those under the direct influence of Stalinism. For example, amongst those who saw a new industrial revolution having taken place in the post-1945 period was Ernest Mandel – in his case this was the 'third industrial revolution' known to history. For Mandel this latest industrial revolution was based on the emergence of a series of new, 'hi-tech' industries alongside the growing involvement of the state in the regulation of the economy. He coined the phrase 'neo-capitalism' to describe this new and distinct state in the evolution of capitalism. Writing in the 1960s he had the following to say:

> With the 1940s appeared the warning signs of a third industrial revolution. The first industrial revolution had been based on the steam engine, the second on the electric motor and the combustion engine. The third industrial revolution is based on the release of nuclear energy and the use of electronic machinery.
>
> (Mandel 1968: 605)[31]

It is this phrase 'based on' that is misleading. The industrial revolution was not 'based on the steam engine'. Certainly the industrial revolution involved the application of steam power to productive processes, but, as we have argued, such applications were possible only because of the transformation of social relations in agriculture that preceded the industrial revolution. The crux of the matter is that the introduction of machinery in the late eighteenth and early nineteenth centuries brought a new class into existence. It seems clear that like many others, Mandel has managed to drain his conception of 'industrial revolution' of its social, class content. His second and third 'industrial revolutions' were in no real sense industrial revolutions for, unlike the first they singularly failed to bring new classes and new class relations into being. In this vital respect, then, the 'first' industrial revolution was the only one that Britain has experienced. In one respect at least Mandel is consistent. For if indeed the post-war period has witnessed a new industrial revolution, then this must mark a new stage in the development of capitalism, what Mandel calls 'neo-capitalism'

> I do not care very much for the term 'neo-capitalism which is ambiguous, to say the least. Nevertheless I am quite convinced that starting either with the great depression of 1929–32 or with the second world war, capitalism entered into a third stage of its development, *which is as different from monopoly capitalism or imperialism as described by Lenin, Hilferding and others as monopoly capitalism was different from classical laissez-faire capitalism*. We have to give this child a name; all other names proposed seem even less acceptable than 'neo-capitalism'. 'State monopoly capitalism', the term used in the Soviet Union and the 'official' communist parties, is very misleading because it implies a degree of independence of the state which, to my mind, does not at all correspond to present-day reality. On the contrary, I would say that today the state is a much more direct instrument for guaranteeing monopoly surplus profit to the strongest private monopolies than it ever was in the past. The German *Spaetkcapitalismus* seems interesting, but simply indicates a time sequence and is difficult to translate into several languages.
>
> (Mandel 1974,[32] emphasis added)

Now if the 'industrial revolution' is narrowed down to a technical phenomenon – as I believe is the case with writers such as Mandel – it is impossible to understand the development of consciousness that took place in the century following 1750. For one outstanding feature of the industrial revolution was that it not only saw the emergence of a new class, the working class, but witnessed a profound development in the consciousness of this class.

In *The Condition* Engels outlines the situation of the worker and what it means for the fight he has to engage against the capitalist:

> He [the worker] is the passive subject of all possible combinations of circumstances, and must count himself fortunate when he has saved his life even for a short time; and his character and way of living are naturally shaped by these conditions. Either he seeks to keep his head above water in this whirlpool, to rescue his manhood, and this he can do solely in rebellion against the class which plunders him so mercilessly and then abandons him to his fate ... or he gives up the struggle against his fate as hopeless.
>
> (Engels 1975a: 413)

Or later

> It must be admitted, even if I had not proved it so often in detail, that the English workers cannot feel happy in this condition; that theirs is not a state in which a man or a whole class of men can think, feel and live as human beings. The workers must therefore strive to escape from this brutalising condition, to secure for themselves a better, more human position; and this they cannot do without attacking the interest of the bourgeoisie which consists in exploiting them. But the bourgeoisie defends its interests with all the power placed at its disposal by the wealth and the might of the State. In proportion as the working-man determines to alter the present state of things, the bourgeois becomes his avowed enemy.
>
> (Engels 1975a: 501)

Commenting on passages such as these Steven Marcus says that their interest lies in the fact that they express the idea that a working-class or labour movement will have to be essentially the activity of the working class itself.

> It represents one of the earliest acknowledgements by a socialist writer of any theoretical standing of this critical historical circumstance, and distinguishes in advance the kind of socialism that Marx and Engels were to develop theoretically from the socialism of their immediate predecessors, the Owenites, Saint-Simonians, and Fourierists and the socialists in Germany.
>
> (Marcus 1974: 226)[33]

Here lies the significance of Lenin's earlier insistence that Engels grasped the fact that the working class was no helpless object, the mere plaything of history but that its very condition forced it to 'help itself'. Engels traces the general path of this development of working class consciousness. Starting in some cases with crime it grows through machine-breaking – in which the working class 'first manifested opposition to the bourgeoisie' (Engels 1975a: 503) through trade unionism, finally to reach Chartism.[34]

One of the legacies of the distortion of Marxism for which Stalinism was principally responsible was the mechanical separation between the struggle of the working class and revolutionary class consciousness. It was Karl Kautsky who rightly said that revolutionary class consciousness was brought into the movement 'from the outside', a proposition which Lenin (1973) strongly supported against those (the 'economists') who conceived of revolutionary class consciousness developing in a purely spontaneous manner. But at the same time Lenin recognised that the working class tended to gravitate towards such a revolutionary consciousness, Marxism, if only because Marxism best explained its historical and objective situation.

In this regard, Engels's comments on the relationship of Chartism to socialist theory are of considerable contemporary significance:

> Hence it is evident that the working-men's movement is divided into two sections, the Chartists and the Socialists. The Chartists are theoretically the more backward, the less developed, but they are genuine proletarians all over, the representatives of their class. The Socialists are more far-seeing, propose practical remedies against distress, but, proceeding originally from the bourgeoisie, are for this reason unable to amalgamate completely with the working class. The union of Socialism with Chartism ... will be the next step, and has already begun. Then only, when this has been achieved, will the working class be the true intellectual leader of England. Meanwhile, political and social development will proceed, and will foster this new party, this new departure of Chartism.
>
> (Engels 1975a: 526–527)[35]

This was written some 150 years ago. Today the working class in Britain stands in need of a 'new party'; the leaders of its traditional party, the Labour Party, have now turned their back explicitly on anything to do with socialism. Clause IV of the Labour Party constitution has been abandoned and Tony Blair and company make no secret of their aim to transform the Labour Party into a version of the US Democratic Party, that is an openly bourgeoisie party. Not only that: the sort of party that is needed is one that follows Engels's conception: not one that stands apart from the working class, preaching from on high to it, but one that is an integral part of its daily struggles.

In this respect, Engels's comments are as fresh today as the day they were written. According to one writer: 'Engels's book remains today, as it was in 1845, by far the best single book on the working class of the period' (Hobsbawm 1969: 17). No doubt the research of the last 150 years has added to our knowledge of the working class. But in its theoretical conceptions, in its grasp of the period and its consequences, in its look into the future, *The Condition* remains unsurpassed. It was a truly revolutionary book. Not only did it assist Marx to become 'a Marxist' but it represented a vital stage in the elaboration of historical materialism. We have drawn attention to the disastrous and stultifying impact which Stalinism had on Marxism. Engels's *The Condition* has nothing whatsoever in common with the crude, mechanical distortions that for decades passed as Marxism in many intellectual circles. In the task of re-appropriating the heritage of Marxism, and in the task of developing it creatively in line with today's requirements the book of the 24-year-old Engels will surely occupy a central place.

[This chapter was first published in J. Lea and G. Pilling (eds) (1996) *The Condition of Britain: Essays on Frederick Engels*, London: Pluto Press, pp. 58–83 – ed.]

Acknowledgements

I should like to thank Terry Brotherstone for some helpful comments on an earlier draft.

Notes

1 In the preface to the English edition (1892) he had the following to say about this earlier position:

> Thus great stress is laid on the dictum that Communism is not a mere party doctrine of the working class, but a theory compassing the emancipation of society at large, including the capitalist class, from its present narrow conditions. This is true enough in the abstract, but absolutely useless, and sometimes worse, in practice. So long as the wealthy classes not only do not feel the want of any emancipation, but strenuously oppose the self-emancipation of the working class, so long the social revolution will have to be prepared and fought out by the working class alone.
>
> (Engels 1990b: 261)

2 This should not lead us to ignore the book as a purely historical piece of work. According to one writer, even today, as an empirical account of the working class and its conditions it stands unrivalled (see Marcus 1974).

3 This was Lenin's estimation: 'Even before Engels, many people had described the sufferings of the proletariat, and had pointed to the necessity of helping it. Engels was the *first* to say that the proletariat is *not only* a suffering class; that it is, in fact, the disgraceful economic conditions of the proletariat that drives it irresistibly forward and compels it to fight for its ultimate emancipation. And the fighting proletariat *will help itself*' (Lenin1972a: 22). The revolutionary role of the working class is a theme strongly present in *The Holy Family*, which was published the year prior to *The Condition*. Marx and Engels speak there of 'the world historic role of the proletariat' which 'executes the sentence that private property pronounces on itself' (Marx and Engels 1975: 36).

4 None of these writers shared Engels's conception that an industrial and social revolution was underway in England, though Gaskell came close when he spoke of, 'one of the most striking revolutions ever produced in the moral and social condition of a moiety of a great nation that which has been consequent to the application of steam to machinery' (Peter Gaskell, *The Manufacturing Population of England*, quoted in D.C. Coleman 1992: 6). For an account of the sources used by Engels see W.O. Henderson (1976) *The Life of Friedrich Engel*, vol. 1, Chapter 2.

5 Explaining the significance of the position of Manchester, Engels says:

> Hence because Manchester is the classic type of a modern manufacturing town, and because I know it as intimately as my own native town, more intimately than most of its residents know it, we shall make a longer stay here.
>
> (Engels 1975a: 345)

6 The 'Marxist' defence of this position found its absurdest expression in the work of Louis Althusser. Cf. Lenin's remarks about Marx's *Capital*: '

> He took one of the social-economic formations – the system of commodity production – *and on the basis of a vast mass of data* which he studied for no less that twenty-five years gave a most detailed analysis of the laws governing the functioning of this formation and its development.
>
> (Lenin 1972b: 141, emphasis added)

7 In the Preface to the German edition (1845) Engels accuses German communism and socialism of having started from theoretical premises alone and of knowing too little of the real world and this 'bad reality' (Engels 1975a: 303). For Marx's and Engels's attitude to the Young Hegelians see *The Holy Family*, their first joint work and published before *The Condition.*

8 At least some of the leading socialists came to recognise the social implications of the momentous changes that had taken place in England. Thus the Owenite James Hole could write in 1851:

> Class stands opposed to class, and so accustomed have men become to pursue their own isolated interests apart from and regardless of that of others, that it has become an acknowledged maxim, that when a man pursues his own interests alone he is most benefiting society – a maxim ... which would justify every crime and folly.... The principle of supply and demand has been extended from commodities to men. These have obtained more liberty, but less bread. They find that in parting with the thraldom of Feudalism they have taken on that of Capital; that slavery has ceased in name but survived in fact.
>
> (James Hole, *Lectures on Social Science*, quoted in Briggs 1963: 140)

9 Compare with:

> Great Britain, of all other countries, has seen developed on the greatest scale, the despotism of Capital and the slavery of Labour. In no other country have the intermediate stations between the millionaire commanding whole industrial armies and the wages-slave living from hand to mouth so gradually been swept away from the soil. There exist here no longer, as in continental countries, large classes of peasants and artisans almost equally dependent on their own property and their own labour. A complete divorce of property from labour has been effected in Great Britain. In no other country, therefore, the war between the two classes that constitute modern society has assumed so colossal dimensions and features so distinct and palpable.
>
> (Marx, Letter to the Labour Parliament, 9 March 1854, in Marx 1980: 57)

10 For a survey of the historiography of the industrial revolution from Toynbee onwards see D. Cannadine (1984: 149–158). Cannadine suggests that the interpretation of the industrial revolution has passed through four distinct phases. Initially its social consequences were stressed, then it was examined as an example of a series of cyclical fluctuations, then as a case of 'economic growth' and finally in terms of the fashionable 'limits to growth' theory.

11 Gertrude Himmelfarb (1984) *The Idea of Poverty*: 282, quoted in D.C. Coleman 1992: 3.

12 We leave aside the cruder attacks that claim that Engels deliberately misused his sources to paint an unnecessarily grim picture of the industrial revolution. The most

notorious of such attacks was that of Henderson and Chaloner in their edition of *The Condition*. For a reply to this sort of attack see E.J. Hobsbawm 'The dark satanic mills' in Hobsbawm's *Labouring Men: Studies in the History of Labour* (1964: 105–119).

13 How Engels's notion of the industrial revolution can be characterised as 'transcendent' when it is sustained with such a mass of concrete empirical material is difficult to comprehend.

14

> The industrial revolution ... [made] the workers machines pure and simple, taking from them the last trace of independent activity, and so forcing them to think and demand a position worthy of men. As in France politics, so in England manufacture and the movement of civil society in general drew into the whirl of history the last classes which had remained sunk in apathetic indifference to the universal interests of mankind.
>
> (Engels 1975a: 309)

It is in this spirit that Engels condemns any idea that there can be a return to some pre-industrial state as Disraeli, Lord Ashley and other members of Young England were at the time proposing. Such an object was quite 'unobtainable' says Engels, 'ridiculous', 'a satire upon all historical development' (Engels 1975a: 578).

15

> Among Engels's English language sources one provided a close link with the world of German Romanticism, itself a vital spring of Engels's historical argument. Thomas Carlyle was himself, of course, greatly influenced by Romanticism ... Carlyle's thunderous rhetorical assault upon the 'condition of England' in *Past and Present* appealed to Engels's revolutionary sentiments as well as seeming to offer support for the evidence of his own eyes on his arrival in England in November 1842.
>
> (Coleman 1992: 6–7)

16 It was at the conclusion of his review of Carlyle's *Past and Present* that Engels declares that he must carry out a more detailed examination of the condition of England: 'The condition of England is of immense importance for history and for all other countries; for as regards social matters England is of course far in advance of all other countries' (Engels 1975d: 468). This was a striking advance on Engels's contention at the end of 1842, when he considered England to be up to its ears in medieval backwardness.

17 It is the working class that has put forward, through its social leaders, the Socialists, the task of destroying capitalism.

> But in any case they [the Socialists] are the only party in England which has a future, relatively weak though they may be. Democracy Chartism must soon be victorious, and then the mass of the English workers will have the choice only between starvation and socialism.
>
> (Engels 1975d: 467)

Engels's appreciation of the position of the working class measures the extent to which he and Marx had finished with the Young Hegelians. Bruno Bauer, for example, thought the masses, far from being a liberating force, were driven by ignorance and passion. Enslaved by the tyranny of 'the practical', by the narrow struggle to improve their lot, they were sunk in preoccupations with their material interests. For a trenchant critique of the revival of similar ideas in the recent past see Ellen Meiksins Wood, *The Retreat from Class: A New 'True' Socialism* (1986).

18 See Maxine Berg and Pat Hudson, 'Rehabilitating the industrial revolution (1992).

19 The industrial revolution has always been a matter for intense ideological debate. It is no accident that for much of the Cold War the apologists for capitalism sought to

show that capitalist industrialisation was not inconsistent with rising living standards. While the matter cannot be entered into fully here, it should be noted that neither Engels nor Marx ever held that the development of capitalism would bring with it an inevitable and irreversible 'immiseration' for the working class, nor that *all* workers had been plunged into poverty as a result of capitalist industrialisation (see, for e.g. Engels 1975a: 372–373). In any case, crucially, Engels did not believe that revolution would occur because of the tendency to absolute impoverishment, but because of the tendency to social polarisation (on this point, see Engels 1975a: 580). In this sense much of the heated controversy about the standard of living of the working class during the period of the industrial revolution was perhaps somewhat misplaced. For a recent survey of where that controversy has now reached see John Rule, *The Labouring Classes in Early Industrial England, 1750–1850* (1986).

20 This was not universally true, as the following statement written in 1927 indicates:

> When, on looking back, we find that the revolution has been going on for two centuries, and had been in preparation for two centuries before that, when we find that both in its causes and consequences it affects the lot of that three-quarters of the human race who are still farmers and peasants as profoundly as it does that of the industrial worker, we may begin to doubt whether the term ... has not by this time served its term.
>
> (George Unwin 'Some economic factors in general history', quoted in M.W. Flinn 1966: 5).

21 The other side of the coin is that the idea of 'industrial revolution' has been greatly expanded. According to which economic historian you consult, you can find 'industrial revolutions' in the Bronze Age, the thirteenth century, the fifteenth century, the period 1540–1640, the late nineteenth and early twentieth centuries. Thus Professor Carus-Wilson saw the mechanisation of the process of fulling in the thirteenth century as constituting an industrial revolution; Nef saw an industrial revolution in the century after 1540 as taking place in the coal industry which brought with it technical changes and the growth of large-scale industry. And this is only England! Germany and Japan in the late nineteenth centuries have their advocates. Walt Rostow claimed to discern no fewer than four industrial revolutions: the first in the period after 1780, associated with the textile industry; the second based on the railway boom of the 1830s; a third based on the steel, machine tools and motor vehicles of the late nineteenth and early twentieth centuries; a fourth is still underway based on electronics and developments in biology. What most of these conceptions share is a concentration on the narrow question of changes in the techniques of production. In any event, so wide is the use of the concept 'industrial revolution' that it loses all meaning.

22 See, for example, Crafts (1989). Crafts, a leading figure in the 'new economic history' school, accepts that there was something called an 'industrial revolution' in Britain. But his understanding of it is far different from that of Engels. He recognises that there was a pronounced structural change in the British economy with resources moving away from agriculture to industry, although, according to his calculations this did not involve rapid changes in productivity in the latter sector.

> The 'industrial revolution' consisted much more in getting a lot of workers into industry than of achieving very high productivity from them once there. It is Britain's agricultural productivity, release of labour from agriculture and triumph in cotton textile exports which emerge as truly remarkable.

Here again, the changes in agriculture that made such gains in per capita output possible were of a *social* character, involving as they did the triumph of capitalist relations in the countryside, a point emphasised below.

23 The whole of the first chapter, 'Peculiarities of Russia's development', deals with this problem.

24 Trotsky suggested that this argument of Bukharin be included in a textbook on dialectics as an example of purely scholastic thinking.

25 It is little wonder that one of our most prominent economic historians, R.M. Hartwell, could admit some years ago that the considerable recent empirical work 'has added little to our understanding of the industrial revolution' (R.M. Hartwell, 'The causes of the industrial revolution: an essay in methodology', quoted in Saville 1969: 249).

26 For the significance of these remarks see Berg and Hudson, 1992. The position of Landes is in sharp contrast to those who, on the basis that as late as 1850 many handicraft industries survived, located in small workshops, maintain that patterns of employment remained dominated by traditional craftsmen, labourers and domestic servants, that there was only a slow diffusion of steam power, and that we cannot properly speak of an 'industrial revolution'. In so doing they simply reveal the narrowness of their conception (see A.E. Musson 1978 and Cannadine 1984).

27 Here again, those who abstract from the *social* content of the industrial revolution are able to argue that the experience of industrial Lancashire was atypical and that it was in fact the mercantile and consumer-dominated Home Counties that provided the main sources and stimulus to economic growth. This misses the point that the industrial revolution cannot be reduced to that of 'economic growth' either slow or rapid. It was the new factory system, with Manchester at its heart, that created the modern working class, and this is the decisive issue here.

28 Saville claims this 'crucial fact of British history' is rarely commented on in contemporary historical writing. Saville's position is echoed in the work of another Marxist:

> It is not incorrect to regard the way in which these conditions were prepared in Britain, especially in England, as being the classic case. It was also a unique one; nowhere else were the conditions precisely reproduced; nowhere else did agrarian relations, by the eighteenth century, conform so exactly with the requirements of industrial capitalism … In England the transformation of feudalism began early and conditions rapidly became favourable for the strengthening of the forces of the market and individual possessiveness. Partly owing to the changes which the feudal class underwent through its internecine conflicts and its ability to strengthen its power in relation to the Crown, it adapted itself to the commercial possibilities which opened up in the sixteenth century. The disintegration of the peasant community began early and its position steadily weakened while the lords were extending their control over their estates and viewing them increasingly as a commercial proposition.
>
> (Kemp 1985: 38)

29 Fetishism arises from the fact that natural objects assume properties which have nothing whatsoever to do with their nature but are entirely the product of the social relations of which these are a part and an expression. That such 'things' do acquire such power is no mere illusion, no simple product of the inadequate thinking of individuals, and therefore something to be 'demystified' by the power of thought alone. For Marx, fetishism arose from the very nature of capitalist production itself – wherein the social relations between individuals and classes take the form of, become attached to, inanimate objects. Thus it wasn't the machine that brought about a social transformation in the eighteenth and early nineteenth century but the fact that such machines took the form of *capital*, that is they were privately owned and confronted a class of wage labourers.

30 For a stinging riposte to such theories and their later development see István Mészáros (1989, especially pp. 60–177).

31 Contrary to what Mandel says, the history of capitalism has been characterised by *continual* changes that have brought first one and then another industrial sector to the fore. Thus it was textiles, cotton in particular that occupied the pioneering role; at a later stage heavy industry – concentrated on iron and steel; it was subsequent

developments in the engineering and chemical industries that later made new means of transportation possible, especially the motor car. Mandel is guilty of more than a smack of 'technological determinism' that was characteristic of 'Marxism' in its Stalinist perversion. Kenneth Smith is certainly nearer the truth when he writes:

> The so-called 'industrial revolution' actually had precious little that was industrial about it in a technological sense: it consisted to a great extent of changes in the organisation and management of work, in new methods of marketing, finance and the control of enterprises.
>
> (Smith 1984)

32 Despite his doubts, this did not prevent Mandel from titling one of his subsequent books *Late Capitalism*!

33 Cf. Engels on the Chartist movement:

> [The workers] demand of every one who presents himself as interested in their welfare, that he should declare himself in favour of the People's Charter as proof of the sincerity of his professions, and in so doing, they protest against all outside help, for the Charter is a demand for the power to help themselves.
>
> (Engels 1975a: 566–567)

34 'Britain gave the world Chartism, the first broad, truly mass and politically organised proletarian revolutionary movement' (Lenin 1974a: 309).

35 These conceptions find more than an echo in Lenin's later statement about the relationship of the Bolshevik party in pre-1917 Russia with the mass movement. In *Left Wing Communism* Lenin (1974b) explained that one of the keys to the success of the Bolsheviks was its ability to merge, 'in a certain measure' with the mass movement.

References

Berg, M. and Hudson, P. (1992) 'Rehabilitating the industrial revolution', *Economic History Review*, 45: 24–50.

Bezanson, A. (1922) 'The early use of the term industrial revolution', *Quarterly Journal of Economics*, 36: 343–349.

Briggs, A. (1963) *Victorian Cities*, Harmondsworth: Penguin.

Cannadine, D. (1984) 'The present and the past in the English industrial revolution, 1880–1980', *Past and Present*, 103: 131–172.

Coleman, D.C. (1992) *Myth, History and the Industrial Revolution*, London: The Hambledon Press.

Crafts, N.F.R. (1989) 'The new economic history and the industrial revolution', in P. Mathias and J.A. Davis (eds) *The First Industrial Revolutions*, Oxford: Blackwell.

Engels, F. (1975a) 'The condition of the working class in England. From personal observation and authentic sources', in *Karl Marx Frederick Engels Collected Works*, vol. 4, Moscow and London: Progress Publishers and Lawrence & Wishart, pp. 295–596.

Engels, F. (1975b) 'Speeches in Elberfeld', in *Karl Marx Frederick Engels Collected Works*, vol. 4, Moscow and London: Progress Publishers and Lawrence & Wishart, pp. 243–264.

Engels, F. (1975c) 'The condition of England', in *Karl Marx Frederick Engels Collected Works*, vol. 3, Moscow and London: Progress Publishers and Lawrence & Wishart, pp. 469–488.

Engels, F. (1975d) 'The condition of England. *Past and Present* by Thomas Carlyle, London, 1843', in *Karl Marx Frederick Engels Collected Works*, vol. 3, Moscow and London: Progress Publishers and Lawrence & Wishart, pp. 444–468.

Engels, F. (1990a) 'Preface to the Second German Edition (1892) of the *Condition of the Working-Class in England*', in *Karl Marx Frederick Engels Collected Works*, vol. 27, Moscow and London: Progress Publishers and Lawrence & Wishart, pp. 307–323.

Engels, F. (1990b) 'Preface to the 1892 English Edition of the *Condition of the Working-Class in England in 1844*', in *Karl Marx Frederick Engels Collected Work*, vol. 27, Moscow and London: Progress Publishers and Lawrence & Wishart, pp. 257–269.

Flinn, M.W. (1966) *Origins of the Industrial Revolution*, London: Longmans.

Galbraith, J.K. (1967) *The New Industrial State*, London: Hamish Hamilton.

Griffin, E. (2010) *A Short History of the British Industrial Revolution*, Basingstoke: Palgrave Macmillan.

Henderson, W.O. (1976) *The Life of Friedrich Engels*, 2 vols, London: Frank Cass.

Hobsbawm, E.J. (1964) 'The dark satanic mills', in Hobsbawm's *Labouring Men: Studies in the History of Labour*, London: Weidenfeld and Nicolson, pp. 105–119.

Hobsbawm, E.J. (1969) 'Introduction' to Engels, F. *The Condition of the Working Class in England: From Personal Observation and Authentic Sources*, London: Panther.

Kemp, T. (1985, second edition) *Industrialization in Nineteenth-Century Europe*, London: Longmans.

Landes, D. (1969) *The Unbound Prometheus: Technological Change and Industrial Development in Western Europe from 1750 to the Present*, London: Cambridge University Press.

Lenin, V.I. (1972a) 'Frederick Engels', in *Collected Works*, vol. 2, Third Printing, Moscow and London: Progress Publishers and Lawrence & Wishart, pp. 15–27.

Lenin, V.I. (1972b) 'What the 'Friends of the People' are and how they fought the Social-Democrats', in *Collected Works*, vol. 1, Third Printing, Moscow and London: Progress Publishers and Lawrence & Wishart, pp. 129–332.

Lenin, V.I. (1973) 'What is to be done?', in *Collected Works*, vol. 5, Third Printing, pp. 347–529, Moscow and London: Progress Publishers and Lawrence & Wishart.

Lenin, V.I. (1974a) 'The Third International and its place in history', in *Collected Works*, vol. 29, Second Printing, Moscow and London: Progress Publishers and Lawrence & Wishart, pp. 305–313.

Lenin, V.I. (1974b) 'Left wing Communism', in *Collected Works*, vol. 31, Moscow and London: Progress Publishers and Lawrence & Wishart, pp. 17–118.

Mandel, E. (1968) *Marxist Economic Theory*, London: Merlin.

Mandel, E. (1974) 'Workers under Neo-Capitalism' in E. Mandel and G. Novak, *The Revolutionary Potential of the Working Class*, New York: Pathfinder.

Marcus, S. (1974) *Engels, Manchester and the Working Class*, London: Weidenfeld and Nicolson.

Marx, K. (1980) 'Letter to the Labour Parliament, 1854', in *Karl Marx Frederick Engels Collected Works*, vol. 13, Moscow and London: Progress Publishers and Lawrence & Wishart, pp. 57–58.

Marx, K. and Engels, F. (1975) 'The Holy Family, or critique of critical criticism. Against Bruno Bauer and Company', in *Karl Marx Frederick Engels Collected Works*, vol. 4, Moscow and London: Progress Publishers and Lawrence & Wishart, pp. 5–211.

Meiksins Wood, E. (1986) *The Retreat from Class: A New 'True' Socialism*, London and New York: Verso.

Mészáros, I. (1989) *The Power of Ideology*, Hemel Hempstead: Harvester Wheatsheaf.

Musson, A.E. (1978) *The Growth of British Industry*, London: Batsford.

Rule, J. (1986) *The Labouring Classes in Early Industrial England, 1750–1850*, London: Longmans.

Saville, J. (1969) 'Primitive accumulation and early industrialisation in Britain', *Socialist Register*, 6: 247–271.

Smith, K. (1984) *The British Economic Crisis: Its Past and Future*, Harmondsworth: Penguin.

Trotsky, L.D. (1974) *The 3rd International After Lenin*, London: New Park Publications. *Militant* (1929) New York edition, online, available at: www.marxists.org/archive/trotsky/1928/3rd/index.htm (accessed 16 December 2011).

Trotsky, L.D. (1980) *History of the Russian Revolution*, New York: Pathfinder Press/Anchor Foundation. 1932 Max Eastman translation, online, available at: http://www.marxists.org/archive/trotsky/1930/hrr/index.htm (accessed 14 May 2012).

Index